Granulomatous Disorders of Adult Skin

Editor

JOSEPH C. ENGLISH III

DERMATOLOGIC CLINICS

www.derm.theclinics.com

Consulting Editor

BRUCE H. THIERS

July 2015 • Volume 33 • Number 3

ELSEVIER

1600 John F. Kennedy Boulevard • Suite 1800 • Philadelphia, Pennsylvania, 19103-2899

http://www.theclinics.com

DERMATOLOGIC CLINICS Volume 33, Number 3
July 2015 ISSN 0733-8635, ISBN-13: 978-0-323-39096-5

Editor: Adrianne Brigido
Developmental Editor: Susan Showalter

Dermatologic Clinics (ISSN 0733-8635) is published quarterly by Elsevier Inc., 360 Park Avenue South, New York, NY 10010-1710. Months of publication are January, April, July, and October. Business and editorial offices: 1600 John F. Kennedy Blvd., Suite 1800, Philadelphia, PA 19103-2899. Customer service office: 11830 Westline Drive, St. Louis, MO 63146. Periodicals postage paid at New York, NY, and additional mailing offices. Subscription prices are USD 365.00 per year for US individuals, USD 559.00 per year for US institutions, USD 425.00 per year for Canadian individuals, USD 681.00 per year for Canadian institutions, USD 495.00 per year for international individuals, USD 681.00 per year for international institutions, USD 165.00 per year for US students/residents, and USD 240.00 per year for Canadian and international students/residents. International air speed delivery is included in all *Clinics* subscription prices. All prices are subject to change without notice. **POSTMASTER:** Send address changes to *Dermatologic Clinics*, Elsevier Health Sciences Division, Subscription Customer Service, 3251 Riverport Lane, Maryland Heights, MO 63043. **Customer Service: 1-800-654-2452 (U.S. and Canada); 314-447-8871 (outside U.S. and Canada). Fax: 314-447-8029. E-mail: journalscustomerservice-usa@elsevier.com (for print support); journalsonlinesupport-usa@elsevier.com (for online support).**

Reprints. For copies of 100 or more, of articles in this publication, please contact the Commercial Reprints Department, Elsevier Inc., 360 Park Avenue South, New York, New York 10010-1710. Tel.: 212-633-3874; Fax: 212-633-3820; Email: repritns@elsevier.com.

The *Dermatologic Clinics* is covered in *MEDLINE/PubMed (Index Medicus)*, *Current Contents/Clinical Medicine*, *Excerpta Medica*, *Chemical Abstracts*, and *ISI/BIOMED*.

Contributors

CONSULTING EDITOR

BRUCE H. THIERS, MD
Professor and Chairman, Department of
Dermatology and Dermatologic Surgery,
Medical University of South Carolina,
Charleston, South Carolina

EDITOR

JOSEPH C. ENGLISH III, MD
Professor of Dermatology, University of
Pittsburgh, Department of Dermatology,
UPMC North Hills Dermatology, Wexford,
Pennsylvania

AUTHORS

MA. LUISA ABAD-VENIDA, MD, FPDS
Head of Training and Research Office,
Department of Dermatology, Jose R.
Reyes Memorial Medical Center, Manila,
Philippines

ARWA AL-HAMAD, PhD
Oral Medicine Unit, UCL Eastman Dental
Institute, University College London,
London, United Kingdom; Dental Services,
Ministry of National Guard, King Abdulaziz
Medical City-Riyadh, Riyadh, Saudi Arabia

AFSANEH ALAVI, MD, MSc, FRCPC
Department of Medicine (Dermatology),
University of Toronto, Toronto, Ontario,
Canada

MARK A. CAPPEL, MD
Department of Dermatology, Mayo Clinic,
Jacksonville, Florida

SARAH S. CHISOLM, MD
Department of Dermatology, UCSF, San
Francisco, California

MARA M. DACSO, MD, MS
Staff Dermatologist and Dermatopathologist,
Center for Dermatology and Cosmetic
Laser Surgery, Plano, Texas; Assistant
Professor of Dermatology, Department of
Dermatology, University of Texas
Southwestern Medical Center, Dallas,
Texas

RONI P. DODIUK-GAD, MD
Division of Dermatology, Department of
Medicine, Sunnybrook Health Sciences
Centre, Toronto, Ontario, Canada; Department
of Dermatology, Ha'emek Medical Center,
Afula, Israel

**SUNIL DOGRA, MD, MAMS, FRCP
(LONDON)**
Additional Professor, Department of
Dermatology, Venereology and Leperology,
Postgraduate Institute of Medical Education
and Research, Chandigarh, India

CHRISTOPHER DOWNING, MD
Center for Clinical Studies, Houston, Texas

LISA A. DRAGE, MD
Fellow, Department of Dermatology, Mayo Clinic College of Medicine, Mayo Clinic, Rochester, Minnesota

JOSEPH C. ENGLISH III, MD
Professor of Dermatology, University of Pittsburgh, Department of Dermatology, UPMC North Hills Dermatology, Wexford, Pennsylvania

STEFANO FEDELE, DDS, PhD
Oral Medicine Unit, UCL Eastman Dental Institute, University College London; Clinical Senior Lecturer/Honorary Consultant in Oral Medicine; Programme Director, MSc in Oral Medicine, Oral Medicine Unit, UCL Eastman Dental Institute, University College London, London, United Kingdom; NIHR University College London Hospitals Biomedical Research Centre

LINDY P. FOX, MD
Department of Dermatology, UCSF, San Francisco, California

PAMELA GANGAR, MD
MD Anderson Cancer Center, Houston, Texas

TANIA M. GONZALEZ-SANTIAGO, MD
Associate Professor of Dermatology, Department of Dermatology, Mayo Clinic College of Medicine, Mayo Clinic, Rochester, Minnesota

LISA M. GRANDINETTI, MD[†]
Assistant Professor, Department of Dermatology, University of Pittsburgh Medical Center, Pittsburgh, Pennsylvania

JACQUELINE A. GUIDRY, MD
Center for Clinical Studies, Houston, Texas

ENRIQUE GUTIÉRREZ-GONZÁLEZ, MD
Department of Dermatology, Faculty of Medicine, Complejo Hospitalario Universitario, Santiago de Compostela, Spain

JOSHUA W. HAGEN, MD, PhD
Department of Dermatology, University of Pittsburgh Medical Center, Pittsburgh, Pennsylvania

ADELE HAIMOVIC, MD
The Ronald O. Perelman Department of Dermatology, New York University School of Medicine, New York, New York

JAMES H. KEELING, MD
Associate Professor, Department of Dermatology, Mayo Clinic, Jacksonville, Florida

EMILY LOUISE KEIMIG, MS, MD
Clinical Instructor, Department of Dermatology, Northwestern University, Chicago, Illinois

JUSTIN KERSTETTER, MD
Department of Pathology and Laboratory Medicine; Assistant Professor of Pathology and Human Anatomy, Loma Linda University Medical Center, Loma Linda, California

INES KEVRIC, MD
Mayo Clinic, Jacksonville, Florida

GRACE L. LEE, MD
Dermatology Resident, The Ohio State University Wexner Medical Center, Columbus, Ohio

DOUGLAS W. LIENESCH, MD
Assistant Professor, Department of Rheumatology, UPMC, University of Pittsburgh, Pittsburgh, Pennsylvania

ANA M. MOLINA-RUIZ, MD, PhD
Associate Professor of Dermatology; Senior Staff Specialist, Department of Dermatology, Fundación Jiménez Díaz, Universidad Autónoma, Madrid, Spain

MANUEL PEREIRO Jr, MD, PhD
Titular Professor, Department of Dermatology, Faculty of Medicine, Complejo Hospitalario Universitario, Santiago de Compostela, Spain

---

† The author is deceased.

STEPHEN PORTER, BSc, MD, PhD, FDSRCS (Edin), FDSRCS (Eng), FHEA
Professor of Oral Medicine, Academic Lead and Institute Director, Oral Medicine Unit, UCL Eastman Dental Institute, University College London, London, United Kingdom

STEVE PRYSTOWSKY, MD
The Ronald O. Perelman Department of Dermatology, New York University School of Medicine, New York, New York

SOPHIA REID, MD
Department of Medicine, University of California, Irvine, Irvine, California

LUIS REQUENA, MD, PhD
Senior Staff Specialist and Head, Department of Dermatology, Fundación Jiménez Díaz, Universidad Autónoma, Madrid, Spain

MISHA ROSENBACH, MD
Assistant Professor of Dermatology and Internal Medicine, Associate Program Director, Dermatology Residency; Director, Dermatology Inpatient Consult Service; Director, Department of Dermatology, Perelman School of Medicine, University of Pennsylvania, Philadelphia, Pennsylvania

MIGUEL SANCHEZ, MD
The Ronald O. Perelman Department of Dermatology, New York University School of Medicine, New York, New York

JOSHUA M. SCHULMAN, MD
Departments of Pathology and Dermatology, UCSF, San Francisco, California

DAVID M. SCOLLARD, MD, PhD
Director, National Hansen's Disease Programs, Baton Rouge, Louisiana

AMAN SHARMA, MD, MAMS, FICP, FACR, FRCP (LONDON)
Assistant Professor, Rheumatology Division, Department of Internal Medicine, Postgraduate Institute of Medical Education and Research, Chandigarh, India

KUSUM SHARMA, MD, MAMS
Additional Professor, Department of Medical Microbiology, Postgraduate Institute of Medical Education and Research, Chandigarh, India

NEIL H. SHEAR, MD, FRCPC
Divisions of Dermatology, Clinical Pharmacology and Toxicology, Faculty of Medicine, Department of Medicine, Sunnybrook Health Sciences Centre, Ontario, Canada

CATHRYN SIBBALD, BScPhm, MD
Department of Medicine (Dermatology), University of Toronto, Toronto, Ontario, Canada

JASON M. SWOGER, MD, MPH
Assistant Professor of Medicine, Department of Gastroenterology, Hepatology and Nutrition, University of Pittsburgh Medical Center, Pittsburgh, Pennsylvania

JEREMY S. TILSTRA, MD, PhD
Department of Rheumatology, UPMC, University of Pittsburgh, Pittsburgh, Pennsylvania

JAIME TORIBIO, MD, PhD
Professor and Chair, Department of Dermatology, Faculty of Medicine, Complejo Hospitalario Universitario, Santiago de Compostela, Spain

STEPHEN K. TYRING, MD, PhD
Center for Clinical Studies; Department of Dermatology, University of Texas Health Science Center, Houston, Texas

SANGEETHA VENKATARAJAN, MD, MBA
MD Anderson Cancer Center, Houston, Texas

JUN WANG, MD
Department of Pathology and Laboratory Medicine; Professor of Pathology and Human Anatomy, Loma Linda University Medical Center, Loma Linda, California

MATTHEW J. ZIRWAS, MD
Associate Clinical Professor, The Ohio State University Wexner Medical Center, Columbus, Ohio

Contents

Granuloma annulare (GA) is a noninfectious granulomatous skin condition that can present with a variety of cutaneous morphologies. It is characterized by collagen degeneration, mucin deposition, and palisaded or interstitial histiocytes. Although the mechanism underlying development of GA is unknown, studies point to a cell-mediated hypersensitivity reaction to an as-yet undetermined antigen. Systemic associations with diabetes, thyroid disorders, lipid abnormalities, malignancy, and infection are described in atypical GA. Treatment is divided into localized skin-directed therapies and systemic immunomodulatory or immunosuppressive therapies. The selected treatment modality should be based on disease severity, comorbid conditions, consideration of potential side effects, and patient preference.

Actinic granuloma and annular elastolytic giant cell granuloma are different terms used to define skin lesions characterized by elastolysis, elastophagocytosis, and multinucleated giant cell infiltrate. The clinical appearance varies from papules to annular plaques. Although elastolytic actinic giant cell granuloma shares some clinical features with granuloma annulare, they can be differentiated by histopathologic findings. The disease is initiated by an immune response triggered by different factors that alter the elastic tissue. The course tends to be chronic, with variable response to treatments, although spontaneous remission may occur. Diabetes mellitus is the systemic disease most frequently associated with this condition.

Necrobiosis lipoidica is a granulomatous condition presenting as indolent atrophic plaques, often on the lower extremities. There is a multitude of case reports suggesting possible associations and documenting different therapeutic alternatives with varied success. Important complications include ulceration and the development of squamous cell carcinoma. The disease course is often indolent and recurrent despite treatment. This article reviews the etiopathogenesis, clinical presentations, and evidence for treatment alternatives of this condition.

Rheumatoid nodules are a common manifestation of rheumatoid arthritis. These lesions are often easily identified based on typical diagnostic features and characteristic locations. When biopsied, nodules have a characteristic histologic appearance. Uncommonly, rheumatoid nodules can occur in systemic locations. There is no evidence that systemic therapy treats underlying rheumatoid nodules. Paradoxically, methotrexate and possibly tumor necrosis factor inhibitors can increase nodule development. Treatment of rheumatoid nodules is often not necessary, unless patients are experiencing pain or there is interference of mechanical function. This review outlines the available data on and associations of rheumatoid nodules.

The terms "palisaded neutrophilic and granulomatous dermatitis," "interstitial granulomatous dermatitis," and the subset "interstitial granulomatous drug reaction" are a source of confusion. There exists substantial overlap among the entities with few strict distinguishing features. We review the literature and highlight areas of distinction and overlap, and propose a streamlined diagnostic workup for patients presenting with this cutaneous reaction pattern. Because the systemic disease associations and requisite workup are similar, and the etiopathogenesis is poorly understood but likely similar among these entities, we propose the simplified unifying term "reactive granulomatous dermatitis" to encompass these entities.

Sarcoidosis is a disease characterized by noncaseating granulomatous infiltration of 1 or more organs. In North America, after the lungs and thoracic lymph nodes, the skin is the next most commonly involved organ. Data from multiple studies indicate a coaction between genetic and environmental factors in immunologically susceptible hosts. The disease's many clinical manifestations and course vary greatly and are influenced by race, ethnicity, and gender. In the skin, the lesions of sarcoidosis are classified as specific when noncaseating granulomas are present, and nonspecific when there is an inflammatory reaction pattern devoid of granulomas.

Awareness of the extraintestinal manifestations of Crohn disease is increasing in dermatology and gastroenterology, with enhanced identification of entities that range from granulomatous diseases recapitulating the underlying inflammatory bowel disease to reactive conditions and associated dermatoses. In this review, the underlying etiopathology of Crohn disease is discussed, and how this mirrors certain skin manifestations that present in a subset of patients is explored. The array of extraintestinal manifestations that do not share a similar pathology, but which are often seen in association with inflammatory bowel disease, is also discussed. Treatment and pathogenetic mechanisms, where available, are discussed.

Orofacial granulomatosis (OFG) is an uncommon chronic inflammatory disorder of the orofacial region. It is characterized by subepithelial noncaseating granulomas and has a spectrum of possible clinical manifestations ranging from subtle oral mucosal swelling to permanent disfiguring fibrous swelling of the lips and face.

Etiopathogenesis is unknown. A range of systemic granulomatous disorders, including Crohn disease and sarcoidosis, may cause orofacial manifestations that cannot be distinguished from those of OFG. Treatment of OFG has proven difficult and unsatisfactory, with no single therapeutic model showing consistent efficacy in reducing orofacial swelling and mucosal inflammation.

nongranulomatous vasculitis, namely, microscopic polyangiitis (MPA). Classic poly-arteritis nodosa (PAN) is a nongranulomatous medium-vessel vasculitis. This review discusses the classification, etiopathogenesis, clinical features, and management of GPA, MPA, EGPA and PAN.

Granulomatous cutaneous T-cell lymphomas (CTCL) and lymphomatoid granuloma-tosis are considered granulomatous lymphoproliferative disorders. The most common types of granulomatous CTCL are granulomatous mycosis fungoides and granulomatous slack skin. Lymphomatoid granulomatosis is a rare Epstein-Barr virus driven lymphoproliferative disorder. This article reviews the etiopathogenesis, clinical presentation, systemic associations, and management of both granuloma-tous slack skin syndrome and lymphomatoid granulomatosis.

A large list of foreign substances may penetrate the skin and induce a foreign body granulomatous reaction. These particles can enter the skin by voluntary reasons or be caused by accidental inclusion of external substances secondary to cutaneous trauma. In these cases, foreign body granulomas are formed around such disparate substances as starch, cactus bristles, wood splinters, suture material, pencil lead, artificial hair, or insect mouthparts. The purpose of this article is to update dermatol-ogists, pathologists, and other physicians on the most recent etiopathogenesis, clinical presentations, systemic associations, evaluation, and evidence-based man-agement concerning foreign body granulomatous reactions of skin.

Granuloma formation is usually regarded as a means of defending the host from persistent irritants of either exogenous or endogenous origin. Noninfectious granu-lomatous disorders of the skin encompass a challenging group of diseases owing to their clinical and histologic overlap. Drug reactions characterized by a granuloma-tous reaction pattern are rare, and defined by a predominance of histiocytes in the inflammatory infiltrate. This review summarizes current knowledge on the various types of granulomatous drug eruptions, focusing on the 4 major types: interstitial granulomatous drug reaction, drug-induced accelerated rheumatoid nodulosis, drug-induced granuloma annulare, and drug-induced sarcoidosis.

Leprosy and tuberculosis are chronic mycobacterial infections that elicit granuloma-tous inflammation. Both infections are curable, but granulomatous injury to cuta-neous structures, including cutaneous nerves in leprosy, may cause permanent damage. Both diseases are major global concerns: tuberculosis for its high preva-lence and mortality, and leprosy for its persistent global presence and high rate of neuropathic disability. Cutaneous manifestations of both leprosy and tuberculosis are frequently subtle and challenging in dermatologic practice and often require a careful travel and social history and a high index of suspicion.

Skin and soft tissue infections caused by nontuberculous mycobacteria are increasing in incidence. The nontuberculous mycobacteria are environmental, acid-fast bacilli that cause cutaneous infections primarily after trauma, surgery and cosmetic procedures. Skin findings include abscesses, sporotrichoid nodules or ulcers, but also less distinctive signs. Important species include *Mycobacterium marinum* and the rapidly growing mycobacterium: *M. fortuitum*, *M. abscessus* and *M. chelonae*. Obtaining tissue for mycobacterial culture and histopathology aids diagnosis. Optimal therapy is not well-established, but is species-dependent and generally dictated by susceptibility studies. Management often includes use of multiple antibiotics for several months and potential use of adjunctive surgery.

Leishmaniasis is a parasitic infection endemic to more than 90 countries worldwide. As travel to endemic areas increases, dermatologists need to keep this entity in the differential for any chronic skin lesion in persons who may have had a possible exposure for any duration. It can be difficult to diagnose because manifestations are varied and sometimes subclinical. This article discusses the current state of epidemiology, pathogenesis, clinical presentation, diagnosis, and treatment options. A special focus is placed on cutaneous manifestations and their treatment.

Granulomatous diseases are caused by multiple infectious and noninfectious causes. Deep fungal infections can present in the skin or extracutaneously, most commonly with lung manifestations. An Azole or amphotericin B is the universal treatment. Blastomycosis-like pyoderma is a clinically similar condition, which is caused by a combination of hypersensitivity and immunosuppression. Successful treatment has been reported with antibiotics and, more recently, the vitamin A analog, acitretin. Granuloma inguinale and lymphogranuloma venereum cause ulcerative genital lesions with a granulomatous appearance on histology. The Centers for Disease Control and Prevention recommens treatment of these genital infections with doxycycline.

DERMATOLOGIC CLINICS

Preface
Granulomatous Disorders of the Adult Skin: Twenty-First Century

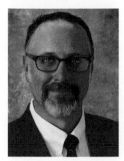

Joseph C. English III, MD
Editor

Granulomatous disorders represent a unique group of diseases, both noninfectious and infectious, that require the utmost clinical pathologic correlation combined with a keen sense of inquiry for underlying systemic disease and immunosuppression. Dermatologists (and others, such as rheumatologists, oncologists, endocrinologists, pulmonologists, oral maxillary surgeons, and infectious disease specialists) need to be able to differentiate these entities, evaluate patients for specific underlying systemic disease (ie, from diabetes to cancer), and treat them with a wide range of immunosuppressant to anti-infectious medications. This issue supplies the readers with a comprehensive, up-to-date, and evidence-based review of multiple granulomatous disorders (ie, palisading, epithelioid, xanthomatous, vasculitic, lymphoproliferative, drug-induced, foreign body reaction, caseating, and suppurative).

This collection of reviews comes from the hard work and passion of hand-selected experts in the realm of granulomatous disorders throughout the world. They have been tasked to provide the reader with the most current information on the etiopathogenesis, clinical/systemic manifestations, and therapeutic modalities of granulomatous disorders. I know you will be pleased with the quality of research, writing, and digital images as much as I am. As most dermatologists are visual learners, I have added a "bonus" supplemental atlas from my own digital image collection to give additional examples of the diseases discussed in this issue.

Joseph C. English III, MD
University of Pittsburgh
Department of Dermatology
UPMC North Hills Dermatology
9000 Brooktree Road, Suite 200
Wexford, PA 15090, USA

E-mail address:
englishjc@upmc.edu

Dermatol Clin 33 (2015) xiii
http://dx.doi.org/10.1016/j.det.2015.05.001
0733-8635/15/$ – see front matter © 2015 Published by Elsevier Inc.

Granuloma Annulare

Emily Louise Keimig, MS, MD

KEYWORDS

- Granuloma annulare (GA) • GA treatment • GA malignancy • GA etiology • GA infection
- GA diabetes • GA thyroid • GA hyperlipidemia

KEY POINTS

- Granuloma annulare (GA) presents with multiple morphologies, including localized, generalized, macular/patch, subcutaneous, perforating, and atypical variants (palmar, mucosal, and photosensitive).
- GA is a cell-mediated hypersensitivity reaction to an unknown antigen resulting in elevated levels of interleukin (IL)-12, interferon (IFN)-γ, and tumor necrosis factor α (TNF-α).
- Many recent studies have failed to find an association between GA and diabetes mellitus (DM).
- Treatment can broadly be divided into localized/skin-directed therapy and systemic immunomodulating therapy.
- Selection of modality should take into consideration disease severity, comorbid conditions, potential side effects, and patient preference.

INTRODUCTION

First described by Colcott and Fox in 1895 and later formally named in 1902 by Radcliffe-Crocker, GA is classified as a noninfectious granulomatous skin condition.[1] The condition is characterized by multiple morphologies, including localized, generalized, subcutaneous, macular or patch, and various atypical morphologies. Histologically, GA shows collagen degradation, mucin deposition, and either a palisaded or interstitial histiocytic infiltrate.[2] Although the exact cause of the condition remains unknown, a cell-mediated hypersensitivity reaction is favored as the mechanism underlying the development of GA.[3–5] There are multiple reports of systemic disease associations with GA, including DM, malignancy, thyroid dysfunction, lipid abnormalities, and infection. Many of these associations are seen with the atypical clinical variants and are discussed in this article. In regard to therapy, a skin-directed or systemic approach can be taken. There are no large randomized controlled trials, however, evaluating the therapies used to treat GA. Consideration for disease severity, comorbid conditions, side effects, and patient preference is imperative.

ETIOPATHOGENESIS

The histologic findings of GA are well known, with focal areas of collagen degeneration surrounded by an inflammatory infiltrate composed of palisaded histiocytes and lymphocytes.[2] The etiology and pathogenesis, however, remain poorly understood. There have been reports of GA appearing after localized subcutaneous trauma for desensitization,[6] bacille Calmette-Guérin vaccination,[7–10] tetanus and diphtheria vaccination,[11,12] hepatitis B vaccination,[13,14] ultraviolet light exposure,[15–17] mesotherapy,[18] and drug exposure.[16,19–23] Studies have pointed to an immunologic mechanism with resultant necrobiosis underlying the development of GA. Various studies have suggested a role of immunoglobulin-mediated vasculitis,[24] lysozyme production,[25] cell-mediated hypersensitivity, and[3] and elastic fibers as targets in GA.[26]

Dr E.L. Keimig is a subinvestigator for Merck, Pfizer, Stiefel, AMGEN, and Lilly. There are no relevant conflicts of interest to disclose.
Department of Dermatology, Northwestern University, 676 North St Clair, Suite 1600, Chicago, IL 60611, USA
E-mail address: ekeimig@nmff.org

Dermatol Clin 33 (2015) 315–329
http://dx.doi.org/10.1016/j.det.2015.03.001
0733-8635/15/$ – see front matter © 2015 Elsevier Inc. All rights reserved.

derm.theclinics.com

Dahl and colleagues[24] examined the vasculature of patients with GA. Immunoglobulin M (IgM) and C3 were found in the vessel walls and IgM, C3, and fibrinogen were all observed along the dermal epidermal junction. Additionally, they found vessel wall necrosis, fibrinoid change, and thickening or occlusion in many specimens. These results suggested that an immunoglobulin-mediated vasculitis may be involved in the pathogenesis of GA. In a study by Umbert and Winkelmann,[2] however, these changes were thought more in response to tissue and vessel changes related to the mononuclear infiltrate characteristic of GA.

Beuchner and colleagues[3] identified the presence of T-cell subsets in lesional skin. Using monoclonal antibodies targeting peripheral T cells, the predominant cell population was identified as activated helper T cells of the T_H1 class. These T-cell populations were found not only within the granulomas but also surrounding the vasculature. Furthermore, the histiocytes in this study demonstrated diffuse activity. The results suggested a cell-mediated response to an unidentified antigen as the dominant pathogenic event in GA.

With the thought that GA represents a delayed-type hypersensitivity reaction resulting in matrix degradation, Fayyazi and colleagues[4] sought to identify the cytokine profile. Specifically, the roles of IFN-γ, matrix metalloproteinases, and TNF-α were investigated. In their study, large numbers of lymphocytes expressed IFN-γ, which subsequently activated macrophages. These activated macrophages in turn produced IL-12, the major cytokine driving differentiation of naïve T cells to the T_H1 subset. Furthermore, a vast majority of both the lymphocytes and the macrophages contained TNF-α. In addition, immunohistochemistry revealed that the macrophages producing the TNF-α additionally coexpress matrix metalloproteinases-2 and -9. These results taken together suggest that in GA, IFN-γ secreting T_H1 cells cause a delayed type of hypersensitivity reaction whereby macrophages are differentiated to aggressive effector cells. The end result of this process is the degradation of the connective tissue matrix characteristic of GA. A recent study by Mempel and colleagues[5] confirmed the presence of T_H1 cells in the granulomas and found high levels of IL-2 within these granulomas, ultimately recruiting more T cells to the sites of activity. Taken together, these 3 studies illustrate that GA is a cell-mediated response to an unknown antigen.

Lastly, the role of genetic predisposition and GA has been examined. Generalized GA was found in association with HLA Bw35.[27] More recently, there has been a case report of generalized GA occurring in monozygotic twins carrying the HLA AH8.1.[28] Further studies are warranted to determine the role of genetics in the development of GA.

CLINICAL PRESENTATIONS

The presentation of GA is variable. Localized GA is the classic variant described in the literature.[29] In this form, flesh-colored to erythematous papules in annular configurations are appreciated (**Fig. 1**). The lesions are commonly found on the dorsal hands or feet. The localized form is the most common presentation of GA, is found in women more often than in men, and tends to appear in patients under the age of 30.[30] Generalized annular GA, by definition, is the presence of 10 or more skin lesions or by widespread annular plaques.[29,31] This form is notable for a later age of onset, a more chronic and relapsing course, rare spontaneous resolution, and, in general, a poorer response to therapy than its localized counterpart.[1]

Subcutaneous GA is a rare presentation that is seen predominantly in children and young adults (**Fig. 2**).[32–34] Lesions appear as firm, asymptomatic, subcutaneous nodules with a tendency to appear on the anterior lower legs, hands, head, and buttocks.[29,33] In 25% of cases, the subcutaneous lesions appear in association with intradermal lesions. These lesions are often biopsied to rule out clinical mimickers, such as rheumatoid nodule, necrobiosis, and epithelioid sarcoma, and sarcoidosis. Macular or patch GA is a rare presentation. In this form, asymptomatic erythematous to brown patches favoring the proximal extremities in women are seen (**Fig. 3**).[35] The differential diagnosis of macular GA includes morphea, parapsoriasis, and cutaneous T-cell lymphoma (CTCL); however, biopsy is diagnostic and in most cases is notable for an interstitial pattern of histiocytes.[35]

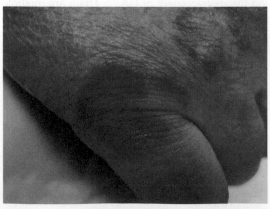

Fig. 1. Localized GA. Erythematous annular plaques on the dorsal hand.

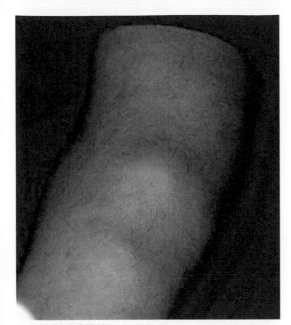

Fig. 2. Subcutaneous nodules on the anterior lower leg in a child. (*Courtesy of* Dr Amy S Paller, Evanston, IL.)

Atypical variants of GA have also been reported. Perforating GA is a rare presentation of disease and represents an atypical variant. This form is notable for a central umbilication with a keratotic core. Within this umbilication, histologically,

elimination of degenerated collagen is seen.[29] These lesions may be pruritic or painful, and, unlike their localized, macular, and generalized counterparts, scar on healing. Additional atypical forms include photosensitive GA (**Fig. 4**),[15–17] palmar GA,[36] disseminated popular,[29] and oral mucosal GA.[37] Generalized GA, disseminated GA, and other atypical GA, as discussed previously, are important to identify because they have been associated with systemic disease.

SYSTEMIC ASSOCIATIONS

The relationship between DM and GA has been controversial. Early studies have suggested a link between the 2 conditions.[30,38,39] More recent studies, however, have called this association into question.[34,40–42] A retrospective study of patients conducted by Studer and colleagues[1] did not find a statistically significant association between GA and DM. Patients with DM and GA tended, however, to have more chronic and relapsing disease than did their nondiabetic counterparts. Gannon and Lynch[40] found an absence of carbohydrate intolerance in patients with GA. Most recently, Nabesio and colleagues[41] conducted a case-control study between patients with GA and matched controls with psoriasis. This study was unable to find a statistically significant relationship between GA and type 2 DM.

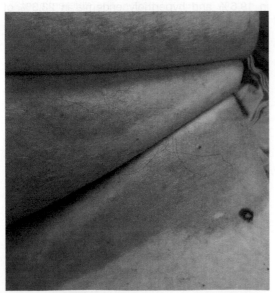

Fig. 3. Patch GA. Erythematous patches on the proximal thigh and lower abdomen. (*Courtesy of* Dr Ahmad Amin, Evanston, IL.)

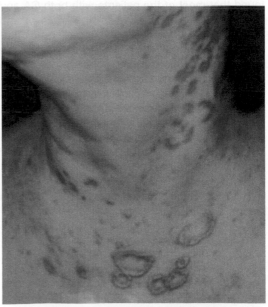

Fig. 4. Photodistributed GA. Erythematous annular plaques photodistributed on the neck and chest. (*Courtesy of* Dr Anne E Laumann, Evanston, IL.)

GA, both generalized[43,44] and localized,[45,46] has been reported to occur in the setting of thyroid disease. Case reports associating localized GA with autoimmune thyroiditis are found in the literature.[45–47] A small, case-controlled study conducted by Vazquez-Lopez and colleagues[48] sought to establish the frequency and type of thyroid disease in adult women with localized GA. In their study, 24 women with localized GA and 100 age-matched female patients with non-GA cutaneous disease were evaluated for underlying thyroid disorders. In the patients with localized GA, 12% demonstrated autoimmune thyroiditis whereas only 1% of the controls were noted to have autoimmune thyroiditis. These statistically significant results ($P = .022$) suggest that a subset of female patients with localized GA may have autoimmune thyroid disease. Therefore, in female patients with localized GA, screening for thyroid disease with thyroid-stimulating hormone and antibodies may be considered.

GA has also been reported to occur in the setting of malignancy. Hematologic malignancies are the most frequently reported. Both Hodgkin[49–54] and non-Hodgkin[49,55–57] lymphoma and leukemias[58–61] have been reported in patients with GA. Solid tumors have also been reported, however, in association with GA. These include cancers of the lung, breast, cervix, colon, prostate, testicles, and thyroid.[51,62–64] Li and colleagues[64] conducted a review of the literature examining the association between GA and malignancy. Their review of 14 case reports and 2 correlation studies found that most of the patients with both GA and malignancy were older (mean age of 54 y) and had atypical clinical presentations of their cutaneous disease and that more than half of the malignancies reported were lymphomas. There was no definitive relationship between GA and malignancy. Although no causative relationship has been established between GA and malignancy, older patients, patients with atypical clinical presentations, and patients with recalcitrant disease should have routine age-appropriate cancer screening for both solid organ and hematologic malignancies.[29,63,65]

There have been multiple reports of GA occurring in a setting of HIV infection.[37,66–70] Presenting morphologies are variable, but often the presentation is atypical. These presentations include photosensitive,[17,71] molluscum contagiousum–like,[72] disseminated papular,[68] generalized,[70] oral mucosal,[37] and perforating.[73] Toro and colleagues[69] conducted a study that illustrated that the most common morphology seen in HIV infection was that of generalized GA and that although GA can occur at all stages of infection, it was slightly more common in patients with AIDS. HIV-infected patients can develop a multitude of mucocutaneous conditions. These have been categorized into 3 groups. Group 1 includes conditions that are nearly always associated with HIV infections in appropriate clinical scenarios. Group 2 conditions are those conditions that occur with increased prevalence in HIV-infected individuals or whose detection in a previously seronegative patient should prompt consideration for testing. Group 3 mucocutaneous conditions occur in patients with HIV but that are not related to the viral infection. GA has been categorized as a group 2 mucocutaneous condition.[74] As a result, in patients with atypical or generalized presentations of GA, HIV screening should be considered, in particular in a setting of appropriate risk factors. In addition, there have been multiple reports of GA resolving with treatment with highly active antiretroviral therapy.[66,75,76]

Infections with hepatitis B and C have also been reported to occur in patients with GA.[29] A recent study examining 10 biopsy specimens found no molecular or culture-based evidence of bacterial, mycobacterial, or fungal infection.[77] With these studies and reports in mind, assessing for risk factors for hepatitis B, hepatitis C, and HIV should be performed in patients with atypical presentations. Follow-up testing with serologies should be performed in the appropriate settings.

The association between lipid abnormalities and GA has been proposed. A study conducted by Dabski and Winkelmann[43] evaluating 100 patients with generalized GA found hypercholesterolemia in 19.6% and hypertriglyceridemia in 23.3% of patients whose levels were tested. More recently, Wu and colleagues[78] conducted a case-control study examining the prevalence of dyslipidemia in patients with GA. The study included 140 patients with GA and 420 matched controls. In patients with GA, dyslipidemia was found in 79.3% of patients compared with 51.9% of the matched controls ($P = .001$). In addition, there were statistically significant differences between the quantitative values for total cholesterol, triglycerides, and low-density lipoprotein cholesterol between the GA group and the control group. Generalized GA had a higher prevalence of dyslipidemia and the annular morphology was associated with dyslipidemia, notably hypercholesterolemia. They found that the odds of finding dyslipidemia among patients with GA were approximately 4 times (odds ratio 4.04; 95% CI, 2.53–6.46) than those seen in matched controls without GA. In a comment to that study,[79] it was recommended that adults and children over age 11 with GA be screened for lipid abnormalities.

In addition to these systemic associations, cases of drug-induced GA have recently been reported in the literature. Allopurinol,[21,80] paroxetine,[16] thalidomide,[81] pegylated IFN-α,[82,83] topiramate,[19,84] TNF-α inhibitors (infliximab, adalimumab, and etanercept),[22,23] and intranasal calcitonin[20] have all been reported to induce lesions clinically and histologically consistent with GA. As a result, for patients with new-onset GA, a detailed drug history should be performed. A trial off of the medication, if possible, can be performed to assess for resolution of cutaneous disease.

In general, a majority of patients with GA are healthy. Dahl[85] conducted a retrospective chart review of 32 patients with GA diagnosed between 1950 and 1970 with a mean follow-up of 35 years and found that most patients had common conditions, such as hypertension, hyperlipidemia, degenerative joint disease, and atherosclerosis. Five patients were noted to have thyroid disorders (not specified). In summary, although a vast majority of patients with GA are healthy, screening for these systemic conditions should be considered in patients with atypical lesions or generalized lesions and in some patients with localized GA.

EVALUATION AND MANAGEMENT

Patients with classic features of localized or generalized annular GA are often diagnosed based on clinical findings alone. But in patients with clinically atypical lesions, or clinical lesions that include other nongranulomatous conditions in the differential diagnosis, biopsy should be performed to confirm the diagnosis. Regardless of clinical presentation, histologically, there is focal degeneration of collagen surrounded by an inflammatory infiltrate composed of lymphocytes and histiocytes. Although this is the classic description of GA, there are 3 patterns of histiocytes that have been described.[2] The most common variant is that of an infiltrative or interstitial pattern. In this form, scattered histiocytes are seen between and surrounding collagen bundles in the upper and the mid-dermis. In a study by Umbert and Winkelmann,[2] this form was found in 71% of reviewed cases. The second pattern is that of the classic palisading granulomas, found in 26% of cases. These palisaded granulomas are scattered within the dermis and show the classic palisaded histiocyties, central degeneration of the connective tissue, and abundant mucin characteristic of GA. The final pattern described in GA is the epithelioid nodule. This was rare and seen in only 3% of studied cases. In the epithelioid form, the histiocytes are aggregated with a nodular appearance with some giant cells. This can be difficult to differentiate from other granulomatous conditions, in particular sarcoidosis; however, the interstitial pattern can often be seen surrounding the epithelioid granuloma, aiding in the diagnosis of GA.

The presence of mucin aids in the diagnosis of GA.[2] The finding of prominent mucin is helpful in the differentiation of GA from other granulomatous conditions, such as necrobiosis lipoidica, sarcoidosis, rheumatoid nodule, and cutaneous Crohn disease. Recently, clonality in sarcoidosis, GA, and granulomatous mycosis fungoides (CTCL) was evaluated.[86] Granulomatous findings in primary cutaneous lymphomas are rare, but their presence histologically can be confused with GA. The presence of a polyclonal T-cell population of cells points to the diagnosis of GA, whereas a monoclonal population of T cells raises the concern for a primary cutaneous lymphoma.[86]

Once a diagnosis of GA has been established, the next challenge facing the clinician and patient is the selection of a treatment modality. Broadly, treatment can be categorized into local, skin-directed therapy and systemic immunomodulatory or immunosuppressive therapy. The treatment selected is often based on severity of disease as well as patient preference.

For localized disease, topical corticosteroids are generally considered first-line therapy.[29] Depending on site, high potency corticosteroids with or without occlusion can be used. Intralesional corticosteroids can be used for localized lesions not responding to topical corticosteroids.[29] Patients must be counseled on risks of corticosteroid use (both topical and intralesional), in particular the risk of atrophy, dyschromia, and striae.[29] Topical tacrolimus has also been reported in the successful treatment of perforating, periorbital, and disseminated GA.[87–91] These results may be related to the recent report of glioma-associated oncogene (gli-1) highly expressed in granulomatous skin disorders, including GA,[92] and may offer future therapeutic options for patients with disseminated and recalcitrant disease.

Various destructive measures have been reported as effective in the treatment of GA. The role of biopsy in resolution of lesions remains controversial. Levin and colleagues[93] reported a case of rapid resolution of biopsied lesions on 2 separate occasions in the same patient with an interstitial pattern seen histologically. Although the mechanism is unclear, it is thought that the induction of wound healing changes the inflammatory milieu with the replacement, rather than the destruction, of extracellular matrix proteins. Contact cryosurgery has also been reported to clear the lesions of GA.[94] A prospective trial of 31 patients with localized GA found resolution in all patients treated with cryosurgery. The patients were treated with one freeze-thaw cycle ranging in duration from 10 to 60 seconds. Blistering occurred in all patients and the therapy was well tolerated. Intralesional therapy with low-dose recombinant human IFN-γ was successfully used to treat 3 patients with GA.[95] In all 3 patients, treated lesions resolved and remained clear at 12 months post-therapy.

Within the past several years, the role of laser therapy in treatment of individual lesions in both localized and generalized GA has been examined; 15 treatments with excimer laser at 300 mJ/cm^2 with 5 doses per treatment session resulted in resolution of GA lesions on the hands with no recurrence at 6-month follow-up.[96] Pulsed dye laser (PDL) therapy has also been examined as a modality to treat isolated lesions in GA. Sliger and colleagues[97] reported near complete clearance using a 595-nm PDL with maintenance of results at 36 weeks. Sniezek and colleagues[98] performed 3 treatments over the course of 13 months with a 585-nm PDL and reported decreased erythema, thickness, and diameter of treated lesions. These results were maintained at 3 years of follow-up. Most recently, fractionated thermolysis has been reported to be helpful in patients with GA. Improvement in lesions treated with the 1550-nm erbium-doped YAG (Er:YAG) laser[99] as well as the 1440-nm Nd:YAG laser[100] have been reported.

Although localized GA or localized lesions of generalized GA may be amenable to these destructive and topical methods, treatment of widespread GA often requires systemic therapy. There are no large studies examining these treatment modalities. Many of the treatments reported include case reports or small case series. These range from ultraviolet light therapy and immunomodulating antiinflammatory drugs to immunosuppressive medications. The modality selected should focus on disease severity, potential side effects, comorbidities, and patient preference.

There have been various reports of skin-directed ultraviolet therapy resulting in improvement and clearance of lesions of GA. Inui and colleagues[101] reported a case of disseminated GA improving after 24 treatments with narrow-band UV-B (NB-UVB) therapy with sustained response 6 months after cessation of therapy. Improvement in 5 patients treated with 16 weeks of thrice-weekly therapy with broadband UV-B was demonstrated by Do and colleagues.[102] The use of various forms of UV-A has also been efficacious. Small studies using UV-A1 have shown improvement in lesions; however, relapses were common after discontinuation of therapy.[103–105]

Psoralen–UV-A (PUVA) has been effective in clearing the lesions of GA in case reports and small case series.[106–109] As in the case of UV-A1 therapy, although many patients showed improvement,[106–109] recurrence was common and maintenance therapy was required.[107,109] One challenge with any form of phototherapy is the need for frequent and consistent office visits. PUVA carries the additional risk of cutaneous malignancy.[29]

Successful treatment of GA lesions with photodynamic therapy (PDT) has been reported. Piaserico and colleagues[110] reported 3 patients successfully treated with methyl aminolevulinate (MAL) and red light PDT. In another study, 7 patients were treated with aminolevulinic acid (ALA) and a red light source with marked improvement in 2 patients and complete clearance in 2 patients.[111] These patients were treated with 2 to 3 sessions at 2- to 4-week intervals. Clazavara-Pinton and colleagues[112] conducted a retrospective analysis of patients treated with MAL and red light PDT. In the 13 patients with GA, there was a marked to moderate response in 9 of the treated patients.

Oral antibiotics, in particular those in the tetracycline family, have been used in the treatment of generalized GA. The tetracyclines are broad-spectrum antibiotics that are additionally antiinflammatory.[113] Duarte reported a patient with generalized GA who cleared with 10 weeks of doxycycline (100 mg daily).[114] This patient remained clear at 1 year of follow-up. Treatment with monthly rifampicin, ofloxacin, and minocycline has been reported effective in the treatment of GA.[115,116] Marcus and colleagues[116] treated 6 patients with recalcitrant biopsy-proved GA with 3 months of monthly rifampicin (600 mg), ofloxacin (400 mg), and minocycline hydrochloride (100 mg) combination therapy. Complete clearance of lesions was noted in all patients 3 to 5 months after therapy. Side effects were mild and some patients developed postinflammatory hyperpigmentation as the lesions resolved. Dapsone therapy has also been reported to result in clearance of generalized and localized GA lesions.[117–119] Reports of dapsone (100–200 mg/d) have shown clearance of lesions within 6 weeks of initiating therapy.[117]

Treatment with fumaric acid esters (FAEs) has been reported effective in the treatment of widespread disease. Weber and colleagues[120] reported a series patients treated with low-dose FAEs for 1 to 18 months. One patient showed complete clearance and 4 were reported to have marked improvement. One patient failed to show any improvement. Kreuter and colleagues[121] reported a female patient with a 25-year history of recalcitrant disseminated disease successfully treated with a combination of low- and high-dose fumaric acids. Therapy was discontinued after 3 months and she remained clear at 6 months. Acharya[122] treated 2 patients with longstanding disseminated GA with FAEs. One patient had clearance after 6 months and was maintained on low-dose FAEs, whereas a second patient had suboptimal clearance of lesions and discontinued therapy after 12 months. Eberlein-Konig and colleagues[123] treated 8 patients with FAEs and noted remission in 3, partial remission in 4, and no change in 1 patient. Breuer and colleagues[124] treated 32 patients with various noninfectious granulomas with FAEs. Of the 13 patients with GA, 8 were noted to have improved. The main side effects associated with FAEs include gastrointestinal, flushing, reversible elevation of transaminases, lymphocytopenia, and eosinophilia.[125]

Antimalarials are often used in the treatment of generalized GA. Chloroquine (250 mg daily) was successfully used in a patient with photodistributed GA.[126] Hydroxychloroquine has been used in the treatment of generalized GA.[127,128] Cannistraci and colleagues[127] treated 9 patients with generalized GA with 4 months of hydroxychloroquine (9 mg/kg/d for 2 months; 6 mg/kg/d for month 3; and 2 mg/kg/d for month 4). In this series of patients, complete remission was seen in all patients within 6 to 7 weeks of initiation of therapy. The 1 child in the study was treated with half of the dosing scheme.

The systemic retinoids isotretinoin[129–136] and etretinate[137,138] have been reported useful in the treatment of generalized GA. Sahin and colleagues[136] reported a case of generalized GA in a diabetic patient successfully treated with isotretinoin (50 mg/d). Their patient had 90% clinical improvement in their lesions. Adams and Hogan[129] also reported a case of longstanding generalized GA showing 90% improvement with oral isotretinoin therapy (40 to 80 mg/d). Additional reports and small case series have shown improvement in generalized GA with the treatment of oral isotretinoin at doses of 0.5 to 1 mg/kg/d.[131–135,139]

In addition to these treatment modalities, there are reports of additional nonimmunosuppressive systemic treatments of generalized GA. These have included calcitriol (0.025 μg daily),[140] niacinamide (1500 mg/d),[141] pentoxifylline (400 mg 3 times daily),[142] potassium iodide,[143] allopurinol (300 mg twice daily),[144] and zileuton (2400 mg daily) combined with vitamin E (400 IU daily).[145,146]

There are a few case reports and small case series evaluating the role for systemic immunosuppression in the treatment of GA. Cyclosporine was used to treat 4 patients with disseminated GA at a starting dose of 4 mg/kg/d for 4 weeks with gradual taper.[147] Resolution was noted within 3 weeks and no relapse was noted either during taper or in the 12 weeks after discontinuation of cyclosporine. There is an additional case report of cyclosporine (5 mg/kg/d) clearing GA in a patient with leukemia.[58] Methotrexate was successfully used to treat 1 patient with disseminated GA.[148] Methotrexate (15 mg weekly) and daily folic acid supplementation resulted in clearance of a majority of lesions in a female patient. With cessation of therapy, lesions recurred and again resolved with reinstitution of therapy. Administration of the alkylating agent chlorambucil in low doses has been reported to result in improvement of GA lesions.[149–152] For any systemic therapy, consideration of both short- and long-term side effects is necessary and close monitoring is required.

Lastly, the role of biologic therapy, specifically anti–TNF-α, has been investigated as a treatment option for patients with recalcitrant generalized or disseminated disease. As discussed previously, TNF-α is important in the formation and maintenance of granulomas and as such may offer a target for therapy. In particular, adalimumab and infliximab have been reported in the treatment of generalized GA. Knoell reported a rapid response of disseminated GA in identical twins with the AH8.1 haplotype.[28] Werchau and colleagues[153] reported a case of generalized GA that resolved after treatment with adalimumab (80 mg initially followed by 40 mg every 2 weeks). Torres and colleagues[154] treated a patient with disseminated GA with adalimumab (80 mg at week 0 followed by 40 mg [starting at week 1] every other week). This patient had complete clearance by week 8. At 6 months, due to sustained response without recurrence, adalimumab was discontinued and at 9 months the patient remained clear. Infliximab has also been used to treat generalized and disseminated GA. Hertl and colleagues[155] reported a case of a patient treated with infliximab (5 mg/kg) at weeks 0, 2, and 6, followed by monthly infusions for 4 months. Improvement was noted within 4 to 6 weeks and no new lesions had appeared at follow-up through 16 months. Murdaca and colleagues[156] treated a patient with disseminated GA with infliximab (5 mg/kg) at weeks 0, 2, and 6 and monthly for 10 months. They also noted improvement within 8 weeks with gradual resolution of lesions over the course of treatment. Most recently, Amy de la Breteque and colleagues[157] reported treatment of recalcitrant GA with infliximab. The dosing in this patient was similar with infliximab (5 mg/kg) administered at 0, 2, and 6 weeks and then every 8 weeks thereafter. After 8 treatments, the lesions had cleared and therapy was discontinued. The patient had mild recurrence of lesions 18 months later and was treated with topical corticosteroids. The results with etanercept are mixed. Although Shupack and Siu[158] reported resolution of generalized GA in 1 patient after 12 weeks of etanercept weekly therapy, Kreuter and colleagues[159] found no improvement in 4 patients with GA treated with etanercept. These recent reports suggest that TNF-α inhibition with adalimumab and infliximab are viable options for patients with severe, recalcitrant disease, or comorbidities contraindicating other therapies previously listed. Caution must be observed, however, because cases of GA induced by TNF-α inhibitors have been reported.[22,23]

SUMMARY

GA is a common noninfectious granulomatous condition that can present with a variety of morphologies. Histologically, it is characterized by central collagen degradation with prominent mucin

deposition and a peripheral histiocytic infiltrate in either a palisaded or interstitial pattern. GA has been associated with several systemic conditions. Recent studies have called into question the association with DM. In patients with chronic, widespread, or relapsing disease, however, screening with hemoglobin A1C is recommended. In female patients with localized disease in particular, screening for thyroid disorders is recommended. The recent association between generalized GA and hyperlipidemia should prompt a lipid panel. Lastly, in patients with acute onset of GA who are over the age of 60 years or in patients with atypical presentations of GA, age-appropriate malignancy work-up, hematologic evaluation, and consideration of screening for HIV, hepatitis B, and hepatitis C is recommended (**Box 1**).

Treatment of GA poses a challenge for both clinician and patient. There are no randomized controlled trials evaluating the different modalities used to treat GA. As discussed, the treatments used stem from case reports or small case series (**Table 1**). For localized disease,

---

Box 1
Recommended evaluations for patients over the age of 60 years or patients with generalized or atypical presentations of granuloma annulare

Complete history and physical examination

Full review of systems

Medication history

Laboratory tests

- Hemoglobin A1C
- Fasting blood glucose
- Fasting lipid panel
- Thyroid-stimulating hormone
- Free thyroxine
- Thyroid antibodies
- HIV studies[a]
- Hepatitis B panel[a]
- Hepatitis C panel[a]

Imaging studies

- Chest radiograph: anterior/posterior and lateral
- CT scan chest, abdomen, pelvis[b]

Age appropriate malignancy screening

- Women: breast examination and mammogram; pelvic examination with Papanicolaou smear; colonoscopy
- Men: prostate examination; prostate specific antigen; colonoscopy

[a] If risk factors identified in history and physical examination.
[b] If clinical suspicion for malignancy.

Table 1
Reported skin-directed and systemic treatments of granuloma annulare

Treatment	Regimen	Outcome	Level of Evidence
Skin-directed therapy			
Cryosurgery[94]	Contact method; 1 freeze-thaw cycle 10–60 s in duration	Resolution of treated lesions	B
Biopsy[93]	Punch biopsy	Resolution of biopsied lesions	D
Topical tacrolimus[87–91]	Topical	Successful	D
Intralesional IFN-γ[95]	2.5×10^5 IU/lesion for 7 consecutive days followed by 3×/wk for 2 wk	Resolution	D
Excimer laser[96]	15 Treatment sessions 300 mJ/cm² with 5 doses per session	Resolution	D
PDL (585–595 nm)[97,98,160]	8 J/cm², 1.5-ms pulse duration, 9 pulses[97]	Resolution	D
	6.75 J/cm², 36–42 pulses at mo 0, 5, 13[98]	Decreased erythema, thickness, diameter	D
	11–15 J/cm², 1.5–2 ms pulse duration, 2–3 sessions at 4–6 wk intervals[160]	Weak improvement for generalized GA with recurrence; notable improvement in localized GA in half of patients treated	C
Er:YAG[99]	5.8–6.8 kJ at 70 J/cm² 8–14 Passes per lesion 11 Treatments q 4 wk	80%–90% Improvement	D
Nd:YAG (1440-nm)[100]	6 J/cm²; 3-ms pulse duration; 2 full passes with 25% overlap at 3-wk intervals	Complete remission	D
NB-UVB[101]	400 mJ/cm² weekly × 24 treatments	Near complete remission	D
BB-UVB[102]	3 × Per wk × 16 wk	Good or excellent response	C
UV-A1[103–105]	High dose and medium dose	Improvement but with relapse	D
PUVA[103–109]	Bath, cream, oral psoralen	Complete clearance in most, significant improvement in 1[108]	C,[107] D[106,108,109]
PDT	MAL + red light[110,112] ALA + red light[111]	Marked to moderate response Marked improvement to complete clearance in 57%	C,[112] D[110] B
Systemic therapy			
Doxycycline[114]	100 mg/d × 10 wk	Near-complete resolution	D
ROM[115,116]	Monthly: R 600 mg O 400 mg M 100 mg	Resolution	D
Dapsone[117–119]	100–200 mg Daily	Partial response to complete remission	D
FAEs[120–124]	Variable dosing schemes	Improvement or complete resolution in most reports	C

(continued on next page)

Table 1
(continued)

Treatment	Regimen	Outcome	Level of Evidence
Chloroquine[126]	250 mg Daily	Successful	D
Hydroxychloroquine[127]	9 mg/kg/d × 2 Mo 6 mg/kg/d Mo 3 2 mg/kg/d Mo 4	Complete remission	D
Isotretinoin[129,130,132–134]	0.5–1 mg/kg/d	Improvement to complete remission	D
Calcitriol[140]	0.025 µg/d	Gradual improvement and resolution	D
Niacinamide[141]	1500 mg/d	Resolution	D
Pentoxifylline[142]	400 mg 3 Times daily	Clearance	D
Allopurinol[144]	300 mg Twice daily	Near-complete clearance	D
5-Lipoxygenase inhibitor + vitamin E[145,146]	Zileuton 600 mg 4 times daily + vitamin E 400 IU daily	Complete clearance in 3 patients; slight improvement in 1 patient	D
Cyclosporine[147]	4 mg/kg/d × 4 wk Decrease 0.5 mg/kg/d every 2 wk	Resolution	D
Methotrexate[148]	15 mg Weekly Folic acid 1 mg daily	Resolution	D
Chlorambucil[150,152]	4–6 mg/d	Resolution	D
Etanercept[158]	50 mg Twice weekly	Improved	D
Adalimumab[28,153,154]	80 mg at Wk 0 40 mg at Wk 1 and every other wk	Clearance	D
Infliximab[155–157]	5 mg/kg at 0, 2, and 6 Wk, then variable	Resolution	D

B, lesser-quality RCT or prospective study; C, case–control study or retrospective study; D, case series or case reports.
Abbreviations: BB-UVB, broadband UV-B; M, minocycline; ms, millisecond; O, ofloxacin; R, rifampicin.
Data from Refs.[28,87–91,93–109,114–124,126,127,129,130,132–134,140–142,144–148,150,152–158]

initiation with skin-directed local therapy is recommended as first-line therapy. This can include topical corticosteroids, topical tacrolimus, intralesional therapy, or destructive methods. For more generalized disease, careful consideration for disease severity, underlying medical conditions and comorbidities, and potential side effects is imperative. Initiation of immunomodulating antiinflammatory therapy is generally safe and notable for mild side effects. Immunosuppression with methotrexate, cyclosporine, and TNF-α inhibitors can be considered in patients with severe disease that has been recalcitrant to other therapies.

REFERENCES

1. Studer EM, Calza AM, Saurat JH. Precipitating factors and associated diseases in 84 patients with granuloma annulare: a retrospective study. Dermatology 1996;193(4):364–8.
2. Umbert P, Winkelmann RK. Histologic, ultrastructural and histochemical studies of granuloma annulare. Arch Dermatol 1977;113(12):1681–6.
3. Buechner SA, Winkelmann RK, Banks PM. Identification of T-cell subpopulations in granuloma annulare. Arch Dermatol 1983;119(2):125–8.
4. Fayyazi A, Schweyer S, Eichmeyer B, et al. Expression of IFNgamma, coexpression of TNFalpha and matrix metalloproteinases and apoptosis of T lymphocytes and macrophages in granuloma annulare. Arch Dermatol Res 2000;292(8):384–90.
5. Mempel M, Musette P, Flageul B, et al. T-cell receptor repertoire and cytokine pattern in granuloma annulare: defining a particular type of cutaneous granulomatous inflammation. J Invest Dermatol 2002;118(6):957–66.
6. Spring P, Vernez M, Maniu CM, et al. Localized interstitial granuloma annulare induced by

subcutaneous injections for desensitization. Dermatol Online J 2013;19(6):18572.

7. Yoon NY, Lee NR, Choi EH. Generalized granuloma annulare after bacillus Calmette-Guerin vaccination, clinically resembling papular tuberculid. J Dermatol 2014;41(1):109–11.

8. Lee SW, Cheong SH, Byun JY, et al. Generalized granuloma annulare in infancy following bacillus calmette-guerin vaccination. Ann Dermatol 2011;23(Suppl 3):S319–21.

9. Kakurai M, Kiyosawa T, Ohtsuki M, et al. Multiple lesions of granuloma annulare following BCG vaccination: case report and review of the literature. Int J Dermatol 2001;40(9):579–81.

10. Houcke-Bruge C, Delaporte E, Catteau B, et al. Granuloma annulare following BCG vaccination. Ann Dermatol Venereol 2001;128(4):541–4 [in French].

11. Baskan EB, Tunali S, Kacar SD, et al. A case of granuloma annulare in a child following tetanus and diphtheria toxoid vaccination. J Eur Acad Dermatol Venereol 2005;19(5):639–40.

12. Baykal C, Ozkaya-Bayazit E, Kaymaz R. Granuloma annulare possibly triggered by antitetanus vaccination. J Eur Acad Dermatol Venereol 2002;16(5):516–8.

13. Wolf F, Grezard P, Berard F, et al. Generalized granuloma annulare and hepatitis B vaccination. Eur J Dermatol 1998;8(6):435–6.

14. Criado PR, de Oliveira Ramos R, Vasconcellos C, et al. Two case reports of cutaneous adverse reactions following hepatitis B vaccine: lichen planus and granuloma annulare. J Eur Acad Dermatol Venereol 2004;18(5):603–6.

15. Gass JK, Todd PM, Rytina E. Generalized granuloma annulare in a photosensitive distribution resolving with scarring and milia formation. Clin Exp Dermatol 2009;34(5):e53–5.

16. Alvarez-Perez A, Gomez-Bernal S, Gutierrez-Gonzalez E, et al. Granuloma annulare photoinduced by paroxetine. Photodermatol Photoimmunol Photomed 2012;28(1):47–9.

17. Cohen PR, Grossman ME, Silvers DN, et al. Generalized granuloma annulare located on sun-exposed areas in a human immunodeficiency virus-seropositive man with ultraviolet B photosensitivity. Arch Dermatol 1990;126(6):830–1.

18. Strahan JE, Cohen JL, Chorny JA. Granuloma annulare as a complication of mesotherapy: a case report. Dermatol Surg 2008;34(6):836–8.

19. Cassone G, Tumiati B. Granuloma annulare as a possible new adverse effect of topiramate. Int J Dermatol 2014;53(2):259–61.

20. Goihman-Yahr M. Disseminated granuloma annulare and intranasal calcitonin. Int J Dermatol 1993;32(2):150.

21. Singh SK, Manchanda K, Bhayana AA, et al. Allopurinol induced granuloma annulare in a patient of lepromatous leprosy. J Pharmacol Pharmacother 2013;4(2):152–4.

22. Viguier M, Richette P, Bachelez H, et al. Paradoxical cutaneous manifestations during anti-TNF-alpha therapy. Ann Dermatol Venereol 2010;137(1):64–71 [in French; quiz: 63, 78–69].

23. Voulgari PV, Markatseli TE, Exarchou SA, et al. Granuloma annulare induced by anti-tumour necrosis factor therapy. Ann Rheum Dis 2008;67(4):567–70.

24. Dahl MV, Ullman S, Goltz RW. Vasculitis in granuloma annulare: histopathology and direct immunofluorescence. Arch Dermatol 1977;113(4):463–7.

25. Padilla RS, Holguin T, Burgdorf WH, et al. Serum lysozyme in patients with localized and generalized granuloma annulare. Arch Dermatol 1985;121(5):624–5.

26. Hanna WM, Moreno-Merlo F, Andrighetti L. Granuloma annulare: an elastic tissue disease? Case report and literature review. Ultrastruct Pathol 1999;23(1):33–8.

27. Friedman-Birnbaum R, Haim S, Gideone O, et al. Histocompatibility antigens in granuloma annulare. Comparative study of the generalized and localized types. Br J Dermatol 1978;98(4):425–8.

28. Knoell KA. Efficacy of adalimumab in the treatment of generalized granuloma annulare in monozygotic twins carrying the 8.1 ancestral haplotype. Arch Dermatol 2009;145(5):610–1.

29. Thornsberry LA, English JC 3rd. Etiology, diagnosis, and therapeutic management of granuloma annulare: an update. Am J Clin Dermatol 2013;14(4):279–90.

30. Muhlemann MF, Williams DR. Localized granuloma annulare is associated with insulin-dependent diabetes mellitus. Br J Dermatol 1984;111(3):325–9.

31. Bansal M, Pandey SS, Manchanda K. Generalized papular granuloma annulare. Indian Dermatol Online J 2012;3(1):74–6.

32. Agrawal AK, Kammen BF, Guo H, et al. An unusual presentation of subcutaneous granuloma annulare in association with juvenile-onset diabetes: case report and literature review. Pediatr Dermatol 2012;29(2):202–5.

33. Requena L, Fernandez-Figueras MT. Subcutaneous granuloma annulare. Semin Cutan Med Surg 2007;26(2):96–9.

34. Grogg KL, Nascimento AG. Subcutaneous granuloma annulare in childhood: clinicopathologic features in 34 cases. Pediatrics 2001;107(3):E42.

35. Mutasim DF, Bridges AG. Patch granuloma annulare: clinicopathologic study of 6 patients. J Am Acad Dermatol 2000;42(3):417–21.

36. Stewart LR, George S, Hamacher KL, et al. Granuloma annulare of the palms. Dermatol Online J 2011;17(5):7.

37. Green TL, Hikado M, Greenspan D. Granuloma annulare of the buccal mucosa in association with

AIDS. Oral Surg Oral Med Oral Pathol 1989;67(3):
319–21.

38. Haim S, Friedman-Birnbaum R, Haim N, et al. Carbohydrate tolerance in patients with granuloma annulare. Study of fifty-two cases. Br J Dermatol 1973;88(5):447–51.

39. Haim S, Friedman-Birnbaum R, Shafrir A. Generalized granuloma annulare: relationship to diabetes mellitus as revealed in 8 cases. Br J Dermatol 1970;83(2):302–5.

40. Gannon TF, Lynch PJ. Absence of carbohydrate intolerance in granuloma annulare. J Am Acad Dermatol 1994;30(4):662–3.

41. Nebesio CL, Lewis C, Chuang TY. Lack of an association between granuloma annulare and type 2 diabetes mellitus. Br J Dermatol 2002;146(1):122–4.

42. Veraldi S, Bencini PL, Drudi E, et al. Laboratory abnormalities in granuloma annulare: a case-control study. Br J Dermatol 1997;136(4):652–3.

43. Dabski K, Winkelmann RK. Generalized granuloma annulare: clinical and laboratory findings in 100 patients. J Am Acad Dermatol 1989;20(1):39–47.

44. Heymann WR. Cutaneous manifestations of thyroid disease. J Am Acad Dermatol 1992;26(6):885–902.

45. Kappeler D, Troendle A, Mueller B. Localized granuloma annulare associated with autoimmune thyroid disease in a patient with a positive family history for autoimmune polyglandular syndrome type II. Eur J Endocrinol 2001;145(1):101–2.

46. Vazquez-Lopez F, Gonzalez-Lopez MA, Raya-Aguado C, et al. Localized granuloma annulare and autoimmune thyroiditis: a new case report. J Am Acad Dermatol 2000;43(5 Pt 2):943–5.

47. Maschio M, Marigliano M, Sabbion A, et al. A rare case of granuloma annulare in a 5-year-old child with type 1 diabetes and autoimmune thyroiditis. Am J Dermatopathol 2013;35(3):385–7.

48. Vazquez-Lopez F, Pereiro M Jr, Manjon Haces JA, et al. Localized granuloma annulare and autoimmune thyroiditis in adult women: a case-control study. J Am Acad Dermatol 2003;48(4):517–20.

49. Barksdale SK, Perniciaro C, Halling KC, et al. Granuloma annulare in patients with malignant lymphoma: clinicopathologic study of thirteen new cases. J Am Acad Dermatol 1994;31(1):42–8.

50. Dadban A, Slama B, Azzedine A, et al. Widespread granuloma annulare and Hodgkin's disease. Clin Exp Dermatol 2008;33(4):465–8.

51. Harman RR. Hodgkin's disease, seminoma of testicle and widespread granuloma annulare. Br J Dermatol 1977;97(Suppl 15):50–1.

52. Mascaro JM Jr. Cutaneous signs of hematologic malignancies: "doctor, is there something wrong with my blood?". Arch Dermatol 2011;147(3):342–4.

53. Schwartz RA, Hansen RC, Lynch PJ. Hodgkin's disease and granuloma annulare. Arch Dermatol 1981;117(3):185–6.

54. Setoyama M, Kerdel FA, Byrnes JJ, et al. Granuloma annulare associated with Hodgkin's disease. Int J Dermatol 1997;36(6):445–8.

55. Bassi A, Scarfi F, Galeone M, et al. Generalized granuloma annulare and non-Hodgkin's lymphoma. Acta Derm Venereol 2013;93(4):484–5.

56. Bhushan M, Craven NM, Armstrong GR, et al. Lymphoepithelioid cell lymphoma (Lennert's lymphoma) presenting as atypical granuloma annulare. Br J Dermatol 2000;142(4):776–80.

57. Martin JE, Wagner AJ, Murphy GF, et al. Granuloma annulare heralding angioimmunoblastic T-cell lymphoma in a patient with a history of epstein-barr virus-associated B-cell lymphoma. J Clin Oncol 2009;27(31):e168–71.

58. Granjo E, Lima M, Lopes JM, et al. Response to cyclosporine in a patient with disseminated granuloma annulare associated with CD4+/CD8+(dim)/CD56+ large granular lymphocytic leukemia. Arch Dermatol 2002;138(2):274–6.

59. Hinckley MR, Walsh SN, Molnar I, et al. Generalized granuloma annulare as an initial manifestation of chronic myelomonocytic leukemia: a report of 2 cases. Am J Dermatopathol 2008;30(3):274–7.

60. Jee MS, Kim ES, Chang SE, et al. Disseminated granuloma annulare associated with chronic myelogenous leukemia. J Dermatol 2003;30(8):631–3.

61. Sokumbi O, Gibson LE, Comfere NI, et al. Granuloma annulare-like eruption associated with B-cell chronic lymphocytic leukemia. J Cutan Pathol 2012;39(11):996–1003.

62. Cohen PR. Granuloma annulare associated with malignancy. South Med J 1997;90(10):1056–9.

63. Cohen PR. Granuloma annulare, relapsing polychondritis, sarcoidosis, and systemic lupus erythematosus: conditions whose dermatologic manifestations may occur as hematologic malignancy-associated mucocutaneous paraneoplastic syndromes. Int J Dermatol 2006;45(1):70–80.

64. Li A, Hogan DJ, Sanusi ID, et al. Granuloma annulare and malignant neoplasms. Am J Dermatopathol 2003;25(2):113–6.

65. Hawryluk EB, Izikson L, English JC 3rd. Non-infectious granulomatous diseases of the skin and their associated systemic diseases: an evidence-based update to important clinical questions. Am J Clin Dermatol 2010;11(3):171–81.

66. Marzano AV, Ramoni S, Alessi E, et al. Generalized granuloma annulare and eruptive folliculitis in an HIV-positive man: resolution after antiretroviral therapy. J Eur Acad Dermatol Venereol 2007;21(8):1114–6.

67. McGregor JM, McGibbon DH. Disseminated granuloma annulare as a presentation of acquired immunodeficiency syndrome (AIDS). Clin Exp Dermatol 1992;17(1):60–2.

68. O'Moore EJ, Nandawni R, Uthayakumar S, et al. HIV-associated granuloma annulare (HAGA): a report of six cases. Br J Dermatol 2000;142(5): 1054–6.

69. Toro JR, Chu P, Yen TS, et al. Granuloma annulare and human immunodeficiency virus infection. Arch Dermatol 1999;135(11):1341–6.

70. Bakos L, Hampe S, da Rocha JL, et al. Generalized granuloma annulare in a patient with acquired immunodeficiency syndrome (AIDS). J Am Acad Dermatol 1987;17(5 Pt 1):844–5.

71. Jones SK, Harman RR. Atypical granuloma annulare in patients with the acquired immunodeficiency syndrome. J Am Acad Dermatol 1989;20(2 Pt 1):299–300.

72. Kapembwa MS, Goolamali SK, Price A, et al. Granuloma annulare masquerading as molluscum contagiosum-like eruption in an HIV-positive African woman. J Am Acad Dermatol 2003;49(2 Suppl Case Reports):S184–6.

73. Huerter CJ, Bass J, Bergfeld WF, et al. Perforating granuloma annulare in a patient with acquired immunodeficiency syndrome. Immunohistologic evaluation of the cellular infiltrate. Arch Dermatol 1987; 123(9):1217–20.

74. Cohen PR. Granuloma annulare: a mucocutaneous condition in human immunodeficiency virus-infected patients. Arch Dermatol 1999;135(11):1404–7.

75. Jacobi D, Rivollier C, Buisson H, et al. Generalized granuloma annulare: remission during treatment of HIV infection. Ann Dermatol Venereol 2005;132(3): 243–5 [in French].

76. Leenutaphong V, Holzle E, Erckenbrecht J, et al. Remission of human immunodeficiency virus-associated generalized granuloma annulare under zidovudine therapy. J Am Acad Dermatol 1988; 19(6):1126–7.

77. Avitan-Hersh E, Sprecher H, Ramon M, et al. Does infection play a role in the pathogenesis of granuloma annulare? J Am Acad Dermatol 2013;68(2): 342–3.

78. Wu W, Robinson-Bostom L, Kokkotou E, et al. Dyslipidemia in granuloma annulare: a case-control study. Arch Dermatol 2012;148(10):1131–6.

79. Dahl MV. Testing lipid levels in granuloma annulare. Arch Dermatol 2012;148(10):1136–7.

80. Brechtel B, Kolde G. Granuloma annulare disseminatum as a rare side effect of allopurinol. Hautarzt 1996;47(2):143 [in German].

81. Ferreli C, Atzori L, Manunza F, et al. Thalidomide-induced granuloma annulare. G Ital Dermatol Venereol 2014;149(3):329–33.

82. Ahmad U, Li X, Sodeman T, et al. Hepatitis C virus treatment with pegylated interferon-alfa therapy leading to generalized interstitial granuloma annulare and review of the literature. Am J Ther 2013; 20(5):585–7.

83. Kluger N, Moguelet P, Chaslin-Ferbus D, et al. Generalized interstitial granuloma annulare induced by pegylated interferon-alpha. Dermatology 2006;213(3):248–9.

84. Lagier L, Dunoyer E, Esteve E. Topiramate: a new inductor of granuloma annulare? Ann Dermatol Venereol 2011;138(2):141–3 [in French].

85. Dahl MV. Granuloma annulare: long-term follow-up. Arch Dermatol 2007;143(7):946–7.

86. Pfaltz K, Kerl K, Palmedo G, et al. Clonality in sarcoidosis, granuloma annulare, and granulomatous mycosis fungoides. Am J Dermatopathol 2011;33(7):659–62.

87. Gomez-Moyano E, Vera-Casano A, Martinez S, et al. Periorbital granuloma annulare successfully treated with tacrolimus 0.1% ointment. Int J Dermatol 2014;53(2):e156–7.

88. Grieco T, Cantisani C, Faina P, et al. Tacrolimus 0.1% and granuloma annulare: description of three cases. J Eur Acad Dermatol Venereol 2009;23(12): 1445–6.

89. Harth W, Linse R. Topical tacrolimus in granuloma annulare and necrobiosis lipoidica. Br J Dermatol 2004;150(4):792–4.

90. Jain S, Stephens CJ. Successful treatment of disseminated granuloma annulare with topical tacrolimus. Br J Dermatol 2004;150(5):1042–3.

91. Lopez-Navarro N, Castillo R, Gallardo MA, et al. Successful treatment of perforating granuloma annulare with 0.1% tacrolimus ointment. J Dermatolog Treat 2008;19(6):376–7.

92. Macaron NC, Cohen C, Chen SC, et al. gli-1 Oncogene is highly expressed in granulomatous skin disorders, including sarcoidosis, granuloma annulare, and necrobiosis lipoidica diabeticorum. Arch Dermatol 2005;141(2):259–62.

93. Levin NA, Patterson JW, Yao LL, et al. Resolution of patch-type granuloma annulare lesions after biopsy. J Am Acad Dermatol 2002;46(3):426–9.

94. Blume-Peytavi U, Zouboulis CC, Jacobi H, et al. Successful outcome of cryosurgery in patients with granuloma annulare. Br J Dermatol 1994; 130(4):494–7.

95. Weiss JM, Muchenberger S, Schopf E, et al. Treatment of granuloma annulare by local injections with low-dose recombinant human interferon gamma. J Am Acad Dermatol 1998;39(1):117–9.

96. Bronfenbrener R, Ragi J, Milgraum S. Granuloma annulare treated with excimer laser. J Clin Aesthet Dermatol 2012;5(11):43–5.

97. Sliger BN, Burk CJ, Alvarez-Connelly E. Treatment of granuloma annulare with the 595 nm pulsed dye laser in a pediatric patient. Pediatr Dermatol 2008;25(2):196–7.

98. Sniezek PJ, DeBloom JR 2nd, Arpey CJ. Treatment of granuloma annulare with the 585 nm pulsed dye laser. Dermatol Surg 2005;31(10):1370–3.

99. Liu A, Hexsel CL, Moy RL, et al. Granuloma annulare successfully treated using fractional photothermolysis with a 1,550-nm erbium-doped yttrium aluminum garnet fractionated laser. Dermatol Surg 2011;37(5):712–5.

100. Karsai S, Hammes S, Rutten A, et al. Fractional photothermolysis for the treatment of granuloma annulare: a case report. Lasers Surg Med 2008; 40(5):319–22.

101. Inui S, Nishida Y, Itami S, et al. Disseminated granuloma annulare responsive to narrowband ultraviolet B therapy. J Am Acad Dermatol 2005; 53(3):533–4.

102. Do TT, Bailey EC, Wang F, et al. Targeted broadband ultraviolet B phototherapy improves disorders characterized by increased dermal matrix. Br J Dermatol 2009;161(6):1405–7.

103. Frigerio E, Franchi C, Garutti C, et al. Multiple localized granuloma annulare: ultraviolet A1 phototherapy. Clin Exp Dermatol 2007;32(6):762–4.

104. Muchenberger S, Schopf E, Simon JC. Phototherapy with UV-A-I for generalized granuloma annulare. Arch Dermatol 1997;133(12):1605.

105. Schnopp C, Tzaneva S, Mempel M, et al. UVA1 phototherapy for disseminated granuloma annulare. Photodermatol Photoimmunol Photomed 2005;21(2):68–71.

106. Batchelor R, Clark S. Clearance of generalized papular umbilicated granuloma annulare in a child with bath PUVA therapy. Pediatr Dermatol 2006; 23(1):72–4.

107. Browne F, Turner D, Goulden V. Psoralen and ultraviolet A in the treatment of granuloma annulare. Photodermatol Photoimmunol Photomed 2011; 27(2):81–4.

108. Grundmann-Kollmann M, Ochsendorf FR, Zollner TM, et al. Cream psoralen plus ultraviolet A therapy for granuloma annulare. Br J Dermatol 2001;144(5): 996–9.

109. Kerker BJ, Huang CP, Morison WL. Photochemotherapy of generalized granuloma annulare. Arch Dermatol 1990;126(3):359–61.

110. Piaserico S, Zattra E, Linder D, et al. Generalized granuloma annulare treated with methylaminolevulinate photodynamic therapy. Dermatology 2009; 218(3):282–4.

111. Weisenseel P, Kuznetsov AV, Molin S, et al. Photodynamic therapy for granuloma annulare: more than a shot in the dark. Dermatology 2008;217(4): 329–32.

112. Calzavara-Pinton PG, Rossi MT, Aronson E, et al, Italian Group For Photodynamic Therapy. A retrospective analysis of real-life practice of off-label photodynamic therapy using methyl aminolevulinate (MAL-PDT) in 20 Italian dermatology departments. Part 1: inflammatory and aesthetic indications. Photochem Photobiol Sci 2013;12(1):148–57.

113. Sapadin AN, Fleischmajer R. Tetracyclines: nonantibiotic properties and their clinical implications. J Am Acad Dermatol 2006;54(2):258–65.

114. Duarte AF, Mota A, Pereira MA, et al. Generalized granuloma annulare–response to doxycycline. J Eur Acad Dermatol Venereol 2009;23(1):84–5.

115. Garg S, Baveja S. Generalized granuloma annulare treated with monthly rifampicin, ofloxacin, and minocycline combination therapy. Indian J Dermatol 2013;58(3):197–9.

116. Marcus DV, Mahmoud BH, Hamzavi IH. Granuloma annulare treated with rifampin, ofloxacin, and minocycline combination therapy. Arch Dermatol 2009;145(7):787–9.

117. Saied N, Schwartz RA, Estes SA. Treatment of generalized granuloma annulare with dapsone. Arch Dermatol 1980;116(12):1345–6.

118. Czarnecki DB, Gin D. The response of generalized granuloma annulare to dapsone. Acta Derm Venereol 1986;66(1):82–4.

119. Steiner A, Pehamberger H, Wolff K. Sulfone treatment of granuloma annulare. J Am Acad Dermatol 1985;13(6):1004–8.

120. Weber HO, Borelli C, Rocken M, et al. Treatment of disseminated granuloma annulare with low-dose fumaric acid. Acta Derm Venereol 2009;89(3): 295–8.

121. Kreuter A, Gambichler T, Altmeyer P, et al. Treatment of disseminated granuloma annulare with fumaric acid esters. BMC Dermatol 2002;2:5.

122. Acharya U. Successful treatment of disseminated granuloma annulare with oral fumaric acid esters. Int J Dermatol 2013;52(5):633–4.

123. Eberlein-Konig B, Mempel M, Stahlecker J, et al. Disseminated granuloma annulare–treatment with fumaric acid esters. Dermatology 2005;210(3): 223–6.

124. Breuer K, Gutzmer R, Volker B, et al. Therapy of noninfectious granulomatous skin diseases with fumaric acid esters. Br J Dermatol 2005;152(6): 1290–5.

125. Wollina U. Fumaric acid esters in dermatology. Indian Dermatol Online J 2011;2(2):111–9.

126. Andreu-Barasoain M, Gomez de la Fuente E, Pinedo F, et al. Long lasting interstitial generalized granuloma annulare on sun-exposed areas. Photodermatol Photoimmunol Photomed 2012;28(4):216–8.

127. Cannistraci C, Lesnoni La Parola I, Falchi M, et al. Treatment of generalized granuloma annulare with hydroxychloroquine. Dermatology 2005;211(2): 167–8.

128. Simon M Jr, von den Driesch P. Antimalarials for control of disseminated granuloma annulare in children. J Am Acad Dermatol 1994;31(6):1064–5.

129. Adams DC, Hogan DJ. Improvement of chronic generalized granuloma annulare with isotretinoin. Arch Dermatol 2002;138(11):1518–9.

130. Ratnavel RC, Norris PG. Perforating granuloma annulare: response to treatment with isotretinoin. J Am Acad Dermatol 1995;32(1):126–7.

131. Schleicher SM, Milstein HJ. Resolution of disseminated granuloma annulare following isotretinoin therapy. Cutis 1985;36(2):147–8.

132. Schleicher SM, Milstein HJ, Lim SJ, et al. Resolution of disseminated granuloma annulare with isotretinoin. Int J Dermatol 1992;31(5):371–2.

133. Tang WY, Chong LY, Lo KK. Resolution of generalized granuloma annulare with isotretinoin therapy. Int J Dermatol 1996;35(6):455–6.

134. Young HS, Coulson IH. Granuloma annulare following waxing induced pseudofolliculitis-resolution with isotretinoin. Clin Exp Dermatol 2000;25(4):274–6.

135. Pasmatzi E, Georgiou S, Monastirli A, et al. Temporary remission of disseminated granuloma annulare under oral isotretinoin therapy. Int J Dermatol 2005; 44(2):169–71.

136. Sahin MT, Turel-Ermertcan A, Ozturkcan S, et al. Generalized granuloma annulare in a patient with type II diabetes mellitus: successful treatment with isotretinoin. J Eur Acad Dermatol Venereol 2006;20(1):111–4.

137. Botella-Estrada R, Guillen C, Sanmartin O, et al. Disseminated granuloma annulare: resolution with etretinate therapy. J Am Acad Dermatol 1992; 26(5 Pt 1):777–8.

138. Asano Y, Saito A, Idezuki T, et al. Generalized granuloma annulare treated with short-term administration of etretinate. J Am Acad Dermatol 2006;54(5 Suppl):S245–7.

139. Baskan EB, Turan A, Tunali S. A case of generalized granuloma annulare with myelodysplastic syndrome: successful treatment with systemic isotretinoin and topical pimecrolimus 1% cream combination. J Eur Acad Dermatol Venereol 2007;21(5):693–5.

140. Boyd AS. Granuloma annulare responsive to oral calcitriol. Int J Dermatol 2012;51(1):120–2.

141. Ma A, Medenica M. Response of generalized granuloma annulare to high-dose niacinamide. Arch Dermatol 1983;119(10):836–9.

142. Rubel DM, Wood G, Rosen R, et al. Generalised granuloma annulare successfully treated with pentoxifylline. Australas J Dermatol 1993;34(3):103–8.

143. Caserio RJ, Eaglstein WH, Allen CM. Treatment of granuloma annulare with potassium iodide. J Am Acad Dermatol 1984;10(2 Pt 1):294–5.

144. Mazzatenta C, Ghilardi A, Grazzini M. Treatment of disseminated granuloma annulare with allopurinol: case report. Dermatol Ther 2010;23(Suppl 1):S24–7.

145. Guardiano RA, Lee W, Norwood C, et al. Generalized granuloma annulare in a patient with adult onset diabetes mellitus. J Drugs Dermatol 2003;2(6):666–8.

146. Smith KJ, Norwood C, Skelton H. Treatment of disseminated granuloma annulare with a 5-lipoxygenase inhibitor and vitamin E. Br J Dermatol 2002;146(4):667–70.

147. Spadino S, Altomare A, Cainelli C, et al. Disseminated granuloma annulare: efficacy of cyclosporine therapy. Int J Immunopathol Pharmacol 2006;19(2): 433–8.

148. Plotner AN, Mutasim DF. Successful treatment of disseminated granuloma annulare with methotrexate. Br J Dermatol 2010;163(5):1123–4.

149. Kossard S, Winkelmann RK. Low-dose chlorambucil in the treatment of generalized granuloma annulare. Dermatologica 1979;158(6):443–50.

150. Mutasim D, Karban AK. Granuloma annulare treated with chlorambucil: an 18-month follow-up. Arch Dermatol 1983;119(6):451–2.

151. Rudolph RI. Disseminated granuloma annulare treated with low-dose chlorambucil. Arch Dermatol 1979;115(10):1212–3.

152. Winkelmann RK, Stevens JC. Successful treatment response of granuloma annulare and carpal tunnel syndrome to chlorambucil. Mayo Clin Proc 1994; 69(12):1163–5.

153. Werchau S, Enk A, Hartmann M. Generalized interstitial granuloma annulare–response to adalimumab. Int J Dermatol 2010;49(4):457–60.

154. Torres T, Pinto Almeida T, Alves R, et al. Treatment of recalcitrant generalized granuloma annulare with adalimumab. J Drugs Dermatol 2011;10(12): 1466–8.

155. Hertl MS, Haendle I, Schuler G, et al. Rapid improvement of recalcitrant disseminated granuloma annulare upon treatment with the tumour necrosis factor-alpha inhibitor, infliximab. Br J Dermatol 2005;152(3):552–5.

156. Murdaca G, Colombo BM, Barabino G, et al. Anti-tumor necrosis factor-alpha treatment with infliximab for disseminated granuloma annulare. Am J Clin Dermatol 2010;11(6):437–9.

157. Amy de la Breteque M, Saussine A, Rybojad M, et al. Infliximab in recalcitrant granuloma annulare. Int J Dermatol 2014;54(5):1–3.

158. Shupack J, Siu K. Resolving granuloma annulare with etanercept. Arch Dermatol 2006;142(3):394–5.

159. Kreuter A, Altmeyer P, Gambichler T. Failure of etanercept therapy in disseminated granuloma annulare. Arch Dermatol 2006;142(9):1236–7 [author reply: 1237].

160. Passeron T, Fusade T, Vabres P, et al. Treatment of granuloma annulare with the 595-nm pulsed dye laser, a multicentre retrospective study with long-term follow-up. J Eur Acad Dermatol Venereol 2013;27(6):785–8.

Elastolytic Actinic Giant Cell Granuloma

Enrique Gutiérrez-González, MD, Manuel Pereiro Jr, MD, PhD*, Jaime Toribio, MD, PhD

KEYWORDS

- Actinic granuloma • Annular elastolytic giant cell granuloma • Elastophagocytosis • Elastosis
- Diabetes mellitus

KEY POINTS

- Elastolytic actinic giant cell granuloma is a distinct condition characterized by annular lesions with erythematous borders and central clearance.
- Actinic damage is recognized as the main triggering factor, although the pathogenesis of cases in sun-covered areas remains unclear.
- A radial ellipse biopsy taken across the ring is recommended for diagnosis. Histologic features are the presence of an inflammatory infiltrate with nonpalisading granulomas and multinucleated giant cells limited to superficial dermis, as well as the absence of mucin and necrobiosis.
- Diabetes mellitus is the most frequently associated systemic disease.

INTRODUCTION

Annular elastolytic giant cell granuloma, also termed actinic granuloma (AG), when it affects sun-exposed skin, is an uncommon granulomatous skin disease. It is characterized clinically by annular plaques with raised erythematous borders that grow centrifugally and leave an atrophic center (**Fig. 1**). On histopathology the lesions show elastophagocytosis by multinucleated giant cells and marked loss of elastic tissue (**Fig. 2**). Elastophagocytosis is the phagocytosis of elastic fibers that can be seen microscopically in the cytoplasm of multinucleated giant cells and histiocytes (**Fig. 3**). This phenomenon is not exclusive to granulomatous disorders; it has been also described in cutaneous malignancies and infections, and can also be drug induced.[1] Although the pathogenesis of elastolytic actinic giant cell granuloma (EAGCG) remains unclear, it is thought that ultraviolet radiation, heat, and other unknown factors might change the antigenicity of elastic fibers.

ETIOPATHOGENESIS

AG was first described by O'Brien[2] in 1975. He postulated that actinically degenerated elastotic tissue was the antigenic basis of this condition, suggesting that elastotic fibers could be the direct stimulus for the development of granulomas and considering it as a phenomenon of repair of the damaged connective tissue. O'Brien[2] considered actinic injury as the primary event, supported by the observation that most of the lesions appear in sun-exposed areas of skin, with a characteristic solar elastosis that manifests as basophilic in sensitive hematoxylin-eosin stains (**Fig. 4**).[3,4]

Whether it should be considered a specific entity or a subtype of granuloma annulare (GA) is a topic of discussion. The original concept was disputed by Ragaz and Ackerman,[5] who thought that the lesions described by O'Brien[2] were variants of GA in sun-damaged skin. Al-Hoqail and colleagues[6] compared the histologic features of AG and GA located both in sun-exposed and

Conflict of Interests: None.
Department of Dermatology, Faculty of Medicine, Complejo Hospitalario Universitario, Santiago de Compostela, Spain
* Corresponding author. Departamento de Dermatología, Facultad de Medicina, C/. San Francisco, s/n, Santiago de Compostela 15782, Spain.
E-mail address: manuel.pereiro.ferreiros@usc.es

derm.theclinics.com

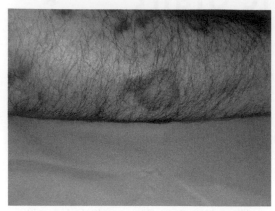

Fig. 1. Annular plaque showing central clearing on the dorsum of the forearm.

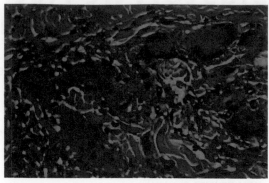

Fig. 3. Foreign body giant cell infiltrate in the mid-dermis (hematoxylin and eosin; original magnification, ×250).

nonexposed areas, concluding that AG was an independent condition that must be differentiated from GA, even in those located in sun-exposed sites. Other investigators supported O'Brien's[2] concept of AG as a distinct entity.[7–10] Cases showing characteristics of both GA and EAGCG have been also reported.[11]

The descriptive term annular elastolytic giant cell granuloma was proposed by Hanke and colleagues[12] for lesions identical to AG but located not only in sun-exposed skin. Under this term he grouped other similar conditions, like Miescher granuloma of the face or atypical necrobiosis lipoidica of the scalp and the face. According to this investigator, the association of solar elastosis and granulomatous inflammation does not imply a cause-effect relationship. They prefer a term that is based on the main histologic features. There have been other descriptions that agree with this concept.[11,13]

O'Brien and Regan[3] refused this term and preferred the original term of AG because "it

conceals the intrinsic and true nature of the lesion, that is, it represents an inflammatory reaction in response to actinically degenerated tissue."

The pathogenesis of EAGCG remains unclear. McGrae[8] suggested an immune response mediated by cells to degenerated elastic tissue, with a predominance of helper T cells in the lymphocytic infiltrate. He also observed differences between the enzymes of the histiocytes of AG and those of GA,[8] supporting that these are different conditions. Elastin peptides are responsible for inducing factor XIIIa(+) cells and macrophages to form granulomas and multinucleated giant cells.[14] Matrix metalloproteinase (MMP)-12, produced by macrophages, is expressed in the infiltrates of EAGCG, explaining the degradation of elastic fibers and inducing the formation of multinucleated giant cells.[15]

Ultraviolet (UV) radiation, especially UVA, because of its longer wavelength, and heat are recognized as causal factors, by changing the antigenicity of elastic fibers and producing an immune response.[2,16] However, collagen is not

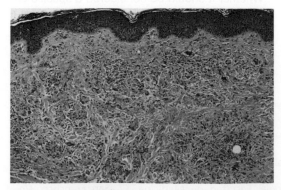

Fig. 2. Interstitial inflammatory infiltrate constituted by giant cell and lymphocytes surrounded by elastotic connective tissue (hematoxylin and eosin; original magnification, ×100).

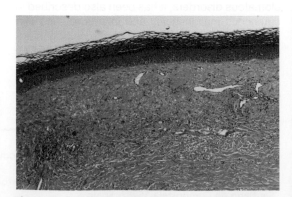

Fig. 4. Basophilic, elastotic degeneration of the dermis: elastic fibers appear thickened, coiled, and bluish (hematoxylin and eosin; original magnification, ×100).

affected by actinic radiation.[17] Development of EAGCG has also been reported after prolonged UVA sun-bed exposure[16] and prolonged doxycycline phototoxicity, highlighting the importance of actinic radiation in the cause of this condition.[18] Heat-damaged skin or repeated skin burns can also favor the development of EAGCG.[19]

A case of widespread EAGCG that spared the area of a burn scar with absent elastic tissue supports the theory that the immune response is directed against elastic fibers.[20] A recent case describing a case of EAGCG sparing the striae distensae, where elastic fibers are also absent, underlines the importance of elastic tissue in the pathogenesis of EAGCG.[21]

CLINICAL PRESENTATIONS

The morphology of AG was initially described as a smooth, elevated, nonscaly, erythematous papule that centrifugally extends to form an annular plaque up to several centimeters in diameter with central clearing, and sometimes atrophy or hypopigmentation.[2] Hair and other skin appendages are preserved. The lesions are usually distributed on sun-exposed areas like the dorsum of the hands, forearms, neck, face, V of neck, and upper back (**Figs. 5–7**).[11] However, other locations, like the legs, especially in women, are common.[13] People with skin phototype I or II seem to be more affected than people with darker phototypes.[2]

These lesions are usually asymptomatic, although some patients complain of mild pruritus or burning sensation.[13] It can last for months or years until spontaneous remission occurs. Although some lesions resolve, new ones may appear, prolonging the condition.

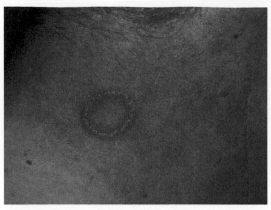

Fig. 6. Annular plaque with raised borders on the side of the neck.

There are also reports of cases of AG-like lesions in sun-protected areas.[12,22–25] O'Brien[17] interpreted these variants as generalized and exaggerated reactions to a minor degree of actinic elastosis.

This condition may present with a single[19] or few lesions[13] or in a generalized fashion.[20,26,27]

Papular (**Fig. 8**)[28–33] and reticular[34,35] variants of EAGCG have been described, and can be observed together in the same patient.[36] An exanthematous form of elastolytic granuloma, presenting as an erythematous macular rash, has also been reported.[37] EAGCG can also present as nonscarring alopecia.[38]

Apart from the skin, the conjunctiva can also be affected by this condition, which differentiates it from GA.[39,40]

Kurose and colleagues[41] reported a case of systemic elastolytic granulomatosis with widespread lesions on the skin and multisystemic involvement with elastolytic granulomas in the uvea lymph nodes, ileum, mesentery, and peritoneum.

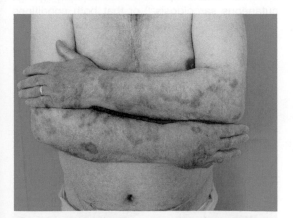

Fig. 5. Annular plaques with erythematous border and central clearing on the dorsal aspect of the forearms and hands.

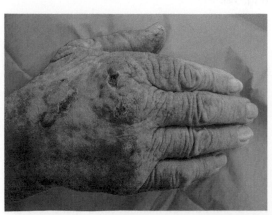

Fig. 7. Erythematous, scaly plaques on the dorsum of the hands.

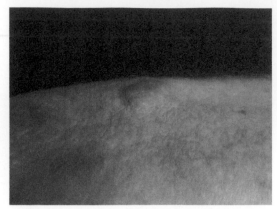

Fig. 8. Papular lesion of elastolytic giant cell granuloma on the dorsum of the forearm.

The age of presentation generally ranges between 40 and 70 years,[2,11,13] although cases in pediatric and young populations have also been documented.[42,43] This condition affects both sexes equally,[2] although a preponderance of female patients has been also reported in other series.[11,13]

Besides the clinical variants than have been reported, O'Brien[17] also described 4 pathologic variants of AG. These patterns are only descriptive and may present alone, together, or sequentially.[13,17]

The giant cell variant is the best known and the most frequent variant of the 4 patterns recognized, accounting for more than 50% of the cases.[13,17] It is characterized by an interstitial infiltrate that is mainly constituted by foreign body giant cells surrounded by diffuse actinic elastosis (**Fig. 9**). These giant cells may be found to be digesting some elastic fibers (**Figs. 10** and **11**). Histiocytes and other inflammatory cells can also be found.[17] In preparations with orcein stain, an absence or scant number of elastic fibers in the residual zone can easily be observed in all the variants (**Fig. 12**).[17,44]

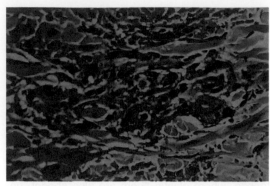

Fig. 10. Phagocytosis of elastic fibers by multinucleated giant cells (hematoxylin and eosin; original magnification, ×400).

The necrobiotic variant, also known as the vascular variant, is the second most frequent pattern. It shows an interstitial infiltrate similar to the giant cell variant (**Fig. 13**) but, in addition, with foci of necrobiosis (**Figs. 14** and **15**). It usually has a palisade constituted mainly by giant cells rather than histiocytes. Actinic damage of surrounding vessels in these cases is noticeable.[17]

The third pattern described by O'Brien[17] is the histiocytic variant. In this subtype, histiocytes are the dominant cells in the infiltrate (**Fig. 16**). These cells also produce elastolysis by releasing elastases. O'Brien[17] postulated that many AGs could begin showing this pattern and then evolve to other histologic variants.

The sarcoid variant is the fourth subtype of AG. The pathologic study usually reveals sarcoid-like granulomas, although cases with only clusters of histiocytes around elastotic fibers can be observed (**Figs. 17** and **18**). Only a few cases with the sarcoid variant of EAGCG have been reported.[13,45] However, some investigators think that this variant represents the annular type of cutaneous sarcoidosis[46] or that both conditions belong to the same disease spectrum.[47]

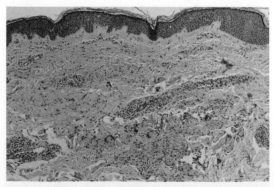

Fig. 9. Infiltrate of multinucleated giant cells and macrophages in the dermis (hematoxylin and eosin; original magnification, ×100).

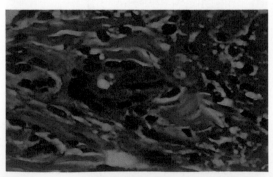

Fig. 11. Giant cell phagocytizing an elastotic fiber (hematoxylin and eosin; original magnification, ×400).

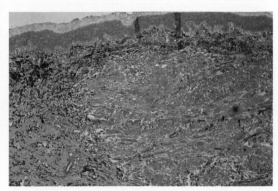

Fig. 12. Loss of elastic fibers within the zone of resolving granulomatous inflammation (orcein; original magnification, ×40).

These patterns may not present individually and features of more than 1 pattern can be observed at the same time.[13]

SYSTEMIC ASSOCIATIONS

Although diabetes mellitus (DM) was not related to this condition in O'Brien's[2] original description, it has been found to be more common in patients affected by EAGCG than in the general population, with estimations that between 37% and 40% of patients affected by this skin condition have DM.[13,48] This higher incidence may be explained by the damage of elastic fibers caused by the hyperglycemia, contributing to triggering the immune response.[25,48] The percentage of patients with diabetes is even higher among patients with the necrobiotic variant of AG.[13] For this reason, DM should be ruled out in patients diagnosed with EAGCG.[11,13]

There are few reports associating EAGCG and malignancies, including hematologic disorders

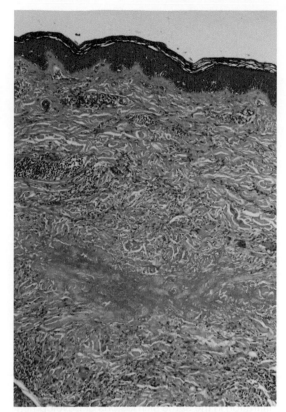

Fig. 14. Focus of necrobiosis surrounded by a lympho-histiocytic infiltrate (hematoxylin and eosin; original magnification, ×400).

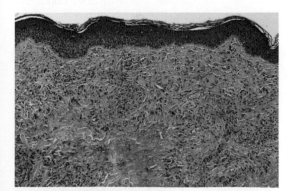

Fig. 13. Granulomatous infiltrate constituted by lymphocytes and macrophages around a focus of necrobiosis (hematoxylin and eosin; original magnification, ×100).

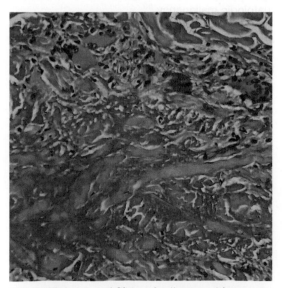

Fig. 15. Degenerated fibers of collagen, with necrobiotic appearance (hematoxylin and eosin; original magnification, ×400).

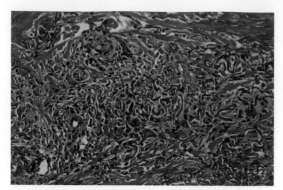

Fig. 16. Intense histiocytic infiltrate scattered among elastotic fibers (hematoxylin and eosin; original magnification, ×250).

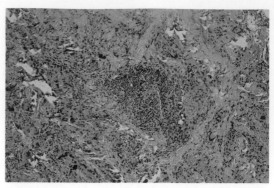

Fig. 18. Giant cells and sarcoid-appearing infiltrates in mid-dermis (hematoxylin and eosin; original magnification, ×250).

like leukemias or lymphomas[49–51] but also solid neoplasias like prostate carcinoma, although this relationship may be incidental.[15] Boussault and colleagues[50] explained this condition as a kind of immune response against a tumor antigen. In 2 of these cases the treatment of the malignancy was followed by the regression of the EAGCG,[49,50] and in 1 of the cases there was a relapse of the granuloma when the leukemia recurred.[49] The coexistence of elastolytic granuloma and leukemia infiltration in the same skin lesions or development in preexisting lymphomatous lesions has been documented.[51,52] Monoclonal gammopathy of unknown significance has also been related to EAGCG.[33] Although the relationship between EAGCG and malignancy has not been confirmed in the literature, some investigators recommend age-appropriate screening tests for solid and hematologic malignancy.[53]

An association between EAGCG and temporal arteritis has been documented, suggesting a common cause of both conditions.[54,55] A similar inflammatory reaction is observed in AG and temporal arteritis. Actinic radiation may injure the elastic tissue not only of the skin but also of superficial arteries, damaging the elastic lamina and becoming antigenic.[3,17] Sorbi and colleagues[56] found increased levels of elastase (MMP-9) in the serum of patients with untreated temporal arteritis. This enzyme was also present in the damaged temporal internal elastic laminae and their vicinity.

The association between EAGCG and sarcoidosis has been also discussed, and some investigators considered this condition to be an underlying factor for developing EAGCG.[12,46] A case of AG associated with erythema nodosum also supports the theory that both conditions belong to the same spectrum of noninfectious granulomatosis.[57]

Our group reported a case of EAGCG on photo-exposed areas in a patient affected by X-linked dominant protoporphyria. It is thought that the increased photosensitivity caused by high levels of porphyrins may contribute to the degeneration of elastic fibers, triggering the development of granulomas (**Fig. 19**).[58]

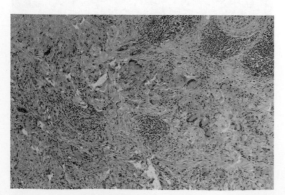

Fig. 17. Giant cells and sarcoid-appearing infiltrates in mid-dermis (hematoxylin and eosin; original magnification, ×100).

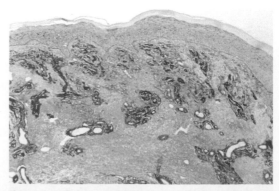

Fig. 19. Deposits positive for periodic acid–Schiff around papillary and mid-dermal blood vessels in a case of giant cell AG associated with protoporphyria (periodic acid schiff staining; original magnification ×40).

A case was recently reported of a patient with EAGCG lesions on the dorsum of the contralateral hand and foot to the hemisphere damaged from a previous ischemic stroke. The investigators suggested that damage of the sensitive fibers may induce a local unbalance of the neuropeptides that control the local immune response.[59]

A case of AGs in a patient with alcoholic cirrhosis of the liver has been described, although the relationship between these conditions is unknown.[60]

Coexistence of EAGCG only in areas affected by vitiligo has also been reported, supporting the importance of sun damage in the cause of this condition.[61,62]

EAGCG can resolve with clinical and histologic features of mid-dermal elastolysis, suggesting that both conditions are different stages in the clinical spectrum of dermal elastolysis.[63] AG has also been associated with pseudoxantoma elasticum in the same patient.[64] Cases with secondary localized amyloidosis[65] or associated with relapsing polychondritis have also been described.[66]

EVALUATION AND MANAGEMENT

Clinically, EAGCG can resemble many other skin conditions, like GA, necrobiosis lipoidica, or annular lichen planus. For this reason, histologic examination remains the gold standard for the diagnosis of this condition. The study of an incisional radial biopsy reveals 3 distinct zones: (1) the area of clinically normal-appearing skin, showing actinic elastosis. Elastic fibers appear thickened, coiled, and bluish, and for this reason solar elastosis is also known as basophilic degeneration of the dermis. (2) The portion corresponding with the annulus of the lesion shows granulomatous inflammation consisting of foreign body–type multinucleated giant cells, histiocytes, lymphocytes, and occasionally epithelioid cells in the upper portion of the dermis. These giant cells may be observed absorbing elastotic fibers. There is no palisading or mucin deposition and necrobiosis is not observed. (3) The central part of the lesion shows minimal granulomatous inflammations, with absent or diminished elastic fibers.[2,12] The epidermis usually is unaffected or shows mild atrophy.

Al-Hoqail and colleagues[6] found some histologic features that can help to distinguish AG from GA, like the presence of multinucleated giant cells and elastophagocytosis, absence of mucin deposition or palisading granulomata, and the location in superficial dermis. The differential diagnosis includes sarcoidosis, GA, and necrobiosis lipoidica

Table 1
Therapeutic agents for the treatment of elastolytic actinic giant cell granuloma

Agents	Response	Level of Evidence
Topical corticosteroids	Good,[30,38,64,69] partial,[15,59] failure[12,18,35,81,82,84]	D
Intralesional corticosteroids	Good,[12,29,70] failure[76]	D
Systemic corticosteroids	Good,[21,41,44] failure[82,84]	D
Phototherapy (nb-UVB, PUVA, Re-PUVA)	Good,[51,71,72] failure[12,69]	D
Cyclosporine A	Good[69,73]	D
Dapsone	Good[74]	D
Topical tacrolimus/pimecrolimus	Good,[33,43] partial,[15] failure[81]	D
Tranilast	Good,[31,43] failure[18,21]	D
Methotrexate	Failure[73]	D
Chloroquine	Good,[12,20,26,63] failure[35,80]	D
Hydroxychloroquine	Good,[12,69,81–84] partial,[67] failure[12]	D
Fumaric acid esters	Good,[79,80] failure[79]	D
Pentoxifylline	Good[75]	D
Isotretinoin	Good,[76] failure[85]	D
Acitretin	Good,[77] partial[78]	D
Cryotherapy	Failure[86]	D
Clofazimine	Failure[20]	D

D, case series or case reports.
Abbreviations: nb-UVB, narrowband UVB; PUVA, psoralen-UVA; Re-PUVA, retinoids-psoralen-UVA.
Data from Refs.[12,18,20,21,26,29–31,33,35,38,41,43,44,51,63,67,69,70,73,75–86]

diabeticorum (NLD). Sarcoidosis usually shows well-defined epithelioid cells tubercles. GA presents with palisading granulomas, mucin deposition, and areas of necrobiosis. NLD tends to affect all the dermis with prominent areas of necrobiosis and absence of multinucleated giant cells.[2,12]

Although UV light is thought to be the main causal factor, Kiken and colleagues[67] tried unsuccessfully to reproduce EAGCG lesions with provocative light exposure in a patient affected by this condition. Phototests showed normal minimal erythema dose both for UVB and UVA.

EAGCG has a chronic course and different treatment modalities have been used with variable success (Table 1). Spontaneous remission of EAGCG may occur,[31,36,68] making the assessment of the efficacy of any treatment difficult. Topical,[18,69] intralesional,[29,70] and systemic[21,44] corticosteroids have been used with some benefit. Topical pimecrolimus[43] and tacrolimus[33] have been reported as an effective therapy. Phototherapy, including narrow band UVB,[71] Psoralen-UVA (PUVA),[72] and Retinoids-Psoralen-UVA (Re-PUVA), can be also an effective treatment.[51] Cyclosporine A,[69,73] dapsone,[74] tranilast,[31,43] pentoxifylline,[75] isotretinoin,[76] and acitretin[77,78] have been reported to be effective in single cases. Fumaric acid esters have also been successfully used, with mild adverse effects.[79,80] Hydroxychloroquine[81–84] and chloroquine[20,26] have also shown positive results, although there are also cases with no response to antimalarials.[12] Failure to isotretinoin,[85] methotrexate,[73] PUVA,[51,69] and cryotherapy[86] has also been reported.

Patients should also be advised to avoid sun exposure and to use sunscreens to prevent development of new lesions.[87]

SUMMARY

EAGCG is an uncommon skin disorder that should be differentiated from other granulomatous skin disorders like GA. Although the giant cell pattern is the most frequent, there are other histologic variants that must be known. The distribution of the lesions in sun-exposed areas suggests that heat and actinic radiation play important roles in the pathogenesis of this condition. However, cases involving sun-protected areas or manifesting in a generalized fashion have also been reported, meaning that sun exposure is not necessary and that further investigations need to be performed. DM is frequently associated, and may be a precipitating factor of EAGCG. For this reason, this possibility should be included in the medical investigations to be performed in patients affected by this condition.

Although EAGCG is not generally associated with malignancy, in case of any suspicious symptom or sign, age-appropriate screening tests for solid and hematologic malignancy should be done.

REFERENCES

1. El-Khoury J, Kurban M, Abbas O. Elastophagocytosis: underlying mechanisms and associated cutaneous entities. J Am Acad Dermatol 2014;70: 934–44.
2. O'Brien JP. Actinic granuloma. An annular connective tissue disorder affecting sun- and heat-damaged (elastotic) skin. Arch Dermatol 1975;111: 460–6.
3. O'Brien JP, Regan W. Actinically degenerate elastic tissue is the likely antigenic basis of actinic granuloma of the skin and of temporal arteritis. J Am Acad Dermatol 1999;40:214–22.
4. Regan W. Actinic radiation plays a significant role in the etiology of actinic granuloma lesions. Int J Dermatol 2006;45:1001.
5. Ragaz A, Ackerman AB. Is actinic granuloma a specific condition? Am J Dermatopathol 1979;1:43–50.
6. Al-Hoqail IA, Al-Ghamdi AM, Martinka M, et al. Actinic granuloma is a unique and distinct entity: a comparative study with granuloma annulare. Am J Dermatopathol 2002;24:209–12.
7. Toribio J, Quinones PA, Perez-Oliva N. Actinic granuloma. Actas Dermosifiliogr 1978;69:289–94.
8. McGrae JD Jr. Actinic granuloma. A clinical, histopathologic, and immunocytochemical study. Arch Dermatol 1986;122:43–7.
9. Moulin G, Moyne G, Franc MP, et al. O'Brien's actinic granuloma, three cases (author's transl). Ann Dermatol Venereol 1982;109:135–49.
10. Steffen C. Actinic granuloma (O'Brien). J Cutan Pathol 1988;15:66–74.
11. Limas C. The spectrum of primary cutaneous elastolytic granulomas and their distinction from granuloma annulare: a clinicopathological analysis. Histopathology 2004;44:277–82.
12. Hanke CW, Bailin PL, Roenigk HH Jr. Annular elastolytic giant cell granuloma. A clinicopathologic study of five cases and a review of similar entities. J Am Acad Dermatol 1979;1:413–21.
13. Gutierrez-Gonzalez E, Gomez-Bernal S, Alvarez-Perez A, et al. Elastolytic giant cell granuloma: clinic-pathologic review of twenty cases. Dermatol Online J 2013;19:20019.
14. Fujimoto N, Akagi A, Tajima S. Expression of 67-kDa elastin receptor in annular elastolytic giant cell granuloma. Elastin peptides induce monocyte-derived dendritic cells or macrophages to form granuloma in vitro. Exp Dermatol 2004;13:179–84.
15. Asahina A, Shirai A, Horita A, et al. Annular elastolytic giant cell granuloma associated with prostate

carcinoma. Demonstration of human metalloelastase (MMP-12) expression. Clin Exp Dermatol 2012;37: 70–2.

16. Davies MG, Newman P. Actinic granulomata in a young woman following prolonged sunbed usage. Br J Dermatol 1997;136:797–8.

17. Brien JP. Actinic granuloma: the expanding significance. An analysis of its origin in elastotic ("aging") skin and a definition of necrobiotic (vascular), histiocytic, and sarcoid variants. Int J Dermatol 1985;24: 473–90.

18. Lim DS, Triscott J. O'Brien's actinic granuloma in association with prolonged doxycycline phototoxicity. Australas J Dermatol 2003;44:67–70.

19. Pestoni C, Pereiro M Jr, Toribio J. Annular elastolytic giant cell granuloma produced on an old burn scar and spreading after a mechanical trauma. Acta Derm Venereol 2003;83:312–3.

20. Ozkaya-Bayazit E, Buyukbabani N, Baykal C, et al. Annular elastolytic giant cell granuloma: sparing of a burn scar and successful treatment with chloroquine. Br J Dermatol 1999;140:525–30.

21. Oka M, Kunisada M, Nishigori C. Generalized annular elastolytic giant cell granuloma with sparing of striae distensae. J Dermatol 2013;40:220–2.

22. Revenga F, Rovira I, Pimentel J, et al. Annular elastolytic giant cell granuloma-actinic granuloma? Clin Exp Dermatol 1996;21:51–3.

23. Campos-Munoz L, Diaz-Diaz RM, Quesada-Cortes A, et al. Annular elastolytic giant cell granuloma: a case report located in non-sun exposed areas. Actas Dermosifiliogr 2006;97:533–5.

24. Ishibashi A, Yokoyama A, Hirano K. Annular elastolytic giant cell granuloma occurring in covered areas. Dermatologica 1987;174:293–7.

25. Muramatsu T, Shirai T, Yamashina Y, et al. Annular elastolytic giant cell granuloma: an unusual case with lesions arising in non-sun-exposed areas. J Dermatol 1987;14:54–8.

26. Klemke CD, Siebold D, Dippel E, et al. Generalised annular elastolytic giant cell granuloma. Dermatology 2003;207:420–2.

27. Sina B, Wood C, Rudo K. Generalized elastophagocytic granuloma. Cutis 1992;49:355–7.

28. Kato H, Kitajima Y, Yaoita H. Annular elastolytic giant cell granuloma: an unusual case with papular lesions. J Dermatol 1991;18:667–70.

29. Kato H, Uyeki Y, Yaoita H. Papular lesions associated with annular elastolytic giant cell granuloma. J Am Acad Dermatol 1989;21:398–400.

30. Fujimura T, Terui T, Tagami H. Disseminated papular interstitial elastolytic giant cell granuloma. Acta Derm Venereol 2003;83:234–5.

31. Morita K, Okamoto H, Miyachi Y. Papular elastolytic giant cell granuloma: a clinical variant of annular elastolytic giant cell granuloma or generalized granuloma annulare? Eur J Dermatol 1999;9:647–9.

32. Marmon S, O'Reilly KE, Fischer M, et al. Papular variant of annular elastolytic giant-cell granuloma. Dermatol Online J 2012;18:23.

33. Rongioletti F, Baldari M, Burlando M, et al. Papular elastolytic giant cell granuloma: report of a case associated with monoclonal gammopathy and responsive to topical tacrolimus. Clin Exp Dermatol 2010;35:145–8.

34. Mielke V, Weber L, Schunter M, et al. Reticular elastolytic giant cell granuloma. A variant of the annular elastolytic giant cell granuloma. Hautarzt 1995;46: 259–62.

35. Hinrichs R, Weiss T, Peschke E, et al. A reticular variant of elastolytic giant cell granuloma. Clin Exp Dermatol 2006;31:42–4.

36. Misago N, Ohtsuka Y, Ishii K, et al. Papular and reticular elastolytic giant cell granuloma: rapid spontaneous regression. Acta Derm Venereol 2007;87: 89–90.

37. Puig L, Moreno A, Garcia P, et al. Exanthematous elastolytic granuloma. J Am Acad Dermatol 1988; 19:564–5.

38. Delgado-Jimenez Y, Perez-Gala S, Penas PF, et al. O'Brien actinic granuloma presenting as alopecia. J Eur Acad Dermatol Venereol 2006;20:226–7.

39. Steffen C. Actinic granuloma of the conjunctiva. Am J Dermatopathol 1992;14:253–4.

40. Gallagher MJ, Roberts F, Osborne S, et al. Actinic granuloma of the conjunctiva. Br J Ophthalmol 2003;87:1044–5.

41. Kurose N, Nakagawa H, Iozumi K, et al. Systemic elastolytic granulomatosis with cutaneous, ocular, lymph nodal, and intestinal involvement. Spectrum of annular elastolytic giant cell granuloma and sarcoidosis. J Am Acad Dermatol 1992;26: 359–63.

42. Boneschi V, Brambilla L, Fossati S, et al. Annular elastolytic giant cell granuloma. Am J Dermatopathol 1988;10:224–8.

43. Lee HW, Lee MW, Choi JH, et al. Annular elastolytic giant cell granuloma in an infant: improvement after treatment with oral tranilast and topical pimecrolimus. J Am Acad Dermatol 2005;53:S244–6.

44. Pock L, Blazkova J, Caloudova H, et al. Annular elastolytic giant cell granuloma causes an irreversible disappearance of the elastic fibres. J Eur Acad Dermatol Venereol 2004;18:365–8.

45. Berliner JG, Haemel A, Leboit PE, et al. The sarcoidal variant of annular elastolytic granuloma. J Cutan Pathol 2013;40:918–20.

46. Gambichler T, Herde M, Hoffmann K, et al. Sarcoid variant of actinic granuloma: is it annular sarcoidosis? Dermatology 2001;203:353–4.

47. Terui T, Tagami H. Annular elastolytic sarcoidosis of the face. Eur J Dermatol 1998;8:127–30.

48. Aso Y, Izaki S, Teraki Y. Annular elastolytic giant cell granuloma associated with diabetes mellitus: a case

report and review of the Japanese literature. Clin Exp Dermatol 2011;36:917–9.

49. Garg A, Kundu RV, Plotkin O, et al. Annular elastolytic giant cell granuloma heralding onset and recurrence of acute myelogenous leukemia. Arch Dermatol 2006;142:532–3.

50. Boussault P, Tucker ML, Weschler J, et al. Primary cutaneous CD4+ small/medium-sized pleomorphic T-cell lymphoma associated with an annular elastolytic giant cell granuloma. Br J Dermatol 2009;160: 1126–8.

51. Kuramoto Y, Watanabe M, Tagami H. Adult T cell leukemia accompanied by annular elastolytic giant cell granuloma. Acta Derm Venereol 1990;70:164–7.

52. Kauffman JA, Ivan D, Cutlan JE, et al. Actinic granuloma occurring in an unusual association with cutaneous B-cell chronic lymphocytic leukemia. J Cutan Pathol 2012;39:294–7.

53. Hawryluk EB, Izikson L, English JC. Non-infectious granulomatous diseases of the skin and their associated systemic diseases: an evidence-based update to important clinical questions. Am J Clin Dermatol 2010;11:171–81.

54. Lau H, Reid BJ, Weedon D. Actinic granuloma in association with giant cell arteritis: are both caused by sunlight? Pathology 1997;29:260–2.

55. Shoimer I, Wismer J. Annular elastolytic giant cell granuloma associated with temporal arteritis leading to blindness. J Cutan Med Surg 2011;15:293–7.

56. Sorbi D, French DL, Nuovo GJ, et al. Elevated levels of 92-kd type IV collagenase (matrix metalloproteinase 9) in giant cell arteritis. Arthritis Rheum 1996; 39:1747–53.

57. Matsuzaki Y, Rokunohe A, Nishikawa Y, et al. Actinic granuloma associated with erythema nodosum. Eur J Dermatol 2011;21:806–7.

58. Garcia-Martinez FJ, Gutierrez-Gonzalez E, Alonso-Gonzalez J, et al. Annular elastolytic giant cell granuloma associated to late-onset X-linked dominant protoporphyria. Dermatology 2013;227: 238–42.

59. Lo Schiavo A, Romano F, Alfano R, et al. Unilateral annular elastolytic giant cell granuloma in a hemiplegic stroke patient. Am J Dermatopathol 2014;36(11): 928–30.

60. Racz I, Berecz M, Harsing J. Actinic granuloma in alcoholic liver disease. Cutis 1992;49:417–9.

61. Watabe D, Akasaka T. Annular elastolytic giant cell granuloma developing on lesions of vitiligo. Int J Dermatol 2013;52:1458–60.

62. de Paz NM, Rodriguez-Martin M, Bustinduy MG, et al. Strict anatomical colocalization of vitiligo and elastolytic granulomas. Case Rep Dermatol 2010;2: 13–7.

63. Muller FB, Groth W. Annular elastolytic giant cell granuloma: a prodromal stage of mid-dermal elastolysis? Br J Dermatol 2007;156:1377–9.

64. Lee HW, Park MA, Lee SC, et al. A case of actinic granuloma associated with periumbilical perforating pseudoxanthoma elasticum. Acta Derm Venereol 1996;76:133–5.

65. Lee YS, Vijayasingam S, Chan HL. Photosensitive annular elastolytic giant cell granuloma with cutaneous amyloidosis. Am J Dermatopathol 1989;11:443–50.

66. Pierard GE, Henrijean A, Foidart JM, et al. Actinic granulomas and relapsing polychondritis. Acta Derm Venereol 1982;62:531–3.

67. Kiken DA, Shupack JL, Soter NA, et al. A provocative case: phototesting does not reproduce the lesions of actinic granuloma. Photodermatol Photoimmunol Photomed 2002;18:315–6.

68. Hermes B, Haas N, Czarnetzki BM. Annular elastolytic giant cell granuloma with a spontaneous healing tendency. Hautarzt 1995;46:490–3.

69. Ventura F, Vilarinho C, da Luz Duarte M, et al. Two cases of annular elastolytic giant cell granuloma: different response to the treatment. Dermatol Online J 2010;16:11.

70. Prendiville J, Griffiths WA, Jones RR. O'Brien's actinic granuloma. Br J Dermatol 1985;113:353–8.

71. Takata T, Ikeda M, Kodama H, et al. Regression of papular elastolytic giant cell granuloma using narrowband UVB irradiation. Dermatology 2006;212:77–9.

72. Perez-Perez L, Garcia-Gavin J, Allegue F, et al. Successful treatment of generalized elastolytic giant cell granuloma with psoralen-ultraviolet A. Photodermatol Photoimmunol Photomed 2012;28:264–6.

73. Tsutsui K, Hirone T, Kubo K, et al. Annular elastolytic giant cell granuloma: response to cyclosporin A. J Dermatol 1994;21:426–9.

74. Igawa K, Maruyama R, Katayama I, et al. Anti-oxidative therapy with oral dapsone improved HCV antibody positive annular elastolytic giant cell granuloma. J Dermatol 1997;24:328–31.

75. Rubio FA, Robayna G, Pizarro A, et al. Actinic granuloma and vitiligo treated with pentoxifylline. Int J Dermatol 1998;37:958–60.

76. Ratnavel RC, Grant JW, Handfield-Jones SE, et al. O'Brien's actinic granuloma: response to isotretinoin. J R Soc Med 1995;88:528P–9P.

77. Stefanaki C, Panagiotopoulos A, Kostakis P, et al. Actinic granuloma successfully treated with acitretin. Int J Dermatol 2005;44:163–6.

78. Lazzarini R, Rotter A, Farias DC, et al. O'Brien's actinic granuloma: an unusually extensive presentation. An Bras Dermatol 2011;86:339–42.

79. Breuer K, Gutzmer R, Volker B, et al. Therapy of noninfectious granulomatous skin diseases with fumaric acid esters. Br J Dermatol 2005;152:1290–5.

80. Gutzmer R, Breuer K, Kiehl P, et al. Successful therapy of annular elastolytic giant cell granuloma with fumaric acid esters. Dermatology 2002;205:421–4.

81. Can B, Kavala M, Turkoglu Z, et al. Successful treatment of annular elastolytic giant cell

granuloma with hydroxychloroquine. Int J Dermatol 2013;52:509–11.

82. de Oliveira FL, de Barros Silveira LK, Machado Ade M, et al. Hybrid clinical and histopathological pattern in annular lesions: an overlap between annular elastolytic giant cell granuloma and granuloma annulare? Case Rep Dermatol Med 2012; 2012:102915.

83. Goncalves RR, Miranda MF, Viana Fde O, et al. Annular elastolytic giant cell granuloma–case report. An Bras Dermatol 2011;86:S69–71.

84. Kelly BJ, Mrstik ME, Ramos-Caro FA, et al. Papular elastolytic giant cell granuloma responding to hydroxychloroquine and quinacrine. Int J Dermatol 2004;43:964–6.

85. Basak PY, Icke I, Akkaya VB, et al. Lack of response to isotretinoin in annular elastolytic giant cell granuloma. J Dermatol 2004;31:678–81.

86. Schwarz T, Lindlbauer R, Gschnait F. Annular elastolytic giant cell granuloma. J Cutan Pathol 1983;10: 321–6.

87. Wee JS, Moosa Y, Misch K, et al. Actinic granuloma: a history of photoexacerbation and the importance of a radial 'three-zone' biopsy. Clin Exp Dermatol 2013;38:219–21.

Necrobiosis Lipoidica

Cathryn Sibbald, BScPhm, MD[a], Sophia Reid, MD[b],
Afsaneh Alavi, MD, MSc, FRCPC[a],*

KEYWORDS

- Necrobiosis lipoidica • Ulcerations • Necrobiosis lipoidica/diagnosis
- Necrobiosis lipoidica/therapy

KEY POINTS

- Necrobiosis lipoidica (NL) typically presents as well-demarcated yellow-brown plaques with violaceous borders with central waxy atrophic appearance and telangiectasias on the lower extremities.
- The pathogenesis likely involves vascular and immunologic mechanisms with impaired neutrophil migration, collagen abnormalities, and granuloma formation.
- Investigations should include screening of underlying disease, especially diabetes and vascular studies when indicated. Biopsies are recommended when alternative diagnoses are considered.
- The disease course is often indolent, and treatment is based on patients' concerns. The most common therapies include topical corticosteroids and calcineurin inhibitors.
- NL lesions should be monitored for transformation to malignancy.

INTRODUCTION

Necrobiosis lipoidica (NL) is a rare idiopathic granulomatous disease of collagen degeneration with risk of ulceration. This disease has typically been associated with diabetes; however, the strength of the association has been questioned over time. Much of the information we know about this disease is from landmark studies performed in the 1960s to 1980s that set the basis for understanding and diagnosing this disease process. Subsequent studies and case reports have helped build the knowledge base about this disease, particularly giving providers an arsenal of treatment options to offer patients. However, at this time, there are no clinical trials to guide the efficacy of treatment options; more research will be needed in this area. The clinical course of this disease is difficult to predict and can vary with individual patients; some will experience a chronic disease process and others will have spontaneous resolution. The effects of other systemic diseases on the clinical process of NL have been debated throughout the literature.[1]

The incidence of NL in individuals with diabetes is only 0.3% to 1.2 %; NL precedes diabetes in up to 14%, appears simultaneously in up to 24%, and occurs after diabetes is diagnosed in 62% of cases.[2,3] Although NL may present in healthy individuals with no underlying disease, the most commonly associated conditions are thyroid disorders and inflammatory diseases, such as Crohn's disease, ulcerative colitis, rheumatoid arthritis, and sarcoidosis. This disease is sometimes confused with other diseases based on clinical presentation and associated locations, such as granuloma annulare, erythema nodosum, necrobiotic xanthogranuloma (NXG), chronic venous stasis ulcers, and sarcoidosis. There are many components of the disease that still require more

Resource funding: none.
Conflict of interest: no relevant conflict of interest to this article.
[a] Department of Medicine (Dermatology), University of Toronto, Toronto, Ontario, Canada; [b] Department of Medicine, University of California, Irvine, Irvine, CA, USA
* Corresponding author. Women's College Hospital (Main Building), Wound Care Center, 76 Grenville Street 5th Floor, Toronto, Ontario M5S 1B2, Canada.
E-mail address: afsaneh.alavi@utoronto.ca

Dermatol Clin 33 (2015) 343–360
http://dx.doi.org/10.1016/j.det.2015.03.003

research to define, such as the pathogenesis and cause as well as treatment options that can prove to be both efficacious and consistent.

ETIOPATHOGENESIS

The cause and pathogenesis of this disease is not well understood, but many theories have been presented. According to published literature, with small center studies, there is a predominance in females affected by the disease.[2,4–7] A study performed by Erfurt-Berge and colleagues[5] in 52 patients with NL found 77% of those affected to be female. This statistic coincides with previous studies that reported a female predominance. Another interesting correlation seen in small trials is that the age of onset in women is younger than men. However, the disease course appears more severe in men as they have a higher likelihood of ulceration in their lesions. The same study by Erfurt-Berge and colleagues[5] found 58% of males to have ulcerations versus only 15% of females. The likelihood of ulceration in NL lesions has been difficult to determine, with the literature reporting a range of 15% to 35% after an inciting incident of trauma.[2,5,8]

The pathogenesis of NL has been speculated for many years with no definitive answer to date. Elements of vascular disturbance involving immune complex deposition or microangiopathic changes leading to collagen degeneration have been the most common theories. Other proposed ideas include collagen production abnormalities and problems with neutrophil migration. Conflicting studies have continued to make the cause and pathogenesis controversial.

Blood Vessels

The most common vascular abnormalities seen in NL lesions are thickening of the vessel walls, fibrosis, and endothelial proliferation leading to occlusion in the deeper dermis.[4] These characteristics were more prominent in diabetic patients than nondiabetics.[9] In a study of 10 idiopathic cases of NL, investigators found that oxygen tension was lower but laser Doppler fluxes were increased around NL lesions in response to hyperemic stimuli.[10] The alterations seen in NL lesions were thought to be caused by glycoprotein deposition, which can be responsible for thickening and occlusion of blood vessels. Increased presence of Glut-1 (human erythrocyte glucose transporter) receptors in fibroblasts detected by immunohistochemical analysis indicates that decreased blood flow is a potential factor. The exact mechanism for increased presence of the receptors is still in debate.[11] A more recent study in persons with

diabetes showed that the blood flow in NL lesions was similar to the blood flow in areas without lesions. Investigators think an inflammatory process is more influential in the pathogenesis than small vessel occlusions.[12]

Collagen

Collagen abnormalities are seen at the level of the collagen fibrils. Absent cross striations are the most prominent finding, with some cases even showing a complete loss of collagen and elastin.[13] Increased cross-linking of collagen caused by the higher levels of lysyl oxidase, typically found in diabetic patients, has been thought to contribute to the thickening of the basement membrane as seen in NL.[14] Anticollagen antibodies have also been reported in patients with NL and other granulomatous disorders, but the levels do not differ from the control population.[15]

Immunoglobulin Deposition

Deposition of fibrin, immunoglobulin M (IgM), and C3 at the dermoepidermal junction of blood vessels has been shown in immunofluorescence studies.[16] Antibody-mediated vasculitis can lead to structural changes in the vasculature leading to occlusion of dermal vessels and result in necrobiosis. However, mild vascular involvement has been noted in only 30% of cases.[17]

Neutrophil Defects

Granuloma formation has been thought to occur as result of defective neutrophil migration allowing macrophages to take on the neutrophil role and accumulate with subsequent granuloma formation.[18] A neutrophil-predominant inflammatory infiltrate can be seen in the early stages of the disease.[3]

Genetics

There have been rare reports of familial cases of NL. In some cases, NL was seen without diabetes or glucose intolerance.[19,20] In other familial cases, diabetes was present.[21] It remains unclear at this time what role genetics may play in the disease etiopathogenesis.[22]

CLINICAL AND HISTOLOGIC PRESENTATION

NL is a rare granulomatous disease that generally has an average age of onset between 30 and 40 years of age; but many factors can alter this age of onset allowing it to present at any age, including birth.[2] The lesions are commonly seen on the bilateral lower extremities, particularly the pretibial surface; however, case reports have identified atypical presentation of lesions on the face, penis, trunk, scalp, and upper extremities. They begin as asymptomatic papules and nodules that erode, in time, to well-demarcated yellow-brown plaques with violaceous borders and have a central waxy atrophic appearance and telangiectasias. Plaques may be less yellow in patients with darker skin color (**Fig. 1**). An erythematous border will be present around each stage of the lesion development. Ulceration is present in up to one-third of patients with NL (**Fig. 2**).[2,3] These lesions have the ability to koebnerize if they are traumatized; therefore, surgical-based treatment options can present a cosmetic challenge.[23–25]

NL can have a similar clinical appearance to other skin diseases particularly granuloma annulare. Histology helps the differentiation based on the appearance of lipids and decreased amount of mucin in NL.[22] Erythema nodosum commonly appears in pretibial areas but as tender erythematous nodules that do not have any epidermal changes, ulceration, or atrophy. NXG is also a chronic granulomatous disease that presents with yellow-red plaques; however, the most common site of involvement is the face and, in particular, the upper and lower eyelids. The trunk and the extremities are far less frequently involved. Most patients have associated paraproteinemia.[26] There are case reports of NXG involving lower extremities with no facial involvement. This case may represent a variant of necrobiotic skin disease in this spectrum not previously characterized (**Fig. 3**).[27] Cutaneous sarcoid lesions will also have a granulomatous appearance, but these lesions also rarely ulcerate or present with atrophy.

Perforating Necrobiosis Lipoidica

This disease is a rare form of NL often associated with a noncomplicated form of NL and not associated with diabetes. The clinical picture consists of keratotic caps on a plaque of NL with a residual small pinpoint depression on removal.[28]

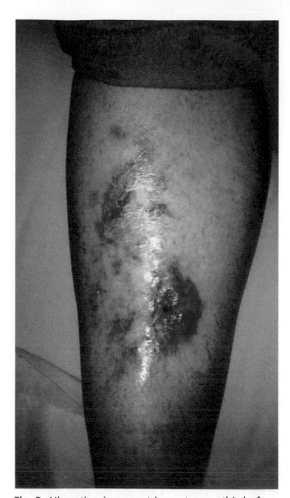

Fig. 2. Ulceration is present in up to one-third of patients with NL.

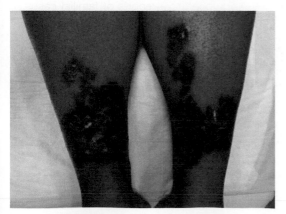

Fig. 1. NL plaques.

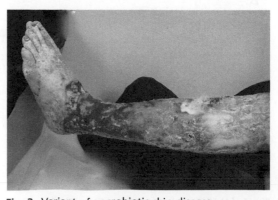

Fig. 3. Variant of necrobiotic skin disease.

Periorbital Necrobiosis Lipoidica

These cases are in the differential diagnosis of NXG that has association with paraproteninemia. Although legs are the most common place for NL, there are cases of reported NL in eyelids.

Surgical Scar Necrobiosis Lipoidica

NL is infrequently found over surgical scars from procedures, including appendectomy and even phlebotomy.[29,30]

Genital Necrobiosis Lipoidica

NL on the glans penis is a rare condition occurring at a mean age of 66 years. It is commonly a differential diagnosis of granuloma annulare (GA) in this area. However, the granulomas in GA are typically more superficial with larger amounts of mucin in their centers.[31–33] NL has also been reported in atypical locations, such as the back and nipple.[34]

Histopathology shows interstitial and palisading necrobiotic granulomas of the subcutaneous tissue and dermis.[4] Newly formed lesions will show small vessel vasculitis that slowly progresses to large vessel vasculitis. With more time, collagen degeneration becomes evident and involves the dermis and subcutaneous fat with a layered granulomatous appearance. There will be a loss of elastic tissue with the presence of multinucleated giant cells and lipid droplets.[22] Blood vessel walls will appear thickened with endothelial cell swelling in the deep dermis.[4] Clinically the appearance of NL lesions is identical in diabetic and nondiabetic patients; however, the histology may vary.

The histology of NL is granulomatous with 2 patterns of palisading, pseudotuberculoid, or a combination of both. The epidermis is usually normal but can be atrophic or even hyperkeratotic. Increased interstitial mucin is commonly found in

GA and subtler in NL lesions. The palisading pattern is more common in cases associated with diabetes.[35,36]

The alteration of connective tissue referred as *necrobiosis*. The altered collagen appears paler with a grayer hue and more impact than normal collagen. The palisading pattern is characterized by single or multiple layers of hyalinized or necrobiotic collagen surrounded by a rim of noninflammatory cells in the lower two-thirds of the dermis producing a sandwich or wedding cake pattern.[35] Vascular alteration, lipid droplets, and giant cells are often present.[36] The pseudotuberculoid pattern of NL consists of less necrobiotic collagen and more epithelioid histiocytes with an increased number of lymphocytes, plasma cells, and giant cells. There is usually no vascular alteration in this pattern with fewer lipids present (**Fig. 4**).[35] Direct immunofluorescence will show deposits in the vasculature consisting of IgM, IgA, C_3, fibrinogen, and only rarely IgG. The immunofluorescence finding in NL is nonspecific and controversial.

SYSTEMIC ASSOCIATIONS

NL has been seen in conjunction with multiple systemic diseases, including sarcoidosis, autoimmune thyroiditis, inflammatory bowel disease, ulcerative colitis, and rheumatoid arthritis.[37] The association with autoimmune disorders, including type 1 diabetes, allows the theory of immune dysregulation to play a more convincing role in the pathogenesis. The true association of NL with these diseases is difficult to determine as most of the literature is guided by case studies.

The most common systemic association related to NL is diabetes. The prevalence rates for NL in all diabetic patients is 0.3% to 1.2% and more commonly seen in patients with type 1 diabetes.[3] The correlation between diabetes and NL was

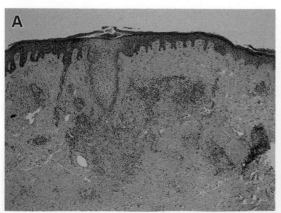 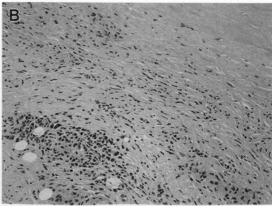

Fig. 4. (A) Histopathology slide of NL. (B) Magnified view.

challenged by studies in the 1990s that showed an only 11% concurrent association of NL and diabetes. It is important to keep in mind that a family history of diabetes as well as a future diagnosis of diabetes may be factors to consider in the epidemiology of NL.[2] Because of all the conflicting statistics garnered in studies, controversy remains in the actual incidence rates of NL in diabetic patients. Debate also exists regarding improved glucose control and the clinical course of NL. Lowitt and Dover[36] assert that necrobiosis lipoidica diabeticorum (NLD) and diabetic control are not related, but a study by Cohen and colleagues[38] challenged this assertation.[36] They performed a review of the literature and included experience with their patients, who demonstrated improvement in the course of nonatrophic NL lesions with improved glycemic control.[38] An interesting association noted is the higher incidence of retinopathy and systemic microvascular disease in patients with both NL and diabetes, so these patients should be monitored closely for additional end organ damage.[39] This association is even seen in pediatric patients.[40]

Thyroid abnormalities have been reported in some patients with NL lesions on the lower extremities, including Graves disease and Hashimoto disease.[41] A more recent study in 2012 revealed that 7 of their 52 participants had thyroid disorders.[5] No causative relationship has been established between the two diseases, but speculation of autoantibodies or autoimmune complex deposition has been present. NL has been reported in patients with inflammatory disorders, such as ulcerative colitis, Crohn disease, rheumatoid arthritis, and sarcoidosis.[5,36,42] These reports have been rare throughout the literature, and no causative relationship has been established with these diseases and NL. Squamous cell carcinoma, although a rare complication, can arise in longstanding NL lesions, even without the presence of ulceration. Case reports have described the appearance of the lesion as an erythematous nodule arising in the NL plaque.[43] The reason for the malignant transformation is unknown, but theories involving loss of UV protection and melanin at the site of the plaque may be contributory.[44] Patients should be adequately surveyed to detect this malignant transformation early so conservative treatment methods can be used.

EVALUATION AND MANAGEMENT

Although the diagnosis is often made based on clinical examination, biopsy should be performed to differentiate NL from conditions with similar clinical appearances, including granuloma annulare,

and NXG. Biopsies should be repeated in cases of nonhealing ulcerated NL to rule out squamous cell carcinoma. Bakos and colleagues[45] reported the presence of arborizing telangiectasias, hairpin vessels, and a yellowish background as suggestive findings in early onset NL.[46]

If there is concern for venous disease or peripheral arterial disease, then further studies should be considered. In patients with diabetes, the calcified arterial vessels may lead to falsely elevated ankle brachial index and measuring toe pressure is warranted.[1] Baseline blood work should include a fasting blood glucose or glycosylated hemoglobin to screen for diabetes or assess glycemic control in patients known to have diabetes. If these are not diagnostic of diabetes, they should be repeated on a yearly basis, as NL can be the first presentation of diabetes. Other blood work and investigations (pregnancy screening, tuberculosis skin tests, blood counts) can be tailored to systemic medications that may be initiated. **Fig. 5** outlines an approach to NL.

Therapy for NL can be challenging, often requiring multiple modalities before achieving a response. Desired cosmesis of lesions is also a concern in many patients. Even when NL heals, remnants of postinflammatory hyperpigmentation and atrophy will linger. Older treatment methods target the micro-occlusion of blood vessels seen on pathology and inflammation associated with active lesions. Newer targets include requisites for the formation and maintenance of granulomas or ulcers, including tumor necrosis factor (TNF) alpha, activated T cells, and other cytokines (**Table 1**).

In the absence of ulceration or symptoms, it is reasonable not to treat NL given that up to 17% of lesions may resolve spontaneously but with sequelae.[2] If patients have diabetes, optimization of glucose should be a goal for overall care of the patients; however, it should be in conjunction with other treatments.[18] Additional lifestyle modifications, including smoking cessation and avoidance of trauma, are equally important to minimize the risk of complications and promote healing.[1,39] Venous disease or lymphedema may complicate NL, especially when ulcerated.[47,48] Compression therapy controls edema and promotes healing in these patients. In addition, nonulcerated lesions on the lower legs can be protected with support stockings to avoid trauma and koebnerization. When ulcerations are present, proper wound care principles are important. Additionally, identifying infection promptly is important. Deep infection needs systemic antimicrobial therapy, but superficial infection can simply be treated with dressings containing antiseptics. Different

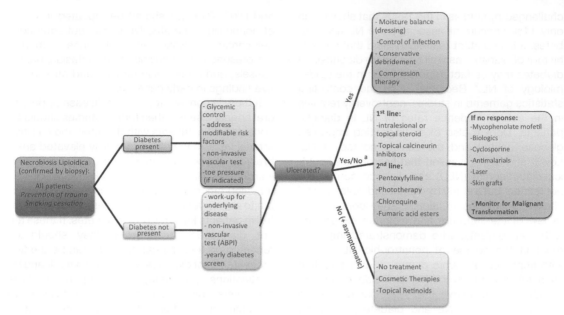

Fig. 5. Approach to NL. [a] Ulcerated or non-ulcerated with symptoms. ABPI, Ankle Brachial Pressure Index.

advanced dressings have been used successfully in case reports, including bovine collagen, protease modulating products, and an ovine forestomach matrix.[49–52] These products target nonspecific local wound factors, such as recruitment of neutrophils, support of angiogenesis and re-epithelialization, and inhibition of harmful metalloproteinases. Granulocyte-macrophage colony-stimulation factor has been used with success to heal ulceration associated with NL lesions, possibly because of its stimulation of macrophages contributing to wound healing, but has not been shown to affect the inflammation or infiltration of NL lesions.[53]

CORTICOSTEROIDS

Topical, intralesional, and systemic corticosteroids have traditionally been used as the first-line treatment.[54–56] Topical steroids decreased inflammation of active lesions. Intralesional and systemic steroids can rapidly halt progression and produce resolution of lesions in most patients.[55] Their efficacy most likely lies in their antiinflammatory properties based on these observations. Most patients treated effectively with steroids have nonulcerated lesions as the efficacy of treatment decreases when the lesions begin to ulcerate. Additionally, for inactive atrophic lesions, topical steroids should be avoided as they may exacerbate the atrophy and increase the risk of new ulcerations. Although systemic steroids can cause hypertension and hyperglycemia, a

short-term course is usually effective in producing resolution of active lesions and is not contraindicated in patients with diabetes or hypertension as long as these parameters are monitored.

Intralesional delivery is preferred in solitary lesions because of decreased side effect profile compared with systemic administration; the border of the plaques should be targeted to avoid atrophic foci.

ULTRAVIOLET LIGHT THERAPY

Phototherapy is used for various inflammatory dermatoses; psoralen-UV-A (PUVA) achieves its effects at the dermal-subdermal junction, where inflammation is evident in NL. In localized applications to lesions, it decreases the active inflamed borders and helps resolve lesions but has no clinical effects on atrophic areas. This finding is supported by a lack of change in ultrasound-determined lesion thickness of atrophic areas in treated lesions.[7]

UVA-1, which supplies a higher proportion of deeper wavelengths, has somewhat similar efficacy to PUVA but a higher risk of erythematous skin reactions, especially with daily treatments.[57] UVA-1 is most beneficial at the early stage of the disease.[57] There are a few cases of successful clearance of NL lesions with photodynamic therapy, which is thought to stimulate apoptosis by activating free oxygen radicals in the skin.[58]

PUVA is used by applying 0.005% psoralen to individual lesions with a UVA dosage of 0.5 J/cm^2

Table 1
NL treatment methods

Type	No. of Patients (Age [Y], Sex)	Treatment Regimen	Diabetes	Ulceration	Results	Reference	Level of Evidence
Nonpharmacological							
Glycemic control	1 (59, F)	Insulin mix BID	Yes	No	Improved lesions after 2 wk of better glycemic control	Kota et al,[18] 2012	D
Wound Care Agents							
Topically applied bovine collagen	1 (46, M)	Gel under occlusive dressing q5 d × 6 wk then collagen sheets × 2 wk then collagen particles × 6 wk then acetic acid soaks daily	No	Yes	Granulation tissue at 8 wk, re-epithelization at 16 wk, healed at 24 wk	Spenceri & Nahass,[51] 1997	D
Ovine forestomach matrix	1	4 Applications	NR	Yes	Complete wound closure at 22 wk	Simcock et al,[50] 2013	D
Protease-modulating dressing	1 (34, F)	—	Yes	Yes	Complete healing at 8 wk	Omugha & Jones,[49] 2003	D
Protease-modulating dressing	1 (21, M)	—	NR	Yes	—	Stewart,[52] 2006	D
GM-CSF	2 (22, F)	100 mcg (2 mL) q1–2 wk	—	Yes	Both: complete healing of ulceration at 10 wk	Remes & Ronnemaa,[53] 1999	D

(continued on next page)

Table 1
(continued)

Type	No. of Patients (Age [Y], Sex)	Treatment Regimen	Diabetes	Ulceration	Results	Reference	Level of Evidence
Phototherapy							
PUVA	30 (27, F), Avg 39 y	Topical PUVA (psoralen) 2×/wk (0.5 J/cm² up to 10 J/cm²)	Yes (43%)	NR	Healing in 17% (n = 5), improvement in 37% (n = 11), no effect in 33% (n = 10), worsening in 13% (n = 4) at an avg of 22 wk	De Rie et al,[7] 2002	C
PUVA	1 (74, M)	Topical PUVA (8-methoxypsoralen) + UVA 2×/wk (0.25 J/cm² initial dose)	Yes	Yes	Decreased pain after 3 sessions, 47% healing at 1 y of treatment Sustained × 1 y after PUVA stopped	Patel et al,[25] 2000	D
UVA-1	6 (5 = F), Avg 32 y	2–5 Treatments/wk × 15–50 sessions	Yes (3/6)	NR	Complete healing in n = 1, moderate improvement in n = 3, minimal effect in n = 2	Beattie et al,[57] 2006	D
UVA-1	1 (54, F)	61–75 W/cm², 3×/wk	No	Yes	Complete healing after 22 treatments Recurrence after 2.5 y: complete healing after 30 treatments, sustained remission at 6 y	Radakovic et al,[94] 2010	D
PDT	1 (60, F)	Methyl aminolevulinate (160 mg/g) application + red light (632 nm) 1/wk × 3 wk	Yes	No	Marked decrease color and size after 3 sessions, complete healing after 6, remission at 2 y follow-up	Heidenheim & Jemec,[95] 2006	D
PDT	1 (31, F)	10% Aminolevulinic acid application + red light (632 nm) q4 wk × 4	Yes	No	Complete healing at 4 applications (16 wk)	De Giorgi et al,[58] 2008	D

Corticosteroids

Medication	Patients (n, age, sex)	Dosage			Outcome	Reference	
Methylprednisolone, Prednisone	6 (5, F), Avg 41 y	1 mg/kg/d × 1 wk then 40 mg/d × 4 wk	Yes (4/6)	No	Rapid resolution in erythema and infiltration, no effect on atrophy, sustained effect at 4–10 mo	Petzelbauer et al,[55] 1992	D
Prednisone	1 (29, F)	55 mg Prednisone daily (1 mg/kg) tapered over 14 wk	Yes	Yes	Decreased erythema, inflammation, and healed ulcerated	Tan et al,[56] 2007	D
Prednisone	1 (F)	High-dose prednisone tapered to maintenance of 6 mg daily	Yes	Yes	Regression of NL lesion	Hocqueloux et al,[54] 1996	D
Calcineurin Inhibitors and other Immunomodulators							
Tacrolimus	2 (26, F; 85, F)	Tacrolimus 0.1% ointment BID	Yes (2/2)	Yes (2/2)	1. Decreased size at 6 wk, healed at 14 wk 2. Healed with scar at 8 wk	Binamer et al,[61] 2012	D
Tacrolimus	1 (70, F)	Tacrolimus 0.1% ointment (with compression)	Yes	Yes	Almost complete clinical resolution at 12 wk	Barth et al,[60] 2011	D
Tacrolimus	1 (62, F)	Tacrolimus 0.1% ointment BID	Yes	Yes	Resolution of ulceration but not plaques at 4 wk	Clayton & Harrison,[59] 2005	D
Tacrolimus	2 (16, F; 23, F)	Tacrolimus 0.1% ointment BID	No (2/2)	No (2/2)	1. Slight reduction of inflammation, no regression of the infiltrate at 8 wk, 2. Complete resolution at 8 wk	Harth & Linse,[62] 2004	D
Cyclosporine	2 (22, F; 31, F)	1. 5 mg/kg/d 2. 3 mg/kg/d	Yes	Yes	1. Improved at 1 mo, healed at 3 mo 2. Healed at 2 mo	Smith,[66] 1997	D
Cyclosporine	2 (52, F; 31, M)	3–4 mg/kg/d	Yes (1/2)	Yes	Healed at 4 mo	Darvay et al,[65] 1999	D
Cyclosporine	1 (44, F)	4 mg/kg/d	No	Yes	Healed at 3 mo, no relapse at 8 mo	Stinco et al,[67] 2003	D

(continued on next page)

Table 1
(continued)

Type	No. of Patients (Age [Y], Sex)	Treatment Regimen	Diabetes	Ulceration	Results	Reference	Level of Evidence
Cyclosporine (+pentoxifylline)	1 (55, F)	3–4 mg/kg/d + 400 mg PO 3 times daily	No	Yes	Edges healing at 1 wk, 80% healed at 4 mo, completely healed at 8 mo	Stanway et al,[8] 2004	D
Cyclosporine	1 (68, F)	2.5 mg/kg/d divided BID	No	Yes	Healed ulceration at 3 mo, recurred with dose decrease	Aslan et al,[64] 2007	D
Methotrexate, cyclosporine + pentoxifylline	1 (53, F)	Cyclosporine 4 then 2 mg/kg/d Methotrexate 15 mg weekly Pentoxifylline 400 mg BID	Yes	Yes	Healing of ulcerations on cyclosporine 4 mg/d, remained stable with taper but flared when methotrexate decreased	West et al,[68] 2007	D
Mycophenolate mofetil	1 (61, F)	500 mg PO BID	No	Yes	Healing of ulceration at 4 wk (recurrence on discontinuing)	Reinhard et al,[69] 2000	D
Biologics							
Intralesional Infliximab	3 (34, F; 65, M; 24, F)	10–20 mg q1 wk × 3 then 1 wk off	Yes (2/3)	Yes (1/3)	Improved erythema, infiltration, and healing in all patients at 3 mo Relapse at 2 mo in 1 patient	Barde et al,[70] 2011	D
Infliximab	1 (84, F)	5 mg/kg IV at 0, 2, 6, 12, and 21 wk	Yes	Yes	Decreased size, pain, drainage after first dose, complete healing at 6 wk	Hu et al,[72] 2009	D
Infliximab	1 (33, M)	5 mg/kg IV q1 mo × 2 mo	Yes	Yes	Decreased erythema, flattening of plaques, healed ulceration at 2 mo	Kolde et al,[73] 2003	D
Infliximab	1 (32, F)	5 mg/kg IV q1 mo × 2 mo	NR	Yes	Marked improvement at 1 mo Complete ulcer healing at 2 mo	Drosou et al,[71] 2003	D

Treatment	n (age, sex)	Dosage			Outcome	Reference	
Etanercept	1 (50, F)	25 mg SC 2×/wk	Yes	Yes	Healed ulcerations at 3 mo	Suarez-Amor et al,[74] 2010	D
Etanercept	1 (35, F)	25 mg SC q1 wk	Yes	No	Decreased size, atrophy, erythema, discoloration at 8 mo	Zeichner et al,[75] 2006	D
Etanercept + adalimumab	1	Etanercept 50 mg SC 2×/wk × 3 mo then q1 wk × 5 mo then adalimumab 40 mg q2 wk × 3 mo then etanercept as initial	Yes	Yes	Decreased erythema and flattening of plaques with etanercept but not adalimumab	Zhang et al,[76] 2009	D
Etanercept	1 (14, M)	Etanercept 25 mg SC 2×/wk + prednisone 30 mg PO daily + surgical debridement, allograft, autograft	No	Yes	Healing at 2 y of follow-up	Cummins et al,[96] 2004	D
Thalidomide	1 (54, F)	150 mg daily × 4 mo then 50 mg daily then tapered to 50 mg 2 times weekly	No	Yes	95% Re-epithelization of ulcer and 50% clearing of other areas at 1 mo Decreased inflammation at 4 mo Stable after 2 y of follow-up	Kukreja & Petersen,[97] 2006	D
Antimalarial							
Hydroxychloroquine	1 (62, F)	200 mg PO BID	—	Yes	Complete healing of ulceration at 10 wk	Kavala et al,[77] 2010	D
Hydroxychloroquine	2 (46, F; 44, F)	400 mg PO daily	No	No	1. No effect at 2 mo then no follow-up 2. Healed at 6 mo, no relapse at 1 y	Durupt et al,[98] 2008	D
Chloroquine	6 (6, F), Avg 38.5 y	200–300 mg PO daily	No	No	Thinned at 3 mo in n = 4, Healed at 6 mo in n = 3, 12 mo in n = 1	Durupt et al,[98] 2008	D
Chloroquine	1 (46, F)	500 mg PO daily	No	No	Decreased pain, erythema at 1 mo Resolution of inflammation at 3 mo	Nguyen et al,[78] 2002	D

(continued on next page)

Table 1
(continued)

Type	No. of Patients (Age [Y], Sex)	Treatment Regimen	Diabetes	Ulceration	Results	Reference	Level of Evidence
Cutaneous Blood Flow Modifiers							
Aspirin	16	ASA 40 mg daily	NR	NR	Healed in 2–4 wk	Beck et al,[85] 1985	B
Pentoxifylline	1 (30, M)	400 mg PO 3 times daily	Yes	Yes	Healed in 8 wk, no relapse at 3 mo	Noz et al,[87] 1993	D
Pentoxifylline	1 (20, F)	400 mg PO 3 times daily	Yes	Yes	Stable size at 1 mo, resolution of lesions at 6 mo	Basaria & Braga-Basaria,[86] 2003	D
Aspirin + dipyridamole	7 (7, M), Avg age 58.7 y	ASA 80 mg daily + dipyridamole 75 mg daily	Yes	Yes	Healed in 2–4 wk	Heng et al,[83] 1989	C
Aspirin + dipyridamole	7	ASA 80 mg daily + dipyridamole 75 mg daily	NR	NR	No significant improvement at 8 wk	Statham et al,[84] 1981	C
Dipyridamole + intralesional triamcinolone	1 (48, F)	25 mg PO TID × 4 wk then 25 mg PO BID × 4 wk then 25 mg PO daily × 10 wk	No	No	Near complete healing at 1 mo	Jiquan et al,[99] 2008	D
Combinations							
Clofazimine + topical tacrolimus + betamethasone	1 (37, F)	Clofazimine 100 mg/d + topical tacrolimus + betamethasone × 4 mo then 200 mg/d × 4 wk	NR	Yes	Improved clinical appearance and healed ulceration at 4 months, complete resolution at 5 mo	Benedix et al,[100] 2009	D
Fumaric Acid Esters							
Fumaric acid esters	1 (50, F)	Dimethyl fumarate 30 mg/d titrated to 240 mg/d over 4 wk	No	No	Complete healing with residual atrophy at 6 months, no relapse at 12 mo	Gambichler et al,[80] 2003	D
Fumaric acid esters	18 (16, F), Avg age 42.8 y	Dimethyl fumarate 30 mg/d titrated to 240 mg/d over 4 wk	Yes (12/18)	Yes (4/18)	Decreased erythema + infiltration in 15 patients at 6 mo, complete ulcer healing in 4/4 patients (3 discontinued therapy)	Kreuter et al,[81] 2005	B

Fumaric acid esters	1 (42, F)	Dimethyl fumarate 30 mg/d titrated to 240 mg/d over 4 wk then decreased to 120 mg/d	No	Yes	Complete ulcer healing at 6 mo No relapse at 12 mo	Eberle et al,[79] 2010	D
Miscellaneous							
Tretinoin	1 (65, F)	0.05% Tretinoin cream every evening × 5 wk	Yes	No	Decreased discoloration, visibility, and atrophy of plaques	Boyd,[101] 1999	D
Tretinoin	1				Decreased atrophy	Heymann,[102] 1996	D
IVIG	1 (63, F)	4 g/kg/d × 5 d	Yes	Yes	Healing of ulcerations at 3 wk (maintained at 2 y follow-up)	Barouti et al,[88] 2013	D
IVIG	1 (54, F)	2 g/kg daily × 5 d (at 0, 1.5, and 3.0 y)	Yes	Yes	Large decrease ulceration + pain at 2 wk, healed at 1 mo, stable × 8 mo Second lesion, minimal improvement × 2 courses, healed after added 3 d of IV prednisone	Batchelor & Todd,[89] 2012	D
Pioglitazone	1 (32, F)	Pioglitazone 7.5 mg PO daily × 1 mo then 15 mg daily	No	No	Improvement in erythema and atrophy at 1 mo, but new lesions at 5 mo	Boyd,[90] 2007	D
Fractional CO_2	11	1–4 Treatments at 30-d intervals	Yes (6/11)	NR	Improved erythema, atrophy, skin texture, and pain in 9/11	Buggiani et al,[92] 2012	C
Hyperbaric O_2 + steroids	1 (28, F)	113 Sessions of hyperbaric oxygen + topical corticosteroids	Yes	Yes	Improvement after 113 sessions	Bouhanick et al,[91] 1998	D

B, lesser quality RCT or prospective study; C, case-control study or retrospective study; D, case series or case reports.

Abbreviations: Avg, average; CO_2, carbon dioxide; F, female; GM-CSF, granulocyte-macrophage colony-stimulating factor; IV, intravenously; IVIG, intravenous immunoglobulin; M, male; N, not reported; O_2, dioxygen; PDT, photodynamic therapy; PUVA, psoralen-UVA; SC, subcutaneously.

twice weekly, titrated to a maximum of 10 J/cm^2. Side effects include possible blistering and subsequent bacterial superinfection, which can be treated with antibiotics. It may be possible to resume therapy at a reduced dose in these cases. A maximum of 4 months or a cumulative dose of 200 J/cm^2 is reasonable.

IMMUNOMODULATOR

Calcineurin inhibitors inhibit T-cell activation by blocking calcineurin and, thus, the production of cytokines, including interleukin 2 (IL-2) by T-helper cells and clonal T-cell proliferation, resulting in both antiinflammatory and immunomodulator effects. Topical tacrolimus has been shown to be effective in resolving ulceration associated with NL.[59–62] Efficacy is variable in NL plaques without ulceration present with the best response seen in early inflammatory stages. The improved effectiveness is thought to be because of enhanced skin penetration in these cases.[62] The lymphocytic infiltrate in the reticular dermis of NL lesions consists of T cells particularly T-helper cells.[63] Systemic cyclosporine has been very effective in resistant ulcerating lesions and usually produces a rapid improvement with complete healing achieved in 2 to 4 months; but on follow-up of these patients, the ulcerations tended to recur when the therapy was discontinued.[8,64–67] Adverse effects include hypertension, hyperkalemia, and nephrotoxicity, of particular importance in patients with preexisting diabetic nephropathy. It is prescribed at a dosage of 2 to 4 mg/kg/d; monitoring includes blood pressure, potassium, and creatinine.

Methotrexate inhibits dihydrofolate reductase, a folate-dependent enzyme. This inhibition leads to decreased activation of TNF alpha, IL-8 and IL-12, and interferon gamma, which likely contribute to the inflammatory element of NL. A combination of cyclosporine, methotrexate, and pentoxifylline was used successfully; but recurrence occurred with withdrawal of methotrexate, and the dose of cyclosporine required was not lower than in other cases of monotherapy.[68] There have not been any cases of monotherapy with methotrexate.

Mycophenolate mofetil, which has a potent cytostatic effect on lymphocytes, was successful in healing an ulcerated lesion in 1 patient; but recurrence occurred when therapy was discontinued.[69] In contrast to calcineurin inhibitors, there is minimal nephrotoxicity, with the main adverse effect being gastrointestinal upset. Although there have been concerns of malignant transformation if using immunomodulatory therapy, there is no evidence to support this theory.

BIOLOGICS

TNF is an important regulator in the formation of granulomas. The monoclonal antibodies adalimumab and infliximab bind directly to soluble TNF alpha to prevent its action. The fusion protein etanercept is a fusion protein consisting of the Fc portion of human IgG1 and TNF receptors that also inhibit soluble TNF function. Both etanercept and infliximab have been repeatedly effective as monotherapy for ulcerating NL.[70–76] From the limited experience, infliximab may produce more rapid response, with healing achieved in a shorter duration of treatment.[74] Adalimumab, a human monoclonal antibody, was not effective in a case report for unknown reasons. These agents are very well tolerated, although there is the potential of reactivating latent tuberculosis. For this reason, a tuberculin skin test and chest radiograph should be performed before initiating treatment.

There is one case report with the use of thalidomide, which suppresses TNF alpha resulting in antiinflammatory effects and inhibits vascular endothelial growth factor resulting in antiangiogenic effects. Its role is limited by its known teratogenicity in addition to adverse effects, including neuropathy manifesting as distal paresthesia and somnolence.

ANTIMALARIAL

Hydroxychloroquine and chloroquine have antiinflammatory actions and inhibit macrophage chemotaxis, which may prevent further granuloma production in NL. Chloroquine additionally inhibits platelet aggregation by blocking conversion of arachidonic acid to prostaglandins, decreasing the risk of occlusion of cutaneous blood vessels. These mechanisms may explain the response of NL to hydroxychloroquine and chloroquine.[77,78] Effects take 1 to 3 months to be fully realized, and long-term data are still lacking. The risk of irreversible retinopathy is rare with courses of less than 5 years, but visual haloes occur more commonly because of rapid deposition of medication in the cornea. Baseline ophthalmology testing and a complete blood count (CBC) are recommended.

FUMARIC ACID ESTERS

Fumaric acid esters inhibit inflammatory cytokines and prevent T lymphocyte proliferation. They have been quite effective in case reports and series, leading to complete resolution or healing of NL in patients continuing treatment for 6 months.[79–81] Unfortunately, they are not currently available in the United States or Canada and can be poorly tolerated because of dose-related nausea. The dose used in NL has been the same as traditionally used for psoriasis, starting with 30 mg of dimethyl-fumarate, which is gradually increased over 3 to 4 weeks to a target of 240 mg.[82] A CBC should be monitored for lymphopenia, observed in as many as 44% of patients.[81]

CUTANEOUS BLOOD FLOW MODULATORS

Medications targeting the thrombosis in cutaneous blood vessels seen in NL were among the first to be tried but seem to have limited success as mono-therapy. Aspirin and dipyridamole inhibit platelet aggregation and decrease blood viscosity. Results are conflicting, with healing of ulcerated NL lesions observed in all 7 patients in 1 case series but not in a subsequent randomized trial compared with placebo.[83,84] Very-low-dose aspirin seemed to have no effect as monotherapy.[85]

Pentoxifylline has additional effects on red blood cell deformity and also decreases produc-tion of TNF alpha. It has been associated with resolution of ulcerated lesions in case reports and had also been used in combination with other systemic medications.[8,86,87] The target dosage of 400 mg 3 times daily is limited by gastrointestinal side effects.

MISCELLANEOUS

Various other treatments have been successful in case reports. Intravenous immunoglobulin (IVIG) has been used to treat a variety inflammatory and granulomatous disorders. IVIG was useful in 2 patients, but 1 patient had an underlying immu-noglobulin deficiency and the other patient required addition of corticosteroids for final heal-ing.[88,89] It is, therefore, not likely to be useful as a first-line agent in the absence of a known deficiency. The use of topical tretinoin led to improvement of atrophy in 2 patients with nonul-cerated NL. Retinoids may work by increasing the type 1 collagen formation that is decreased in lesions of NL and could represent a good alter-native in nonulcerated plaques where atrophy is a prominent feature.

Pioglitazone, a potent agonist for peroxisome proliferator activator receptor gamma (PPAR γ), was used in a case with nonulcerated NL; but despite some improvement in the initial lesions, new plaques developed while on therapy.[90] It is a PPAR γ activator, leading to suppression of TNF alpha and inflammatory cytokines, in addition to having antiatherosclerotic properties.

Hyperbaric oxygen and fractionated carbon dioxide have also been used successfully. Hyperbaric oxygen was only used in 1 case and required 113 sessions, whereas fractional carbon dioxide achieved improvement in 9 of 11 patients in a case series with only 2 to 4 sessions.[91,92] Pulsed dye should likely be avoided as it was un-successful at a low dose in 1 patient and produced skin breakdown at higher doses.[93]

SUMMARY

NL is often indolent, and the decision on the treat-ment is individualized and based on patients' con-cerns. There is no gold standard treatment of NL, due to an incomplete understanding of the patho-genesis. The most common treatments of NL are potent topical steroids and calcineurin inhibitors. Physical therapies and immunomodulators are beneficial in some cases. Ulceration is a common complication, and patients need to be monitored for less common sequelae like transition to malignancy.

REFERENCES

1. Reid SD, Ladizinski B, Lee K, et al. Update on nec-robiosis lipoidica: a review of etiology, diagnosis, and treatment options. J Am Acad Dermatol 2013;69:783–91.
2. Muller SA, Winkelmann RK. Necrobiosis lipoidica diabeticorum. A clinical and pathological investiga-tion of 171 cases. Arch Dermatol 1966;93:272–81.
3. Peyri J, Moreno A, Marcoval J. Necrobiosis lipoid-ica. Semin Cutan Med Surg 2007;26:87–9.
4. Muller SA, Winkelmann RK. Necrobiosis lipoidica diabeticorum histopathologic study of 98 cases. Arch Dermatol 1966;94:1–10.
5. Erfurt-Berge C, Seitz AT, Rehse C, et al. Update on clinical and laboratory features in necrobiosis lip-oidica: a retrospective multicentre study of 52 pa-tients. Eur J Dermatol 2012;22:770–5.
6. Berking C, Hegyi J, Arenberger P, et al. Photody-namic therapy of necrobiosis lipoidica–a multi-center study of 18 patients. Dermatology 2009; 218:136–9.
7. De Rie MA, Sommer A, Hoekzema R, et al. Treat-ment of necrobiosis lipoidica with topical psoralen plus ultraviolet A. Br J Dermatol 2002;147:743–7.
8. Stanway A, Rademaker M, Newman P. Healing of severe ulcerative necrobiosis lipoidica with cyclo-sporin. Australas J Dermatol 2004;45:119–22.
9. Quimby SR, Muller SA, Schroeter AL. The cuta-neous immunopathology of necrobiosis lipoidica diabeticorum. Arch Dermatol 1988;124:1364–71.
10. Boateng B, Hiller D, Albrecht HP, et al. Cutaneous microcirculation in pretibial necrobiosis lipoidica. Comparative laser Doppler flowmetry and oxygen partial pressure determinations in patients and

healthy probands. Hautarzt 1993;44:581–6 [in German].

11. Holland C, Givens V, Smoller BR. Expression of the human erythrocyte glucose transporter Glut-1 in areas of sclerotic collagen in necrobiosis lipoidica. J Cutan Pathol 2001;28:287–90.

12. Ngo B, Wigington G, Hayes K, et al. Skin blood flow in necrobiosis lipoidica diabeticorum. Int J Dermatol 2008;47:354–8.

13. Oikarinen A, Mortenhumer M, Kallioinen M, et al. Necrobiosis lipoidica: ultrastructural and biochemical demonstration of a collagen defect. J Invest Dermatol 1987;88:227–32.

14. Markey AC, Tidman MJ, Rowe PH, et al. Aggressive ulcerative necrobiosis lipoidica associated with venous insufficiency, giant-cell phlebitis and arteritis. Clin Exp Dermatol 1988;13:183–6.

15. Evans CD, Pereira RS, Yuen CT, et al. Anti-collagen antibodies in granuloma annulare and necrobiosis lipoidica. Clin Exp Dermatol 1988;13:252–4.

16. Ullman S, Dahl MV. Necrobiosis lipoidica. An immunofluorescence study. Arch Dermatol 1977;113:1671–3.

17. O'Toole EA, Kennedy U, Nolan JJ, et al. Necrobiosis lipoidica: only a minority of patients have diabetes mellitus. Br J Dermatol 1999;140:283–6.

18. Kota SK, Jammula S, Kota SK, et al. Necrobiosis lipoidica diabeticorum: a case-based review of literature. Indian J Endocrinol Metab 2012;16:614–20.

19. Roche-Gamon E, Vilata-Corell JJ, Velasco-Pastor M. Familial necrobiosis lipoidica not associated with diabetes. Dermatol Online J 2007;13:26.

20. Ho KK, O'Loughlin S, Powell FC. Familial nondiabetic necrobiosis lipoidica. Australas J Dermatol 1992;33:31–4.

21. Shimanovich I, Erdmann H, Grabbe J, et al. Necrobiosis lipoidica in monozygotic twins. Arch Dermatol 2008;144:119–20.

22. Hawryluk EB, Izikson L, English JC 3rd. Non-infectious granulomatous diseases of the skin and their associated systemic diseases: an evidence-based update to important clinical questions. Am J Clin Dermatol 2010;11:171–81.

23. Gebauer K, Armstrong M. Koebner phenomenon with necrobiosis lipoidica diabeticorum. Int J Dermatol 1993;32:895–6.

24. Schumacher F, Schnyder UW. Necrobiosis lipoidica and Koebner phenomenon. Hautarzt 1991;42:587–8 [in German].

25. Patel GK, Harding KG, Mills CM. Severe disabling Koebnerizing ulcerated necrobiosis lipoidica successfully managed with topical PUVA. Br J Dermatol 2000;143:668–9.

26. Wee SA, Shupack JL. Necrobiotic xanthogranuloma. Dermatol Online J 2005;11:24.

27. Ghiasi N, Alavi A, Coutts PM, et al. Necrobiotic xanthogranuloma as an unusual cause of refractive chronic bilateral leg ulceration. Int J Low Extrem Wounds 2012;11:293–5.

28. Vanhooteghem O, Andre J, de la Brassinne M. Epidermoid carcinoma and perforating necrobiosis lipoidica: a rare association. J Eur Acad Dermatol Venereol 2005;19:756–8.

29. Acebo E, Gardeazabal J, Marcellan M, et al. Necrobiosis lipoidica over appendectomy scar in a patient with morphea of the breast. Actas Dermosifiliogr 2006;97:52–5 [in Spanish].

30. Vion B, Burri G, Ramelet AA. Necrobiosis lipoidica and silicotic granulomas on Muller's phlebectomy scars. Dermatology 1997;194:55–8.

31. Alonso ML, Rios JC, Gonzalez-Beato MJ, et al. Necrobiosis lipoidica of the glans penis. Acta Derm Venereol 2011;91:105–6.

32. Sawada Y, Mori T, Nakashima D, et al. Necrobiosis lipoidica of the scrotum. Eur J Dermatol 2011;21:98–9.

33. Tokura Y, Mizushima Y, Hata M, et al. Necrobiosis lipoidica of the glans penis. J Am Acad Dermatol 2003;49:921–4.

34. Kavanagh GM, Novelli M, Hartog M, et al. Necrobiosis lipoidica–involvement of atypical sites. Clin Exp Dermatol 1993;18:543–4.

35. Lynch JM, Barrett TL. Collagenolytic (necrobiotic) granulomas: part II–the 'red' granulomas. J Cutan Pathol 2004;31:409–18.

36. Lowitt MH, Dover JS. Necrobiosis lipoidica. J Am Acad Dermatol 1991;25:735–48.

37. Magro CM, Crowson AN, Regauer S. Granuloma annulare and necrobiosis lipoidica tissue reactions as a manifestation of systemic disease. Hum Pathol 1996;27:50–6.

38. Cohen O, Yaniv R, Karasik A, et al. Necrobiosis lipoidica and diabetic control revisited. Med Hypotheses 1996;46:348–50.

39. Kelly WF, Nicholas J, Adams J, et al. Necrobiosis lipoidica diabeticorum: association with background retinopathy, smoking, and proteinuria. A case controlled study. Diabet Med 1993;10:725–8.

40. Verrotti A, Chiarelli F, Amerio P, et al. Necrobiosis lipoidica diabeticorum in children and adolescents: a clue for underlying renal and retinal disease. Pediatr Dermatol 1995;12:220–3.

41. Murray CA, Miller RA. Necrobiosis lipoidica diabeticorum and thyroid disease. Int J Dermatol 1997;36:799–800.

42. Berkson MH, Bondi EE, Margolis DJ. Ulcerated necrobiosis lipoidica diabeticorum in a patient with a history of generalized granuloma annulare. Cutis 1994;53:85–6.

43. Lim C, Tschuchnigg M, Lim J. Squamous cell carcinoma arising in an area of long-standing necrobiosis lipoidica. J Cutan Pathol 2006;33:581–3.

44. Beljaards RC, Groen J, Starink TM. Bilateral squamous cell carcinomas arising in long-standing necrobiosis lipoidica. Dermatologica 1990;180:96–8.

45. Bakos RM, Cartell A, Bakos L. Dermatoscopy of early-onset necrobiosis lipoidica. J Am Acad Dermatol 2012;66:e143–4.

46. Conde-Montero E, Aviles-Izquierdo JA, Mendoza-Cembranos MD, et al. Dermoscopy of necrobiosis lipoidica. Actas Dermosifiliogr 2013;104:534–7.

47. Nakajima T, Tanemura A, Inui S, et al. Venous insufficiency in patients with necrobiosis lipoidica. J Dermatol 2009;36:166–9.

48. Morihara K, Takenaka H, Morihara T, et al. Atypical form of necrobiosis lipoidica associated with lymphoedema. J Eur Acad Dermatol Venereol 2007; 21:831–3.

49. Omugha N, Jones AM. The management of hard-to-heal necrobiosis with PROMOGRAN. Br J Nurs 2003;12:S14–20.

50. Simcock JW, Than M, Ward BR, et al. Treatment of ulcerated necrobiosis lipoidica with ovine forestomach matrix. J Wound Care 2013;22:383–4.

51. Spenceri EA, Nahass GT. Topically applied bovine collagen in the treatment of ulcerative necrobiosis lipoidica diabeticorum. Arch Dermatol 1997;133: 817–8.

52. Stewart E. Using a protease-modulating dressing to treat necrobiosis lipoidica diabeticorum. J Wound Care 2006;15:74–7.

53. Remes K, Ronnemaa T. Healing of chronic leg ulcers in diabetic necrobiosis lipoidica with local granulocyte-macrophage colony stimulating factor treatment. J Diabetes Complications 1999;13: 115–8.

54. Hocqueloux L, Gautier JF, Lebbe C, et al. Ulcerated necrobiosis lipoidica associated with insulin-dependent diabetes mellitus. Beneficial effect of corticosteroid therapy by oral administration. Presse Med 1996;25:25–7 [in French].

55. Petzelbauer P, Wolff K, Tappeiner G. Necrobiosis lipoidica: treatment with systemic corticosteroids. Br J Dermatol 1992;126:542–5.

56. Tan E, Patel V, Berth-Jones J. Systemic corticosteroids for the outpatient treatment of necrobiosis lipoidica in a diabetic patient. J Dermatolog Treat 2007;18:246–8.

57. Beattie PE, Dawe RS, Ibbotson SH, et al. UVA1 phototherapy for treatment of necrobiosis lipoidica. Clin Exp Dermatol 2006;31:235–8.

58. De Giorgi V, Buggiani G, Rossi R, et al. Successful topical photodynamic treatment of refractory necrobiosis lipoidica. Photodermatol Photoimmunol Photomed 2008;24:332–3.

59. Clayton TH, Harrison PV. Successful treatment of chronic ulcerated necrobiosis lipoidica with 0.1% topical tacrolimus ointment. Br J Dermatol 2005; 152:581–2.

60. Barth D, Harth W, Treudler R, et al. Topical tacrolimus in necrobiosis lipoidica. Hautarzt 2011;62: 459–62 [in German].

61. Binamer Y, Sowerby L, El-Helou T. Treatment of ulcerative necrobiosis lipoidica with topical calcineurin inhibitor: case report and literature review. J Cutan Med Surg 2012;16:458–61.

62. Harth W, Linse R. Topical tacrolimus in granuloma annulare and necrobiosis lipoidica. Br J Dermatol 2004;150:792–4.

63. Alegre VA, Winkelmann RK. A new histopathologic feature of necrobiosis lipoidica diabeticorum: lymphoid nodules. J Cutan Pathol 1988;15:75–7.

64. Aslan E, Korber A, Grabbe S, et al. Successful therapy of ulcerated necrobiosis lipoidica non diabeticorum with cyclosporine A. Hautarzt 2007;58: 684–8 [in German].

65. Darvay A, Acland KM, Russell-Jones R. Persistent ulcerated necrobiosis lipoidica responding to treatment with cyclosporin. Br J Dermatol 1999;141: 725–7.

66. Smith K. Ulcerating necrobiosis lipoidica resolving in response to cyclosporine-A. Dermatol Online J 1997;3:2.

67. Stinco G, Parlangeli ME, De Francesco V, et al. Ulcerated necrobiosis lipoidica treated with cyclosporin A. Acta Derm Venereol 2003;83:151–3.

68. West EA, Warren RB, King CM. A case of recalcitrant necrobiosis lipoidica responding to combined immunosuppression therapy. J Eur Acad Dermatol Venereol 2007;21:830–1.

69. Reinhard G, Lohmann F, Uerllch M, et al. Successful treatment of ulcerated necrobiosis lipoidica with mycophenolate mofetil. Acta Derm Venereol 2000; 80:312–3.

70. Barde C, Laffitte E, Campanelli A, et al. Intralesional infliximab in noninfectious cutaneous granulomas: three cases of necrobiosis lipoidica. Dermatology 2011;222:212–6.

71. Drosou A, Kirsner RS, Welsh E, et al. Use of infliximab, an anti-tumor necrosis alpha antibody, for inflammatory dermatoses. J Cutan Med Surg 2003;7: 382–6.

72. Hu SW, Bevona C, Winterfield L, et al. Treatment of refractory ulcerative necrobiosis lipoidica diabeticorum with infliximab: report of a case. Arch Dermatol 2009;145:437–9.

73. Kolde G, Muche JM, Schulze P, et al. Infliximab: a promising new treatment option for ulcerated necrobiosis lipoidica. Dermatology 2003;206:180–1.

74. Suarez-Amor O, Perez-Bustillo A, Ruiz-Gonzalez I, et al. Necrobiosis lipoidica therapy with biologicals: an ulcerated case responding to etanercept and a review of the literature. Dermatology 2010;221: 117–21.

75. Zeichner JA, Stern DW, Lebwohl M. Treatment of necrobiosis lipoidica with the tumor necrosis factor

antagonist etanercept. J Am Acad Dermatol 2006; 54:S120–1.

76. Zhang KS, Quan LT, Hsu S. Treatment of necrobiosis lipoidica with etanercept and adalimumab. Dermatol Online J 2009;15:12.

77. Kavala M, Sudogan S, Zindanci I, et al. Significant improvement in ulcerative necrobiosis lipoidica with hydroxychloroquine. Int J Dermatol 2010;49:467–9.

78. Nguyen K, Washenik K, Shupack J. Necrobiosis lipoidica diabeticorum treated with chloroquine. J Am Acad Dermatol 2002;46:S34–6.

79. Eberle FC, Ghoreschi K, Hertl M. Fumaric acid esters in severe ulcerative necrobiosis lipoidica: a case report and evaluation of current therapies. Acta Derm Venereol 2010;90:104–6.

80. Gambichler T, Kreuter A, Freitag M, et al. Clearance of necrobiosis lipoidica with fumaric acid esters. Dermatology 2003;207:422–4.

81. Kreuter A, Knierim C, Stucker M, et al. Fumaric acid esters in necrobiosis lipoidica: results of a prospective noncontrolled study. Br J Dermatol 2005; 153:802–7.

82. Mrowietz U, Christophers E, Altmeyer P. Treatment of severe psoriasis with fumaric acid esters: scientific background and guidelines for therapeutic use. The German Fumaric Acid Ester Consensus Conference. Br J Dermatol 1999;141:424–9.

83. Heng MC, Song MK, Heng MK. Healing of necrobiotic ulcers with antiplatelet therapy. Correlation with plasma thromboxane levels. Int J Dermatol 1989; 28:195–7.

84. Statham B, Finlay AY, Marks R. A randomized double blind comparison of an aspirin dipyridamole combination versus a placebo in the treatment of necrobiosis lipoidica. Acta Derm Venereol 1981; 61:270–1.

85. Beck HI, Bjerring P, Rasmussen I, et al. Treatment of necrobiosis lipoidica with low-dose acetylsalicylic acid. A randomized double-blind trial. Acta Derm Venereol 1985;65:230–4.

86. Basaria S, Braga-Basaria M. Necrobiosis lipoidica diabeticorum: response to pentoxiphylline. J Endocrinol Invest 2003;26:1037–40.

87. Noz KC, Korstanje MJ, Vermeer BJ. Ulcerating necrobiosis lipoidica effectively treated with pentoxifylline. Clin Exp Dermatol 1993;18:78–9.

88. Barouti N, Cao AQ, Ferrara D, et al. Successful treatment of ulcerative and diabeticorum necrobiosis lipoidica with intravenous immunoglobulin in a patient with common variable immunodeficiency. JAMA Dermatol 2013;149:879–81.

89. Batchelor JM, Todd PM. Treatment of ulcerated necrobiosis lipoidica with intravenous immunoglobulin and methylprednisolone. J Drugs Dermatol 2012;11:256–9.

90. Boyd AS. Treatment of necrobiosis lipoidica with pioglitazone. J Am Acad Dermatol 2007;57: S120–1.

91. Bouhanick B, Verret JL, Gouello JP, et al. Necrobiosis lipoidica: treatment by hyperbaric oxygen and local corticosteroids. Diabetes Metab 1998;24: 156–9.

92. Buggiani G, Tsampau D, Krysenka A, et al. Fractional CO2 laser: a novel therapeutic device for refractory necrobiosis lipoidica. Dermatol Ther 2012;25:612–4.

93. Currie CL, Monk BE. Pulsed dye laser treatment of necrobiosis lipoidica: report of a case. J Cutan Laser Ther 1999;1:239–41.

94. Radakovic S, Weber M, Tanew A. Dramatic response of chronic ulcerating necrobiosis lipoidica to ultraviolet A1 phototherapy. Photodermatol Photoimmunol Photomed 2010;26(6):327–9.

95. Heidenheim M, Jemec GB. Successful treatment of necrobiosis lipoidica diabeticorum with photodynamic therapy. Arch Dermatol 2006;142(12): 1548–50.

96. Cummins DL, Hiatt KM, Mimouni D, et al. Generalized necrobiosis lipoidica treated with a combination of split-thickness autografting and immunomodulatory therapy. Int J Dermatol 2004; 43(11):852–4.

97. Kukreja T, Petersen J. Thalidomide for the treatment of refractory necrobiosis lipoidica. Arch Dermatol 2006;142(1):20–2.

98. Durupt F, Dalle S, Debarbieux S, et al. Successful treatment of necrobiosis lipoidica with antimalarial agents. Arch Dermatol 2008;144(1):118–9.

99. Jiquan S, Khalaf AT, Jinquan T, et al. Necrobiosis lipoidica: a case with histopathological findings revealed asteroid bodies and was successfully treated with dipyridamole plus intralesional triamcinolone. J Dermatolog Treat 2008; 19(1):54–7.

100. Benedix F, Geyer A, Lichte V, et al. Response of ulcerated necrobiosis lipoidica to clofazimine. Acta Derm Venereol 2009;89(6):651–2.

101. Boyd AS. Tretinoin treatment of necrobiosis lipoidica diabeticorum. Diabetes Care 1999;22(10): 1753–4.

102. Heymann WR. Necrobiosis lipoidica treated with topical tretinoin. Cutis 1996;58(1):53–4.

Rheumatoid Nodules

Jeremy S. Tilstra, MD, PhD*, Douglas W. Lienesch, MD

KEYWORDS

- Rheumatoid nodules • Accelerated nodulosis • Palisading macrophages • Benign nodulosis
- Methotrexate • Rheumatoid arthritis • Pulmonary rheumatoid nodules

KEY POINTS

- Rheumatoid nodules are the common extra-articular manifestation of rheumatoid arthritis (RA).
- Systemic RA medications are not proven therapy for rheumatoid nodules; paradoxically, methotrexate and possibly other systemic therapies can induce or exacerbate nodule formation.
- Regardless of location, rheumatoid nodules have a consistent histologic appearance with a central area of fibrinoid necrosis, surrounded by palisading macrophages that are CD68+ and enclosed by a granulation layer.
- Subcutaneous nodules with typical clinical characteristics require neither biopsy for diagnosis nor specific treatment unless they are causing pain, interference in mechanical function, nerve compression, or other local phenomena.
- Pulmonary rheumatoid nodules require a more aggressive diagnostic evaluation to exclude malignancy, infection, or other causes of lung nodules.

INTRODUCTION

Rheumatoid nodules are the most common extra-articular manifestation of RA. RA is a chronic inflammatory arthritis that affects nearly 1.5 million adults in the United States[1] and 2 million in Europe.[2] It was traditionally a debilitating disease, but with advances in treatment, RA is now a manageable chronic disease state. The predominant feature of RA is synovial inflammation manifested as swelling and tenderness of small, medium, and large joints in a symmetric pattern, with a predilection for the smaller joints of the hands and feet.

RA is classified by the combined American College of Rheumatology (ACR) and European League Against Rheumatism (EULAR) criteria (**Table 1**), which encompass joint swelling, elevated levels of serum rheumatoid factors (RFs) and anti–cyclic citrullinated peptide antibodies (anti-CCP), inflammatory markers, and symptom duration.[3] Prior classification criteria have included the presence of symmetric arthritis, rheumatoid nodules, and typical radiographic changes.

Patients with RA produce an array of auto-antibodies, including RF CCP. Although elevation of RF and CCP levels is not necessary for diagnosis, it helps to differentiate RA from other inflammatory arthropathies. In a 700-patient retrospective study, the sensitivity and specificity for anti-CCP was 74.0% and 94%, respectively, whereas RF had a sensitivity of 69.7% and specificity of 81%. Differences in specificity were largely due to the increased prevalence of RF in primary Sjögren syndrome, chronic viral hepatitis, and systemic lupus erythematosus (SLE).[4] Detection of antibody with anti-CCP2 antibody, the commonly used assay, resulted in improved sensitivity (64%–89%) and specificity (88%–99%). RF sensitivity ranged from 59% to 79% and specificity from 80% to 84% in the same groups.[5] Patients who meet classification criteria for RA as outlined in **Table 1**, but present without

Department of Rheumatology, UPMC, University of Pittsburgh, S700 Biomedical Center, 3500 Terrace Street, Pittsburgh, PA 15261, USA
* Corresponding author.
E-mail address: tilstraj@upmc.edu

Dermatol Clin 33 (2015) 361–371
http://dx.doi.org/10.1016/j.det.2015.03.004
0733-8635/15/$ – see front matter

Table 1
ACR/EULAR classification criteria for rheumatoid arthritis

Criteria	Points
A. Joint Involvement	
1 Large joint	0
2–10 Large joints	1
1–3 Small joints	2
4–10 Small joints	3
>10 Joints (at least 1 small joint)	5
B. Serology	
Neg RF and neg CCP	0
Low pos RF or low pos CCP	2
High pos RF or high pos CCP	3
C. Acute phase reactant	
Normal CRP and ESR	0
Abnormal CRP or ESR	1
D. Duration of symptoms	
<6 wk	0
≥6 wk	1

Score of ≥6 is diagnostic criteria for rheumatoid arthritis.
Abbreviations: CCP, cyclic citrullinated peptide; CRP, C-reactive protein; ESR, erythrocyte sedimentation rate; neg, negative; pos, positive; RF, rheumatoid factor.
Adapted from Aletaha D, Neogi T, Silman AJ, et al. 2010 Rheumatoid arthritis classification criteria: an American College of Rheumatology/European League Against Rheumatism collaborative initiative. Ann Rheum Dis 2010;69(9):2574; with permission.

Box 1
Extra-articular manifestation of rheumatoid arthritis

Skin manifestations
    Rheumatoid nodules
    Rheumatoid small-vessel vasculitis
    Pyoderma gangrenosum
Ocular manifestations
    Keratoconjunctivitis sicca
    Episcleritis
    Scleritis
    Peripheral ulcerative keratitis
Pulmonary manifestations
    Interstitial lung disease
    Parenchymal pulmonary nodules
    Pulmonary effusion
Cardiac manifestations
    Pericarditis
    Myocarditis
    Increased cardiovascular disease
Renal manifestations
    Glomerulonephritis due to amyloid
Neurologic manifestations
    Peripheral neuropathy
    Mononeuritis multiplex
    Central nervous system vasculitis
Hematologic manifestations
    Felty syndrome
    Pancytopenia (in any combination)

Adapted from Cojocaru M, Cojocaru IM, Silosi I, et al. Extra-articular manifestations in rheumatoid arthritis. Maedica (Buchar) 2010; 5(4):286–91.

RF or anti-CCP antibodies, and who do not fulfill criteria for other diseases are considered to have seronegative RA.

RA is a systemic disease with an array of extra-articular manifestations (**Box 1**) Extra-articular manifestation of the skin are common and usually occur in RF-positive patients and early in disease course.[6] The most frequent cutaneous manifestation is rheumatoid nodules. Other rare skin lesions include cutaneous ulcers from medium vasculitis, nail fold infarcts or palpable purpura from small vessel vasculitis, pyoderma gangrenosum, and granulomatous dermatitis.[7] The remainder of this article further defines the pathogenesis, histology, and treatment of rheumatoid nodules.

RHEUMATOID NODULES

Rheumatoid nodules are one of the most common extra-articular manifestations noted in RA. These nodules are usually encountered on extensor surfaces and areas of pressure or repetitive trauma, most notably the olecranon and dorsal aspect of the hand (**Fig. 1**). However, they can develop on any tendon/ligament-like structures such as the Achilles tendon and vocal cords. In bedbound patients, these nodules can also be seen on the occiput and ischium. The prevalence is estimated at 10%, although the 10-year occurrence rate in any single individual may be as high as 30% over 10 years.[8] The most common noncutaneous location for rheumatoid nodules is the lung (see section Systemic Location of Rheumatoid Nodules). Rarely rheumatoid nodules can be associated with other diseases such as rheumatic fever, and there are case reports of nodules in

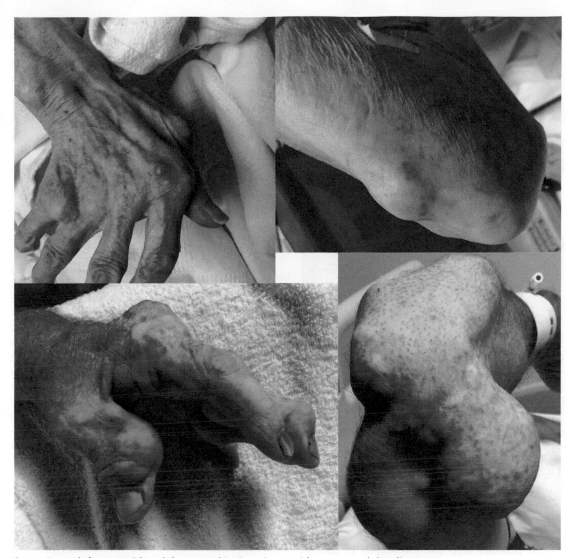

Fig. 1. Several rheumatoid nodules, noted in 2 patients with severe nodular disease.

other connective tissue diseases, although these cases are rare. The size of the nodules varies from 2 to 5 cm; they are firm, nontender, and moveable in subcutaneous planes.[9] Diagnosis is usually determined clinically. When seen in early or aggressive disease and located on extensor or pressure point surfaces, the differential is usually limited. The lesions are often firm, painless, and have no characteristic features on radiography (**Fig. 2**) Nodules can be mobile or bound down to soft tissue, fascia, or periostium. No additional diagnostic testing is warranted for nodules with typical clinical characteristics. However, in cases of diagnostic uncertainty, rheumatoid nodules have a distinct histologic appearance on excision biopsy (see section on Histopathology and Pathogenesis).

PREVALENCE OF RHEUMATOID NODULES

Studies indicate that rheumatoid nodule incidence is highest during initial RA presentation, with approximately 7% of patients demonstrating nodules at the time of diagnosis.[10] The overall occurrence rates have been reported in as many as 35% of individuals,[6] In a study examining Asian and Hispanic populations placing overall prevalence at approximately 17%, prevalence was higher in the Hispanic population.[11] Most patients with rheumatoid nodules have positive RF factor.[12] In patients with Felty syndrome, a disorder defined by neutropenia and splenomegaly associated with RA, nodular development has been reported in nearly 75% of patients.[13] The prevalence of systemic (noncutaneous) sites of rheumatoid

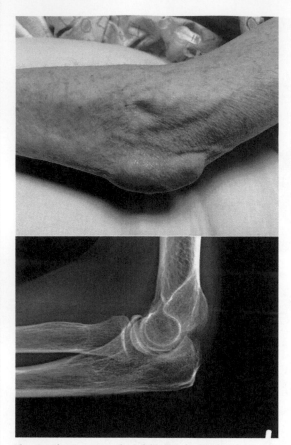

Fig. 2. Classic example of large rheumatoid nodule overlying olecranon bursa. These nodules are radiolucent with no defining features on imaging as shown in the corresponding radiograph.

central fibrinoid necrosis.[17] These HLA-DR+ antigen-presenting cells were found to secrete large amounts of interleukin (IL)-1.[16] Other studies examining cytokine production from rheumatoid nodules have shown increased levels of tumor necrosis factor (TNF), interferon, IL-10, IL-15, IL-18, and IL-12 (but not IL-2, IL-4, and IL-17).[18] In addition, a focal vasculitis has been observed in one-third of all rheumatoid nodules.[9] Deposits of RF and the terminal components of complement are also found on the endothelium of small vessels within nodules.[19]

Although subcutaneous nodules are the most common presentation of rheumatoid nodule, systemic nodules are also noted particularly in lung parenchyma. The histology of these pulmonary nodules is similar to that of subcutanous nodules, with irregular central necrosis surrounded by palisading CD68-positive macrophages with additional surrounding inflammatory infiltrate including lymphocytes, as described earlier.[14,20] Nearly 50% of lung nodules are cavitary in appearance likely because of the response in the surrounding parenchymal lung tissues.[20] In one study, albeit comprising only 2 cases, there were aggregates of CD20 B lymphocytes and CD3 T-cells with CD21-positive follicular dendritic cells situated at their center, consistent with germinal center formation, which is not described with subcutaneous nodules[14]; however, this is not a commonly reported phenomenon.

nodules is much lower, documented in less than 1% of patients with RA (discussed in section Systemic Location of Rheumatoid Nodules).

HISTOPATHOLOGY

The histologic appearance of rheumatoid nodules is specific and representative of an immune-mediated granulomatous process, which exhibits a central area of necrosis surrounded by palisading epithelioid macrophages enclosed by granulation tissue containing lymphocytes and histiocytes.[14–16] The area of central necrosis contains a large population of HLA-DR+ staining material likely from necrosing endothelial cells and macrophages. Of the surrounding palisading cells, the vast majority stain intensely positive for HLA-DR+ and are noted to be a monocyte/macrophage antigen-presenting population with phagocytic properties.[15,16] Later studies defined these macrophages as a combination of CD64+ ± C4d cells, with the C4d+ cells localizing closer the

RISK FACTORS AND PATHOGENESIS

Numerous studies have evaluated the risk factors and associations for the development of rheumatoid nodules. The one clear modifiable risk factor is smoking. In a study of 420 consecutive patients with RA, smoking conferred an odds ratio (OR) of 1.8 (confidence interval [CI], 1.0–2.9) for rheumatoid nodules.[21] Additional studies show that ever smokers had an OR of 7.3 (CI, 2.3–24.6) of developing rheumatoid nodules, with no difference noted between men and women.[22]

The presence of elevated level of serum RF was also an independent risk factor for developing rheumatoid nodules with reported OR of 2.2 to 4.0.[10,21,22] Anti-CCP antibodies were more frequent in rheumatoid patients with nodules.[10] Rheumatoid nodules also seem to be a hallmark of more aggressive disease. Nodular patients with RA showed worsened radiographic progression during a 5-year period compared with their nonnodular counterparts.[10]

Numerous studies in populations of patients with RA have investigated potential genetic associations for rheumatoid nodule development. A meta-analysis of more than 3000 patients did not identify any strong associations but did show a weak association with nodule development in patients with HLA-DRB1.[23] A smaller study identified HLA-DRB1 as a possible associated gene, and HLA-DRB1*0401 homozygotes had worse nodular disease. The number of patients (6) was too small to determine significance of these findings.[21] Although there are scattered reports that there is a male predominance of rheumatoid nodules, a large cohort review of more than 600 patients did not support this theory.[24] This prior observation was likely due to historical higher smoking rates in men, which has equalized over time. Overall, it is unlikely that genetics plays a major role in conferring risk for rheumatoid nodules.

The pathogenesis of the rheumatoid nodule development remains obscure, although there are several hypotheses. Rheumatoid nodules commonly form over extensor surfaces and other sites prone to repetitive trauma.[7] Trauma to small vessels causes an aggregation of inflammatory products, specifically RF complexes, leading to macrophage activation and IL-1 release. This secondary inflammatory reaction then leads to fibrin deposition, subsequent necrosis due to slow cytolytic and enzymatic degradation, and finally containment by surrounding palisading macrophages.[25]

A similar theory implicates RF in the nodule formation process onset. In this case, localized vasculitis results in complement activation. Activated complement components then cause vesiculation of the endothelial cells with accompanying IgM RF deposition, which subsequently leads to accumulation of fibrin deposits. However, it is unclear from this study whether this is a primary or secondary process in rheumatoid nodule formation.[19] Other studies suggest that the nodule is merely a Th1 granuloma,[26] although, if this were the case, these nodules should be amenable to current disease-modifying antirheumatic drug (DMARD)/biologic treatment strategies. A recent study showed that microchimerisms are found in 47% of 33 rheumatoid nodules, suggesting that there could be an allogenic source within rheumatoid nodules stimulating a localized inflammatory response.[27]

Unfortunately, these theories do not explain why only portions of patients with RA develop rheumatoid nodules. In addition, these theories are less convincing in cases of systemic rheumatoid nodule involvement. For instance, in the lung one would expect tissue trauma to occur proximally rather than peripherally near the pleura where these lesions more often occur.

SYSTEMIC LOCATION OF RHEUMATOID NODULES

Rheumatoid nodules rarely occur in the lung or cardiac structures. The radiographic prevalence of pulmonary rheumatoid nodules is less than 1% on radiologic studies[20,22,28] but have been reported at nearly 30% on autopsy specimens.[20] Predisposing risk factors are similar to those of subcutaneous nodules, including smoking and RF positivity.[29] Multiple nodules are more common than single nodules and are predominantly located in middle and superior peripheral lobes. Approximately 50% of these lesions are cavitary (Fig. 3). These cavitary lesions may rupture,

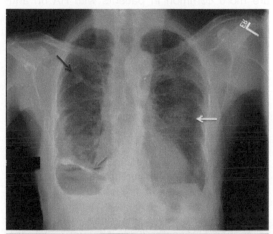

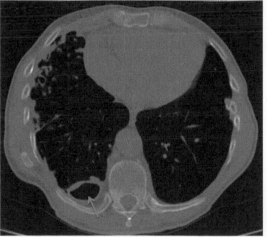

Fig. 3. Pulmonary rheumatoid nodule. Radiograph shows 1.1 cm nodular density with a central lucency in the right upper lobe (*red arrow*), a masslike opacity in the left mid lung (*yellow arrow*), and R sided pneumothorax (*blue arrow*). The corresponding computed tomographic scan shows pulmonary nodules throughout the periphery, some of which are cavitating throughout the periphery as well as the loculated pneumothorax (*blue arrow*). (*Courtesy of Rayford June, MD, Penn State, Hershey, PA.*)

resulting in pneumothoracies, pleural effusions, or hemoptysis.[29] A study of 5 cases highlights the unpredictable nature of pulmonary rheumatoid nodules, which can evolve, regress, or remain unchanged despite lack of any therapeutic changes.[28] They do not seem to trend with clinical disease course, as has been noted with subcutaneous nodules, and can worsen after initiation of anti-TNF therapy[30] (see section Accelerated Nodulosis).

Rheumatoid pulmonary nodules often present a diagnostic challenge to differentiate them from infection or neoplasm, particularly in patients who are exposed to immunosuppressant therapies. Tuberculosis or invasive fungal infections are more common in patients with RA on anti-TNF inhibitor therapy and may mimic cavitary or noncavitary pulmonary rheumatoid nodules. Bronchogenic carcinoma and rheumatoid nodules, sharing risk factors (smoking) and radiographic characteristics, must be differentiated. A case series from 1989 exemplifies this diagnostic dilemma, reporting 7 cases of patients with RA presenting with new pulmonary nodules proved malignant on biopsy.[29] Given these concerns, biopsies are performed at higher rates in pulmonary rheumatoid nodules than in subcutaneous nodules. The histologic findings are similar to subcutaneous nodules with the exception of germinal center–like formations on the periphery in lung nodules reported in a single case study[14] (refer to section Histopathology). Although pulmonary nodules present a more rare extra-articular manifestation of RA, they pose more of a diagnostic dilemma, and the authors recommend a thorough evaluation for infection and malignancy in these cases.

The heart is another important rheumatoid nodule location. There are reports of rheumatoid nodular lesions forming in the pericardium, myocardium, and most notably valves. Although cardiac involvement of RA is high in autopsy case studies (often reported 30% range), clinical manifestations are uncommon (<3% of cases), most frequently pericarditis.[31,32] As with pulmonary lesions, the histopathology of cardiac nodules mimics the description of subcutaneous nodules. It is defined by a central zone of necrosis, surrounded by palisading histiocytes, and an outer layer of inflammatory infiltrate.[32] A study of 37 patients suggests that valvular nodules occur in the following order: mitral 57%, aortic 48%, tricuspid 13%, and pulmonic 11%.[32] Another series of 22 patients with aortic valve lesions found that two-thirds of these patients had concomitant mitral valve nodular involvement and both were associated with subcutaneous nodules (75%).

The most common complication of valvular disease in this study was congestive heart failure, followed by pericarditis.[33] Rheumatoid patients with nodular disease also had a higher degree of valvular abnormalities than their nonnodular counterparts.[31] Consistent with other forms of rheumatoid nodule disease, traditional therapies do not seem to be effective.[34]

There are scattered reports of rheumatoid nodules occurring in the central nervous system. These cases are extremely rare and are often reported in patients with long-standing nodular disease. Sequelae include nerve root and spinal cord compression and leptomeningitis. As with rheumatoid nodules in other systemic locations, these nodules have the same histologic appearance.[35,36] Most reports occurred before 1980, and since the advent of aggressive DMARD and biologics therapy, reported cases are few. The most recent report from 2014 responded to corticosteroid therapy.[37]

RHEUMATOID NODULES IN OTHER DISEASES

With initial descriptions dating back to the 1870s, there are long-standing reports of rheumatoid-like nodules documented in rheumatic fever. However, an early comparative study from 1933 provides an excellent review of these conditions. The nodules were more commonly found at the extensor surface of the knees and elbows, similar to those seen in RA, and were associated with more severe disease, including cardiac complications.[38] This finding was supported by a study that showed that 90.4% of patients with nodules had concomitant carditis.[39] Unlike rheumatoid nodules, they were often short lived with most resolving in several weeks.[38,39] Histologically, these lesions are remarkably similar with areas of central fibrinoid necrosis surrounded by a layer of cellular infiltrates.[38] Later studies suggested that there is less fibrosis, necrosis, and palisading associated with rheumatic fever nodules compared with RA-associated nodules,[40] but it remains unclear if this is due a time-dependent process in nodule development or a difference in pathogenesis. The surrounding macrophages, referred to as Aschoff bodies in rheumatic fever, are similar to the $CD68^+$ macrophages found in RA nodules.[41]

There are case reports of patients with other forms of systemic autoimmune disease developing rheumatoid nodules, but the patients' diagnosis in these cases is often confounded by the lack of specificity in rheumatologic classification criteria. For instance, patients who meet classification criteria for SLE may also meet criteria for

RA and could therefore be considered to have an overlap of both diseases. This problem is exemplified in a small case series reporting 3 patients with rheumatoid nodules who met criteria for both SLE and RA, 2 of whom had elevated levels of RF and CCP antibodies.[42] Additional cases include laryngeal nodules fitting histologic criteria for rheumatoid nodules in a patient later found to have Sjögren syndrome and SLE overlap. RF and CCP status were not reported in this patient.[43] Although there have been reports of rheumatoid nodules in spondyloarthritis, most rheumatologists would argue that the presence of nodules in these cases would suggest that seronegative RA is a more accurate diagnosis.

There have been reviews suggesting that hepatitis C can be associated with rheumatoid nodules. However, in a review of 28 patients with hepatitis C and arthritis, none of the patients had subcutaneous nodules even though many would have met criteria for RA if they had not had underlying hepatitis.[44]

ACCELERATED NODULOSIS

Methotrexate is considered the first-line therapy for moderate or severe RA and is highly effective as monotherapy or in combination with other DMARDs or biologic agents. Although methotrexate is usually well tolerated, methotrexate-induced accelerated nodulosis, characterized by the rapid onset or worsening of rheumatoid nodules in association with methotrexate, has been recognized as a rare side effect. Other DMARDs and biologic agents have also been implicated. A systematic review of accelerated nodulosis from 2002 comprising a total of 58 cases from 3 case series found that 76% of cases had finger involvement.[45] These nodules were clinically and histologically indistinguishable from standard rheumatoid nodules.[45]

A study of 79 patients with RA reported an increased frequency of the HLA-DRB1*0401 allele in patients with accelerated nodulosis. Of affected patients, 71% carried this allele compared with only 17.8% of RA controls without accelerated nodulosis and 17% of healthy controls.[46]

Owing to the lack of clinical trials and a paucity of complete case reports and case series of accelerated nodulosis, no clear treatment recommendations can be made. Common practice is to discontinue methotrexate, and pre–biologic era reports suggest a response to colchicine, hydroxychloroquine, and D-penicillamine.[45,46]

Biologic agents have also been implicated. There is a single case report that accelerated nodulosis occurred after 1 year of infliximab therapy in a patient with excellent control of joint inflammation.[47] Accelerated nodulosis with formation of both subcutaneous and new lung nodules was reported after initiation of etanercept.[48,49] Discontinuation of the etanercept or addition of leflunomide led to regression of lesions. In cases in which isolated pulmonary rheumatoid nodules following long-standing anti-TNF therapy have been reported, it remains unclear whether the nodules reflected uncontrolled disease or a direct effect of the biologic therapy.[30] As with methotrexate-induced accelerated nodulosis, the pathophysiology of anti-TNF therapy–related nodule formation is unknown.

In isolated reports, aromatase inhibitors and azathioprine have been associated with accelerated nodulosis. With the former, a 71-year-old woman with controlled RA developed breast cancer and was administered letrozole, an aromatase inhibitor, and subsequently developed nodulosis, which resolved with discontinuation of the agent.[50] Azathioprine was reported to cause accelerated nodulosis in a patient with active RA; in this instance, the accelerated nodulosis occurred within 1 month of starting therapy.[51]

In most of the described cases, there was improved arthritis control with concomitant worsening of nodularity, suggesting a different mechanism between synovitis and nodule formation. Some studies have postulated that the higher levels of IL-1 and lower levels of TNF produced by nodules than synovia may suggest one of the mechanisms.

RHEUMATOID NODULOSIS

Rheumatoid nodulosis is characterized by the development of rheumatoid nodules in patients without chronic synovitis. This condition was initially described in 1949,[7] and Couret and colleagues[52] established the diagnostic criteria in 1988. The criteria require multiple biopsy proven nodules, recurrent joint symptoms without chronic synovitis or radiographic findings, and no or mild systemic manifestations. A modified criteria presented in 2003 included these criteria, adding positive RF and a poor response to standard treatment.[53] In the 11 cases reported before 1981, all patients were men.[54] Subsequent studies support the observation that men are predominately effected, comprising nearly 82% of all reported cases in the literature.[7,51]

In a review of 16 patients initially diagnosed with rheumatoid nodulosis, 6 went on to develop frank RA. Most (14 of 16) had large subchondral bone cysts, which frequently demonstrated cholesterol crystals within the joint.[53] Although early reports suggested that nonsteroidal anti-inflammatory drugs (NSAIDs) were sufficient for treatment of rheumatoid nodulosis,[54] the condition was successfully controlled in only 5 of 16 patients with NSAID alone and only 1 had complete remission with NSAID therapy. Methotrexate was associated with worsening of nodulosis[53] (see section Accelerated Nodulosis). Therefore, methotrexate should be used with caution in patients with rheumatoid nodulosis.

In children, a benign rheumatoid nodulosis variant, pseudorheumatoid nodules or benign rheumatoid nodules, may occur. Histologically, these skin lesions are similar to rheumatoid nodules but occur in a different distribution, with pretibial, dorsum of the foot, and scalp involvement. They can be large, but there is no systemic disease or positive result on serology,[55] and most regress within 2 years. In a report describing clinical features of 174 prior cases, only 2 developed systemic disease.[56]

TREATMENT OF RHEUMATOID NODULES

During the past 23 to 30 years, advances in RA treatment have led to a remarkable improvement in patient's symptoms, function, outcomes, and quality of life, particularly in patients with moderate to severe disease. Aggressive therapy with DMARDs such as methotrexate, along with biologic agents that specifically target key inflammatory cytokines and pathways, has dramatically changed the prognosis for this patient group. However, there are little data to support the impression that rheumatoid nodules are less prevalent in this era.

Frequently, nodules are asymptomatic, present no major clinical problems, and require no specific therapy. Indications for specific treatment include pain, nerve entrapment, or interference in function. For example, a nodule overlying a bony structure on the plantar surface of the foot may be painful during weight bearing, resulting in altered gait, and lead to pressure ulceration. In this or similar situations, treatment options include direct injection with corticosteroid preparations or surgical excision.

Several small studies demonstrate that local injection of glucocorticoids can reduce the size of rheumatoid nodules.[57,58] A 2006 study of 20 patients showed that triamcinolone injection reduced the size of nodules, with a mean change from 130 to 8 mm in diameter.[57] An older study demonstrated a greater than 50% size reduction in most nodules (75%) injected with methylprednisolone, compared with less than 7% of lesions in the placebo group.[58] In both these small studies, the only adverse event noted was pain,

seen at similar rates in treatment and control groups.[57,58] However, because of concern for infection, recurrence of nodules, and persistent drainage, this procedure is not a common practice.[7]

Surgical excision is generally avoided unless the rheumatoid nodule is causing severe pain, nerve compression, skin ulceration, or recurrent infections. There are few studies noting the efficacy of this treatment. A small study of 3 patients suggests that excision may be effective,[59] but it is commonly noted that nodules can recur in the area of excision.[60] Although data supporting surgical excision of nodules are scarce, in the proper clinical situation it is considered standard practice.

Use of aggressive systemic therapy in RA, including DMARDs and biologic agents, has been proved to reduce joint inflammation and damage and is believed to decrease some of the other extra-articular manifestations as well. However, the effectiveness of systemic therapy for rheumatoid nodules is less clear. In a study of a cohort of patients with RA receiving etanercept, 10 of 87 had a total of 22 nodules. After 180 days of treatment, there were no new nodules but there was also no regression or clearance of previously formed lesions.[61] The lack of new nodules suggests that early aggressive therapy reduces nodule formation thereby lowering prevalence. However, other studies do not support this hypothesis. A small study examined nodule formation during infliximab therapy. Of 5 patients with RA treated with infliximab, all demonstrated clinical improvement in musculoskeletal symptoms. Three patients with pretreatment nodules had no increase in the number of nodules, 1 patient had an increase in the number of nodules, and 1 patient who was without nodules before therapy developed them while receiving infliximab.[62] Nodule histology was similar in the infliximab-treated patients and controls.[62] The increased rheumatoid nodule formation during infliximab therapy noted in this study coincides with numerous reports of onset or worsening pulmonary rheumatoid nodules after initiation of anti-TNF therapy.[30] Holding TNF inhibitor therapy resulted in a 30% reduction in pulmonary nodules.[63] In contrast to TNF inhibitors, B-cell depletion with rituximab has shown potential benefits. At a mean follow-up of 13 months, 10 patients with RA and rheumatoid lung nodules treated with rituximab showed a reduction in the total number and size of nodules, from 26 to 19 and 15 to 9.8 mm, respectively. There is a report of subcutaneous nodulosis after etanercept therapy that responded to rituximab therapy with no

Table 2
Treatment recommendations and level of evidence

Disease	Treatment	Level of Evidence
Rheumatoid nodules	Local steroid injection	B
	Surgical excision	E
Accelerated nodulosis	Stop offending agent, ie, methotrexate or anti-TNF and switch to another agent	C
	Colchicine, hydroxychloroquine	D
	Rituximab (lung nodules only)	D

B, lesser quality RCT or prospective study; C, case-control study or retrospective study; D, case series or case reports; E, expert opinion.

further nodule formation and slow regression of previously formed nodules.[64]

There are isolated case reports of unproven but potentially efficacious nonsystemic therapies. Following failure with treatment with topical corticosteroids, a man with rheumatoid nodulosis had reduction in the size of rheumatoid nodules with topical tacrolimus 0.1% applied twice daily.[65] Another case study suggests that injection of fluorouracil leads to regression of rheumatoid nodules.[66] Controlled clinical trials are necessary to evaluate the efficacy and safety of these therapies.

In summary, local corticosteroid injection remains the best studied therapy for rheumatoid nodules (grade 1B). Surgical excision is rarely indicated except in the specific situations indicated earlier. Without formal clinical trials, the data are insufficient to make other clear treatment recommendations; however, **Table 2** outlines the level of evidence for several of the treatments discussed earlier.

REFERENCES

1. Myasoedova E, Crowson CS, Kremers HM, et al. Is the incidence of rheumatoid arthritis rising? Results from Olmsted County, Minnesota, 1955–2007. Arthritis Rheum 2010;62(6):1576–82.
2. Ndosi M, Lewis M, Hale C, et al. The outcome and cost-effectiveness of nurse-led care in people with rheumatoid arthritis: a multicentre randomised controlled trial. Ann Rheum Dis 2014;73:1975–82.
3. Aletaha D, Neogi T, Silman AJ, et al. 2010 Rheumatoid arthritis classification criteria: an American College of Rheumatology/European League against Rheumatism collaborative initiative. Ann Rheum Dis 2010;69(9):1580–8.
4. Sauerland U, Becker H, Seidel M, et al. Clinical utility of the anti-CCP assay: experiences with 700 patients. Ann N Y Acad Sci 2005;1050:314–8.
5. Niewold TB, Harrison MJ, Paget SA. Anti-CCP antibody testing as a diagnostic and prognostic tool in rheumatoid arthritis. QJM 2007;100(4):193–201.
6. Cojocaru M, Cojocaru IM, Silosi I, et al. Extra-articular manifestations in rheumatoid arthritis. Maedica (Buchar) 2010;5(4):286–91.
7. Sayah A, English JC 3rd. Rheumatoid arthritis: a review of the cutaneous manifestations. J Am Acad Dermatol 2005;53(2):191–209 [quiz: 210–2].
8. Young A, Koduri G. Extra-articular manifestations and complications of rheumatoid arthritis. Best Pract Res Clin Rheumatol 2007;21(5):907–27.
9. Garcia-Patos V. Rheumatoid nodule. Semin Cutan Med Surg 2007;26(2):100–7.
10. Nyhall-Wahlin BM, Turesson C, Jacobsson LT, et al. The presence of rheumatoid nodules at early rheumatoid arthritis diagnosis is a sign of extra-articular disease and predicts radiographic progression of joint destruction over 5 years. Scand J Rheumatol 2011;40(2):81–7.
11. Richman NC, Yazdany J, Graf J, et al. Extraarticular manifestations of rheumatoid arthritis in a multiethnic cohort of predominantly Hispanic and Asian patients. Medicine (Baltimore) 2013;92(2):92–7.
12. Kaye BR, Kaye RL, Bobrove A. Rheumatoid nodules. Review of the spectrum of associated conditions and proposal of a new classification, with a report of four seronegative cases. Am J Med 1984;76(2):279–92.
13. Turesson C, McClelland RL, Christianson T, et al. Clustering of extraarticular manifestations in patients with rheumatoid arthritis. J Rheumatol 2008;35(1):179–80.
14. Highton J, Hung N, Hessian P, et al. Pulmonary rheumatoid nodules demonstrating features usually associated with rheumatoid synovial membrane. Rheumatology (Oxford) 2007;46(5):811–4.
15. Hedfors E, Klareskog L, Lindblad S, et al. Phenotypic characterization of cells within subcutaneous rheumatoid nodules. Arthritis Rheum 1983;26(11):1333–9.
16. Miyasaka N, Sato K, Yamamoto K, et al. Immunological and immunohistochemical analysis of rheumatoid nodules. Ann Rheum Dis 1989;48(3):220–6.
17. Knoess M, Krukemeyer MG, Kriegsmann J, et al. Co-localization of C4d deposits/CD68+ macrophages in rheumatoid nodule and granuloma annulare: immunohistochemical evidence of a complement-mediated mechanism in fibrinoid necrosis. Pathol Res Pract 2008;204(6):373–8.
18. Stamp LK, Easson A, Lehnigk U, et al. Different T cell subsets in the nodule and synovial membrane: absence of interleukin-17A in rheumatoid nodules. Arthritis Rheum 2008;58(6):1601–8.

19. Kato H, Yamakawa M, Ogino T. Complement mediated vascular endothelial injury in rheumatoid nodules: a histopathological and immunohistochemical study. J Rheumatol 2000;27(8):1839–47.

20. Kitamura A, Matsuno T, Narita M, et al. Rheumatoid arthritis with diffuse pulmonary rheumatoid nodules. Pathol Int 2004;54(10):798–802.

21. Mattey DL, Dawes PT, Fisher J, et al. Nodular disease in rheumatoid arthritis: association with cigarette smoking and HLA-DRB1/TNF gene interaction. J Rheumatol 2002;29(11):2313–8.

22. Shannon TM, Gale ME. Noncardiac manifestations of rheumatoid arthritis in the thorax. J Thorac Imaging 1992;7(2):19–29.

23. Gorman JD, David-Vaudey E, Pai M, et al. Lack of association of the HLA-DRB1 shared epitope with rheumatoid nodules: an individual patient data meta-analysis of 3,272 Caucasian patients with rheumatoid arthritis. Arthritis Rheum 2004;50(3):753–62.

24. Turesson C, O'Fallon WM, Crowson CS, et al. Extraarticular disease manifestations in rheumatoid arthritis: incidence trends and risk factors over 46 years. Ann Rheum Dis 2003;62(8):722–7.

25. Ziff M. The rheumatoid nodule. Arthritis Rheum 1990;33(6):761–7.

26. Hessian PA, Highton J, Kean A, et al. Cytokine profile of the rheumatoid nodule suggests that it is a Th1 granuloma. Arthritis Rheum 2003;48(2):334–8.

27. Chan WF, Atkins CJ, Naysmith D, et al. Microchimerism in the rheumatoid nodules of patients with rheumatoid arthritis. Arthritis Rheum 2012;64(2):380–8.

28. Gomez Herrero H, Arraiza Sarasa M, Rubio Marco I, et al. Pulmonary rheumatoid nodules: presentation, methods, diagnosis and progression in reference to 5 cases. Reumatol Clin 2012;8(4):212–5.

29. Jolles H, Moseley PL, Peterson MW. Nodular pulmonary opacities in patients with rheumatoid arthritis. A diagnostic dilemma. Chest 1989;96(5):1022–5.

30. Toussirot E, Berthelot JM, Pertuiset E, et al. Pulmonary nodulosis and aseptic granulomatous lung disease occurring in patients with rheumatoid arthritis receiving tumor necrosis factor-alpha-blocking agent: a case series. J Rheumatol 2009;36(11):2421–7.

31. Kitas G, Banks MJ, Bacon PA. Cardiac involvement in rheumatoid disease. Clin Med 2001;1(1):18–21.

32. Chand EM, Freant LJ, Rubin JW. Aortic valve rheumatoid nodules producing clinical aortic regurgitation and a review of the literature. Cardiovasc Pathol 1999;8(6):333–8.

33. Iveson JM, Thadani U, Ionescu M, et al. Aortic valve incompetence and replacement in rheumatoid arthritis. Ann Rheum Dis 1975;34(4):312–20.

34. Anaya JM. Severe rheumatoid valvular heart disease. Clin Rheumatol 2006;25(5):743–5.

35. Bathon JM, Moreland LW, DiBartolomeo AG. Inflammatory central nervous system involvement in rheumatoid arthritis. Semin Arthritis Rheum 1989;18(4):258–66.

36. Jackson CG, Chess RL, Ward JR. A case of rheumatoid nodule formation within the central nervous system and review of the literature. J Rheumatol 1984;11(2):237–40.

37. Takahashi M, Yamamoto J, Idei M, et al. Multiple intracranial nodules associated with rheumatoid arthritis: case report. Neurol Med Chir (Tokyo) 2014;54(4):317–20.

38. Dawson MH. A comparative study of subcutaneous nodules in rheumatic fever and rheumatoid arthritis. J Exp Med 1933;57(5):845–58.

39. Behera M. Subcutaneous nodules in acute rheumatic fever–an analysis of age old dictums. Indian Heart J 1993;45(6):463–7.

40. Bywaters EG, Glynn LE, Zeldis A. Subcutaneous nodules of Still's disease. Ann Rheum Dis 1958;17(3):278–85.

41. Chopra P, Ray R. Recent trends in cardiac pathology. In: Deodhar K, editor. Recent advances in pathology. New Delhi (India): Jaypee Brothers Medical Publishers; 2002. p. 98.

42. Rothfield NF, Lim AA. Systemic lupus erythematosus evolving into rheumatoid arthritis. J Rheumatol 2006;33(1):188–90.

43. Schwartz IS, Grishman E. Rheumatoid nodules of the vocal cords as the initial manifestation of systemic lupus erythematosus. JAMA 1980;244(24):2751–2.

44. Zuckerman E, Keren D, Rozenbaum M, et al. Hepatitis C virus-related arthritis: characteristics and response to therapy with interferon alpha. Clin Exp Rheumatol 2000;18(5):579–84.

45. Patatanian E, Thompson DF. A review of methotrexate-induced accelerated nodulosis. Pharmacotherapy 2002;22(9):1157–62.

46. Ahmed SS, Arnett FC, Smith CA, et al. The HLA-DRB1*0401 allele and the development of methotrexate-induced accelerated rheumatoid nodulosis: a follow-up study of 79 Caucasian patients with rheumatoid arthritis. Medicine (Baltimore) 2001;80(4):271–8.

47. Mackley CL, Ostrov BE, Ioffreda MD. Accelerated cutaneous nodulosis during infliximab therapy in a patient with rheumatoid arthritis. J Clin Rheumatol 2004;10(6):336–8.

48. Cunnane G, Warnock M, Fye KH, et al. Accelerated nodulosis and vasculitis following etanercept therapy for rheumatoid arthritis. Arthritis Rheum 2002;47(4):445–9.

49. Kekow J, Welte T, Kellner U, et al. Development of rheumatoid nodules during anti-tumor necrosis factor alpha therapy with etanercept. Arthritis Rheum 2002;46(3):843–4.

50. Chao J, Parker BA, Zvaifler NJ. Accelerated cutaneous nodulosis associated with aromatase inhibitor

therapy in a patient with rheumatoid arthritis. J Rheumatol 2009;36(5):1087–8.

51. Langevitz P, Maguire L, Urowitz M. Accelerated nodulosis during azathioprine therapy. Arthritis Rheum 1991;34(1):123–4.

52. Couret M, Combe B, Chuong VT, et al. Rheumatoid nodulosis: report of two new cases and discussion of diagnostic criteria. J Rheumatol 1988;15(9): 1427–30.

53. Maldonado I, Eid H, Rodriguez GR, et al. Rheumatoid nodulosis: is it a different subset of rheumatoid arthritis? J Clin Rheumatol 2003;9(5):296–305.

54. Wisnieski JJ, Askari AD. Rheumatoid nodulosis. A relatively benign rheumatoid variant. Arch Intern Med 1981;141(5):615–9.

55. Simons FE, Schaller JG. Benign rheumatoid nodules. Pediatrics 1975;56(1):29–33.

56. Rush PJ, Bernstein BH, Smith CR, et al. Chronic arthritis following benign rheumatoid nodules of childhood. Arthritis Rheum 1985;28(10):1175–8.

57. Baan H, Haagsma CJ, van de Laar MA. Corticosteroid injections reduce size of rheumatoid nodules. Clin Rheumatol 2006;25(1):21–3.

58. Ching DW, Petrie JP, Klemp P, et al. Injection therapy of superficial rheumatoid nodules. Br J Rheumatol 1992;31(11):775–7.

59. Arnold C. The management of rheumatoid nodules. Am J Orthop (Belle Mead NJ) 1996;25(10):706–8.

60. Hasham S, Burke FD. Diagnosis and treatment of swellings in the hand. Postgrad Med J 2007; 83(979):296–300.

61. Kaiser M, Bozonnat M, Jorgensen C, et al. Effect of etanercept on tenosynovitis and nodules in rheumatoid arthritis. Arthritis Rheum 2002;46(2):559–60.

62. Baeten D, De Keyser F, Veys EM, et al. Tumour necrosis factor alpha independent disease mechanisms in rheumatoid arthritis: a histopathological study on the effect of infliximab on rheumatoid nodules. Ann Rheum Dis 2004;63(5):489–93.

63. Glace B, Gottenberg JE, Mariette X, et al. Efficacy of rituximab in the treatment of pulmonary rheumatoid nodules: findings in 10 patients from the French AutoImmunity and Rituximab/Rheumatoid Arthritis registry (AIR/PR registry). Ann Rheum Dis 2012; 71(8):1429–31.

64. Sautner J, Rintelen B, Leeb BF. Rituximab as effective treatment in a case of severe subcutaneous nodulosis in rheumatoid arthritis. Rheumatology (Oxford) 2013;52(8):1535–7.

65. Garrido-Rios A, Sánchez-Velicia L, Sanz-Muñoz C, et al. Rheumatoid nodulosis: successful response to topical tacrolimus. Clin Rheumatol 2009;28(11): 1341–2.

66. Amini S, Baum B, Weiss E. A novel treatment for rheumatoid nodules (RN) with intralesional fluorouracil. Int J Dermatol 2009;48:4.

Reactive Granulomatous Dermatitis

A Review of Palisaded Neutrophilic and Granulomatous Dermatitis, Interstitial Granulomatous Dermatitis, Interstitial Granulomatous Drug Reaction, and a Proposed Reclassification

Misha Rosenbach, MD[a],*, Joseph C. English III, MD[b]

KEYWORDS

- Interstitial granulomatous dermatitis • Palisaded neutrophilic and granulomatous dermatitis
- Reactive granulomatous dermatitis • Interstitial granulomatous drug reaction
- Granuloma annulare • Granulomatous dermatitis • Granulomatous drug reaction

KEY POINTS

- Palisaded neutrophilic and granulomatous dermatitis, interstitial granulomatous dermatitis, and interstitial granulomatous drug reaction represent cutaneous reaction patterns that occur in the setting of a systemic trigger.
- Systemic triggers include connective tissue diseases (lupus, vasculitis, other), arthritides (rheumatoid arthritis, other inflammatory and reactive arthritides), malignancy (hematologic more often than solid organ), and medications.
- We suggest the unifying term "reactive granulomatous dermatitis" to encompass these entities, guide clinical management, and coordinate scientific literature regarding this group of reactive skin diseases.

INTRODUCTION

In this article, we review a number of reactive granulomatous processes. Patients may present with a cutaneous granulomatous eruptions in response to medications, autoimmune disease, arthritides, and internal malignancies. There is a wide spectrum of clinical morphologic patterns, and a broad array of histologic subtypes that may occur. We will review palisaded neutrophilic and granulomatous dermatitis (PNGD), interstitial granulomatous dermatitis (IGD), and interstitial granulomatous drug reaction (IGDR), with a focus on the potential distinctions between these entities, and the areas of overlap.[1] We attempt a clear and concise review of each entity, associated diseases or medications, systemic evaluation, and management. Finally, in an attempt to clarify some of the

Conflict of interest: No relevant conflicts.

[a] Department of Dermatology, Perelman School of Medicine, University of Pennsylvania, Philadelphia, PA, USA; [b] University of Pittsburgh, Department of Dermatology, UPMC North Hills Dermatology, Wexford, PA, USA

* Corresponding author.

E-mail address: Misha.rosenbach@uphs.upenn.edu

derm.theclinics.com

confusion surrounding these cutaneous reaction patterns, we propose a new, unifying term: reactive granulomatous dermatitis (RGD).

PALISADED NEUTROPHILIC AND GRANULOMATOUS DERMATITIS

Palisaded neutrophilic and granulomatous dermatitis is a term originally coined by Chu and colleagues in 1994[2] to encompass a cutaneous reaction pattern seen in association with a number of systemic diseases. These authors described characteristic symmetric skin colored to erythematous smooth, umbilicated, or crusted papules primarily on the elbows and extremities with a spectrum of histologic findings ranging from frank leukocytoclastic vasculitis to dense neutrophilic infiltrates and scattered areas of collagen degeneration to sparse palisades of histiocytes and small granulomas to histiocytes around dermal fibrosis.[2] Previous terms for this entity include Churg–Strauss granuloma, cutaneous extravascular necrotizing granuloma, rheumatoid papules, and Winkelmann granuloma; some authors include IGD within this entity. In 1983, Finan and Winkelmann[3] performed a thorough review of the literature describing cases of Churg–Strauss granuloma and systemic disease associations, and in 1990 Finan[4] suggested this entity further encompassed that which had been termed "rheumatoid papules," which later were all grouped by Chu and colleagues under the umbrella of PNGD. The complex, evolving nomenclature and expanding clinical spectrum of this disease is a source of confusion to both clinicians and readers of the scientific literature.

Etiopathogenesis

The etiology of this disease is unknown. PNGD rarely occurs in the absence of a systemic disease,[5] and many feel it represents a cutaneous reaction pattern owing to underlying internal inflammation. Theories as to the etiopathogenesis of PNGD include abnormal neutrophil activation, circulating immune complex deposition,[3,5] a delayed-type hypersensitivity reaction,[6] or a low-grade small vessel vasculitis.[3,7] Because a subset of PNGD demonstrates features of vasculitis, and many of the associated diseases can affect the vasculature, some feel PNGD may begin as a leukocytoclastic vasculitis[2,5] and then progress through stages of collagen degradation[5] and chronic inflammation and fibrosis, leading to the spectrum of clinical and histologic features reported.[2]

Clinical and Histologic Presentation

Patients of all ages may develop PNGD, although reports in childhood are rare.[8–10] Women are affected more frequently (approximately 3:1 ratio), likely owing to the systemic diseases associated with PNGD.[8] The classic clinical presentation of PNGD is that of flesh-colored to erythematous papules, which may be umbilicated or crusted, appearing symmetrically on the extremities particularly around the elbows (**Fig. 1**).[2,3,8,9] Over time, the clinical spectrum of PNGD has continued to expand, with numerous recent reports describing multiple morphologic lesion types diagnosed as PNGD by histology. There exist reports of urticarial plaques,[11] erythematous nodules[11,12] with scale,[12,13] papulonodules,[14] pink-to-red papules and plaques,[15] erythematous edematous plaques,[12,14,16] violaceous patches and plaques,[17] annular papules and plaques,[11,18–20] annular gyrate plaques[21] and even linear bands,[8,11] with lesion locations reported to extend beyond the classic elbows and hands to include the legs,[6] nose,[22] cheek, and scalp.[8] A review of the reported distribution of lesions in PNGD noted that 51% of cases involve the upper extremities and 27% the lower extremities; trunk, head, and neck lesions are reported less commonly (21%).[8] Some authors suggest that the clinical spectrum reported may represent lesions of the same process seen at different stages of temporal evolution.[2,11]

The histologic findings of PNGD may be varied, possibly depending on the lesion's age or associated underlying disease.[2] Early lesions may display intense neutrophilic inflammation, karyorrhectic debris, and frank leukocytoclastic vasculitis (10%–30%; **Fig. 2**).[3,5,11,23,24] There are typically more neutrophils, nuclear dust, and fibrinoid

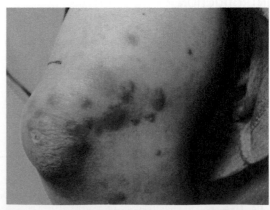

Fig. 1. Palisaded and neutrophilic granulomatous dermatitis, clinical. Classic presentation of erythematous papules around the elbows, some with slight umbilication and central crusting.

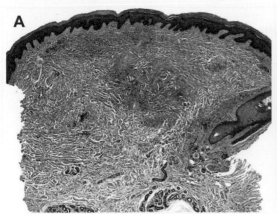
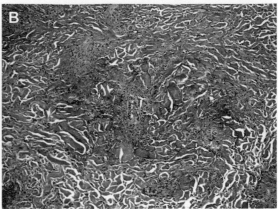

Fig. 2. Palisaded and neutrophilic granulomatous dermatitis, histopathology. Histologic specimen demonstrating perivascular and interstitial neutrophilic inflammation and karyorrhexis (A; stain: hematoxylin and eosin; original magnification, ×40) and altered collagen with surrounding palisaded granulomas (B; stain: hematoxylin and eosin; original magnification, ×100). (*Courtesy of* Dr. Adam Rubin, MD.)

change than in pure vasculitis. As the lesions evolve, there are piecemeal areas of collagen degeneration and palisades of histiocytes and small granulomas, eventually accompanied by areas of fibrosis.[2,11] The presence of vasculitis is felt to distinguish PNGD from IGD (see below). Granuloma annulare generally contains more mucin and less intense neutrophilic infiltrate and nuclear debris.

Systemic Associations

Palisaded neutrophilic and granulomatous dermatitis is reported rarely in the absence of an underlying systemic disease. The diseases most commonly reported with PNGD include connective tissue diseases—particularly systemic lupus erythematosus—as well as inflammatory arthritis, hematologic disorders, and rarely infections or medications (**Table 1**). Most case reports of medication-induced PNGD have occurred in the setting of medications used to treat diseases previously reported to occur with PNGD, such as tumor necrosis factor inhibitors for rheumatoid arthritis[17,21,22] and allopurinol in a patient with quiescent chronic myelogenous leukemia.[15]

Evaluation and Management

Patients with PNGD should be evaluated for underlying internal systemic diseases. All patients warrant serologic testing, including antinuclear antibody, antineutrophilic cytoplasmic antibodies, rheumatoid factor, cyclic citrullinated peptide, complete blood count with differential, chest radiography, and consideration should be given to checking for paraproteinemias in select cases. Individual patients may warrant extended, targeted workup depending on their other systemic manifestations including potential evaluation for

occult infections or medication-induced disease. The differential diagnosis often includes other reactive skin findings, such as small vessel vasculitis, neutrophilic dermatoses, granuloma annulare, and IGD. In cases where those entities cannot be excluded confidently, a broader systemic workup may be indicated, including in particular urinalysis, complement levels, and thorough workup for extracutaneous vasculitis in cases of potential leukocytoclastic vasculitis.

Approximately 20% of cases may resolve spontaneously, sometimes as quickly as in 1 week.[8] The main principle of PNGD management is to identify the underlying disease and target therapy to control that disorder. Most treatments reported in the literature are aimed at controlling the underlying systemic disease (nonsteroidal antiinflammatory drugs, colchicine, hydroxychloroquine, methotrexate, cyclosporine, cyclophosphamide, systemic corticosteroids, etanercept, infliximab),[6,25] and are likely too potent to use if treating PNGD alone. PNGD-specific treatments include intralesional kenalog,[13,26] dapsone,[12,26–29] and systemic corticosteroids.[8] Topical medications are not effective generally, although rare reports note improvement.[22]

Summary

Classic PNGD consists of symmetric erythematous papules on the extremities and histology that includes neutrophilic inflammation with possible frank vasculitis, cellular debris, altered collagen, and variable palisaded histiocytes and granulomas. It is seen in the setting of systemic diseases, such as connective tissue diseases, inflammatory arthritis, hematologic disorders, and rarely with infections or medications.

Table 1
Diseases reported in association with palisaded neutrophilic and granulomatous dermatitis (PNGD)

Disease	Strength of Association
Connective tissue disease	+++
Systemic lupus erythematosus[3,20,76,81]	
Limited systemic sclerosis[8]	
Undifferentiated connective tissue disease[23]	
ANCA-associated vasculitis[3,9]	
Erythema elevatum diutinum[14]	
Sjögren's syndrome[8]	
Mixed cryoglobulinemia[8]	
Takayasu's aortitis[82]	
Arthritides	++
Rheumatoid arthritis[3,11,14,17,22,23]	
Ankylosing spondylitis[83]	
Lymphoproliferative disease	++
Acute myelogenous leukemia,[3] multiple myeloma,[3] lymphoma[3,84]	
Other	+
Sarcoidosis[18,19,25]	
Ulcerative colitis[3,12]	
Celiac disease and type I diabetes[85]	
Behçet's[6]	
Multiple sclerosis[8]	
Cellulitis (in patient with SLE), subacute bacterial endocarditis,[3] hepatitis,[3] streptococcal infection,[3,86] AIDS[87]	
Medications	+
TNF inhibitors,[17,21,22] allopurinol[15]	

Abbreviations: ANCA, antineutrophilic cytoplasmic antibodies; SLE, systemic lupus erythematosus; TNF, tumor necrosis factor.

INTERSTITIAL GRANULOMATOUS DERMATITIS

The first use of the term IGD is attributed to Ackerman in 1993.[30] Over the years, IGD has alternately been referred to as IGD with arthritis, IGD with cords and arthritis,[31] linear subcutaneous bands of rheumatoid arthritis,[32] linear rheumatoid nodules,[33] linear granuloma annulare,[34] railway track dermatitis,[35] and Ackerman syndrome.[36,37] The initial descriptions were of patients with inflammatory arthritis and a pathognomonic linear band on the upper trunk, which was firm, palpable, and generally asymptomatic. The histologic findings include variably dense interstitial histiocytes often surrounding foci of abnormal collagen leading to "clefting" away of the altered collagen and histiocyte section, termed the "floating sign."[38] As with PNGD, the clinical (and to a lesser extent the histologic) spectrum of IGD has expanded, and coupled with the complex, evolving nomenclature and confusion over whether IGD represents a distinct entity or a subset of PNGD, has proven a source of confusion to both clinicians and readers of the scientific literature.

Etiopathogenesis

The etiopathogenesis of IGD is poorly understood. Because almost all cases are associated with an underlying inflammatory condition, IGD has been interpreted as a nonspecific sign of immune dysfunction.[39] A true understanding of the pathophysiology of IGD is complicated by many authors referring to the overlap between IGD and PNGD, and declaring that IGD is likely a disease that begins as a cutaneous reaction to some form of vascular injury or immune complex deposition, as with PNGD. Most authors relay that the theory is that immune complexes in dermal vessels leads to inflammation, damaged collagen, and a resultant granulomatous infiltrate.[40]

Clinical and Histologic Presentation

IGD has been reported in children[10,41] and adults of all ages, although it is less common in the pediatric age group.[42] Similar to PNGD, there is a 3:1 female to male predominance,[38] again likely owing to the association with underlying autoimmune diseases. The initial description of IGD was that of linear subcutaneous cords or bands on the proximal trunk,[32] although over time the clinical morphologic spectrum has expanded and many feel that other presentations are in fact more common with cords reported in less than 10% of cases.[38] Beyond the ropelike, linear cord lesions,[32,43] erythematous to violaceous patches or plaques symmetrically on the upper trunk and proximal limbs are a frequent manifestation (**Fig. 3**).[38] Other clinical morphologies reported include small skin colored papules,[38,44] papules and plaques,[45] diffuse macular erythema,[38] annular plaques,[40,45–47] polycyclic indurated plaques,[37] "cockades" of color with violaceous centers surrounded by erythema,[39] annular scaly plaques,[48] subcutaneous nodules,[31,46] large atrophic hyperpigmented plaques,[49] disseminated indurated violaceous plaques and papules,[50] periungual and mucosal erythema,[51] and even elbow papules and nodules similar to those of PNGD.[52] The skin lesions are generally symmetric on the lateral upper trunk and proximal inner arms and proximal thighs (although reports exist of lesions on the buttocks, abdomen, breast, and umbilicus[53]), and are usually asymptomatic.

The histology of IGD is characterized by histiocytes scattered throughout the dermis in varying densities, frequently arranged around foci of degenerated collagen (**Fig. 4**). The inflammatory infiltrate is composed of CD68$^+$ epithelioid histiocytes in the majority of cases.[38] The histiocytes may form small granulomas, and often clusters of histiocytes can rim abnormal collagen and lead to visible clefting, which has been termed the "floating sign," reported in two-thirds of cases.[38] Although rare, eosinophils and neutrophils may be seen,[54] and vasculitis is generally absent in IGD (1 case reported vasculitis, albeit with no histologic image,[36] with more than 35 other reports lacking vasculitis).[38,54] Lymphocytes abutting the epidermis with basal vacuolization are rare, and could represent a distinguishing feature of IGDR differentiating that from pure IGD. Mucin deposition is generally minimal to absent.[38] Beyond the absence of mucin, the infiltrate tends to be more diffuse and include the deeper dermis, helping to distinguish IGD from interstitial granuloma annulare.[30,38] Altered elastic fibers have been seen, and 1 case of IGD resolved with features acquired cutis laxa.[55]

Systemic Associations

IGD is generally seen in the setting of an underlying systemic disease, similar to PNGD (**Table 2**). The diseases most commonly reported with IGD are inflammatory arthritides, particularly rheumatoid arthritis, along with connective tissue diseases, such as systemic lupus erythematosus, and malignancies. IGD has been reported in the setting of both hematologic disorders and solid organ internal malignancies. Beyond those common associations, IGD has been reported to occur with a variety of other diseases, including rarely infections (*Borrelia burgdorferi* and pulmonary coccidioidomycosis in particular).

Drug-induced IGD has been reported in association with a number of medications. There exists substantial confusion in the literature between drug-induced IGD, and IGDR. Most lists of medications reported in association with IGD[39,44,49,56] actually refer to papers describing cases of IGDR. A number of reports of drug-induced IGD include histologic descriptions with mucin[57] (more consistent with granuloma annulare) or interface dermatitis and dermal eosinophils[58] (more consistent with IGDR). This potential confusion is appropriately highlighted by Perrin and colleagues[59] in their article entitled "Interstitial granulomatous drug reaction with a

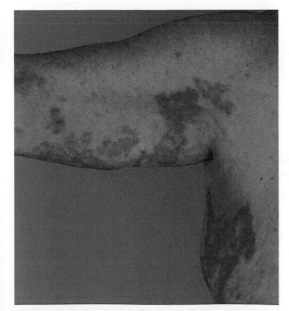

Fig. 3. Interstitial granulomatous dermatitis, clinical. Erythematous annular patches with slightly indurated borders symmetrically on the trunk and inner proximal extremity.

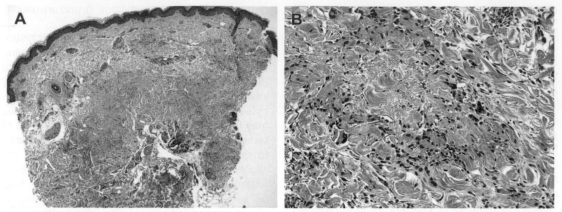

Fig. 4. Interstitial granulomatous dermatitis, histopathology. Histologic specimen demonstrating diffuse interstitial histiocytes (*A*; stain: hematoxylin and eosin; original magnification, ×40) and areas of piecemeal collagen alteration with surrounding histiocytes and small granulomas with areas clefting (*B*; stain: hematoxylin and eosin; original magnification, ×100).

histologic pattern of interstitial granulomatous dermatitis." These authors reported 3 cases of true drug-induced IGD, one owing to candesartan, fluindione, or furosemide, the second owing to enalapril, and the third owing to furosemide.[59] There are rare reports consistent with true IGD with apparent drug associations, particularly with tumor necrosis factor inhibitors[60]; another case noted IGD owing to soy.[56]

Interstitial granulomatous drug reaction

The entity "interstitial granulomatous drug reaction (IGDR)" deserves separate discussion, because some authors view IGDR as a separate and distinct entity from drug-induced forms of IGD. Many publications, however, use the term "interstitial granulomatous drug reaction" in describing cases of "drug-induced IGD," although the reports often lack the key, defining features attributed to true IGDR.

Table 2
Diseases reported in association with interstitial granulomatous dermatitis (IGD)

Disease	Strength of Association
Connective tissue disease	++
SLE[36,39,40,88,89]	
Undifferentiated connective tissue disease[37]	
Inflammatory arthritides	+++
Rheumatoid arthritis[38,40,43,47,50,73,90]	
Seronegative arthritis[38,49,55,70,91,92]	
Hematologic disorders	++
IgA gammopathy,[38] anemia and thrombocytopenia,[38,40] lymphoma,[38,93,94] myelodysplastic syndrome,[95] myelodysplasia with leukemic progression,[96] leukemia[97]	
Solid organ malignancies	+
Breast,[38,46] endometrial,[38] lung,[98] esophageal[99]	
Other	+
Autoimmune hepatitis,[52] uveitis,[42] chronic inflammatory demyelinating polyneuropathy,[48] autoimmune thyroiditis,[40,100,101] antiphospholipid antibody syndrome,[102] diabetes,[40] vitiligo,[40] pulmonary coccidiodomycosis,[103] pulmonary silicosis,[104] *Borrelia burgdorferi* infection[105]	
Medications[a]	+
TNF inhibitors,[60] soy,[56] angiotensin converting enzyme inhibitors,[59] furosemide[59]	

Abbreviations: IgA, immunoglobulin A; SLE, systemic lupus erythematosus; TNF, tumor necrosis factor.
  [a] Because some authors do not draw a distinction between IGD and IGDR, identifying pure cases of drug-induced IGD is challenging. This list includes only those medications with publications documenting histology consistent with IGD and a triggering medication.

IGDR was first described by Magro and colleagues[61] in 1998. They reported 20 patients with erythematous to violaceous plaques, often annular, concentrated on the inner arms, proximal medial thighs, proximal trunk, and intertriginous sites, with distinctive histologic features (**Fig. 5**). The key histologic features of IGDR include diffuse interstitial histiocytes with granulomas including rare giant cells, surrounding piecemeal fragmentation of collagen, similar to IGD. Mucin was scant and vasculitis absent, similar to IGD. Magro and colleagues[61] further noted that cases of IGDR should include an interface dermatitis with basal vacuolar degeneration and areas of dyskeratotic keratinocytes and prominent tissue eosinophilia (**Fig. 6**); lymphoid atypia was noted in many cases with large cells with hyperchromatic nuclei and occasional convoluted nuclear contours. These 3 histologic features were felt to distinguish the entity IGDR from IGD owing to medications. In this initial description, calcium channel blockers, β-blockers, lipid-lowering agents, and angiotensin-converting enzyme inhibitors were the most common offending agents.[61]

Since the initial description of IGDR, a number of reports have described cases of "IGDR" with a growing list of offending agents implicated in inducing this reaction, with an expanded spectrum of clinical manifestations (isolated plaque,[62,63] erythroderma,[64] scalp involvement,[58] cheeks and extensor forearms,[65] subcutaneous nodules on the palms and soles,[66] erythema nodosum-like lesions,[67] and more). Unfortunately, many publications use the term "IGDR" when referring to "drug-induced IGD," where a medication is implicated in inducing classic findings of IGD, but lacking the histologic features described by Magro and colleagues as characteristic of IGDR. Some authors have continued to draw distinctions between the 2 entities, and the lack of consensus has led to

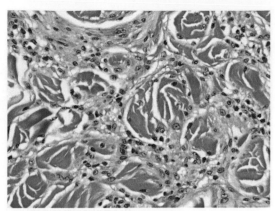

Fig. 6. Interstitial granulomatous drug reaction, histopathology. Histologic specimen demonstrating diffuse interstitial histiocytes and prominent eosinophils, with rare lymphoid atypia and areas of piecemeal collagen alteration with surrounding histiocytes and small granulomas (stain: hematoxylin and eosin; original magnification, ×400). Basal vacuolar degeneration with a mild interface reaction is another classic feature (not shown). (*Courtesy of* Dr. Andras Schaffer, MD, PhD.)

confusion in the medical literature. **Table 3** lists medications that have been reported to induce IGD or IGDR. If the publication included a histologic description consistent with true IGDR, it is classified as IGDR; if the publication reported a reaction as IGDR but it lacked features of IGDR as described by Magro and colleagues,[61] it is classified as IGD; if the publication reported partial features of IGDR, it was classified as borderline/indeterminate. In some cases, numerous medications were potential culprits; **Table 3** lists medications that were associated temporally with the rash and, when discontinued, were associated with resolution (some but not all were exposed to rechallenge and led to recurrence of the eruption). There are reports of interstitial granulomatous T-cell dyscrasia[68] and cases of severe systemic drug reactions (drug reaction with eosinophilia and systemic symptoms[69]), which may show similar features; whether these share a similar pathophysiology and should be considered within this entity is a matter of debate.

Given the extensive confusion and overlap, and the fact that ultimately patients with either drug-induced IGD or IGDR require a thorough evaluation of potential triggering medications and a trial of medication cessation, we feel that practicing clinicians and the scientific community may be better served by grouping these entities together as drug-induced forms of a RGD.

Evaluation and Management

Patients with IGD should be evaluated for underlying internal systemic diseases. There is a strong

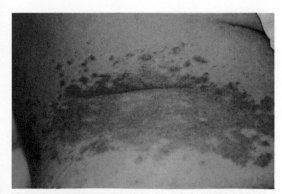

Fig. 5. Interstitial granulomatous drug reaction, clinical. A large erythematous-to-violaceous roughly annular thin plaque shown here on the waist; lesions are generally symmetric.

Table 3
Medications associated with interstitial granulomatous drug reaction (IGDR) or drug-induced interstitial granulomatous dermatitis (IGD)

Reaction	Drug
Interstitial granulomatous drug reaction	Calcium channel blockers[61]
	β-Blockers[61]
	ACE inhibitors[61,63,64]
	Lipid-lowering agents (gemfibrozil, statin medications)[61]
	Brompheniramine[61]
	Ranitidine[61]
	Bupropion[61]
	Furosemide[61]
	Sennoside[106]
	Chinese herbal medication[62]
	Trastuzumab[58]
	Thalidomide[65]
	Allopurinol[69]
Drug-induced interstitial granulomatous dermatitis	TNF inhibitors[60]
	Soy[56]
	ACE inhibitors[59]
	Furosemide[59]
Borderline/ indeterminate	Atorvastatin[107]
	Sorafenib[108]
	Anakinra[109]
	Adalimumab[110]
	Ganciclovir[66]
	Chinese herbal medication[67]
	Febuxostat[111]
	Strontium ranelate[112]

If publication included histologic description consistent with true IGDR, classified as IGDR; if publication reported a reaction as IGDR but it lacked features of IGDR as described by Magro and colleagues,[61] classified as IGD; if publication reported partial features of IGDR, classified as borderline/indeterminate.

Abbreviations: ACE inhibitor, angiotensin converting enzyme inhibitor; TNF, tumor necrosis factor.

association with inflammatory arthritis, and patients should be evaluated thoroughly for potential joint disease with physical examination, history, serologic testing (rheumatoid factor, cyclic citrullinated peptide), and possibly joint imaging or rheumatology referral. Given the spectrum of disease associations reported, all patients warrant further serologic testing, including antinuclear antibody, antineutrophilic cytoplasmic antibodies, complete blood count with differential, chest radiography, serum and urine protein electrophoresis and immunofixation for paraproteinemias in most cases. IGD has been reported in connection with solid organ malignancies as well, and all patients warrant age-appropriate malignancy screening. Individual patients may warrant extended, targeted workup depending on their other systemic manifestations, including potential evaluation for occult infections or medication-induced disease. Given the rare reports of infections associated with IGD, appropriate serologic testing may be indicated. All patients with IGD should undergo a thorough evaluation for potential medication triggers, and if features of IGDR are present (tissue eosinophils, interface dermatitis with basal vacuolar alteration, or lymphoid atypia), this possibility should be explored thoroughly, including trials of medication cessation. Drug-induced forms of granulomatous dermatitis may be slow to develop, and when the implicated agents are stopped, may take weeks to months to resolve.[61]

IGD may self-resolve without treatment.[38,70] Given the more numerous reports of drug-induced forms, a thorough medication review and drug cessation trial is often indicated. If no medication culprit is found, similar to PNGD, the guiding principle of IGD management is to identify an underlying disease and target therapy to control that disorder; as with PNGD, most treatments reported in the literature are aimed at controlling the underlying systemic disease. As such, reported treatments include aggressive systemic agents geared toward controlling the IGD-associated systemic disease, which may also clear the IGD (systemic steroids,[38] etanercept,[38,47] methotrexate,[36,38] cyclosporine,[46] intravenous immunoglobulin,[71] tocilizumab,[72] and ustekinumab[50]). There are reports of improvement with topical steroids,[38,42,46] nonsteroidal antiinflammatory drugs,[46,73] systemic corticosteroids,[43,46] dapsone, and hydroxychloroquine.[46] Infliximab was used for a recalcitrant case.[74]

Summary

Classic IGD consists of palpable linear cords on the trunk and histologic findings of interstitial epithelioid histiocytes surrounding small foci of altered collagen, often leading to the "floating sign," with absent mucin and no vasculitis. It is seen in the setting of systemic diseases, such as arthritis, connective tissue diseases, hematologic disorders, malignancies, and rarely with infections or medications. IGDR may be a subtype of IGD associated with a drug; the response can take weeks to months to develop and a similar timeframe to resolve. Clues may be histologic findings of tissue eosinophilia, an interface reaction, and occasional lymphoid atypia, in addition to features of classic IGD.

Table 4
Classic descriptions of PNGD, IGD, and IGDR

	PNGD	IGD	IGDR
Clinical morphology	Symmetric umbilicated papules on the elbows	Linear erythematous cords on the trunk	Erythematous macules and patches symmetrically on the trunk and proximal extremities
Histology	Intense neutrophilic inflammation, ± leukocytoclastic vasculitis, degenerated collagen, palisading granulomas, minimal mucin	Spares interstitial histiocytes, rosettes of degenerated collagen ± "floating" sign, absent vasculitis and no mucin	Similar to IGD with addition of a vacuolar interface reaction and prominent dermal eosinophils, variable lymphoid atypia
Associations	Connective tissue diseases, inflammatory arthritis, hematologic disorders	Inflammatory arthritis, connective tissue diseases, hematologic disorders, medications	Medications (CCBs, BB, ACE inhibitors, statins, other)

Abbreviations: ACE inhibitor, angiotensin converting enzyme inhibitor; BB, β-blockers; CCB, calcium channel blocker; IGD, interstitial granulomatous dermatitis, IGDR, interstitial granulomatous drug reaction; PNGD, palisaded neutrophilic and granulomatous dermatitis.

REACTIVE GRANULOMATOUS DERMATITIS

As detailed, there exists substantial overlap between PNGD, IGD, and IGDR. The terms are at times used interchangeably in the literature,[1,23] and some authors view drug-induced IGD and IGDR as the same entity with authors viewing IGD as a subset of PNGD, whereas other authors draw strict distinctions. The confusing nomenclature dates back to the earliest report, by Dykman and colleagues[32] in 1965, who are credited with the first report of PNGD while describing patients with rheumatoid arthritis with linear subcutaneous bands, although that report was later the basis for further reports by Ackerman in 1993,[30] which led to the term Ackerman dermatitis, which is felt by many to represent what is currently known as IGD.[1,11] With the initial strictest definitions and descriptions of these entities, there may be clear differences between them—such as elbow papules in PNGD and trunk cords in IGD (although now both IGD with elbow papules[75] and PNGD with cords have been reported[76])—particularly histologically (vasculitis and neutrophilic dust in PNGD; floating sign of histiocytes around collagen in IGD; interface dermatitis, numerous dermal eosinophils, and lymphocyte atypia in IGDR; **Table 4**). However, these entities share substantial overlap, both in the reported spectrum of clinical morphologies, histologic findings, underlying etiologies, and response to treatment, and may be better considered as subtypes of a common process.

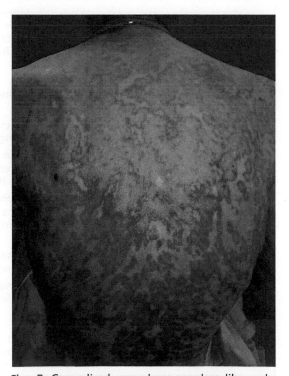

Fig. 7. Generalized granuloma-annulare–like polymorphic reactive granulomatous dermatitis. There are diffuse annular thin plaques resembling granuloma annulare, with absent mucin on histology, suggesting granuloma-annulare–like interstitial granulomatous dermatitis. (*Courtesy of* Joseph C. English III, MD, Wexford, PA.)

There remain types of reactive cutaneous granulomatous dermatitis that are not encapsulated by the aforementioned entities, including granuloma annulare and sarcoidosis-like cutaneous reactions, which are beyond the spectrum of this review. However, there exist clinical eruptions that resemble PNGD, IGD, or IGDR, either clinically or histologically, and occur in response to inciting systemic processes similar to those entities, such as generalized/erythrodermatous granulomatous dermatitis in the setting of myelodysplastic syndrome,[77] or generalized granuloma-annulare-like polymorphic eruptions (**Fig. 7**), which may warrant consideration within the umbrella of diseases described in this review. Furthermore, there are subtypes of drug-induced granulomatous dermatitides that have hitherto not been considered to represent drug-induced IGD or IGDR, but that may best be captured under a broader umbrella term as well (enfuvirtide granulomatous injection site reactions,[78] BRAF-inhibitor granulomatous eruption,[79] and drug-induced granulomatous T-cell dyscrasias[68]).

We propose the term "reactive granulomatous dermatitis" (RGD) to encompass the group of cutaneous reactive eruptions hitherto classified as PNGD, IGD, or IGDR. These entities may have similar clinical and histologic features (albeit occurring along a spectrum), and share same systemic associations. Medication-induced forms exist. The etiopathogenesis is unclear, whether related to immune complex deposition, delayed hypersensitivity, or another process. Treatment is geared at controlling the underlying trigger, which may entail

Table 5
Summary of initial evaluation and management of patients with reactive granulomatous dermatitis (RGD; includes PNGD, IGD, IGDR)

			Level of Evidence[a]
Evaluate for drug-induced disease	Review of medications	Including supplements, diet, herbal medications Including medications present for weeks to months Focus on CCBs, BBs, ACE inhibitors, statins	D
Evaluate for systemic disease	Connective tissue disease	ANA ANCA Additional testing dictated by systemic symptomatology	D
	Arthritis	RF/CCP Rheumatology evaluation Consider imaging	D
	Malignancy	Age appropriate malignancy screen CBC with differential SPEP/UPEP with IFE	D
	Other	Chest radiography Occult infections (endocarditis, hepatitis, pulmonary fungal infection)	D
Management	General	Skin biopsy Medication cessation trial when indicated Control underlying systemic disease	D
	RGD specific	Watchful waiting Topical or intralesional corticosteroids NSAIDs Dapsone Hydroxychloroquine Systemic corticosteroids Consider additional agents in extensive/recalcitrant cases	D

Abbreviations: ACE inhibitor, angiotensin converting enzyme inhibitor; ANA, antinuclear antibody; ANCA, antineutrophilic cytoplasmic antibodies; BB, β-blocker; CBC, complete blood count; CCB, calcium channel blocker; CCP, cyclic citrullinated peptide; IFE, immunofixation electrophoresis; IGD, interstitial granulomatous dermatitis, IGDR, interstitial granulomatous drug reaction; NSAIDs, nonsteroidal antiinflammatory drugs; PNGD, palisaded neutrophilic and granulomatous dermatitis; RF, rheumatoid factor; SPEP, serum protein electrophoresis; Statins, 3-hydroxy-3-methyl-glutaryl-coenzyme A reductase inhibitors; UPEP, urine protein electrophoresis.
[a] D, case series or case reports.

removing a culprit medication, removing an underlying malignancy, or controlling a systemic autoimmune disease (**Table 5**). Acknowledging that there may be some variation among the subtypes of RGD, it may be appropriate to consider this umbrella term with subtle variations, such as "RGD, PNGD-type; RGD, IGD type; RGD, drug induced; and RGD, granuloma annulare-like/polymorphous" (**Table 6**). Furthermore, the group of diseases discussed herein and collected under the term RGD may be further confused by potential overlap with neutrophilic dermatoses (such rheumatoid neutrophilic dermatosis[2] and some forms of Sweet syndrome[5,12]) which may further cloud the picture. It is not inconceivable to think of a future classification of RGD, including variants, such as RGD, neutrophil predominant (potentially

bridging what is currently PNGD, erythema elevatum diutinum [EED], some forms of Sweet syndrome and perhaps some tumor necrosis factor-induced dermatitides); RGD, histiocyte predominant (what is currently IGD, and perhaps some forms of histiocytoid Sweet syndrome[80]), RGD, eosinophil predominant (what is currently IGDR, drug-induced forms of IGD, and perhaps some cases of urticarial vasculitis may in fact fall more in this category), and RGD, mucinous type (with perhaps some forms of atypical granuloma annulare or interstitial granuloma annulare may be better classified under this umbrella term).

Granulomatous dermatitis is not a diagnosis per se in most cases. It is instead a reaction pattern in the skin that occurs in response to a systemic process, such as an underlying autoimmune disease,

Table 6
Spectrum of reactive granulomatous dermatitis (RGD)

Type	Predominant Clinical Presentation[a]	Predominant Histopathologic Findings	Predominant Disease Associations
RGD, PNGD type	Erythematous papules around the elbows	Intense neutrophilic inflammation, degenerated collagen, palisading granulomas, with or without leukocytoclastic vasculitis; minimal mucin	Connective tissue disease Arthritides Other (hematologic malignancy, drug)
RGD, IGD type	Erythematous cords on the trunk Annular erythematous-to-violaceous patches on proximal limbs and trunk	Spares interstitial histiocytes, rosettes of degenerated collagen, "floating" sign, absent vasculitis and no mucin	Arthritides Connective tissue disease Malignancy (hematologic, solid organ) Other (infection, drug)
RGD, drug induced	Annular erythematous-to-violaceous patches on proximal limbs and trunk	Spares interstitial histiocytes, rosettes of degenerated collagen, vacuolar interface reaction and prominent dermal eosinophils, variable lymphoid atypia; absent vasculitis and no mucin	Medications
RGD, polycyclic/diffuse[b]	Polycyclic, annular, erythematous-to-violaceous plaques with indurated border Red-brown diffuse mildly infiltrated erythroderma	Spares interstitial histiocytes, rosettes of degenerated collagen surrounded by predominantly histiocytes, relatively scant neutrophils, rare eosinophils; absent vasculitis and nil-to-scant mucin	Connective tissue disease Arthritides Malignancy

Abbreviations: IGD, interstitial granulomatous dermatitis, PNGD, palisaded neutrophilic and granulomatous dermatitis.
[a] All RGD teds to be symmetric.
[b] Diffuse RGD includes polycyclic, granuloma annulare-like, polymorphous, and erythrodermatous RGD.

malignancy, or medication reaction. The nomenclature currently surrounding these entities is a source of confusion. Given the extent of clinical and histologic overlap, similar underlying triggers, and overlapping approach to patient care, we propose a unifying umbrella term, reactive granulomatous dermatitis (RGD), to clarify these entities. Rather than trying to decide which type it is, clinicians may be better served simply recognizing the process and identifying the underlying trigger.

REFERENCES

1. Hawryluk EB, Izikson L, English JC 3rd. Non-infectious granulomatous diseases of the skin and their associated systemic diseases: an evidence-based update to important clinical questions. Am J Clin Dermatol 2010;11:171–81.
2. Chu P, Connolly MK, LeBoit PE. The histopathologic spectrum of palisaded neutrophilic and granulomatous dermatitis in patients with collagen vascular disease. Arch Dermatol 1994;130:1278–83.
3. Finan MC, Winkelmann RK. The cutaneous extravascular necrotizing granuloma (Churg-Strauss granuloma) and systemic disease: a review of 27 cases. Medicine (Baltimore) 1983;62:142–58.
4. Finan MC. Rheumatoid papule, cutaneous extravascular necrotizing granuloma, and Churg-Strauss granuloma: are they the same entity? J Am Acad Dermatol 1990;22:142–3.
5. Misago N, Shinoda Y, Tago M, et al. Palisaded neutrophilic granulomatous dermatitis with leukocytoclastic vasculitis in a patient without any underlying systemic disease detected to date. J Cutan Pathol 2010;37:1092–7.
6. Kim SK, Park CK, Park YW, et al. Palisaded neutrophilic granulomatous dermatitis presenting as an unusual skin manifestation in a patient with Behçet's disease. Scand J Rheumatol 2005;34:324–7.
7. Al-Daraji WI, Coulson IH, Howat AJ. Palisaded neutrophilic and granulomatous dermatitis. Clin Exp Dermatol 2005;30:578–9.
8. Hantash BM, Chiang D, Kohler S, et al. Palisaded neutrophilic and granulomatous dermatitis associated with limited systemic sclerosis. J Am Acad Dermatol 2008;58:661–4.
9. Hunt RD, Hartman RD, Molho-Pessach V, et al. Palisaded neutrophilic and granulomatous dermatitis in an adolescent girl with perinuclear antineutrophil cytoplasmic antibody-positive pauci-immune glomerulonephritis and arthritis. J Am Acad Dermatol 2012;67:e164–6.
10. Kwon EJ, Hivnor CM, Yan AC, et al. Interstitial granulomatous lesions as part of the spectrum of presenting cutaneous signs in pediatric sarcoidosis. Pediatr Dermatol 2007;24:517–24.
11. Sangueza OP, Caudell MD, Mengesha YM, et al. Palisaded neutrophilic granulomatous dermatitis in rheumatoid arthritis. J Am Acad Dermatol 2002;47:251–7.
12. Asahina A, Fujita H, Fukunaga Y, et al. Early lesion of palisaded neutrophilic granulomatous dermatitis in ulcerative colitis. Eur J Dermatol 2007;17:234–7.
13. Brecher A. Palisaded neutrophilic and granulomatous dermatitis. Dermatol Online J 2003;9:1.
14. Muscardin LM, Cota C, Amorosi B, et al. Erythema elevatum diutinum in the spectrum of palisaded neutrophilic granulomatous dermatitis: description of a case with rheumatoid arthritis. J Eur Acad Dermatol Venereol 2007;21:104–5.
15. Gordon K, Miteva M, Torchia D, et al. Allopurinol-induced palisaded neutrophilic and granulomatous dermatitis. Cutan Ocul Toxicol 2012;31:338–40.
16. Heidary N, Mengden S, Pomeranz MK. Palisaded neutrophilic and granulomatous dermatosis. Dermatol Online J 2008;14:17.
17. Stephenson SR, Campbell SM, Drew GS, et al. Palisaded neutrophilic and granulomatous dermatitis presenting in a patient with rheumatoid arthritis on adalimumab. J Cutan Pathol 2011;38:644–8.
18. Gordon EA, Schmidt AN, Boyd AS. Palisaded neutrophilic and granulomatous dermatitis: a presenting sign of sarcoidosis? J Am Acad Dermatol 2011;65:664–5.
19. Mahmoodi M, Ahmad A, Bansal C, et al. Palisaded neutrophilic and granulomatous dermatitis in association with sarcoidosis. J Cutan Pathol 2011;38:365–8.
20. Germanas JP, Mehrabi D, Carder KR. Palisaded neutrophilic granulomatous dermatitis in a 12-year-old girl with systemic lupus erythematosus. J Am Acad Dermatol 2006;55:S60–2.
21. Singh M, Comfere N. Palisaded neutrophilic and granulomatous dermatitis. N Engl J Med 2012;366:e33.
22. Collaris EJ, van Marion AM, Frank J, et al. Cutaneous granulomas in rheumatoid arthritis. Int J Dermatol 2007;46:33–5.
23. Bremner R, Simpson E, White CR, et al. Palisaded neutrophilic and granulomatous dermatitis: an unusual cutaneous manifestation of immune-mediated disorders. Semin Arthritis Rheum 2004;34:610–6.
24. Wilmoth GJ, Perniciaro C. Cutaneous extravascular necrotizing granuloma (Winkelmann granuloma): confirmation of the association with systemic disease. J Am Acad Dermatol 1996;34:753–9.
25. Pastar Z, Radoš J, Pavic I, et al. Palisaded neutrophilic and granulomatous dermatitis in association with subcutaneous nodular and systemic sarcoidosis. Acta Dermatovenerol Croat 2013;21:245–9.

26. He Y, Maverakis E, Ramirez-Maverakis D, et al. Combination therapy with intralesional triamcinolone and oral dapsone for management of palisaded neutrophilic and granulomatous dermatitis. Dermatol Online J 2013;19:17.

27. Fett N, Kovarik C, Bennett D. Palisaded neutrophilic granulomatous dermatitis without a definable underlying disorder treated with dapsone. J Am Acad Dermatol 2011;65:e92–3.

28. Martin JA, Jarrett P. Rheumatoid papules treated with dapsone. Clin Exp Dermatol 2004;29:387.

29. Lee MW, Jang KA, Lim YS, et al. Cutaneous extravascular necrotizing granuloma (Churg Strauss granuloma). Clin Exp Dermatol 1999;24:193–5.

30. Ackerman AB. Histologic diagnosis of inflammatory skin diseases: interstitial granulomatous dermatitis with arthritis. In: Ackerman AB, Guo Y, Vitale P, et al, editors. Clues to diagnosis in dermatopathology. 1st edition. Chicago: ASCP Press; 1993. p. 309–12.

31. Verneuil L, Dompmartin A, Comoaz F, et al. Interstitial granulomatous dermatitis with cutaneous cords and arthritis: a disorder associated with autoantibodies. J Am Acad Dermatol 2001;45:286–91.

32. Dykman CJ, Galens GJ, Good AE. Linear subcutaneous bands in rheumatoid arthritis. Ann Intern Med 1965;63:134–40.

33. Betloch I, Moragon M, Jorda E, et al. Linear rheumatoid nodule. Int J Dermatol 1988;27:645–56.

34. Harpster EF, Mauro T, Barr RJ. Linear granuloma annulare. J Am Acad Dermatol 1989;21:1138–41.

35. Aloi FG, Tomasini CF, Molinero A. Railway track-like dermatitis: an atypical Mondor's disease. J Am Acad Dermatol 1989;20:920–3.

36. Dubey S, Merry P. Interstitial granulomatous dermatitis (Ackerman's syndrome) in SLE presenting with the rope sign. Rheumatology 2007;46:80.

37. Flecht M, Faulhaber J, Gottmann U, et al. Interstitial granulomatous dermatitis (Ackerman's syndrome). Eur J Dermatol 2010;20:661–2.

38. Peroni A, Colato C, Schena D, et al. Interstitial granulomatous dermatitis: a distinct entity with characteristic histological and clinical pattern. Br J Dermatol 2011;166:775–83.

39. Blaise S, Salameire D, Carpentier PH. Interstitial granulomatous dermatitis: a misdiagnosed cutaneous form of systemic lupus erythematosus. Clin Exp Dermatol 2008;33:712–4.

40. Tomasini C, Pippione M. Interstitial granulomatous dermatitis with plaques. J Am Acad Dermatol 2002;46:892–9.

41. Moon HR, Lee JH, Won CH, et al. A child with IGD and juvenile idiopathic arthritis. Pediatr Dermatol 2013;30:e272–3.

42. Warycha MA, Fangman W, Kamino H, et al. Interstitial granulomatous dermatitis in a child with chronic uveitis. J Am Acad Dermatol 2008;58:S100–2.

43. Worsnop FS, Ostlere L. Interstitial granulomatous dermatitis with arthritis presenting with the rope sign. Clin Exp Dermatol 2013;38:564–5.

44. Johnson H, Mengden S, Brancaccio RR. Interstitial granulomatous dermatitis. Dermatol Online J 2008; 14:18.

45. Long D, Thiboutot DM, Majeski JT, et al. Interstitial granulomatous dermatitis with arthritis. J Am Acad Dermatol 1996;34:957–61.

46. Busquets-Perez N, Narvaez J, Valverde-Garcia J. Interstitial granulomatous dermatitis with arthritis (Ackerman syndrome). J Rheumatol 2006;33: 1207–9.

47. Zoli A, Massi G, Pinelli M, et al. Interstitial granulomatous dermatitis in rheumatoid arthritis responsive to etanercept. Clin Rheumatol 2010;29: 99–101.

48. Walling HW, Swick BL. Interstitial granulomatous dermatitis associated with chronic inflammatory demyelinating polyneuropathy. Cutis 2012;90:30–2.

49. Jabbari A, Cheung W, Kamino H, et al. Interstitial granulomatous dermatitis with arthritis. Dermatol Online J 2009;15:22.

50. Leloup P, Aubert H, Causse S, et al. Usteklnumab therapy for severe interstitial granulomatous dermatitis with arthritis. JAMA Dermatol 2013;149: 626–7.

51. Nakamura N, Asai J, Daito J, et al. Interstitial granulomatous dermatitis? An unusual presentation in the mucosa and periungual skin. J Dermatol 2011;38:382–5.

52. Lee KJ, Lee ES, Lee DY, et al. Interstitial granulomatous dermatitis associated with autoimmune hepatitis. J Eur Acad Dermatol Venereol 2007;21: 684–5.

53. Patsatsi A, Kyriakou A, Triantafyllidou E, et al. Interstitial granulomatous dermatitis: another clinical variant. Case Rep Dermatol 2011;3:195–200.

54. Altaykan A, Erkin G, Boztepe G, et al. Interstitial granulomatous dermatitis with arthritis. Hum Pathol 2004;35:892–4.

55. Lucas A, Bañuls J, Mataix J, et al. Localized acquired cutis laxa secondary to interstitial granulomatous dermatitis. Clin Exp Dermatol 2009;34: e102–5.

56. Dyson SW, Hirsch A, Jaworsky C. Interstitial granulomatous dermatitis secondary to soy. J Am Acad Dermatol 2004;51:S105–7.

57. Mason HR, Swanson JK, Ho J, et al. Interstitial granulomatous dermatitis associated with darifenacin. J Drugs Dermatol 2008;7:895–7.

58. Martin G, Cañueto J, Santos-Briz A, et al. Interstitial granulomatous dermatitis with arthritis associated with trastuzumab. J Eur Acad Dermatol Venereol 2010;24:493–501.

59. Perrin C, Lacour JP, Castanet J, et al. Interstitial granulomatous drug reaction with a histological

pattern of interstitial granulomatous dermatitis. Am J Dermatopathol 2001;23:295–8.

60. Deng A, Harvey V, Sina B, et al. Interstitial granulomatous dermatitis associated with the use of tumor necrosis factor inhibitors. Arch Dermatol 2006;142:198–202.

61. Magro CM, Crowson AN, Schapiro BL. The interstitial granulomatous drug reaction: a distinctive clinical and pathological entity. J Cutan Pathol 1998;25:72–8.

62. Lee HW, Yun WJ, Lee MW, et al. Interstitial granulomatous drug reaction caused by Chinese herbal medication. J Am Acad Dermatol 2005;52:712–3.

63. Siami K, Wilkerson M, Clark SH, et al. An indurated plaque on the ankle of a 74-year-old woman. Arch Pathol Lab Med 2004;128:e129–30.

64. Chen YC, Hsiao CH, Tsai TF. Interstitial granulomatous drug reaction presenting as erythroderma: remission after discontinuation of enalapril maleate. Br J Dermatol 2008;158:1143–4.

65. Yazgano KD, Tambay E, Mete O, et al. Interstitial granulomatous drug reaction due to thalidomide. J Eur Acad Dermatol Venereol 2009;23:490–3.

66. Marcollo Pini A, Kerl K, Kamarachev J, et al. Interstitial granulomatous drug reaction following intravenous ganciclovir. Br J Dermatol 2008;158:1391–2.

67. Lee MW, Choi J, Sung KJ, et al. Interstitial and granulomatous drug reaction presenting as erythema nodosum-like lesions. Acta Derm Venereol 2002;82:473–4.

68. Magro CM, Cruz-Inigo AE, Votava H, et al. Drug-associated reversible granulomatous T cell dyscrasia: a distinct subset of the interstitial granulomatous drug reaction. J Cutan Pathol 2010;37:96–111.

69. Kim MS, Lee JH, Park K, et al. Allopurinol-induced DRESS syndrome with a histologic pattern consistent with interstitial granulomatous drug reaction. Am J Dermatopathol 2014;36:193–5.

70. Aloi F, Tomasini C, Pippione M. Interstitial granulomatous dermatitis with plaques. Am J Dermatopathol 1999;21:320–3.

71. Alghamdi R, Bejar C, Steff M, et al. Intravenous immunoglobulins as a treatment of interstitial granulomatous dermatitis with arthritis. Br J Dermatol 2012;167:218–20.

72. Schanz S, Schmalzing M, Guenova E, et al. Interstitial granulomatous dermatitis with arthritis responding to tocilizumab. Arch Dermatol 2012;148:17–20.

73. Banuls J, Betlloch I, Botella R, et al. Interstitial granulomatous dermatitis with plaques and arthritis. Eur J Dermatol 2003;13:308–10.

74. Kreuter A, Gambichler T, Altmeyer P. Infliximab therapy for interstitial granulomatous dermatitis. J Eur Acad Dermatol Venereol 2007;21:251–2.

75. Szepetiuk G, Lesuisse M, Pierard GE, et al. Auto-immunity-related granulomatous dermatitis in association with hepatitis. Case Rep Dermatol 2012;4:80–4.

76. Gulati A, Paige D, Yagoob M, et al. Palisaded neutrophilic granulomatous dermatitis associated with systemic lupus erythematosus presenting with the burning rope sign. J Am Acad Dermatol 2009;61:711–4.

77. Balin SJ, Wetter DA, Kurtin PJ, et al. Myelodysplastic syndrome presenting as generalized granulomatous dermatitis. Arch Dermatol 2011;147:331–5.

78. Ball RA, Kinchelow T, ISR Substudy Group. Injection site reactions with the HIV-1 fusion inhibitor enfuvirtide. J Am Acad Dermatol 2003;49:826–31.

79. Park JJ, Hawryluk EB, Tahan SR, et al. Cutaneous granulomatous eruption and successful response to potent topical steroids in patients undergoing targeted BRAF inhibitor treatment for metastatic melanoma. JAMA Dermatol 2014;150:307–11.

80. Requena L, Kutzner H, Palmedo G, et al. Histiocytoid Sweet syndrome: a dermal infiltration of immature neutrophilic granulocytes. Arch Dermatol 2005;141:834–42.

81. Misago N, Inoue H, Inoue T, et al. Palisaded neutrophilic granulomatous dermatitis in systemic lupus erythematosus with a butterfly rash-like lesion. Eur J Dermatol 2010;20:128–9.

82. Perniciaro C, Winkelmann RK. Cutaneous extravascular necrotizing granuloma in a patient with Takayasu's aortitis. Arch Dermatol 1986;122:201.

83. de Unamuno Bustos B, Rabasco AG, Sanhez RB, et al. Palisaded neutrophilic and granulomatous dermatitis associated with ankylosing spondylitis. Am J Dermatopathol 2013;35:847–50.

84. Calonje JE, Greaves MW. Cutaneous extravascular necrotizing granuloma (Churg-Strauss) as a paraneoplastic manifestation of non-Hodgkin's B-cell lymphoma. J R Soc Med 1993;86:549–50.

85. Biswas A, Chittari K, Gey van Pittius D, et al. Palisaded neutrophilic and granulomatous dermatitis in a child with type I diabetes mellitus and coeliac disease. Br J Dermatol 2008;159:488–9.

86. Misago N, Narisawa Y, Tada Y, et al. Palisaded neutrophilic granulomatous dermatitis caused by cellulitis in a patient with systemic lupus erythematosus. Int J Dermatol 2011;50:1583–5.

87. Golden BD, Wong DC, Dicostanzo D, et al. Rheumatoid papules in a patient with acquired immune deficiency syndrome and symmetric poylarthritis. J Rheumatol 1996;23:760.

88. Wong HK, Kaffenberger BH, Zirwas M. A palpable erythematous cord over the trunk in a patient with systemic lupus erythematosus. JAMA Dermatol 2013;149:609–14.

89. Marmon S, Robinson M, Meehan SA, et al. Lupus-erythematosus-associated interstitial granulomatous dermatitis. Dermatol Online J 2012;18:31.

90. Comte C, Guillot B, Durand L, et al. Dermatite granulomateuse interstitielle avec arthritis: quatre cas. Ann Dermatol Venereol 2008;135:38–43 [in French].

91. Chen DL, Chong AH, Green J, et al. A novel case of polyfibromatosis and interstitial granulomatous dermatitis with arthritis. J Am Acad Dermatol 2006;55:S32–7.

92. Wollina U, Schönlebe J, Unger L, et al. Interstitial granulomatous dermatitis with plaques and arthritis. Clin Rheumatol 2003;22:347–9.

93. Choi MJ, Shin D, Kim YC, et al. Interstitial granulomatous dermatitis with arthritis accompanied by anaplastic large cell lymphoma. J Dermatol 2014; 41:363–4.

94. Michailidou D, Voulgarelis M, Pikazis D. Exacerbation of IGD with arthritis by anakinra in a patient with diffuse large B-cell lymphoma. Clin Exp Rheumatol 2014;32:259–61.

95. Patsinakidis N, Susok L, Hessam S, et al. IGD associated with myelodysplastic syndrome - complete clearance under therapy with 5-azacytidine. Acta Derm Venereol 2014;94(6):725–6.

96. Cornejo KM, Lum CA, Izumi AK. A cutaneous interstitial granulomatous dermatitis-like eruption arising in myelodysplasia with leukemic progression. Am J Dermatopathol 2013;35:e26–9.

97. Swing DC Jr, Sheehan DJ, Sangueza OP, et al. Interstitial granulomatous dermatitis secondary to acute promyelocytic leukemia. Am J Dermatopathol 2008;30:197–9.

98. Schreckenberg C, Asch PH, Sibilia J, et al. Interstitial granulomatous dermatitis and paraneoplastic rheumatoid polyarthritis disclosing cancer of the lung. Ann Dermatol Venereol 1998;125:585–8 [in French].

99. Moyano Almagro B, López Navarro N, Contreras Steyls M, et al. IGD and arthritis revealing oesophageal carcinoma. Clin Exp Dermatol 2013;38:501–3.

100. Sakaizawa K, Hasegawa J, Kawachi S, et al. Interstitial granulomatous dermatitis with plaques. Eur J Dermatol 2008;18:600–1.

101. Antunes J, Pacheco D, Travassos AR, et al. Autoimmune thyroiditis presenting as interstitial granulomatous dermatitis. An Bras Dermatol 2012;87:748–51.

102. Lee HW, Chang SE, Lee MW, et al. Interstitial granulomatous dermatitis with plaques associated with antiphospholipid syndrome. Br J Dermatol 2005; 152:814–6.

103. DiCaudo DJ, Connolly SM. Interstitial granulomatous dermatitis associated with pulmonary coccidioidomycosis. J Am Acad Dermatol 2001;45:840–5.

104. Kroesen S, Itin PH, Hasler P. Arthritis and interstitial granulomatous dermatitis (Ackerman syndrome) with pulmonary silicosis. Semin Arthritis Rheum 2003;32:334–40.

105. Moreno C, Kutzner H, Palmedo G, et al. Interstitial granulomatous dermatitis with histiocytic pseudorosettes: a new histopathologic pattern in cutaneous borreliosis. J Am Acad Dermatol 2003;48:376–84.

106. Fujita Y, Shimizu T, Shimizu H. A case of interstitial granulomatous drug reaction due to sennoside. Br J Dermatol 2004;150:1035–7.

107. Hernandez N, Peñate Y, Borrego L. Generalized erythematous-violaceous plaques in a patient with a history of dyslipidemia. Int J Dermatol 2013;52: 393–4.

108. Martinez-Moran C, Nájera L, Ruiz-Casado AI, et al. Interstitial granulomatous drug reaction to sorafenib. Arch Dermatol 2011;147:1118–9.

109. Regula CG, Hennessy J, Clarke LE, et al. Interstitial granulomatous drug reaction to anakinra. J Am Acad Dermatol 2008;59:S25–7.

110. Martorell-Calatayud A, Balmer N, Cardona LF, et al. Interstitial granulomatous drug reaction to adalimumab. Am J Dermatopathol 2010;32:408–9.

111. Atzori L, Luca P, Pinna AL. Interstitial granulomatous drug reaction due to febuxostat. Indian J Dermatol Venereol Leprol 2014;80:182–4.

112. Groves C, McMenamin ME, Casey M, et al. Interstitial granulomatous reaction to strontium ranelate. Arch Dermatol 2008;144:268–9.

Sarcoidosis

Miguel Sanchez, MD*, Adele Haimovic, MD, Steve Prystowsky, MD

KEYWORDS

- Sarcoidosis • Cutaneous sarcoidosis • Erythema nodosum • Lupus pernio
- Extracutaneous sarcoidosis • Granuloma • Therapy

KEY POINTS

- Sarcoidosis is a multisystemic granulomatous disease of unknown cause that affects the skin in 20% to 30% of cases.
- Sarcoidosis skin lesions may be specific, which tend to be chronic, or nonspecific, which tend to be acute.
- Lupus pernio is associated with chronic disease, whereas erythema nodosum is associated with acute disease and spontaneous resolution.
- Systemic treatment of the skin is reserved for symptomatic, widespread, disfiguring, and/or quality of life–altering disease and includes oral corticosteroids, methotrexate, antimalarials, minocycline, and some tumor necrosis factor inhibitors.
- The diagnosis of sarcoidosis requires a multimodal approach that comprises clinical findings, histologic presence of noncaseating granulomas, demonstration of organ involvement radiologically or through other tests, and exclusion of other diseases.

INTRODUCTION

Sarcoidosis is a chronic but frequently self-resolving disease of unknown cause characterized histologically by the formation of noncaseating epithelioid cell granulomas in one or more organs. The protean skin manifestations can confound even experienced dermatologists, and, in some cases, effective treatment is challenging. A reasonable diagnosis can be made in most cases from the appearance of skin lesions, confirmatory histology, involvement of other organ systems, and exclusion of other noncaseating granulomatous diseases. It must always be remembered that sarcoidosis is a potentially lethal and disabling disease with a broad spectrum of heterogeneous anatomic involvement leading to a remarkable range of possible symptoms that can mimic those of many other diseases. Therefore, sarcoidosis should be included in many clinical differential diagnoses (see **Table 2**). Evaluation of extracutaneous involvement should be performed at the initial presentation of sarcoidosis on any organ (**Box 1**),[1] and a review of systems should be part of follow-up visits. Collaborative communication between specialists and primary care physicians engenders better patient care.

Depending on study design and selected population, cutaneous disease has been reported to occur in 9% to 37% of all cases,[2,3] but in the ACCESS (A Case-control Etiologic Study of Sarcoidosis) study, specific lesions were present in 16%, similarly to the 17% reported in a recent study from Barcelona, Spain.[4] Cutaneous sarcoidosis is the initial manifestation of the disease in nearly one-third of patients.[5] The skin (as well as the liver, spleen, and lymph nodes) is most often involved in African Americans.

Disclosure: The work reported in this article has not received financial support from any pharmaceutical company or other commercial source.
Conflicts of interest: The authors have no significant conflicts of interest to declare.
The Ronald O. Perelman Department of Dermatology, New York University School of Medicine, New York, NY 10016, USA
* Corresponding author. The Ronald O. Perelman Department of Dermatology, New York University School of Medicine, 240 East 38th Street, 11th floor, New York, NY 10016.
E-mail address: MiguelR.Sanchez@nyumc.org

Dermatol Clin 33 (2015) 389–416
http://dx.doi.org/10.1016/j.det.2015.03.006
0733-8635/15/$ – see front matter © 2015 Elsevier Inc. All rights reserved.

EPIDEMIOLOGY

Sarcoidosis has been reported from practically all countries and in every race, but its prevalence varies by geographic location, ethnicity, gender, and age. In the United States, the lifetime risk for developing sarcoidosis was estimated to be 2.4% in African Americans and 0.84% in white people and the adjusted annual incidence is more than 3 times higher in the former (35.5 per 100,000) than the latter (10.9 per 100,000).[6,7] Women develop sarcoidosis more often than men,[8,9] but in both genders the incidence peaks between the ages of 25 and 45 years.[10] In Scandinavia, where the annual incidence is the highest in

the world (64 cases per 100,000 people), incidence rates in women are bimodal with peaks occurring at 25 to 29 and 65 to 69 years of age.[1,8,11] In Japan, where the annual incidence is only 1 to 2 cases per 100,000 people, incidence rates peak between the ages of 20 and 34 years but a second peak occurs in women aged 50 to 60 years.[12] In a recent study, 35% of cases had skin involvement.[12] Alarmingly, the age-adjusted, sarcoidosis-related mortality in the United States increased 50.5% in women and 30.1% in men from 1988 to 2007.[13] The prognosis is especially grave in black women in whom sarcoidosis-related complications are the cause of death in 25% of those with the disease.[14]

ETIOPATHOGENESIS

Despite considerable effort, the cause of sarcoidosis has eluded investigators. The disease has been described as an immune paradox because peripheral anergy is present despite a brisk tissue inflammatory response.[15] Studies suggest that development of sarcoidosis involves an interplay between extrinsic antigens, genetic factors, and immune responses.[16,17] The regulation of immune mechanisms is more complex and extensive than can be discussed in this article,[18] but researchers have suggested that poorly degraded antigen is engulfed by antigen-presenting cells (APCs) and displayed on the APCs' major histocompatibility complex (MHC).[10,18] A CD4+ T-cell receptor attaches to this antigen-MHC complex and becomes activated. The result is a release of cytokines, including interleukin (IL)-2, which induce clonal proliferation of activated, strongly Th1 polarized T-helper cells that secrete proinflammatory cytokines, such as IL-2, IL-12, and IL-18 (interferon-gamma–inducing factor), which facilitate granuloma formation. Some selectins, integrins, cytokines (such as CXCL-8), and cellular adhesion molecules promote diapedesis of monocytes from blood vessels to activated tissue macrophages. Further release of cytokines and chemokines causes macrophage aggregation into granulomas.[10,18] Granulomas are composed of epithelioid cells, mononuclear cells, and CD4+ T cells with a few CD8+ T cells around the periphery. Recently, serum amyloid A was found to be present in granulomas and to amplify Th1 responses by interacting with Toll-like receptor 2. If Th1 immune responses predominate, upregulation of interferon-gamma, IL-10, and other cytokines results in antigen clearance and granuloma resolution. In more than 60% of sarcoidosis cases, the granulomas resolve within 2 to 5 years.[19] If Th-2 immune responses predominate, upregulation of tumor necrosis factor (TNF) and granulocyte-macrophage colony-stimulating factor secretion, together with secretion of fibroproliferative cytokine IL-13, transforming growth factor (TGF)-β, and CCL-18, sustain the persistence of granulomas, resulting in chronic disease and fibrosis.[18] Natural killer T cells have been reported to be decreased in cases with chronic active sarcoidosis.[18]

Chronic fibrosis with permanent tissue damage occurs in 10% to 30% of patients.[19]

The role of Th17 immunity in sarcoidosis is being investigated.[18,20] Th17-helper cells are prominently present in and around granulomas early in the disease, as well as during progression toward fibrosis, and have been found in the blood of patients with sarcoidosis. These cells are involved in the disease's progression.[18] In a recent study, upregulated expression of IL-23, a main cytokine in the Th17 pathway, and TGF-β, which together with IL-23 promotes differentiation of naive T-cell receptors into Th17 cells, was shown in skin sarcoidosis lesions. In addition IL-17R and IL-21, which promote communication with other immune system cells, were also present in skin granulomas.[20] Although IL-17A, IL-17F, and IL-22 were not detected, IL-21 and Il-23 can act independently of IL-17.[20] Overproduction of IL-21 may also interfere with dendritic cell activation and maturation, which could potently regulate T-cell responses in granulomas.[21] STAT3 (signal transducer and activator of transcription 3), which is important in the development of Th17 cells, was also found.[20] In contrast, there seems to be an imbalance between Th17 and regulatory T cells (T_reg) cells, as has been described in several inflammatory and autoimmune diseases.[22] T_reg cells are decreased in patients with sarcoidosis and do not effectively suppress the development of granulomas.[22]

It is possible that several agents can serve as antigenic nidi for sarcoidosis granulomas but the development of the disease is influenced by the host's immune system and genetic composition. Environmental exposures and infectious organisms have long been considered disease promoters (Table 1).[16,23–25] In a multicentric case-controlled trial that compared 706 newly diagnosed cases of sarcoidosis with matched control subjects, exposure to numerous occupational agents, including insecticides, mold, metal fumes, and industrial organic dust, was reported to modestly increase the risk of acquiring the disease.[25] Notably, World Trade Center firefighters and other rescue and recovery workers exposed to aerosolized debris dust developed a sarcoidlike pulmonary disease. However, most of these patients have not developed extrapulmonary disease. No environmental or infectious antigens

Table 1
Some environmental factors and infectious agents that have been implicated most commonly as causal triggers of sarcoidosis

Environmental and Occupational	Infectious
Mold	Mycobacteria
Mildew	*Propionibacterium acnes*
Industrial organic dusts	*Propionibacterium granulosum*
Pesticides/ insecticides	Viruses (Herpes simplex, Epstein-Barr, Coxsackie B, retrovirus)
Wood burning	Mycoplasma
Firefighting materials	*Borrelia burgdorferi*
Building materials	—
Gardening materials	—
Solvents	—

Adapted from Haimovic A, Sanchez M, Judson MA, et al. Sarcoidosis: a comprehensive review and update for the dermatologist: part I. Cutaneous disease. J Am Acad Dermatol 2012;66(5):699.e1–18; [quiz: 717–8]; with permission.

have been identified.[26,27] Sporadic cases of sarcoidosis have also been reported in World Trade Center rescuers, with exposed African Americans having twice the risk of developing pulmonary disease.[28]

Among the many implicated infectious agents, scientific data involving mycobacteria has been the most compelling (**Box 2**).[29–35] A recently found, nonpigmented, rapidly growing strain, called *Mycobacterium immunogenum* has received attention as a potential cause of sarcoidosis because of its capacity to grow in degraded metalworking fluid and isolation from cases of hypersensitivity pneumonitis and keratitis.[36] A less persuasive case can be made for *Propionibacterium acnes*, the only microorganism isolated from sarcoidosis lesions by culture.[37] As discussed later, a recent study found that itraconazole was as effective as prednisone in pulmonary sarcoidosis, supporting previous reports that have implicated a fungal pathogenesis because of the beneficial therapeutic effect of antifungals.[38] Also, sarcoidosis affecting several organs, including the skin, has been triggered by medications including interferon and TNF-α antagonists.[39,40]

Evidence supporting genetic influences on the development and course of sarcoidosis include increased concordance in monozygotic twins compared with dizygotic twins, presence of familial

---

Box 2
Findings implicating mycobacteria as a cause of sarcoidosis

- A poorly soluble antigen derived from mycobacteria, called catalase-peroxidase G (mKatG), is demonstrable in sarcoidal granulomas and about half of patients mount cellular and humoral immune responses against this antigen.
- Mycobacterial proteins, such as mKatG and superoxide dismutase A, are present in sarcoidosis granulomas more often than in other types of granulomas.[29,30]
- Peripheral blood mononuclear cells and diagnostic bronchoalveolar lavage fluid show specific Th1 cytokine responses directed at mKatG and other mycobacterial proteins similar to those responses observed in active mycobacterial infection.[31]
- Serum samples often contain antibodies to mycobacterial heat-shock protein 70 and *Mycobacterium tuberculosis* mycolyl transferase antigen 85A.[32]
- In 22 of 31 cases of bronchoalveolar lavage samples, CD4 and CD8 responded to 1 or more mycobacterial epitopes. The responses seemed to wane as clinical disease improved.[33] Using matrix-assisted laser desorption ionization imaging mass spectrometry, immune responses against mycobacteria are present within sarcoidosis bronchoalveolar lavage, which, unlike those of *Propionibacterium acnes*, are distinct from disease controls.[34]
- In a study of 15 cases of pulmonary sarcoidosis, antituberculoid therapy resulted in increases in forced vital capacity.[35]

---

aggregation, and difference in disease prevalence and severity among various racial groups.[7,41,42] In the ACCESS study, patients with sarcoidosis reported having a parent or sibling with the disease 5 times more often than control subjects.[43] Six genome-wide association studies have been conducted (5 in Europeans and 1 in African Americans).[44] Several genes (**Box 3**) and haplotypes (**Box 4**) that have a protective effect or enhance susceptibility or influence the course of the disease have been identified. In African Americans, a novel sarcoidosis-associated locus, *NOTCH4*, was recently found to be associated with sarcoidosis.[45] In this racial group, a gene on chromosome 5q11.2 increases risk for sarcoidosis, whereas another gene on 5p15.2 is protective.[46] A single nucleotide polymorphism within the butyrophilin-like 2 (BTNL2) gene, which regulates T-cell activation, increases the risk of developing sarcoidosis in Europeans, with BTNL2 16071A doubling the risk of progression to persistent and progressive disease,[47] whereas a different polymorphism of this gene enhances the risk in African Americans.[48] In German patients, a protective effect was found for the annexin A11 gene, which regulates calcium signaling, cell division, and apoptosis, and the presence of the TNF-A2 allele was associated with Löfgren syndrome.[49]

CLINICAL MANIFESTATIONS
Cutaneous Sarcoidosis

Specific sarcoidosis lesions (**Table 2**) have, on histologic examination, granulomas and, on diascopy, often show the apple-jelly coloration characteristic of granulomatous skin lesions.[16] Depending on skin color, specific lesions range from flesh tinted to brown, to pink or violaceous. Nonspecific skin lesions lack granulomas and are caused by inflammatory reactions to sarcoidosis.[16,50,71] Although most lesions have distinct features that allow recognition or at least impart a high level of suspicion, the skin manifestations are protean and can mimic nearly any skin disease (**Table 3**). In the Barcelona study, skin lesions were present prior to or simultaneous with the diagnosis of systemic sarcoidosis in 80% of the cases.[4] Some skin lesions are valuable predictors of disease course.[51,72,73] Recently, dermoscopic findings for sarcoid skin lesions were reported. Areas of translucent orange globules and structureless whitish areas with linear vessels are present dermoscopically in sarcoidosis but also in other granulomatous diseases, and no specific pattern has been described yet.[74,75]

Specific Cutaneous Sarcoidosis

Maculopapular sarcoidosis
Although maculopapular lesions and eruptions have been reported to be common and associated with spontaneous resolution and favorable prognosis, the frequency of this type may be misrepresented in the medical literature, because many of the lesions for which photographs are included are papular. However, Mañá and colleagues[52] found that 23% of 86 cases of specific lesions were maculopapular and provided photographic documentation of a case. Maculopapular lesions consist of pink to brown, discrete patches studded with tiny papules.[16] The lesions are most often found on the face, especially on the nasal folds, eyelids, and

Box 3
Gene associations in sarcoidosis

Enhance susceptibility

  CR1 in Italians

  IL-1A in British, Czech, and Dutch

  BTNL2 in German and US Americans

  HSPA1L in Polish

  Interferon (IFN)-α in Japanese

  IFN-γ in Japanese

  TNF-α/β in Germans, Dutch, and British

  ANXA11 in African Americans and Europeans

Associated with chronic course

  TLR4 in Germans

  CC10/SCGB1A1: progressive disease in Japanese from Hokkaido

  TGF-β: development of pulmonary fibrosis in Dutch

  CCR5Δ32: severe disease in Czech, Dutch, and British

Protect against development

  SLC11A1 (formerly NRAMP1) in African Americans

  Vascular endothelial growth factor in Japanese

  IκBα in British

  CCR2-641 allele in Japanese

Löfgren association

  CCR2 in Dutch

  TNF-α*2 allele in Germans and Polish

Abbreviations: ANXA, annexin; BTNL - butyrophilin-like protein; CC10, clara cell 10-kDa protein; CCR – chemokine receptor; CR, complement receptor; IFN, interferon; IL, interleukin; SCGB, secretoglobin; SLC, solute carrier; TGF, tumor growth factor; TNF, tumor necrosis factor; TLR, toll like receptor.

Box 4
Human lymphocyte antigen associations in sarcoidosis

Worsen prognosis

  HLA-DRB1*1501-DQB1*0602 (severe pulmonary disease)

  HLA-DRB1*0301-DRB3*0101 (lung disease in Scandinavians)

Protective

  HLA-DRB1*04-DQB1*0301

Associated with disease resolution

  HLA-DRB1*0401-DPB1*0401

Associated with Löfgren syndrome

  HLA-DRB1*0301-DQB1*0201

Abbreviation: HLA, human leukocyte antigen.

without scarring, even without treatment.[9,71] The papules may be lichenoid and resemble lichen planus. Papules on the knees have been reported to have an association with acute disease and erythema nodosum (EN).[52]

Plaque sarcoidosis This type consists of single or multiple round, oval, or annular plaques. The face, back, buttocks, and extensor surface of the extremities are the most frequently involved areas (**Fig. 2**).[71] The plaques are thick and indurated, characteristically described as having a granulomatous feel, and often heal with scarring or pigmentary changes, especially hypopigmentation in African Americans.[16,50] These lesions are associated with chronic pulmonary disease, uveitis, and lymphadenopathy that usually requires systemic treatment.[60,77] Verrucous (**Fig. 3**), lichenoid, and psoriasiform types may require histopathologic diagnosis to differentiate them from viral warts, lichen planus, and psoriasis, respectively.[16,56]

Lupus pernio This type predominantly but not exclusively develops in African Americans. Reddish purple to violaceous brown, shiny, indurated plaques over the central face, especially on the nasal alae, cheeks, lips, and ears (**Fig. 4**). Lupus pernio lesions enlarge and are progressively disfiguring. In his original descriptions, Besnier emphasized the infiltrative, chilblainlike appearance of lupus pernio, which should not be confused with papular, papulonodular, or nodular sarcoidosis lesions, which can also involve the nose and cheeks but are significantly less destructive and usually more treatment responsive. Lupus pernio lesions not only can ulcerate and scar but may

orbits but also on the nape of neck, back, buttocks, and extremities. The papules can enlarge and become confluent into plaques, which concern patients but resolution within 2 years occurs in most cases, especially those with acute sarcoidosis.[51] The papules are occasionally pruritic.

Papular sarcoidosis

The lesions are discrete papules measuring 1 cm or less that are commonly present on the face, especially around the eyelids and nasolabial folds.[71,76] They can coalesce into plaques (**Fig. 1**).[2] The papules are often associated with minimal to no systemic disease and may resolve spontaneously

Table 2
Specific cutaneous sarcoidosis

Specific Lesions of Cutaneous Sarcoidosis	Frequency	DDX	Prognosis[a]
Papular	Very common	Syringomas and other appendageal tumors, adenoma sebaceum, xanthelasma, xanthomas, acne, granulomatous rosacea[2,50]	Associated with an acute form of sarcoidosis (hilar lymphadenopathy, peripheral lymphadenopathy, parotid enlargement, EN, and acute uveitis); usually resolves within 2 y[51]
Plaque	Very common	Psoriasis, lupus vulgaris, morphea, LP, LE, leishmaniasis, nummular eczema, secondary or tertiary syphilis, granuloma annulare, Kaposi sarcoma, plaque-stageMF[2,50]	Persistent lesions and commonly associated with chronic forms of systemic sarcoidosis[52]
Annular	Uncommon	Granuloma annulare, elastolytic actinic cell granuloma, leprosy, tinea, reactive granulomatous dermatitis	Chronic systemic disease
Angiolupoid	Uncommon	Rosacea, discoid LE, morphea, large basal cell carcinoma[53]	Lesions usually do not spontaneously resolve[52]
Verrucous	Rare	Warts, prurigo nodularis, hypertrophic LP, hypertrophic DLE, SCC[54,55]	Reports are in patients with systemic disease, particularly respiratory involvement[56,57]
Lichenoid	Rare	Lichen planus, lichen nitidus, lichenoid drug eruption, popular mucinosis	Most reports are in young children with eye and joint complications, and no respiratory involvement[58,59]
Psoriasiform	Uncommon	Psoriasis, SCC, tinea, dermatomyositis	May resolve with scarring[9]
Nodular	Common	Foreign body reaction, lipoma, cyst, rheumatoid nodule, lymphocytoma cutis, nodular lymphoma, pseudolymphoma, cutaneous metastasis, dermatofibrosarcoma, reticulohistiocytosis, atypical mycobacteria infection	Chronic systemic disease
Lupus pernio	Common	Lupus vulgaris, DLR, scar, nodular rosacea, superficial Wegener granulomatosis, paracoccidioidomycosis, nasal NK/T-cell lymphoma, granuloma faciale, rhinoscleroma, nodular amyloidosis	Associated with chronic progressive systemic sarcoidosis, including pulmonary fibrosis, chronic uveitis, bone cysts, upper respiratory disease.[51,52,60,61] LP is difficult to treat and may lead to severe disfigurement
Subcutaneous (Darier-Roussy)	Common	Lipodermatosclerosis, tuberculosis, nodular lymphoma, deep mycoses, epidermoid cysts, lipomas, cutaneous metastases, cellulitis, foreign body granuloma[2,50]	Association with bilateral hilar lymphadenopathy and nonsevere systemic disease has been reported[62,63]
Scar	Common	Keloid, hypertrophic scar, granulomatous foreign body reaction	Controversial; some reports suggest an association with systemic disease,[60,64] whereas others have not found any prognostic significance[4]

Variant	Frequency	Differential diagnosis	Comments
Hypopigmented	Uncommon	Hypopigmented MF, leprosy, pityriasis alba, pityriasis lichenoides chronica, pityriasis versicolor, vitiligo, postinflammatory hypopigmentation, idiopathic guttate hypomelanosis	—
Atrophic	Uncommon	Discoid lupus erythematosus, necrobiosis lipoidica diabeticorum	Lesions may progress to ulcers
Ulcerative	Uncommon	Venous stasis ulcers, necrobiosis lipoidica, necrobiotic xanthogranuloma, mycobacterial and deep fungal infection, vasculitic ulcers, superficial pyoderma gangrenosum, superficial ulcerative rheumatoid necrobiosis[50]	May be the presenting sign of sarcoidosis.[65] Extracutaneous disease developed in many of the reported cases[65,66]
Ichthyosiform	Rare	Ichthyosis vulgaris, acquired ichthyosis, pityriasis rotunda	One study estimated that 95% of patients with ichthyosiform sarcoidosis will develop systemic involvement[67]
Erythrodermic	Rare	Erythroderma caused by psoriasis, eczema, pityriasis rubra pilaris, drug eruption, lymphoma/leukemia, or dermatomyositis, chronic graft-vs-host disease	Systemic symptoms such as fever, weight loss, arthralgias, uveitis, and dyspnea may be present[68]
Morpheaform	Rare	Morphea, lichen sclerosus, nephrogenic sclerosing dermopathy	—
Photodistributed	Rare	Polymorphous light eruption, acute LE, photocontact dermatitis, phototoxic eruption, systemic photoallergy, hydroa vacciniforme, chronic actinic dermatitis	—
Sarcoidal alopecia	Rare	Discoid lupus erythematosus, lichen planopilaris, pseudopelade, acne keloidalis, central centrifugal cicatricial alopecia, morphea	Systemic sarcoidosis is present in nearly all reported cases[69]
Oral	Uncommon	Orofacial granulomatosis, Crohn disease, granulomatous infections, foreign body granulomas, perioral dermatitis, granulomatous rosacea[50]	—
Genital sarcoidosis	Rare	Syphilis, lymphogranuloma venereum, Crohn disease, condyloma, genital cancer, foreign body reactions	—
Nail	Rare	Psoriasis, lichen planus, fungal infection, drug eruption, subungual verruca vulgaris	Often signifies chronic systemic sarcoidosis. Nail involvement has been associated with lupus pernio, dactylitis, and bone cysts[70]

Abbreviations: DDX, differential diagnosis; DLE, discoid lupus erythematosus; EN, erythema nodosum; LE, lupus erythematosus; LP, lichen planus; MF, mycosis fungoides; NK, natural killer; SCC, squamous cell carcinoma.

[a] Associations between specific lesions and systemic involvement have been suggested; however, the exact relationship is not fully defined.

Data from Statement on sarcoidosis. Joint Statement of the American Thoracic Society (ATS), the European Respiratory Society (ERS) and the World Association of Sarcoidosis and Other Granulomatous Disorders (WASOG) adopted by the ATS Board of Directors and by the ERS Executive Committee, February 1999. Am J Respir Crit Care Med. 1999;160: 736–55.

Table 3
Some symptoms and manifestations in sarcoidosis

- Constitutional
  - Fatigue
  - Weight loss
  - Fever
  - Night sweats
- Respiratory
  - Chest pain
  - Cough (usually persistent and dry)
  - Dyspnea
  - Wheezing
  - Hemoptysis
  - Clubbing
- Reticuloendothelial
  - Lymphadenopathy, especially hilar
- Upper respiratory
  - Nasal congestion
  - Hoarseness
  - Epistaxis
  - Nasal perforation
- Ocular
  - Burred vision
  - Eye pain
  - Redness
  - Teary eyes
  - Photosensitivity
- Neurologic
  - Headache
  - Cranial nerve (especially VII nerve) palsy
  - Hearing loss
  - Meningitis
  - Seizures
  - Ataxia
  - Cognitive dysfunction
  - Optic neuritis with partial loss of vision and color acuity
- Rheumatologic
  - Osseous sarcoidosis
  - Acute arthritis (most commonly in ankles)
  - Chronic arthritis
  - Psoriaticlike arthritis
  - Axial sarcoidosis
  - Sacroiliitis
  - Periarthritis
  - Costochondritis
  - Myopathy
  - Lupus erythematosus
  - Sjögren syndrome
- Neurologic
  - Headache
  - Cranial nerve (especially VII nerve) palsy
  - Hearing loss
  - Meningitis
  - Seizures
  - Ataxia
  - Cognitive dysfunction
  - Optic neuritis with partial loss of vision and color acuity
- Cardiac
  - Palpitations
  - Arrhythmias
  - Chest pain
  - Congestive heart failure
  - Complete or bundle branch heart block
  - Syncope
  - Pericarditis
  - Orthopnea
  - Sudden death
  - Cardiomyopathy
- Endocrine/metabolic
  - Hypercalcemia
  - Thyroid disease (usually autoimmune)
  - Amenorrhea
  - Bleeding of uterus or cervix
  - Epididymo-orchitis
  - Testicular swelling
  - Adrenal insufficiency
  - Polyuria/polydipsia
- Psychiatric
  - Memory loss
  - Brain fog
  - Depression
  - Psychosis
- Renal
  - Nephrolithiasis
  - Obstructive disease
- Gastrointestinal
  - Hepatomegaly
  - Portal hypertension
  - Cirrhosis
  - Splenomegaly

Note that sarcoid granulomas could develop on any organ tissue.

infiltrate the upper respiratory tract and cause nasal ulceration, septal perforation, and obstruction.[61,78] Less commonly, lupus pernio develops on the dorsal hands, fingers, and toes where it is associated with bone cysts, dystrophic nails, and lytic bone lesions,[2,52] but some cases with exclusive involvement in these have been chilblains pernio. The eruption can be recalcitrant to even aggressive systemic treatment. Patients with lupus pernio invariably have an increased risk of chronic disease lasting more than 2 years[60,77] and progressive systemic disease.[16,77] A clinicoradiologic study found involvement of the intrathoracic area in 74%, upper respiratory tract in 54%, reticuloendothelial system in 54%, eyes in 37%, as well as bone cysts in 43% of lupus pernio cases.[61]

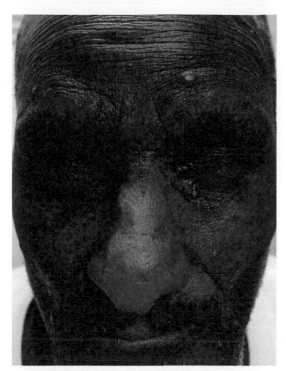

Fig. 1. Papular sarcoidosis presenting with papules on the eyelids, malar cheeks and forehead, some of which coalesce into plaques.

Angiolupoid sarcoidosis is a type of lupus pernio characterized by livid pink to light orange-brown color and numerous, prominent telangiectasias (**Fig. 5**).[53] However, in some reports the term has been loosely used to describe other types of sarcoidosis lesions with telangiectasias.

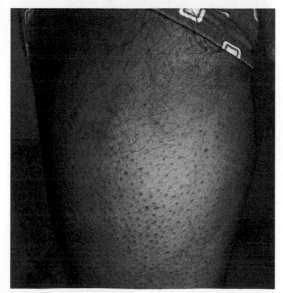

Fig. 2. Annular sarcoidosis plaque resembling tinea corporis and granuloma annulare.

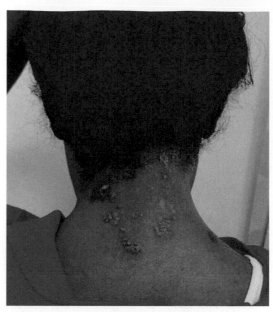

Fig. 3. Verrucous sarcoidosis on the posterior neck.

Unusually high incidences of angiolupoid lesions in some series may have been caused by telangiectatic formation induced by high-potency topical steroid use in regular plaques of sarcoidosis.

Subcutaneous sarcoidosis Subcutaneous sarcoidosis (Darier-Roussy disease) is caused by infiltration of adipose tissue. Single to multiple, asymptomatic to mildly tender, indurated skin colored, panniculitic plaques or nodules characteristically develop on the extremities, particularly the forearms.[62] Subcutaneous sarcoidosis is associated with bilateral hilar lymphadenopathy and nonsevere systemic disease.[4,63] Progression to chronic fibrotic sarcoidosis is rare.[4,63]

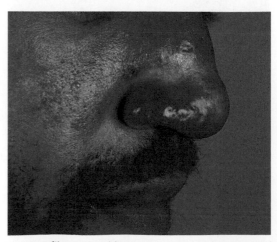

Fig. 4. Infiltrated red-brown plaques on the nose and cheek. Note scars from ulcerations.

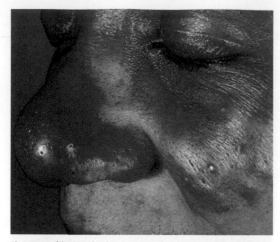

Fig. 5. Infiltrated plaque on the nose with multiple telangiectasias.

Scar sarcoidosis Sarcoidosis may cause granulomatous infiltration of surgical scars, tattoos (**Fig. 6**), skin piercings, acne keloidalis, herpes zoster lesions, and other sites of trauma. This type constitutes between 5.4% and 13.8% of skin sarcoidosis cases.[73,79] Although usually not associated with symptoms other than scar enlargement, rarely scars become painful or itchy. A changing scar in a patient with inactive sarcoidosis may suggest disease reactivation.[79] Scar sarcoidosis may precede or accompany systemic disease.[3] Some studies reported chronic systemic disease in patients with scar sarcoidosis, whereas others have failed to corroborate this finding.[64,80]

Hypopigmented sarcoidosis Hypopigmented sarcoidosis mainly affects dark-skinned patients.[50,81]

Patches and thin papules or plaques with decreased pigmentation are present on physical examination (**Fig. 7**). Erythematous or skin-colored papules near the center of the patch impart a fried-egg appearance. The lesions need to be distinguished from vitiligo, hypopigmented cutaneous T-cell lymphoma, and leprosy. Biopsy of early lesions may fail to reveal typical granulomas but raised hypopigmented lesions show well-formed dermal granulomas.[82,83]

Atrophic and ulcerative sarcoidosis Intact morpheaform hypopigmented, shiny patches, or thin plaques with cigarette paper–like central atrophy is a rare manifestation of skin sarcoidosis.[84] Although usually round or oval, the lesions may also be linear. Differentiation from localized scleroderma may require histopathologic demonstration of epithelioid granulomas within the dermal sclerosis. In the pretibial aspects of the legs, atrophic sclerodermatous plaques with depressed centers assume a necrobiosis lipoidica–like appearance and ulcerate, presumably because of trauma.[65] In one retrospective series, 4.8% of 147 skin sarcoidosis cases had atrophic-ulcerative necrobiosis lipoidica–like plaques.[66] All patients were African American.[66] Papulonodules and other nonatrophic sarcoidosis lesions can become ulcerated. Altogether, between 1% and 5% of skin

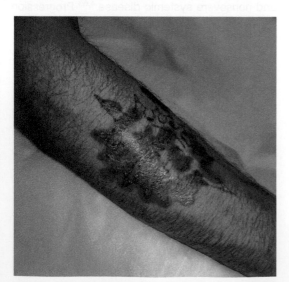

Fig. 6. Sarcoidosis infiltration of a tattoo resulting in induration.

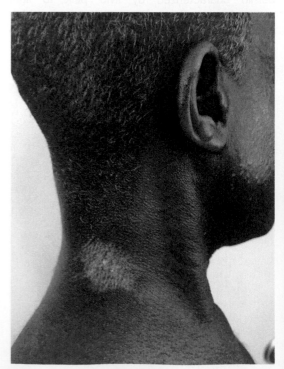

Fig. 7. Hypopigmented sarcoidosis of the posterior neck.

sarcoidosis lesions are ulcerative, predominating in African Americans and Japanese,[16,52] and these lesions can be the presenting manifestation of sarcoidosis.[65,66] Most patients with this type of sarcoidosis have chronic systemic disease.

Ichthyosiform sarcoidosis This rare variant presents with large skin-colored to tan patches with adherent, polygonal, gray or brown thin scale (**Fig. 8**). The skin lesions are usually found on the lower extremities and asymptomatic. Nearly all cases have or develop systemic involvement.[67,85]

Rare variants Other rare types of cutaneous sarcoidosis include the erythrodermic[86] and photodistributed[87] forms.

Scalp sarcoidosis Sarcoidosis alopecia is nearly always scarring and can be patchy or diffuse. Scalp lesions include skin-colored or erythematous patches and plaques that may be mistaken for discoid lupus (especially when follicular plugging is present) and lichen planopilaris (**Fig. 9**).[76] Hypopigmented and atrophic patches that resemble morphea have also been reported. The scalp lesions can also be papules, nodules, and ulcerations.[69] One review of 28 scalp sarcoidosis

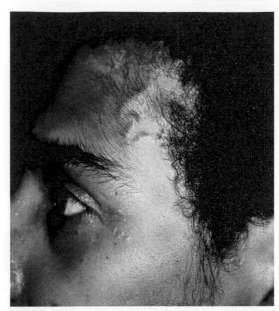

Fig. 9. Frontal band of alopecia with indurated borders.

cases found that 91% were African American and 92% were women.[69] Nearly all cases had lesions in other skin areas as well as systemic disease.[69] The presence of orange spots on trichoscopy has been reported as a possible diagnostic clue for sarcoidosis.[88]

Mucosal sarcoidosis Sarcoidosis may involve the oral, nasal, and genital mucosa. Granulomatous lesions, usually papules or papulonodules, develop on any part of the oral mucosa and presentations vary from infiltrated papules to firm nodules to ulcers (**Fig. 10**).[89,90] Anogenital sarcoidosis, although rare, may manifest with tender indurated papules and nodules, pruritic scaly plaques, or swelling.[91–94]

Nail sarcoidosis Nail manifestations caused by sarcoidosis include subungual hyperkeratosis, pitting, clubbing, onychorrhexis, trachyonychia, splinter hemorrhages, paronychia, pterygium,

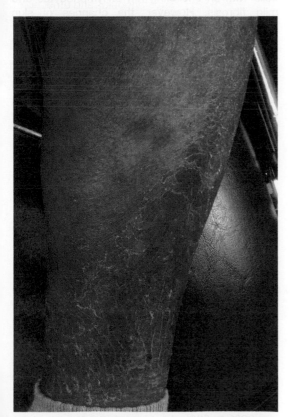

Fig. 8. Biopsy-proven ichthyosiform sarcoidosis with adherent polygonal brown scales on the lower extremity.

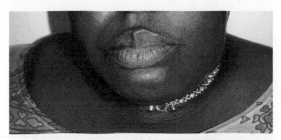

Fig. 10. Sarcoidosis involving the labial vermillion border.

onycholysis, nail plate thinning, dactylitis, longitudinal ridging, and nail bed discoloration.[95–97] A review of 33 cases of nail sarcoidosis reported that bone cysts were present on radiographic imaging in almost half of the cases and that all had systemic involvement.[95] Therefore, radiologic examination and evaluation for systemic disease is warranted in individuals with sarcoidosis nail dystrophy.[70]

NONSPECIFIC CUTANEOUS SARCOIDOSIS
Erythema Nodosum

Occurring in approximately 10% of sarcoidosis cases, EN is the most common nonspecific skin manifestation (**Fig. 11**). On histology, the lesions show a septal panniculitis without granulomas. Patients often experience systemic symptoms such as fever, arthritis, and malaise. In one study, EN was the presentation in 88% of 49 cases of Löfgren syndrome, an acute form of sarcoidosis, characterized by EN, polyarthritis/arthralgias, and bilateral hilar adenopathy with or without parenchymal infiltrates.[98] Notably, some patients with Löfgren syndrome do not develop EN. The prevalence varies according to the population studied, the syndrome being most common in Europeans, especially Scandinavians. Löfgren syndrome

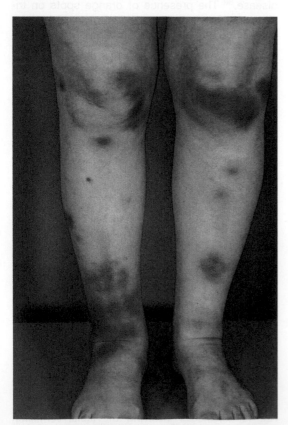

Fig. 11. EN in a patient with Löfgren syndrome.

indicates a favorable prognosis, with studies reporting resolution within 2 years in more than 80% of patients. In a study of 186 patients, the mean age of presentation of Löfgren syndrome was 37 years.[99] Nearly 85% of the cases were in women, and 49% presented in the spring.[99] Standardized high-resolution musculoskeletal ultrasonography shows that the ankle swelling is caused by soft tissue edema and tenosynovitis and that articular synovitis is rare.[100]

Other Nonspecific Cutaneous Eruptions

Sweet syndrome, erythema multiforme, pyoderma gangrenosum, prurigo, calcinosis cutis, vasculitis, and digital clubbing have all been reported to be nonspecific manifestations of sarcoidosis or sarcoidosis-induced organ disease.[50,52]

Histopathology

The histopathologic changes of skin sarcoidosis are characterized by the presence of multiple, discrete, naked, predominantly epithelioid granulomas in the dermis (**Fig. 12**). These granulomas are composed of central collections of epithelioid cells with an encircling rim of lymphocytes and mild fibrosis. However, the changes of skin sarcoidosis are more diverse than was previously recognized and can include tuberculoid granulomas, interstitial granulomas, focal necrosis, elastophagocytosis, linear perineural granulomas resembling leprosy, increased dermal mucin, and lichenoid inflammation, sometimes with plasma cells.[101] Asteroid and Schumann bodies are not specific for sarcoidosis. Also, the presence of birefringent material does not exclude sarcoidosis because foreign bodies may serve as nidi for sarcoidosis granulomas.

SYSTEMIC MANIFESTATIONS

In a recent review of 120 patients with cutaneous sarcoidosis, 64% and 60% of patients with specific and nonspecific skin lesions, respectively, had systemic involvement.[5] Clinical manifestations of systemic sarcoidosis are diverse (see **Table 3**) Approximately one-third of patients present with vague constitutional symptoms such as fatigue, fever, nights sweats, and weight loss.[102]

Pulmonary sarcoidosis is clinically and pathologically the most common manifestation of the disease. At some point, 90% of patients have abnormal chest radiographs (**Table 4**). About two-thirds of cases develop restrictive disease and 30% to 50% also have obstructive changes, but in 80% spirometric findings return to normal within 2 years.[103–105] Pulmonary hypertension is

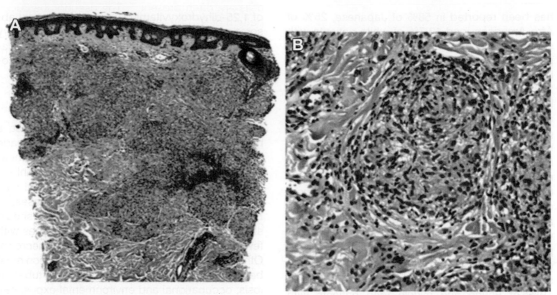

Fig. 12. Typical noncaseating granulomas in a case of sarcoidosis of the skin. (*A*) H&E ×40. (*B*) H&E ×200. (*Courtesy of* Shane Meehan, MD, New York, NY.)

a serious complication that occurs in 1% to 6% of patients overall, usually in symptomatic cases of pulmonary disease.[106] About half of patients with intrathoracic sarcoidosis present with hilar adenopathy (stage I disease) that is bilateral in nearly all cases.[107] In the United States and Europe, respiratory failure accounts for the largest number of sarcoidosis-related deaths.[108,109]

Ocular sarcoidosis occurs in approximately one-third of sarcoidosis cases but 70% of cases with Japanese ancestry.[110,111] At least two-thirds of ocular sarcoidosis cases have anterior uveitis,[112,113] which may be acute or chronic and

insidious. Posterior uveitis occurs in up to 28% of sarcoidosis cases[114,115] and is associated with central nervous system (CNS) involvement.[116] Glaucoma and vision loss are complications of uveitis. Other ocular lesions include lacrimal gland enlargement, conjunctival granulomas, and scleritis.[113] Heerfordt-Waldenström syndrome is characterized by anterior uveitis, parotic gland enlargement, fever, and occasionally facial nerve palsy.[16]

Cardiac sarcoidosis is clinically evident in approximately 5% of sarcoidosis cases,[117] but granulomatous infiltration of the heart

Table 4
Staging of pulmonary sarcoidosis

Stage	Chest Radiograph Finding	CT Scan Finding
Stage I	Hilar lymphadenopathy without lung infiltrate	Lymphadenopathy
Stage II	Lymphadenopathy plus lung infiltrates	Lymphadenopathy with: • Bronchovascular bundles • Reticular patterns • Mass densities infiltrates • Mosaic pattern • Subpleural nodules
Stage III	Only lung infiltrates	Any of the changes listed earlier without lymphadenopathy
Stage IV	Pulmonary fibrosis	Traction bronchiectasis Honeycombing Cysts

Abbreviation: CT, computed tomography.

Adapted from Scadding JG. Prognosis of intrathoracic sarcoidosis in England. A review of 136 cases after five years' observation. Br Med J 1961;2(5261):1165–72.

has been reported in 58% of Japanese, 25% of Afro-American, and 13.7% of white patients with sarcoidosis.[11] Although only 50% to 60% of patients with cardiac sarcoidosis at autopsy have been diagnosed during their lifetimes, 13% to 25% and up to 85% of sarcoidosis-related deaths in the United States and Japan, respectively, are attributed to myocardial involvement.[118,119] Using gadolinium delayed-enhancement cardiovascular magnetic resonance, cardiac involvement was identified in 21 (26%) of 81 prospectively and randomly selected subjects with sarcoidosis (73% African American), in whom coronary disease was excluded by x-ray angiography, although none of the detected abnormalities were specific for cardiac sarcoidosis. Eight of the patients had serious adverse effects, including 5 deaths, within 21 months.[120] A recent Swedish study diagnosed sarcoidosis by cardiac biopsy in 19% of young and middle-aged patients with atrioventricular block in whom no cause could be found.[121] The evaluation and management of cardiac sarcoidosis is outside the scope of this article but excellent reviews have been published recently.[122–124]

CNS sarcoidosis symptoms that are attributable to the disease occur in only 5% to 13% of patients.[125] Any part of the nervous system may be affected.[126] The most common manifestation of neurosarcoidosis is facial nerve palsy.[127] Other presentations include neuroendocrine dysfunction, mass lesions, encephalopathy, seizures, peripheral neuropathy, and cognitive dysfunction.[128,129] Optic neuritis is an emergency that results in permanent blindness.[130] MRI with gadolinium is the preferred imaging modality to diagnose and evaluate the response to treatment of neurosarcoidsois.[129,131]

Hepatic sarcoidosis is at least twice as common in black as in white Americans.[132,133] By computed tomography, 5% of sarcoidosis cases have hepatic lesions and 15% have splenic lesions,[134] but symptomatic liver disease is rare and barely more than 10% of cases have high serum aminotransferase and alkaline phosphatase levels.[17] However, a cholestasis syndrome can be the cause of pruritus with or without jaundice. The presence of constitutional symptoms should prompt consideration of liver involvement.[17] Rare cases of pruritus caused by primary biliary cirrhosis in patients with sarcoidosis have been reported.

Calcium dysregulation is common in sarcoidosis, with hypercalciuria occurring in 40% to 62% and hypercalcemia in 5% to 10% of cases.[135–137] Activated macrophages in sarcoidal granulomas promote conversion of 25-hydroxyvitamin D to 1,25-dihydroxyvitamin D.[17,130] Increased levels of 1,25-dihydroxyvitamin D increase intestinal absorption of calcium, bone resorption, and urinary calcium excretion. This impaired calcium regulation and hypercalciuria can result in nephrocalcinosis and nephrolithiasis.

EVALUATION AND MANAGEMENT

Despite the lack of a specific diagnostic test, a reasonable diagnosis of sarcoidosis can be made with the following 3 criteria: presence of noncaseating granulomas on histology, clinical manifestations and radiographic findings consistent with sarcoidosis, and exclusion of other diseases.[138] Biopsy of a specific cutaneous lesion should show the presence of epithelioid granulomas with few surrounding lymphocytes and absent necrosis. Other causes of granulomatous inflammation must be excluded, including infections such as tuberculosis; occupational and environmental exposures, such as beryllium, zirconium, drug-induced granulomatosis; and cancers with sarcoidal reactions.[10] When no specific skin lesions are present, bronchoalveolar lavage, endobronchial biopsy, or/and transbronchial biopsy are usually necessary to establish a diagnosis of pulmonary sarcoidosis.[10] A biopsy is not required in patients who present with asymptomatic bilateral hilar adenopathy or classic Löfgren syndrome.[10,17] Molecular imaging techniques such as fluorodeoxyglucose PET and MRI are useful tools in the assessment of sarcoidosis.[139] Angiotensin-converting enzyme (ACE) levels have shown to be increased in up to 60% of cases,[17] but serum ACE levels also are increased in other granulomatous diseases and are influenced by genetic polymorphisms, so the value of the test as a diagnostic test and prognostic marker remains limited. Even after correcting for polymorphisms the sensitivity and specificity for a diagnosis of sarcoidosis was 70% and 80%, respectively.[140]

Sarcoidosis has a variable course and organ involvement may occur at any point in the disease. There are no guidelines delineating the extent and frequency of systemic assessment in cases of cutaneous sarcoidosis but, in addition to treating skin disease, evaluation for the development of systemic disease through a review of systems during every visit is warranted.[130] **Box 1** lists the recommended initial evaluation of patients with sarcoidosis.[1]

Treatment

Support for most treatments of skin sarcoidosis is based often on observational studies, uncontrolled prospective studies, small case series, individual case reports, and opinions of respected authorities (**Table 5**). However, results of studies with well-conceived methodologies evaluating therapeutic effect on the pulmonary system have been adopted to support the use of pharmacologic agents in other organs, including the skin. In general, treatment is directed at abolishing, or at least limiting, the inflammatory response, especially the effect of TNF-α, which is integral in the formation and organization of granulomas.[170] Some immunosuppressive agents, including methotrexate, leflunomide, and thalidomide, indirectly inhibit TNF-α release. Biologic TNF-α antagonists, in particular infliximab, have been effective even in corticosteroid-resistant cases.[143] A therapeutic algorithm for the treatment of cutaneous sarcoidosis based on the limited published literature, reviewed later, and personal experience is included in **Fig. 13**.[16]

TOPICAL AND INTRALESIONAL THERAPY

Topical and intralesional corticosteroids are considered the treatment of choice for limited cutaneous sarcoidosis, although data showing their efficacy are limited. Medium-potency to high-potency corticosteroids can be effective, although the best clinical results are obtained with intralesional injections. Ultrapotent topical corticosteroids can be applied to lesions twice daily, carefully observing for atrophy. Thin papules and plaques may respond to corticosteroids of lesser potency. Intralesional corticosteroids offer the advantage of higher drug concentration in the dermis where granulomas are present and are especially valuable for nodules and lesions resistant to topical medications.[144,171] Improvement in lupus pernio without atrophy or dyschromia was achieved with halobetasol proprionate 0.05% ointment twice daily[141] and in 3 patients with papulonodules using clobetasol proprionate 0.05% cream under hydrocolloid dressing occlusion weekly.[142]

Tacrolimus ointment has also been reported to be effective in several case reports and may be used as monotherapy or, based on the disparate mechanisms of action, together with topical/intralesional corticosteroids, although such use is not supported by clinical trials.[172]

Systemic Agents

Systemic treatment of skin sarcoidosis may not be necessary unless the disease is symptomatic, rapidly progressive, disfiguring, or unresponsive to topical therapy, especially if psychological stability or quality of life is compromised.[1,16] The disease may spontaneously remit.

Oral Glucocorticosteroids

Systemic corticosteroids serve as the mainstay of therapy. However, trials evaluating their effects on lung function have yielded mixed results.[145,146] In a study of lupus pernio, the most therapeutically recalcitrant among the common skin types, in which a dose of 20 to 40 mg/d of prednisone equivalent was administered, Stagaki and colleagues[147] reported improvement in 72% and 56% of cases treated with steroid monotherapy and steroid plus either hydroxychloroquine or methotrexate, respectively, and resolution or near resolution in 20% and 29% of cases treated with steroid monotherapy and steroid plus another agent, respectively.[147] However, it is surprising that only 39% of cases had nasal lesions. No controlled study has examined the optimal dose, duration, or tapering method. In our practice prednisone at 0.5 mg/kg/d or methylprednisolone at 0.4 mg/kg/d is initiated generally but the dose is influenced by factors, such as comorbidities; if satisfactory improvement has not occurred after 2 weeks the dose is escalated to 1 mg/kg/d of prednisone equivalent, while simultaneously initiating another agent that is individually effective in skin sarcoidosis and has steroid-sparing effects (see later discussion). Once improvement occurs, the dose of prednisone is decreased by 5 to 10 mg per week to the lowest dose of prednisone that prevents recurrence. Although systemic glucocorticoids usually effect swift improvement of most cases of systemic sarcoidosis, relapse commonly occurs.[65,145] However, these agents should be avoided unless absolutely necessary or administered for short periods because, even at low doses, corticosteroids result in weight gain, skin thinning, sleep disturbance, osteoporosis, and neuropsychiatric disorders.[2,16,173]

Methotrexate

Methotrexate, a folate analogue, is the preferred agent for steroid sparing and one of 2 for monotherapy for systemic treatment of skin disease.[146] Anti-inflammatory effects probably stem from release of adenosine, which in low doses not only inhibits lymphocyte proliferation but also suppresses TNF-α release from monocytes, macrophages, and neutrophils. Methotrexate is effective alone or combined with either steroids or other therapies,[52,150,174] such as antimalarials, although these agents reduce methotrexate bioavailability. A Delphi study of sarcoidosis experts found that methotrexate was the preferred second-line therapy for pulmonary sarcoidosis.[175] In one nonrandomized interventional study of 50 subjects treated with 10 mg of methotrexate weekly for 2 or more years,

Table 5
Therapies for cutaneous sarcoidosis

Treatment	Usual Dose	Indications	Main Potential Side Effects	Level of Evidence
Topical corticosteroids[141,142]	Twice daily application	Limited and discrete papules, plaques, and nodules	Atrophy, striae, purpura, hypopigmentation, telangiectasias, acne-folliculitis, suppression of the hypothalamic-pituitary-adrenal axis	C
Intralesional triamcinolone[143,144]	5–10 mg/mL, every 3–4 wk until resolution	Limited and discrete papules, plaques, and nodules	Same as listed earlier	C
Oral corticosteroid[145–147]	Initial: 0.5 – 1 mg/kg/d of prednisone equivalent; gradually taper to the lowest effective dose	Widespread, disfiguring, chronic, or lesions refractory to local therapy	Steroid folliculitis, weight gain, mood disturbance, gastrointestinal upset, hypertension, diabetes mellitus, osteoporosis, aseptic vascular necrosis	C
Chloroquine[148]	250–750 mg daily dose Maximum dose is 3.5 mg/kg/d	Steroid-sparing agent or monotherapy Effective in most lesions	Corneal deposits, retinopathy (risk decreases if doses are <3.5 mg/kg/d and no renal disease is present), gastrointestinal distress, neurologic and hematologic abnormalities	C
Hydroxychloroquine[149]	200–400 mg daily dose Maximum dose is 6.5 mg/kg/d	Same as for chloroquine	Same as listed earlier but less corneal, lenticular, and uveal toxicity than chloroquine. The risk of retinopathy decreases if doses are <6.5 mg/kg/d and no renal disease is present	C
Methotrexate[150–152]	7.5–25 mg/wk orally, SQ or IM. May taper dose once improvement occurs. Maintenance dose may be administered biweekly	Corticosteroid-sparing agent or as a monotherapy in patients unable to take steroid	Hepatotoxicity, pulmonary fibrosis, hematologic abnormalities, immunosuppression, teratogenic, mucositis, and nausea Folic acid supplementation may reduce toxicity	C

Drug	Dose	Indication	Adverse effects	Evidence
Minocycline[153,154]	Minocycline, 200 mg/d; Tetracycline, 1000 mg/d	May be helpful in selected cases	Phototoxicity, dizziness, gastrointestinal upset, hypersensitivity reactions, vulvovaginal candidiasis, tooth discoloration, and bone deposition; contraindicated for children <8 y old and pregnant women	D
Leflunomide[155,156]	20 mg/d. Some start with loading dose of 100 mg/d for 3 d	Refractory skin disease	Gastrointestinal disturbance, hematologic abnormalities, hypersensitivity skin reactions, and immunosuppression	D
Thalidomide[157-160]	50-400 mg/d (usually 50-150 mg)	Refractory skin disease	Teratogenicity, peripheral neuropathy, sedation, nausea, neutropenia, and venous thrombosis	D
Infliximab[147,161-163]	3-7 mg/kg IV at 0, 2, and 6 wk (3-10 mg/kg) and then every 6 wk. Dose and interval may then be adjusted depending on the response	Widespread disease, disfiguring and/or refractory lesions. We recommend it as second-line therapy in steroid-unresponsive lupus pernio	Infection, including tuberculosis reactivation and those caused by opportunistic organisms, allergic reactions (including anaphylaxis), lymphoma, solid organ malignancy, and demyelinating diseases	C
Adalimumab[164-166]	40 mg every 1-2 wk	Widespread disease, disfiguring and/or refractory lesions	Infection, including tuberculosis reactivation and those caused by opportunistic organisms, headache, nausea, injection site reaction, lymphoma, solid organ malignancy, and demyelinating diseases	C
Golimumab	200 mg at week 0, 100 mg every 4 wk thereafter	Widespread disease, disfiguring and/or refractory lesions	Infection, including tuberculosis reactivation and those caused by opportunistic organisms, lymphoma	D
Azathioprine	50-200 mg daily	Cutaneous disease refractory to standard therapy	Liver and renal abnormalities, skin carcinoma, infections, gastrointestinal effects, and neutropenia	D

(continued on next page)

Table 5
(continued)

Treatment	Usual Dose	Indications	Main Potential Side Effects	Level of Evidence
Fumaric acid esters	2 tablets (30 mg dimethyl fumarate; 75 mg monoethyl fumarate) increasing over next 8 wk to maximum of 6 tablets divided into 3 doses daily	Cutaneous disease unresponsive to topical therapy	In two-thirds, diarrhea, stomach cramps, fullness and flatulence; flushing in one-third	D
Mycophenolate mofetil[167]	30 to 45 mg/kg divided into 3 doses per day (MMF plasma trough 1–3 mg/L)	Cutaneous disease refractory to corticosteroids and standard therapy	Hyperglycemia, gastrointestinal upset, bone marrow suppression, and hypercholesterolemia	D
Pentoxifylline[168]	400 mg 3 times daily	Cutaneous disease refractory to corticosteroids and standard therapy	Nausea, arrhythmia, and hypersensitivity reaction	D
Apremilast[169]	20 mg twice daily then decrease to 20 mg daily	Efficacy and safety of apremilast in chronic cutaneous sarcoidosis	Gastrointestinal upset, headache, cough, and hypersensitivity reaction	D

C, case-control study or retrospective study; D, case series or case reports.

Abbreviations: IM, intramuscular; IV, intravenous; MMF, mycophenolate mofetil; SQ, subcutaneous.

Adapted from Lodha S, Sanchez M, Prystowsky S. Sarcoidosis of the skin: a review for the pulmonologist. Chest. 2009;136(2):583–96; and Haimovic A, Sanchez M, Judson MA, et al. Sarcoidosis: a comprehensive review and update for the dermatologist: part I. Cutaneous disease. J Am Acad Dermatol. 2012;66(5):699.e1–18.

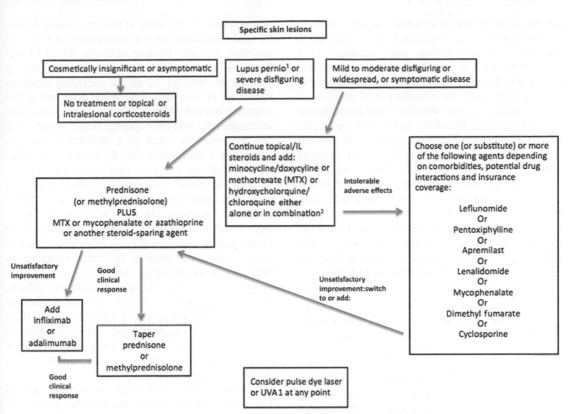

Fig. 13. Suggested algorithm for the treatment of cutaneous sarcoidosis. A study suggested that lupus pernio responds poorly to regimens that do not contain systemic corticosteroids or infliximab. If lupus pernio is moderate to severe (disfiguring, ulcerating), expedite treatment with systemic corticosteroids plus steroid-sparing agent and, if response is not satisfactory, administer infliximab. In the rheumatologic literature, studies have suggested that these combinations achieve improve results compared with monotherapy with either agent. UVA, ultraviolet A. (*Data from* Dale J, Alcom N, Capell H, et al. Combination therapy for rheumatoid arthritis: methotrexate and sulfasalazine together or with other DMARDs. Nat Clin Pract Rheumatol 2007;3(8):450–8.)

skin lesions regressed in 16 of the 17 patients.[151] A more recent retrospective analysis of 26 cases analyzed the efficacy of low-dose methotrexate monotherapy. Of the 11 patients with cutaneous sarcoidosis treated with 7.5 mg of methotrexate weekly, 37% reported improvement in skin lesions.[152] A drawback to methotrexate use is that a therapeutic response takes 4 to 8 weeks and occasionally as long as 6 months.[150] Relapse frequently occurs after discontinuation so low-dose maintenance therapy is often necessary.[52,151]

Antimalarial Agents

Antimalarial agents, such as chloroquine and hydroxychloroquine, are the other favored agents when systemic treatment is required. In cases in which a prompt response is not required, treatment with an antimalarial is begun. Antimalarials are also used in patients treated with glucocorticoids to reduce the dose. Improvement with

antimalarials is not seen for 4 to 6 weeks[149] and the effect is predominantly suppressive.[148] An open-label study in 14 patients treated with chloroquine showed improvement in skin lesions; 9 of the 13 patients available for follow-up relapsed.[148] Although some patients are unable to tolerate these drugs because of nausea (which may improve by taking the medication with food), other gastrointestinal symptoms, hematologic abnormalities, and neurologic disease, serious side effects are rare.[52,146] Routine ophthalmologic examinations are needed to evaluate for corneal deposits and retinopathy, which are rare with doses of chloroquine less than 3.5 mg/kg/d and hydroxychloroquine less than 6.5 mg/kg/d.

Minocycline

Tetracycline derivatives may be effective[52,146] alone or combined with corticosteroids[146,153,174] in the treatment of cutaneous sarcoidosis by suppressing granuloma formation or through an antimicrobial effect on infectious agents such as propionibacteria or mycobacteria.[176] Complete resolution of skin lesions was achieved in 8 patients (67%) and partial resolution in 2 patients (17%) with skin lesions treated with minocycline, 100 mg twice daily for a median of 12 months.[153] In 3 patients who had relapsed after discontinuation of treatment, the skin lesions improved again with readministration of minocycline.[153] In a recent retrospective review, 20 of 27 (74%) patients with non–lupus pernio cutaneous sarcoidosis responded to minocycline treatment.[154] Of these, 2 were being treated with concomitant oral corticosteroids for pulmonary disease, 18 received minocycline as first-line therapy, and 9 received minocycline as second-line treatment.[154] The advantage of tetracycline derivatives is their low side effect profile over long periods of time.

Leflunomide

Reports have heralded the efficacy of leflunomide, a pyrimidine synthetase inhibitor, alone or in combination with methotrexate, as a therapy for recalcitrant cutaneous sarcoidosis.[145,155,156] Some clinicians recommend a loading dose of 100 mg daily followed by 20 mg daily, but this loading dose significantly increases the rate of adverse events.[145] Leflunomide is thought to have a superior side effect profile to methotrexate and may be a promising nonsteroidal agent.[145,155]

TUMOR NECROSIS FACTOR ALPHA INHIBITORS

Small case series and case reports have described beneficial responses in corticosteroid-resistant cutaneous sarcoidosis, usually between 1 to 5 months after initiation of treatment with doses of 100 to 200 mg of thalidomide.[157–160,177] Often, responders relapse after thalidomide discontinuation.[159,160] A more recently published, multicenter, randomized, double-blind, placebo-controlled investigator-masked study that included an intent-to-treat population of 39 subjects with clinical and biopsy confirmed cutaneous sarcoidosis did not achieve complete responses after 3 months of thalidomide at a dose of 100 mg daily and, similarly to the control group, 21% had partial responses.[178] Despite this disappointing outcome, it is possible that more prolonged and/or higher doses of thalidomide may achieve better results, particularly since a non-controlled study with less precise methodology found that the percentage of complete responses induced by thalidomide in the subjects with cutaneous sarcoidosis rose from 32% at 3 months to 67% at 6 months, respectively.[160] Notably, in the open-label follow up trial conducted at the conclusion of the prospective 3 month Droitcourt study, 11 of 14 patients who remained on thalidomide for 6 months as well as 10 of 14 receiving placebo improved or very well improved, suggesting the possible benefit of time. Besides concern about teratogenicity and neuropathy, major drawbacks are the need to enroll in a restricted program under the Thalidomide Risk Evaluation and Mitigation Strategy program and reluctance for insurance to cover because the drug does not have regulatory approval for sarcoidosis. After 3 months, lenalidomide, a thalidomide analogue, significantly improved a patient with ulcerative lupus pernio unresponsive to high-dose prednisone who was unable to take thalidomide because of neuropathy. This analogue is promising because its immunomodulatory effects and downregulation of TNF secretion exceed those of thalidomide with a safer adverse effect profile.[179] No studies have been conducted with the other US Food and Drug Administration (FDA)–approved analogue pomalidomide, which is an even more potent analogue.

Biologics with TNF-inhibiting activity are a welcome addition to the therapeutic armamentarium of sarcoidosis. However, because this agent has not received FDA approval for sarcoidosis, obtaining insurance coverage can be challenging. Small series and cases reports have described encouraging results for infliximab in cutaneous disease.[161–163,180] Inflammatory serum proteins (macrophage inflammatory protein 1 beta [MIP-1β] and TNF-RII) that remained at increased levels during steroid treatment normalized with infliximab. In one open trial of 10 patients with systemic sarcoidosis, all 5 cases with lupus pernio had dramatic improvement of the lesions.[181] In 5 of the 6 patients who were simultaneously receiving corticosteroids, the prednisone dose was reduced.[181] A larger retrospective study of 54 patients with lupus pernio showed that therapeutic regimens containing infliximab were superior to corticosteroids at a prednisone-equivalent dose of 20 to 40 mg alone or combined with methotrexate or hydroxychloroquine for the treatment of lupus pernio.[147] Remissions are often induced but patients relapse after discontinuation of treatment, therefore continuation of infliximab at an adjusted dose is recommended.[182] Adalimumab, a humanized monoclonal antibody, was evaluated for safety and efficacy in a double-blind, randomized, placebo-controlled study of cutaneous sarcoidosis.[164] Select patients were on other systemic agents during the trial. The first 12 weeks of the study were blinded and 10 patients received adalimumab and 5 received placebo. Although not statistically significant, 5 of 10 patients in the adalimumab group versus 1 of 5 patients in the placebo group showed improvement in their skin lesions. During the open-label portion of the trial, 10 of the 13 remaining participants received adalimumab and reported benefit.[164] Etanercept, a soluble TNF receptor, is less effective in sarcoidosis than infliximab and adalimumab[183,184] and is the most likely TNF-α antagonist to induce sarcoidosislike granulomatosis (**Table 6**).[40,185,186] Golimumab, a chimeric monoclonal antibody against CD20, was reported to help ocular disease but was disappointing in pulmonary disease. Neither golimumab nor ustekinumab produced beneficial effects in chronic pulmonary sarcoidosis but improvement in the Skin Physician Global Assessment of patients with cutaneous sarcoidosis with or without pulmonary involvement was recorded at 28 weeks in subjects treated with golimumab, suggesting that this agent should be further investigated in skin sarcoidosis.[187]

ANTIBIOTICS

By choosing antimycobacterial agents that target genes encoding mycobacterial products within sarcoidosis (rpoB [rifampin] and DNA gyrase A [levofloxacin]), Drake and colleagues[35,188] devised a broad antimycobacterial regimen of 4 concomitantly administered antibiotics (levofloxacin, ethambutol, azithromycin, and rifampin). The favorable results reported in 2 recent studies provide indirect but intriguing support for a role of microorganisms in the cause of sarcoidosis. In an open-label, single-center study of 15 cases with pulmonary sarcoidosis, the investigators reported forced vital capacity improvement in the 8 patients who were able to tolerate the treatment without adverse effects requiring discontinuation.[35] The same investigators conducted a placebo-controlled, single-masked trial that randomized 30 subjects with symptomatic chronic cutaneous sarcoidosis to receive 8 weeks of the antimycobacterial regimen or placebo. Immunosuppressive agents were continued in 4 of the subjects in the antimycobacterial group and 8 in the placebo group. In the intention-to-treat analysis, the mean reduction in diameter of the antimycobacterial group index lesions was 8.4 mm, compared with a mean increase of 0.07 mm in the placebo group. The disease severity, measured by erythema, induration, and desquamation, also decreased in the antimycobacterial group.[188]

OTHER PHARMACOLOGIC AGENTS

Five patients refractory to standard therapies improved on mycophenolate mofetil and the dose of prednisone was decreased.[167] Pentoxifylline, a phosphodiesterase type 4 (PDE4) inhibitor, has been used to manage pulmonary sarcoidosis. Apremilast, a novel PDE4 inhibitor, prevents the synthesis of proinflammatory cytokines and chemokines, including TNF-α.[169] Significant reduction of lesion induration in 15 patients with chronic refractory cutaneous sarcoidosis was reported after 12 weeks of treatment with apremilast. However, treatment had no effect on erythema, desquamation, or scaling. Three patients relapsed within 3 months of apremilast discontinuation.[169] Anecdotal reports documenting improvement of cutaneous sarcoidosis with isotretinoin[189,190] and with allopurinol have been published.[191] Case reports have described improvement of steroid-refractory lung function during cyclosporine therapy but a randomized trial found no benefit as a steroid-sparing agent and increased complications.[192] Cyclophosphamide resulted in improvement of cardiac and CNS sarcoidosis, as well as some pulmonary patients in case reports. Mycophenolate mofetil may have a beneficial effect as a steroid-sparing agent and possibly alone, although documentation of its effects in cutaneous sarcoidosis is scant.[193] In an international retrospective cohort study, azathioprine was as effective a steroid-sparing agent as methotrexate in cases of pulmonary sarcoidosis, although it had

Table 6			
Skin sarcoidosis during TNF inhibitor therapy			
TNF Inhibitor	**Etanercept**	**Adalimumab**	**Infliximab**
Number of Cases	5 cases	1 case	3 cases
Type of Lesion	3 nodules, 2 plaques	EN, nodules	2 nodules, 1 plaque
Duration of Therapy	1–21 mo	21 mo	14–23 mo
Outcome	Resolution	Clinical but not radiologic resolution	Resolution

a higher rate of infection.[194] Dimethyl fumarate was recently approved by the FDA for multiple sclerosis, and has been reported to improve or clear cutaneous sarcoidosis cases, some of which were recalcitrant to other therapies.[195]

In few but noteworthy case reports, phototherapy had a beneficial effect. After a total dose of 2640 J/cm^2 of medium dose ultraviolet A1 (UVA1) given over 50 sessions, nearly complete resolution of plaque sarcoidosis involving 70% of the body surface was achieved without systemic medications,[196] whereas improvement but no resolution of papulonodular sarcoidosis in the forehead resulted from a UVA1 dose of 2460 J/cm^2 administered during 25 treatments.[197] In a small case series of 6 patients unresponsive to topical and systemic medications, there was complete resolution in 3 cases and 50% improvement in another 3 with a mean dose of 58.8 J/cm^2 given over a mean of 50 sessions. All patients received systemic steroids at the start of phototheapy.[198]

Case reports have described improvement or resolution of skin lesions, especially popular and nodular sarcoidosis, scar sarcoidosis, and lupus pernio,[199] with several lasers, including pulsed dye laser (PDL),[200–202] carbon dioxide (CO_2),[203,204] neodymium:yttrium aluminum garnet,[205] and Q-switched ruby lasers.[206] In one of these reports, significant improvement of lupus pernio recalcitrant to systemic steroids and steroid-sparing agents was achieved with PDL therapy followed by nonablative fractional resurfacing.[207] However, ulceration after PDL treatment[208] and induction of sarcoidal lesions after CO_2 laser ablation[209] have also been reported.

Surgery is usually not recommended for the treatment of cutaneous sarcoidosis because of the potential for recurrence, graft loss, and poor cosmetic results. However, there have been sporadically reported cases of surgical excision with acceptable results, especially in destructive or disfiguring lesions affecting the nose.[210–212]

SUMMARY

The diverse manifestations of sarcoidosis and its expansive scope of disease severity rank it as one of medicine's most convincing imitators. Although significant advances have been made in genetics, immunology, and treatment of sarcoidosis, physicians and scientists remain baffled by the etiopathogenesis of the disease. TNF inhibitors are a promising addition to the disease armamentarium but optimal therapeutic management remains unstandardized, and randomized, double-blind, controlled trials are needed to better guide management. In addition to treating skin disease that can be widespread, disfiguring, symptomatic, and quality of life impairing, dermatologists facilitate the diagnosis of systemic sarcoidosis through skin biopsy, thus eliminating the potential complications incurred in more invasive diagnostic procedures. It must always be remembered that sarcoidosis is a systemic disease and the absence of symptoms does not preclude organ damage, therefore dermatologists caring for patients with sarcoidosis should perform systemic evaluation or collaborate with internists or pulmonologists with experience in sarcoidosis. We have seen several patients in whom the skin disease was successfully treated and the patient developed life-threatening systemic disease after failing to keep appointments. Also, several patients divulged symptoms, such as palpitations, increasing fatigue, cough, and visual changes, but delayed contacting their internists. Dermatologists are essential members of the team in cases with multisystem disease and can provide sole care for patients with only cutaneous sarcoidosis as long as development of systemic disease is regularly evaluated.

REFERENCES

1. Hunninghake GW, Costabel U, Ando M, et al. ATS/ERS/WASOG statement on sarcoidosis. American Thoracic Society/European Respiratory Society/World Association of Sarcoidosis and other Granulomatous Disorders. Sarcoidosis Vasc Diffuse Lung Dis 1999;16(2):149–73.
2. Lodha S, Sanchez M, Prystowsky S. Sarcoidosis of the skin: a review for the pulmonologist. Chest 2009;136(2):583–96.
3. English JC 3rd, Patel PJ, Greer KE. Sarcoidosis. J Am Acad Dermatol 2001;44(5):725–43 [quiz: 744–6].
4. Marcoval J, Mañá J, Rubio M. Specific cutaneous lesions in patients with systemic sarcoidosis: relationship to severity and chronicity of disease. Clin Exp Dermatol 2011;36(7):739–44.
5. Yanardag H, Tetikkurt C, Bilir M, et al. Diagnosis of cutaneous sarcoidosis; clinical and the prognostic significance of skin lesions. Multidiscip Respir Med 2013;8(1):26.
6. Bresnitz EA, Strom BL. Epidemiology of sarcoidosis. Epidemiol Rev 1983;5:124–56.
7. Rybicki BA, Major M, Popovich J Jr, et al. Racial differences in sarcoidosis incidence: a 5-year study in a health maintenance organization. Am J Epidemiol 1997;145(3):234–41.
8. Hillerdal G, Nöu E, Osterman K, et al. Sarcoidosis: epidemiology and prognosis. A 15-year European study. Am Rev Respir Dis 1984;130(1):29–32.
9. Marchell RM, Judson MA. Cutaneous sarcoidosis. Semin Respir Crit Care Med 2010;31(4):442–51.

10. Valeyre D, Prasse A, Nunes H, et al. Sarcoidosis. Lancet 2014;383(9923):1155–67.

11. Iwai K, Sekiguti M, Hosoda Y, et al. Racial difference in cardiac sarcoidosis incidence observed at autopsy. Sarcoidosis 1994;11(1):26–31.

12. Morimoto T, Azuma A, Abe S, et al. Epidemiology of sarcoidosis in Japan. Eur Respir J 2008;31(2): 372–9.

13. Swigris JJ, Olson AL, Huie TJ, et al. Sarcoidosis-related mortality in the United States from 1988 to 2007. Am J Respir Crit Care Med 2011;183(11): 1524–30.

14. Cozier YC, Berman JS, Palmer JR, et al. Sarcoidosis in black women in the United States: data from the Black Women's Health Study. Chest 2011;139(1):144–50.

15. Miyara M, Amoura Z, Parizot C, et al. The immune paradox of sarcoidosis and regulatory T cells. J Exp Med 2006;203(2):359–70.

16. Haimovic A, Sanchez M, Judson MA, et al. Sarcoidosis: a comprehensive review and update for the dermatologist: part I. Cutaneous disease. J Am Acad Dermatol 2012;66(5):699.e1–18 [quiz: 717–8].

17. Iannuzzi MC, Rybicki BA, Teirstein AS. Sarcoidosis. N Engl J Med 2007;357(21):2153–65.

18. Loke WJ, Herbert C, Thomas PS. Sarcoidosis: immunopathogenesis and immunological Markers. International Journal of Chronic Diseases 2013; vol. 2013, Article ID 928601, 13 pages, 2013. http://dx. doi.org/10.1155/2013/928601.

19. Baughman RP, Lower EE, du Bois RM. Sarcoidosis. Lancet 2003;361(9363):1111–8.

20. Judson MA, Marchel RM, Maschelli MA, et al. Molecular profiling and gene expression analysis in cutaneous sarcoidosis: the role of interleukin-12, interleukin-23, and the T-helper 17 pathway. J Am Acad Dermatol 2012;66(6):901–10.

21. Zaba LC, Smith GP, Sanchez M, et al. Dendritic cells in the pathogenesis of sarcoidosis. Am J Respir Cell Mol Biol 2010;42(1):32–9.

22. Huang H, Lu Z, Jiang C, et al. Imbalance between Th17 and regulatory T-Cells in sarcoidosis. Int J Mol Sci 2013;14(11):21463–73.

23. Newman KL, Newman LS. Occupational causes of sarcoidosis. Curr Opin Allergy Clin Immunol 2012; 12(2):145–50.

24. Chen ES, Moller DR. Etiology of sarcoidosis. Clin Chest Med 2008;29(3):365–77, vii.

25. Barnard J, Rose C, Newman L, et al. Job and industry classifications associated with sarcoidosis in A Case-Control Etiologic Study of Sarcoidosis (ACCESS). J Occup Environ Med 2005;47(3):226–34.

26. Jordan HT, Stellman SD, Prezant D, et al. Sarcoidosis diagnosed after September 11, 2001, among adults exposed to the World Trade Center disaster. J Occup Environ Med 2011;53(9):966–74.

27. Crowley LE, Herbert R, Moline JM, et al. "Sarcoid like" granulomatous pulmonary disease in World Trade Center disaster responders. Am J Ind Med 2011;54(3):175–84.

28. Morgenthau AS, Iannuzzi MC. Recent advances in sarcoidosis. Chest 2011;139(1):174–82.

29. Song Z, Marzilli L, Greenlee BM, et al. Mycobacterial catalase-peroxidase is a tissue antigen and target of the adaptive immune response in systemic sarcoidosis. J Exp Med 2005;201(5): 755–67.

30. Allen SS, Evans W, Carlisle J, et al. Superoxide dismutase A antigens derived from molecular analysis of sarcoidosis granulomas elicit systemic Th-1 immune responses. Respir Res 2008;9:36.

31. Chen ES, Wahlström J, Song Z, et al. T cell responses to mycobacterial catalase-peroxidase profile a pathogenic antigen in systemic sarcoidosis. J Immunol 2008;181(12):8784–96.

32. Brownell I, Ramírez-Valle F, Sanchez M, et al. Evidence for mycobacteria in sarcoidosis. Am J Respir Cell Mol Biol 2011;45(5):899–905.

33. Oswald-Richter KA, Beachboard DC, Zhan X, et al. Multiple mycobacterial antigens are targets of the adaptive immune response in pulmonary sarcoidosis. Respir Res 2010;11:161.

34. Oswald-Richter KA, Beachboard DC, Seeley EH, et al. Dual analysis for mycobacteria and propionibacteria in sarcoidosis BAL. J Clin Immunol 2012; 32(5):1129–40.

35. Drake W, Richmond BW, Oswald-Richter K, et al. Effects of broad-spectrum antimycobacterial therapy on chronic pulmonary sarcoidosis. Sarcoidosis Vasc Diffuse Lung Dis 2013;30(3):201–11.

36. Tillie-Leblond I, Grenouillet F, Reboux G, et al. Hypersensitivity pneumonitis and metalworking fluids contaminated by mycobacteria. Eur Respir J 2011;37(3):640–7.

37. Eishi Y. Etiologic link between sarcoidosis and Propionibacterium acnes. Respir Investig 2013;51(2): 56–68.

38. Tercelj M, Salobir B, Zupancic M, et al. Antifungal medication is efficient in the treatment of sarcoidosis. Ther Adv Respir Dis 2011;5(3):157–62.

39. Lamrock E, Brown P. Development of cutaneous sarcoidosis during treatment with tumour necrosis alpha factor antagonists. Australas J Dermatol 2012;53(4):e87–90.

40. Tong D, Manolios N, Howe G, et al. New onset sarcoid-like granulomatosis developing during anti-TNF therapy: an under-recognised complication. Intern Med J 2012;42(1):89–94.

41. Smith G, Brownell I, Sanchez M, et al. Advances in the genetics of sarcoidosis. Clin Genet 2008;73(5): 401–12.

42. Familial Associations in Sarcoidosis. A report to the Research Committee of the British Thoracic

and Tuberculosis Association. Tubercle 1973;54(2): 87–98.

43. Rybicki BA, Iannuzzi MC, Frederick MM, et al. Familial aggregation of sarcoidosis. A Case-Control Etiologic Study of Sarcoidosis (ACCESS). Am J Respir Crit Care Med 2001;164(11):2085–91.

44. Kishore A, Petrek M. Immunogenetics of sarcoidosis. Int Trends Immun 2013;1(4):43–53.

45. Adrianto I, Lin CP, Hale JJ, et al. Genome-wide association study of African and European Americans implicates multiple shared and ethnic specific loci in sarcoidosis susceptibility. PLoS One 2012;7: e43907.

46. Rybicki BA, Levin AM, McKeigue P, et al. A genome-wide admixture scan for ancestry-linked genes predisposing to sarcoidosis in African-Americans. Genes Immun 2011;12(2):67–77.

47. Wijnen PA, Voorter CE, Nelemans PJ, et al. Butyrophilin-like 2 in pulmonary sarcoidosis: a factor for susceptibility and progression? Hum Immunol 2011;72(4):342–7.

48. Rybicki BA, Walewski JL, Maliarik MJ, et al, ACCESS Research Group. The BTNL2 gene and sarcoidosis susceptibility in African Americans and Whites. Am J Hum Genet 2005;77(3):491–9.

49. Hofmann S, Franke A, Fischer A, et al. Genome-wide association study identifies ANXA11 as a new susceptibility locus for sarcoidosis. Nat Genet 2008;40(9):1103–6.

50. Fernandez-Faith E, McDonnell J. Cutaneous sarcoidosis: differential diagnosis. Clin Dermatol 2007;25(3):276–87.

51. Mañá J, Marcoval J, Graells J, et al. Cutaneous involvement in sarcoidosis. Relationship to systemic disease. Arch Dermatol 1997;133(7):882–8.

52. Mañá J, Marcoval J. Skin manifestations of sarcoidosis. Presse Med 2012;41(6 Pt 2):e355–74.

53. Arias-Santiago S, Santiago SA, Fernández-Pugnaire MA, et al. Recurrent telangiectasias on the cheek: angiolupoid sarcoidosis. Am J Med 2010; 123(1):e7–8.

54. Glass LA, Apisarnthanarax P. Verrucous sarcoidosis simulating hypertrophic lichen planus. Int J Dermatol 1989;28(8):539–41.

55. Pezzetta S, Zarian H, Agostini C, et al. Verrucous sarcoidosis of the skin simulating squamous cell carcinoma. Sarcoidosis Vasc Diffuse Lung Dis 2013;30(1):70–2.

56. Stockman DL, Rosenberg J, Bengana C, et al. Verrucous cutaneous sarcoidosis: case report and review of this unusual variant of cutaneous sarcoidosis. Am J Dermatopathol 2013;35(2):273–6.

57. Smith HR, Black MM. Verrucous cutaneous sarcoidosis. Clin Exp Dermatol 2000;25(1):98–9.

58. Tsuboi H, Yonemoto K, Katsuoka KA. 14-year-old girl with lichenoid sarcoidosis successfully treated with tacrolimus. J Dermatol 2006;33(5):344–8.

59. Seo SK, Yeum JS, Suh JC, et al. Lichenoid sarcoidosis in a 3-year-old girl. Pediatr Dermatol 2001; 18(5):384–7.

60. Veien NK, Stahl D, Brodthagen H. Cutaneous sarcoidosis in Caucasians. J Am Acad Dermatol 1987;16(3 Pt 1):534–40.

61. Spiteri MA, Matthey F, Gordon T, et al. Lupus pernio: a clinico-radiological study of thirty-five cases. Br J Dermatol 1985;112(3):315–22.

62. Marcoval J, Moreno A, Mañá J, et al. Subcutaneous sarcoidosis. Dermatol Clin 2008;26(4):553–6, ix.

63. Ahmed I, Harshad SR. Subcutaneous sarcoidosis: is it a specific subset of cutaneous sarcoidosis frequently associated with systemic disease? J Am Acad Dermatol 2006;54(1):55–60.

64. Chudomirova K, Velichkova L, Anavi B, et al. Recurrent sarcoidosis in skin scars accompanying systemic sarcoidosis. J Eur Acad Dermatol Venereol 2003;17(3):360–1.

65. Albertini JG, Tyler W, Miller OF 3rd. Ulcerative sarcoidosis. Case report and review of the literature. Arch Dermatol 1997;133(2):215–9.

66. Yoo SS, Mimouni D, Nikolskaia OV, et al. Clinico-pathologic features of ulcerative-atrophic sarcoidosis. Int J Dermatol 2004;43(2):108–12.

67. Cather JC, Cohen PR. Ichthyosiform sarcoidosis. J Am Acad Dermatol 1999;40(5 Pt 2):862–5.

68. Wirth FA, Gould WM, Kauffman CL. Erythroderma in a patient with arthralgias, uveitis, and dyspnea. Arch Dermatol 1999;135(11):1411–4.

69. Katta R, Nelson B, Chen D, et al. Sarcoidosis of the scalp: a case series and review of the literature. J Am Acad Dermatol 2000;42(4):690–2.

70. Momen SE, Al-Niaimi F. Sarcoid and the nail: review of the literature. Clin Exp Dermatol 2013; 38(2):119–24 [quiz: 125].

71. Elgart ML. Cutaneous sarcoidosis: definitions and types of lesions. Clin Dermatol 1986;4(4):35–45.

72. Marchell RM, Judson MA. Chronic cutaneous lesions of sarcoidosis. Clin Dermatol 2007;25(3):295–302.

73. Yanardağ H, Pamuk ON, Karayel T. Cutaneous involvement in sarcoidosis: analysis of the features in 170 patients. Respir Med 2003;97(8):978–82.

74. Pellicano R, Tiodorovic-Zivkovic D, Gourhant JY, et al. Dermoscopy of cutaneous sarcoidosis. Dermatology 2010;221(1):51–4.

75. Lallas A, Argenziano G, Apalla Z, et al. Dermoscopic patterns of common facial inflammatory skin diseases. J Eur Acad Dermatol Venereol 2014;28(5): 609–14.

76. Katta R. Cutaneous sarcoidosis: a dermatologic masquerader. Am Fam Physician 2002;65(8): 1581–4.

77. Mañá J, Marcoval J, Rubio M, et al. Granulomatous cutaneous sarcoidosis: diagnosis, relationship to systemic disease, prognosis and treatment. Sarcoidosis Vasc Diffuse Lung Dis 2013;30(4):268–81.

78. Paller AS, Surek C, Silva-Walsh I, et al. Cutaneous sarcoidosis associated with sarcoidosis of the upper airway. Arch Dermatol 1983;119(7):592–6.

79. Singal A, Thami GP, Goraya JS. Scar sarcoidosis in childhood: case report and review of the literature. Clin Exp Dermatol 2005;30(3):244–6.

80. James DG. Dermatological aspects of sarcoidosis. QJM 1959;28(109):108–24.

81. Jacyk WK. Cutaneous sarcoidosis in black South Africans. Int J Dermatol 1999;38(11):841–5.

82. Mayock RL, Bertrand P, Morrison CE, et al. Manifestations of sarcoidosis. Analysis of 145 patients, with a review of nine series selected from the literature. Am J Med 1963;35:67–89.

83. Hall RS, Floro JF, King LE Jr. Hypopigmented lesions in sarcoidosis. J Am Acad Dermatol 1984;11(6):1163–4.

84. Dogra S, De D, Radotra BD, et al. Atrophic sarcoidosis: an unusual presentation of cutaneous sarcoidosis. Skinmed 2010;8(1):59–60.

85. Feind-Koopmans AG, Lucker GP, van de Kerkhof PC. Acquired ichthyosiform erythroderma and sarcoidosis. J Am Acad Dermatol 1996;35(5 Pt 2):826–8.

86. Yoon CH, Lee CW. Case 6. Erythrodermic form of cutaneous sarcoidosis. Clin Exp Dermatol 2003;28(5):575–6.

87. Wong S, Pearce C, Markiewicz D, et al. Seasonal cutaneous sarcoidosis: a photo-induced variant. Photodermatol Photoimmunol Photomed 2011;27(3):156–8.

88. Torres F, Tosti A, Misciali C, et al. Trichoscopy as a clue to the diagnosis of scalp sarcoidosis. Int J Dermatol 2011;50(3):358–61.

89. Kasamatsu A, Kanazawa H, Watanabe T, et al. Oral sarcoidosis: report of a case and review of literature. J Oral Maxillofac Surg 2007;65(6):1256–9.

90. Bouaziz A, Le Scanff J, Chapelon-Abric C, et al. Oral involvement in sarcoidosis: report of 12 cases. QJM 2012;105(8):755–67.

91. Vera C, Funaro D, Bouffard D. Vulvar sarcoidosis: case report and review of the literature. J Cutan Med Surg 2013;17(4):287–90.

92. McLaughlin SS, Linquist AM, Burnett JW. Cutaneous sarcoidosis of the scrotum: a rare manifestation of systemic disease. Acta Derm Venereol 2002;82(3):216–7.

93. Wei H, Friedman KA, Rudikoff D. Multiple indurated papules on penis and scrotum. J Cutan Med Surg 2000;4(4):202–4.

94. Watkins S, Ismail A, McKay K, et al. Systemic sarcoidosis with unique vulvar involvement. JAMA Dermatol 2014;150:666–7.

95. Patel KB, Sharma OP. Nails in sarcoidosis: response to treatment. Arch Dermatol 1983;119(4):277–8.

96. Santoro F, Sloan SB. Nail dystrophy and bony involvement in chronic sarcoidosis. J Am Acad Dermatol 2009;60(6):1050–2.

97. Wakelin SH, James MP. Sarcoidosis: nail dystrophy without underlying bone changes. Cutis 1995;55(6):344–6.

98. Gran JT, Bøhmer E. Acute sarcoid arthritis: a favourable outcome? A retrospective survey of 49 patients with review of the literature. Scand J Rheumatol 1996;25(2):70–3.

99. Mañá J, Gómez-Vaquero C, Montero A, et al. Löfgren's syndrome revisited: a study of 186 patients. Am J Med 1999;107(3):240–5.

100. Le Bras E, Ehrenstein B, Fleck M, et al. Evaluation of ankle swelling due to Lofgren's syndrome: a pilot study using B-mode and power Doppler ultrasonography. Arthritis Care Res (Hoboken) 2014;66(2):318–22.

101. Ball NJ, Kho GT, Martinka M. The histologic spectrum of cutaneous sarcoidosis: a study of twenty-eight cases. J Cutan Pathol 2004;31(2):160–8.

102. Costabel U, Guzman J, Baughman RP. Systemic evaluation of a potential cutaneous sarcoidosis patient. Clin Dermatol 2007;25(3):303–11.

103. Baughman RP. Pulmonary sarcoidosis. Clin Chest Med 2004;25(3):521–30, vi.

104. Lynch JP 3rd, Kazerooni EA, Gay SE. Pulmonary sarcoidosis. Clin Chest Med 1997;18(4):755–85.

105. Judson MA, Baughman RP, Thompson BW, et al. Two year prognosis of sarcoidosis: the ACCESS experience. Sarcoidosis Vasc Diffuse Lung Dis 2003;20(3):204–11.

106. Fisher KA, Serlin DM, Wilson KC, et al. Sarcoidosis-associated pulmonary hypertension: outcome with long-term epoprostenol treatment. Chest 2006;130(5):1481–8.

107. Mihailovic-Vucinic V, Jovanovic D. Pulmonary sarcoidosis. Clin Chest Med 2008;29(3):459–73. viii-ix.

108. Nardi A, Brillet PY, Letoumelin P, et al. Stage IV sarcoidosis: comparison of survival with the general population and causes of death. Eur Respir J 2011;38(6):1368–73.

109. Gideon NM, Mannino DM. Sarcoidosis mortality in the United States 1979-1991: an analysis of multiple-cause mortality data. Am J Med 1996;100(4):423–7.

110. Pietinalho A, Ohmichi M, Hiraga Y, et al. The mode of presentation of sarcoidosis in Finland and Hokkaido, Japan. A comparative analysis of 571 Finnish and 686 Japanese patients. Sarcoidosis Vasc Diffuse Lung Dis 1996;13(2):159–66.

111. Ohara K, Okubo A, Sasaki H, et al. Intraocular manifestations of systemic sarcoidosis. Jpn J Ophthalmol 1992;36(4):452–7.

112. Baughman RP, Lower EE, Kaufman AH. Ocular sarcoidosis. Semin Respir Crit Care Med 2010;31(4):452–62.

113. Bradley D, Baughman RP, Raymond L, et al. Ocular manifestations of sarcoidosis. Semin Respir Crit Care Med 2002;23(6):543–8.

114. Silver MR, Messner LV. Sarcoidosis and its ocular manifestations. J Am Optom Assoc 1994;65(5): 321–7.

115. Obenauf CD, Shaw HE, Sydnor CF, et al. Sarcoidosis and its ophthalmic manifestations. Am J Ophthalmol 1978;86(5):648–55.

116. Rothova A, Alberts C, Glasius E, et al. Risk factors for ocular sarcoidosis. Doc Ophthalmol 1989; 72(3–4):287–96.

117. Sharma OP, Maheshwari A, Thaker K. Myocardial sarcoidosis. Chest 1993;103(1):253–8.

118. Matsui Y, Iwai K, Tachibana T, et al. Clinicopathological study of fatal myocardial sarcoidosis. Ann N Y Acad Sci 1976;278:455–69.

119. Sekhri V, Sanal S, Delorenzo LJ, et al. Cardiac sarcoidosis: a comprehensive review. Arch Med Sci 2011;7(4):546–54.

120. Patel MR, Cawley PJ, Heitner JF, et al. Detection of myocardial damage in patients with sarcoidosis. Circulation 2009;120(20):1969–77.

121. Kandolin R, Lehtonen J, Kupari M. Cardiac sarcoidosis and giant cell myocarditis as causes of atrioventricular block in young and middle-aged adults. Circ Arrhythm Electrophysiol 2011;4(3):303–9.

122. Mehta D, Lubitz SA, Frankel Z, et al. Cardiac involvement in patients with sarcoidosis: diagnostic and prognostic value of outpatient testing. Chest 2008;133(6):1426–35.

123. Yodogawa K, Seino Y, Ohara T, et al. Effect of corticosteroid therapy on ventricular arrhythmias in patients with cardiac sarcoidosis. Ann Noninvasive Electrocardiol 2011;16(2):140–7.

124. Chapelon-Abric C. Cardiac sarcoidosis. Curr Opin Pulm Med 2013;19(5):493–502.

125. Ricker W, Clark M. Sarcoidosis; a clinicopathologic review of 300 cases, including 22 autopsies. Am J Clin Pathol 1949;19(8):725–49.

126. James DG, Sharma OP. Neurosarcoidosis. Proc R Soc Med 1967;60(11 Part 1):1169–70.

127. Nowak DA, Widenka DC. Neurosarcoidosis: a review of its intracranial manifestation. J Neurol 2001;248(5):363–72.

128. Lower EE, Weiss KL. Neurosarcoidosis. Clin Chest Med 2008;29(3):475–92, ix.

129. Terushkin V, Stern BJ, Judson MA, et al. Neurosarcoidosis: presentations and management. Neurologist 2010;16(1):2–15.

130. Haimovic A, Sanchez M, Judson MA, et al. Sarcoidosis: a comprehensive review and update for the dermatologist: part II. Extracutaneous disease. J Am Acad Dermatol 2012;66(5):719.e1–10 [quiz: 729–30].

131. Pawate S, Moses H, Sriram S. Presentations and outcomes of neurosarcoidosis: a study of 54 cases. QJM 2009;102(7):449–60.

132. Baughman RP, Teirstein AS, Judson MA, et al. Clinical characteristics of patients in a case control study of sarcoidosis. Am J Respir Crit Care Med 2001;164(10 Pt 1):1885–9.

133. Vatti R, Sharma OP. Course of asymptomatic liver involvement in sarcoidosis: role of therapy in selected cases. Sarcoidosis Vasc Diffuse Lung Dis 1997;14(1):73–6.

134. Scott GC, Berman JM, Higgins JL. CT patterns of nodular hepatic and splenic sarcoidosis: a review of the literature. J Comput Assist Tomogr 1997; 21(3):369–72.

135. Lebacq E, Desmet V, Verhaegen H. Renal involvement in sarcoidosis. Postgrad Med J 1970;46(538): 526–9.

136. Conron M, Young C, Beynon HL. Calcium metabolism in sarcoidosis and its clinical implications. Rheumatology (Oxford) 2000;39(7):707–13.

137. Sharma OP. Vitamin D, calcium, and sarcoidosis. Chest 1996;109(2):535–9.

138. Judson MA. The diagnosis of sarcoidosis. Clin Chest Med 2008;29(3):415–27, viii.

139. Mañá J, Gámez C. Molecular imaging in sarcoidosis. Curr Opin Pulm Med 2011;17(5):325–31.

140. Stokes GS, Monaghan JC, Schrader AP, et al. Influence of angiotensin converting enzyme (ACE) genotype on interpretation of diagnostic tests for serum ACE activity. Aust N Z J Med 1999;29(3): 315–8.

141. Khatri KA, Chotzen VA, Burrall BA. Lupus pernio: successful treatment with a potent topical corticosteroid. Arch Dermatol 1995;131(5):617–8.

142. Volden G. Successful treatment of chronic skin diseases with clobetasol propionate and a hydrocolloid occlusive dressing. Acta Derm Venereol 1992;72(1):69–71.

143. Bargagli E, Olivieri C, Rottoli P. Cytokine modulators in the treatment of sarcoidosis. Rheumatol Int 2011;31(12):1539–44.

144. Callen JP. Intralesional corticosteroids. J Am Acad Dermatol 1981;4(2):149–51.

145. Beegle SH, Barba K, Gobunsuy R, et al. Current and emerging pharmacological treatments for sarcoidosis: a review. Drug Des Devel Ther 2013; 7:325–38.

146. Badgwell C, Rosen T. Cutaneous sarcoidosis therapy updated. J Am Acad Dermatol 2007;56(1): 69–83.

147. Stagaki E, Mountford WK, Lackland DT, et al. The treatment of lupus pernio: results of 116 treatment courses in 54 patients. Chest 2009;135(2):468–76.

148. Siltzbach LE, Teirstein AS. Chloroquine therapy in 43 patients with intrathoracic and cutaneous sarcoidosis. Acta Med Scand Suppl 1964;425:302–8.

149. Jones E, Callen JP. Hydroxychloroquine is effective therapy for control of cutaneous sarcoidal granulomas. J Am Acad Dermatol 1990;23(3 Pt 1):487–9.

150. Baughman RP, Lower EE. A clinical approach to the use of methotrexate for sarcoidosis. Thorax 1999;54(8):742–6.

151. Lower EE, Baughman RP. Prolonged use of methotrexate for sarcoidosis. Arch Intern Med 1995; 155(8):846–51.

152. Isshiki T, Yamaguchi T, Yamada Y, et al. Usefulness of low-dose methotrexate monotherapy for treating sarcoidosis. Intern Med 2013;52(24):2727–32.

153. Bachelez H, Senet P, Cadranel J, et al. The use of tetracyclines for the treatment of sarcoidosis. Arch Dermatol 2001;137(1):69–73.

154. Steen T, English JC. Oral minocycline in treatment of cutaneous sarcoidosis. JAMA Dermatol 2013; 149(6):758–60.

155. Baughman RP, Lower EE. Leflunomide for chronic sarcoidosis. Sarcoidosis Vasc Diffuse Lung Dis 2004;21(1):43–8.

156. Bohelay G, Bouaziz JD, Nunes H, et al. Striking leflunomide efficacy against refractory cutaneous sarcoidosis. J Am Acad Dermatol 2014;70(5): e111–3.

157. Carlesimo M, Giustini S, Rossi A, et al. Treatment of cutaneous and pulmonary sarcoidosis with thalidomide. J Am Acad Dermatol 1995;32(5 Pt 2):866–9.

158. Lee JB, Koblenzer PS. Disfiguring cutaneous manifestation of sarcoidosis treated with thalidomide: a case report. J Am Acad Dermatol 1998;39(5 Pt 2): 835–8.

159. Baughman RP, Judson MA, Teirstein AS, et al. Thalidomide for chronic sarcoidosis. Chest 2002; 122(1):227–32.

160. Fazzi P, Manni E, Cristofani R, et al. Thalidomide for improving cutaneous and pulmonary sarcoidosis in patients resistant or with contraindications to corticosteroids. Biomed Pharmacother 2012;66(4): 300–7.

161. Meyerle JH, Shorr A. The use of infliximab in cutaneous sarcoidosis. J Drugs Dermatol 2003;2(4): 413–4.

162. Saleh S, Ghodsian S, Yakimova V, et al. Effectiveness of infliximab in treating selected patients with sarcoidosis. Respir Med 2006;100(11):2053–9.

163. Mallbris L, Ljungberg A, Hedblad MA, et al. Progressive cutaneous sarcoidosis responding to anti-tumor necrosis factor-alpha therapy. J Am Acad Dermatol 2003;48(2):290–3.

164. Pariser RJ, Paul J, Hirano S, et al. A double-blind, randomized, placebo-controlled trial of adalimumab in the treatment of cutaneous sarcoidosis. J Am Acad Dermatol 2013;68(5):765–73.

165. Philips MA, Lynch J, Azmi FH. Ulcerative cutaneous sarcoidosis responding to adalimumab. J Am Acad Dermatol 2005;53(5):917.

166. Judson MA. Successful treatment of lupus pernio with adalimumab. Arch Dermatol 2011;147(11): 1332–3.

167. Kouba DJ, Mimouni D, Rencic A, et al. Mycophenolate mofetil may serve as a steroid-sparing agent for sarcoidosis. Br J Dermatol 2003;148(1):147–8.

168. Zabel P, Entzian P, Dalhoff K, et al. Pentoxifylline in treatment of sarcoidosis. Am J Respir Crit Care Med 1997;155(5):1665–9.

169. Baughman RP, Judson MA, Ingledue R, et al. Efficacy and safety of apremilast in chronic cutaneous sarcoidosis. Arch Dermatol 2012;148(2):262–4.

170. Baughman RP, Iannuzzi M. Tumour necrosis factor in sarcoidosis and its potential for targeted therapy. BioDrugs 2003;17(6):425–31.

171. Verbov J. The place of intralesional steroid therapy in dermatology. Br J Dermatol 1976;94(Suppl 12): 51–8.

172. Katoh N, Mihara H, Yasuno H. Cutaneous sarcoidosis successfully treated with topical tacrolimus. Br J Dermatol 2002;147(1):154–6.

173. McDonough AK, Curtis JR, Saag KG. The epidemiology of glucocorticoid-associated adverse events. Curr Opin Rheumatol 2008;20(2):131–7.

174. Doherty CB, Rosen T. Evidence-based therapy for cutaneous sarcoidosis. Drugs 2008;68(10):1361–83.

175. Schutt AC, Bullington WM, Judson MA. Pharmacotherapy for pulmonary sarcoidosis: a Delphi consensus study. Respir Med 2010;104(5):717–23.

176. Marshall TG, Marshall FE. Sarcoidosis succumbs to antibiotics–implications for autoimmune disease. Autoimmun Rev 2004;3(4):295–300.

177. Nguyen YT, Dupuy A, Cordoliani F, et al. Treatment of cutaneous sarcoidosis with thalidomide. J Am Acad Dermatol 2004;50(2):235–41.

178. Droitcourt C, Rybojad M, Porcher R, et al. A randomized, investigator-masked, double-blind, placebo-controlled trial on thalidomide in severe cutaneous sarcoidosis. Chest 2014;146(4): 1046–54.

179. Dalm VA, van Hagen PM. Efficacy of lenalidomide in refractory lupus pernio. JAMA Dermatol 2013; 149(4):493–4.

180. Wanat KA, Rosenbach M. Case series demonstrating improvement in chronic cutaneous sarcoidosis following treatment with TNF inhibitors. Arch Dermatol 2012;148(9):1097–100.

181. Doty JD, Mazur JE, Judson MA. Treatment of sarcoidosis with infliximab. Chest 2005;127(3): 1064–71.

182. Panselinas E, Rodgers JK, Judson MA. Clinical outcomes in sarcoidosis after cessation of infliximab treatment. Respirology 2009;14(4):522–8.

183. Thielen AM, Barde C, Saurat JH, et al. Refractory chronic cutaneous sarcoidosis responsive to dose escalation of TNF-alpha antagonists. Dermatology 2009;219(1):59–62.

184. Utz JP, Limper AH, Kalra S, et al. Etanercept for the treatment of stage II and III progressive pulmonary sarcoidosis. Chest 2003;124(1):177–85.

185. Louie GH, Chitkara P, Ward MM. Relapse of sarcoidosis upon treatment with etanercept. Ann Rheum Dis 2008;67(6):896–8.

186. Chaowattanapanit S, Aiempanakit K, Silpa-Archa N. Etanercept-induced sarcoidosis presented with scrotal lesion: a rare manifestation in genital area. J Dermatol 2014;41(3):267–8.

187. Judson MA, Baughman RP, Costabel U, et al. Safety and efficacy of ustekinumab or golimumab in patients with chronic sarcoidosis. Eur Respir J 2014;44:1296–307.

188. Drake WP, Oswald-Richter K, Richmond BW, et al. Oral antimycobacterial therapy in chronic cutaneous sarcoidosis: a randomized, single-masked, placebo-controlled study. JAMA Dermatol 2013; 149(9):1040–9.

189. Georgiou S, Monastirli A, Pasmatzi E, et al. Cutaneous sarcoidosis: complete remission after oral isotretinoin therapy. Acta Derm Venereol 1998; 78(6):457–9.

190. Chong WS, Tan HH, Tan SH. Cutaneous sarcoidosis in Asians: a report of 25 patients from Singapore. Clin Exp Dermatol 2005;30(2):120–4.

191. Voelter-Mahlknecht S, Benez A, Metzger S, et al. Treatment of subcutaneous sarcoidosis with allopurinol. Arch Dermatol 1999;135(12):1560–1.

192. Wyser CP, van Schalkwyk EM, Alheit B, et al. Treatment of progressive pulmonary sarcoidosis with cyclosporin A. A randomized controlled trial. Am J Respir Crit Care Med 1997;156(5): 1371–6.

193. Brill AK, Ott SR, Geiser T. Effect and safety of mycophenolate mofetil in chronic pulmonary sarcoidosis: a retrospective study. Respiration 2013;86(5):376–83.

194. Vorselaars AD, Wuyts WA, Vorselaars VM, et al. Methotrexate vs azathioprine in second-line therapy of sarcoidosis. Chest 2013;144(3):805–12.

195. Nowack U, Gambichler T, Hanefeld C, et al. Successful treatment of recalcitrant cutaneous sarcoidosis with fumaric acid esters. BMC Dermatol 2002;2:15.

196. Mahnke N, Medve-Koenigs K, Berneburg M, et al. Cutaneous sarcoidosis treated with medium-dose UVA1. J Am Acad Dermatol 2004;50(6):978–9.

197. Graefe T, Konrad H, Barta U, et al. Successful ultraviolet A1 treatment of cutaneous sarcoidosis. Br J Dermatol 2001;145(2):354–5.

198. Gleeson CM, Morar N, Staveley I, et al. Treatment of cutaneous sarcoid with topical gel psoralen and ultraviolet A. Br J Dermatol 2011;164(4):892–4.

199. Brauer JA, Gordon Spratt EA, Geronemus RG. Laser therapy in the treatment of connective tissue diseases: a review. Dermatol Surg 2014;40(1):1–13.

200. Roos S, Raulin C, Ockenfels HM, et al. Successful treatment of cutaneous sarcoidosis lesions with the flashlamp pumped pulsed dye laser: a case report. Dermatol Surg 2009;35(7):1139–40.

201. Holzmann RD, Astner S, Forschner T, et al. Scar sarcoidosis in a child: case report of successful treatment with the pulsed dye laser. Dermatol Surg 2008;34(3):393–6.

202. Cliff S, Felix RH, Singh L, et al. The successful treatment of lupus pernio with the flashlamp pulsed dye laser. J Cutan Laser Ther 1999;1(1):49–52.

203. O'Donoghue NB, Barlow RJ. Laser remodelling of nodular nasal lupus pernio. Clin Exp Dermatol 2006;31(1):27–9.

204. Young HS, Chalmers RJ, Griffiths CE, et al. CO2 laser vaporization for disfiguring lupus pernio. J Cosmet Laser Ther 2002;4(3–4):87–90.

205. Ekbäck M, Molin L. Effective laser treatment in a case of lupus pernio. Acta Derm Venereol 2005; 85(6):521–2.

206. Grema H, Greve B, Raulin C. Scar sarcoidosis–treatment with the Q-switched ruby laser. Lasers Surg Med 2002;30(5):398–400.

207. Emer J, Uslu U, Waldorf H. Improvement in lupus pernio with the successive use of pulsed dye laser and nonablative fractional resurfacing. Dermatol Surg 2014;40(2):201–2.

208. Green JJ, Lawrence N, Heymann WR. Generalized ulcerative sarcoidosis induced by therapy with the flashlamp-pumped pulsed dye laser. Arch Dermatol 2001;137(4):507–8.

209. Kormeili T, Neel V, Moy RL. Cutaneous sarcoidosis at sites of previous laser surgery. Cutis 2004;73(1): 53–5.

210. Lesavoy MA, Shirvanian VN, Grimes P. Surgical reconstruction of nasal sarcoidosis: a case report. Ann Plast Surg 2010;64(6):800–2.

211. Preminger BA, Hiltzik DH, Segal J, et al. An operative approach to the treatment of refractory cutaneous nasal sarcoid: a case report and review of the literature. Ann Plast Surg 2009;63(6):685–7.

212. Goldin JH, Jawad SM, Reid AP. Cutaneous nasal sarcoidosis–treatment by excision and split-skin grafting. J Laryngol Otol 1983;97(11):1053–6.

Cutaneous Manifestations of Crohn Disease

Joshua W. Hagen, MD, PhD[a], Jason M. Swoger, MD, MPH[b],
Lisa M. Grandinetti, MD[a,†,*]

KEYWORDS

- Extraintestinal manifestations • Crohn disease • Inflammatory bowel disease
- Cutaneous Crohn disease

KEY POINTS

- Cutaneous manifestations of inflammatory bowel disease (IBD) can often be the presenting sign of underlying gastrointestinal disease, and clinicians should have a low threshold to initiate evaluation for underlying gastrointestinal (GI) disease when patients present with representative skin lesions.
- In patients with known IBD, dermatologic manifestations are common, occurring in up to one-third of patients.
- Cutaneous extraintestinal manifestations are traditionally divided into 3 categories: (1) disease-specific lesions that show the same histopathologic findings as the underlying GI disease, (2) reactive lesions that are inflammatory lesions that do not share the GI pathology, and (3) associated conditions believed caused by HLA linkage phenomenon.
- For many extraintestinal manifestations, the cutaneous disease course does not always mirror the GI disease course, presenting a therapeutic challenge.
- Consultation and coordination of care with gastroenterology are essential for optimal patient benefit.

CROHN DISEASE

Introduction

Crohn disease (CD) is an inflammatory condition of the gastrointestinal (GI) tract, characterized by unpredictable periods of symptomatic relapses and remissions. The incidence of CD in the United States is approximately 3.1 to 14.6 per 100,000 person-years.[1,2] CD can affect any location in the GI tract, from the mouth to the anus, but most commonly presents in the terminal ileum (30%), colon (20%), or small bowel and colon (45%).[3] In addition, CD can affect other organs, including the eyes, skin, and liver, and joints, which are termed extraintestinal manifestations (EIMs).

Etiopathogenesis

The underlying cause of CD is not known, although several factors have been identified that contribute to disease onset.[1] These factors include genetic, microbial, environmental (smoking), immunologic, vascular, and psychosocial factors.[1,4,5] Medications such as nonsteroidal antiinflammatory drugs (NSAIDs) and oral contraceptives have also been implicated in the onset and worsening of CD, although this remains controversial.[6–8] The chronic inflammation in CD is driven by a dysregulated immune system and is dependent on both the Th-1 and Th-17 pathways.[9] Although there is a component of genetic susceptibility in the cause of CD, it

Disclosures: The authors have no relevant financial disclosures.
[a] Department of Dermatology, University of Pittsburgh Medical Center, Medical Arts Building, 3708 Fifth Avenue, 5th Floor, Pittsburgh, PA 15213, USA; [b] Department of Gastroenterology, Hepatology and Nutrition, University of Pittsburgh Medical Center, 200 Lothrop street, C-Wing, Mezzanine, Pittsburgh, PA 15213, USA
† The author is deceased.
* Corresponding author.
E-mail address: grandinettilm@upmc.edu

Dermatol Clin 33 (2015) 417–431
http://dx.doi.org/10.1016/j.det.2015.03.007
0733-8635/15/$ – see front matter © 2015 Elsevier Inc. All rights reserved.

does not follow a Mendelian inheritance pattern, and disease onset is likely triggered by exposure to 1 or more triggers in a genetically susceptible individual.[5] Most of the CD-related genes that have been found help to regulate the interaction of gut microbiota and the mucosal immune system.

Clinical Presentations

The clinical presentation of CD can be variable, although most patients present with abdominal pain, diarrhea, rectal bleeding, weight loss, fatigue, fevers, and malnutrition.[2] CD can present at any age, from pediatrics to patients in the sixth or seventh decades of life, but most commonly presents in early adulthood.[1] Complications of CD are also common, because of the transmural inflammation associated with the disease, and patients may present with symptoms caused by these complications.[2] The fibrostenotic phenotype of CD leads to the development of small bowel or colonic strictures, and patients often present with bowel obstructions. In addition, fistulae may form between the GI tract and other organs, including the bladder, skin, vagina, or other locations in the bowel. A subset of patients with CD present with perianal manifestations of the disease, including perianal fistulae and abscesses.

Diagnosis and treatment

The diagnosis of CD is made by a combination of laboratory studies, radiographic imaging, and ileocolonoscopy with biopsy.[2] Several different classes of medications are used to treat both the inflammation and symptoms associated with CD, including mesalamine products, short-term corticosteroids, immunomodulators (azathioprine, 6-mercaptopurine, methotrexate), biological therapies (infliximab, adalimumab, certolizumab pegol, natalizumab, vedolizumab), antibiotics, antidiarrheals, and bile-acid sequestrants. The goals of treatment are to achieve mucosal healing, avoid the development of complications and surgery, and to optimize quality of life. Approximately 70% of patients with CD require surgery during their lifetime, and many have postoperative recurrence and require additional surgical interventions.[2,10,11]

Systemic/Extraintestinal Associations

As mentioned earlier, multiple EIMs of CD have been described (**Table 1**).[2] Arthritis and arthralgias are most common, occurring in up to 50% of patients in some studies.[12,13] Ophthalmologic manifestations are rarely seen (<5% of cases), including episcleritis and anterior uveitis, and tend to occur when the GI disease is active.[14] Hepatobiliary abnormalities may be related either to CD itself or, often, to the medications used to treat it.[15] Common hepatobiliary manifestations of CD include granulomatous hepatitis, amyloidosis, fatty liver, pericholangitis, cholelithiasis, primary sclerosing cholangitis (PSC), portal vein thrombosis, and cholangiocarcinoma.[16] Patients with CD are also at an increased risk of developing venous thromboembolic disease, with a 3-fold higher risk than control patients.[17,18]

In addition to these EIMs, dermatologic manifestations of CD are common, occurring in up to one-third of patients; the remainder of this article is devoted to these cutaneous manifestations of CD.

CUTANEOUS MANIFESTATIONS OF CROHN DISEASE

The skin and oral mucosa represent easily accessible sites to monitor for development of EIMs of inflammatory bowel disease (IBD) and, consequently, there is a growing appreciation for the number of associated skin findings that occur. Estimates of prevalence vary widely for each EIM, but some range as high as 43% of patients, indicating that an understanding of these entities is critical to the effective care of patients with IBD in both the gastroenterology and dermatology settings.[12,19] Cutaneous lesions of IBD have traditionally been divided into 3 categories reflective of their etiopathology: (1) specific lesions (those that have the same histopathologic findings as the underlying GI disease), (2) reactive lesions (those in which the inflammatory process does not share the GI pathology), and (3) associated conditions (believed to be caused by HLA linkage phenomenon and sequelae of chronic inflammation).[20] In the current era of ever-expanding therapeutic options for IBD, some investigators have proposed a fourth category of EIMs, namely those that are therapy related. These EIMs are discussed in connection with the disease-associated conditions in light of certain skin findings that have potential overlap between these last 2 categories.

DISEASE-SPECIFIC CUTANEOUS MANIFESTATIONS
Perianal Fissures/Fistulae and Acrochordae

Perianal fissures and fistulae (**Fig. 1**) are one of the specific lesions of CD and are a commonly encountered finding in up to one-third of patients.[20] This finding is strongly associated with colonic involvement of CD compared with those patients with small bowel disease only. Chronic inflammation in the setting of fissures and fistulae promotes development of cutaneous abscesses and acrochordae.

Metastatic (Cutaneous) Crohn Disease

Metastatic CD refers to inflammatory lesions that extend to involve areas not typically considered as part of the spectrum of the underlying IBD. Clinically, this manifests as erythematous and violaceous plaques, nodules, and ulcerations with epithelioid granulomatous inflammation primarily localized on the extremities or intertriginous skin (**Fig. 2**). The face and genitalia are less commonly involved. A tissue biopsy is usually necessary to establish the diagnosis, because the clinical appearance of the lesions can have overlapping features with several other disorders. As the name suggests, metastatic CD is, by definition, separated from the GI tract by normal tissue and thereby excludes classic perianal CD. According to previously published data, metastatic Crohn is one of the rarer cutaneous manifestations of CD.[21] The timing to

Table 1
Level of evidence for therapies of cutaneous EIMs

Skin Finding	Therapy	Highest Level of Evidence Cited
Vulvoperineal CD	Metronidazole	D
	Azathioprine with topical steroid	D
	Infliximab	D
	Infliximab with hyperbaric O_2	E
	Intralesional steroids	E
Genital lymphedema	Metronidazole	D
	Topical steroid with support	D
	Surgery	D
Lymphangioma circumscripta	Surgery/laser	D
Orofacial granulomatosis	Mesalamine/prednisolone	D
	Diet modification	B
	Steroid mouthwash/gels	E
	Infliximab	B
	Adalimumab	B
Erythema nodosum	Prednisone	D
	TNF inhibitors	D
	Colchicine	D
	Hydroxychloroquine	D
	Dapsone	D
Pyoderma gangrenosum	Intralesional steroids	E
	Topical potent corticosteroids	E
	Topical calcineurin inhibitors	D
	Topical dapsone	D
	Cromolyn sodium	D
	Topical 5-aminosalicylic acid	D
	Prednisone	C
	Azathioprine	D
	6-mercaptopurine	D
	Cyclosporine	D
	Methotrexate	D
	Mycophenolate mofetil	D
	Infliximab	C
	Adalimumab	C
Peristomal pyoderma gangrenosum	Topical potent corticosteroids	D
	Intralesional steroids	D
	Crushed dapsone	D
	Dapsone gel	E
	Corticosteroid inhalers	D
	TNF inhibitors	D
	Ustekinumab	D
	Stoma closure	D

(continued on next page)

Table 1
(continued)

Skin Finding	Therapy	Highest Level of Evidence Cited
Pyostomatitis vegetans	Topical steroids	D
	Antiseptic mouthwashes	D
	Azathioprine	D
	Dapsone	D
	Prednisolone	D
	Infliximab	D
Oral aphthous ulcers	Viscous lidocaine	NA
	Topical steroids	NA
Sweet syndrome	Prednisone	D
	Colchicine	D
	Dapsone	D
	Cyclosporine	D
	Cyclophosphamide	D
	Indomethacin	D
	Clofazimine	D
Leukocytoclastic vasculitis	Prednisone	D
Epidermolysis bullosa acquisita	Dapsone	D
	Sulfapyridine	D
	Colchicine	D
	Cyclosporine	D
	Mycophenolate mofetil	D
	Rituximab	D
	Intravenous immunoglobulin	D
	Extracorporeal phototherapy	D

B, lesser-quality RCT or prospective study; C, case-control study or retrospective study; D, case series or case reports; E, expert opinion; NA, not available.

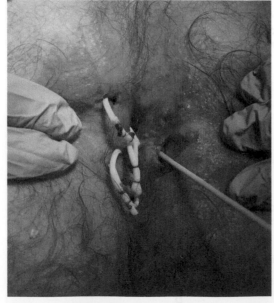

Fig. 1. Perianal fistulae with setons in place in a patient with severe CD.

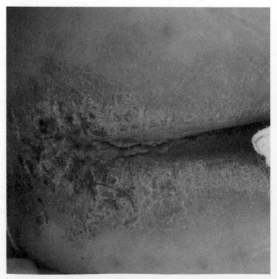

Fig. 2. Hyperplastic folds in the gluteal cleft consistent with cutaneous (metastatic) CD.

development of metastatic lesions varies widely but has been reported to occur after the initial diagnosis of CD in most adults and around the same time as diagnosis of CD in approximately half of childhood cases of CD.[22] These lesions can be particularly frustrating to the clinician, because surgical correction of the affected portion of bowel does not always improve metastatic CD, highlighting the observation that skin and intestinal disease do not always mirror each other in this setting.[23,24] Several specific manifestations of cutaneous CD are discussed in greater detail in the following sections.

Vulvoperineal Crohn disease

Granulomatous infiltration of the skin of the vulva and perineum in CD is a rarely reported finding that may precede the development of GI manifestations by months to years. The initial presentation may be highlighted by vulvar or perineal pain.[25] This pain can progress to cutaneous ulcerations and fistulas in some cases (**Fig. 3**). There have been reported cases of adolescent vulvoperineal Crohn that initially presented as lesions suspicious for sexual abuse.[26] Involvement of the perineum is seen more frequently in women and at a younger age, with noted predominance of colonic over small bowel involvement of the GI tract. Without a history of previous GI symptoms, a skin biopsy showing epithelioid granulomas is the finding

most likely to lead to a diagnosis of vulvoperineal CD. A poorer prognosis for these patients has been documented in terms of surgical healing as well as need for proctectomy.[27] Because surgical outcomes are poor, selected cases have been successfully medically managed with a variety of approaches, including metronidazole,[28,29] azathioprine plus topical steroid,[30] and infliximab.[31,32] Several investigators have recently suggested that a combination of infliximab and hyperbaric oxygen may provide synergistic benefit in managing this presentation of CD, although clinical evidence is still lacking.[33] Anecdotally, we have noted success with serial intralesional corticosteroid injections into the vulva and perineal skin (L.M.G., personal observation).

Genital lymphedema and lymphangiomata

Another related and similarly rare presentation of metastatic CD is genital tumefaction secondary to lymphedema of the genital skin.[34-41] Although this finding is rare, most young patients with noninfectious genital skin granulomas and genital lymphedema have an associated diagnosis of CD, most frequently with anal involvement but also with occasional orofacial granulomatosis (OFG).[37] This disease has been treated successfully with metronidazole, which led to resolution of edema over a several-month course[34] or a combination of topical steroids and physical support.[37] Surgical correction has also been pursued in some cases.[36] Because of the strong associations noted earlier, granulomatous lymphangitis of the genitalia has been considered a forme fruste of CD and warrants close clinical follow-up for development of GI symptoms, which may be absent at the initial onset of skin disease.[37]

Impaired lymphatic drainage of the vulvar area, as can be seen in a variety of settings including metastatic Crohn, has been hypothesized to underlie the development of vulvar lymphangioma circumscripta (LC)[42,43] and should be in the differential for individuals with a history of genital tumefaction or questionable appearing genital warts[44] in the setting of CD. Surgical excision followed by laser ablation has been reported as a successful means of treatment of vulvar LC.[43]

Similar to OFG, anogenital granulomatosis has been suggested as a diagnostic term that encompasses the triad of vulvitis granulomatosa, posthitis granulomatosa, and anoperineitis granulomatosa. The disease findings include lymphedema and noncaseating granulomas that are indistinguishable from those of either CD or sarcoidosis. Therefore, providers should initiate appropriate clinical workup for either or both diseases in the appropriate clinical contexts.[45]

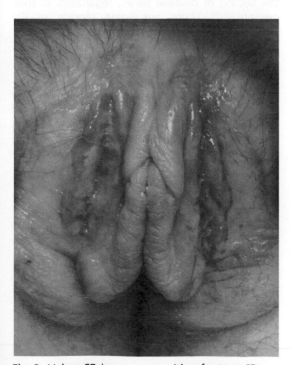

Fig. 3. Vulvar CD in a woman with refractory CD.

Oral Crohn Disease

Oral lesions are commonly encountered in patients with CD, with certain manifestations falling under the designation of disease-specific lesions and others representing reactive EIMs (such as aphthous ulcers). The incidence of true, disease-specific oral CD has been estimated to affect approximately 6% of patients with CD overall.[46,47] A more detailed dissection of the oral disease-specific manifestations can be found in the following paragraphs.

Orofacial granulomatosis

OFG (which is discussed in more detail in another article by Al-Hamad and colleagues elsewhere in this issue) is a rare and heterogeneous diagnosis characterized by chronic swelling of oral and facial tissues secondary to granulomatous inflammation. It has been proposed in some cases to be a precursor of, or initial presentation for, CD and has shown response to mesalamine and prednisolone.[48] A Swedish study of OFG with or without coincident CD[49] showed a higher incidence of an NOD2 gene polymorphism in those patients with CD. However, this association has not been found in other geographic cohorts. OFG is not always associated with CD. Although OFG does not predict development of CD, the progression to CD (when it does occur) is more commonly seen in children. Approximately half are diagnosed with CD before OFG, and the remaining half in the reverse order.[50] To further add to the potential confusion regarding the association between OFG and CD, some investigators suggest that OFG with granulomatous inflammation in the GI tract may be a clinicopathologic entity distinct from CD.[51] It has recently been suggested that there is an association of an oral allergy syndrome and findings of OFG either alone or in conjunction with CD.[52] In addition to the treatment options mentioned earlier, diet modification directed at avoiding cinnamon and benzoates has shown efficacy in reducing oral inflammation.[53] Steroid-containing mouthwash or gel preparations may aid in symptomatic relief. Anti–tumor necrosis factor (TNF) therapy with infliximab and adalimumab has also proved useful in treating OFG; however, long-term outcomes were not favorable in the case of infliximab.[54]

REACTIVE CUTANEOUS MANIFESTATIONS
Erythema Nodosum

Erythema nodosum (EN) is a form of septal panniculitis without attendant vasculitis most commonly seen on the pretibial skin and is the most common cutaneous manifestation of CD, estimated to occur in 4% to 6% of patients with CD.[20] It falls within the category of reactive lesions and is seen more commonly in young, female patients with CD at rates up to 3 to 6 times higher than in male patients.[55] Clinically, it manifests as painful, indurated, erythematous to violaceous plaques (Fig. 4). The sites of involvement are typically the extensor surface of the lower extremities, but other sites have been reported, including thighs, arms, trunk, neck, and face.[55,56] Lesions of EN frequently occur in the setting of systemic symptoms of malaise, fatigue, and arthralgias. Patients with colonic CD involvement are more likely to develop EN than those patients with more proximal GI involvement.[57] Biopsy is often not required, because the diagnosis can often be made from clinical clues alone. However, ruling out an infectious process (eg, *Streptococcus*), drug reaction (eg, sulfonamides or oral contraceptives), underlying malignancy or other systemic inflammatory process (eg sarcoidosis, Sjögren syndrome, Behçet disease) is important when in doubt. Ulceration, if present, should prompt a biopsy to rule out a distinct vasculitic or malignant process.

Treatment centers on rest, elevation, and compression in mild EN. For more severe EN, success has been reported with oral steroid tapers or anti-TNF biologics, as well as scattered reports of colchicine, hydroxychloroquine, and dapsone.[58] Individual nodules can last for several weeks and then resolve with little to no residual scar formation; however, new lesions are not uncommon in the setting of disease flares, regardless of their severity.[55,59] There are some reports of EN induced by biological therapies used for CD, such as certolizumab.[60]

Pyoderma Gangrenosum

Pyoderma gangrenosum (PG), first described by Brocq, constitutes a cutaneous manifestation of ongoing immune dysregulation and represents one of the reactive skin lesions seen in the setting

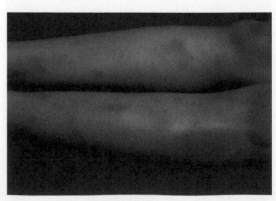

Fig. 4. Multiple EN in a woman with IBD.

of IBD. The prevalence of PG in patients with CD has been estimated to be 0.7% of patients and almost one-third of patients with PG have an underlying IBD.[20] Much like reactive EN lesions, PG lesions are more common in patients with colonic involvement of their underlying CD.[23] The timing for appearance of PG lesions extends along the entire spectrum with relation to the diagnosis of the associated IBD.[55] Clinically, the lesions appear first as erythematous pustules or nodules that progress to ulceronecrotic lesions with granulation tissue, pus, and rolled, violaceous, undermined borders, and are found classically as single or multiple distinct lesions on the lower extremities in either a unilateral or a bilateral distribution (**Fig. 5**).[61] Cribriform scars are common after the resolution of PG lesions.

Four distinct subtypes of PG are recognized, with pustular and ulcerative forms more heavily represented in patients with IBD. The etiopathogenesis of PG is poorly understood but is believed to involve aberrant neutrophil activity and altered cellular immunity.[62,63] Recent hypotheses for the cause of PG focus on the potential role of coexisting autoinflammatory disorders and the possibility of using interleukin 1 (IL-1) inhibitors to modulate disease activity.[64] Although the diagnosis is frequently made using clinical information alone, skin biopsies show perivascular lymphocyte-rich infiltrates and endothelial swelling with an accompanying florid dermal neutrophilic infiltrate and may be helpful in ruling out infectious, vasculitic, or neoplastic mimickers.[65] The pathergy phenomenon recognized in patients with PG explains the

occasional worsening of disease after biopsies or other site manipulations.

Local therapy with weekly intralesional triamcinolone, potent topical corticosteroid ointments, topical calcineurin inhibitors, topical dapsone, cromolyn sodium, and topical 5-aminosalicylic acid have all reportedly been effective in treating early/mild lesions.[66] Oral steroid therapy represents the classic first-line systemic therapy for more extensive PG that is associated with CD, but clearance rates have reportedly been low.[67] In addition to oral prednisone, various reports indicate some success with azathioprine, 6-mercaptopurine, cyclosporine, methotrexate, and mycophenolate mofetil.[68,69] Cyclosporine in particular has shown notable efficacy as a systemic immunomodulator, with complete healing times averaging 7 months.[70] However, the limitations of long-term cyclosporine administration must be considered. Biological agents such as infliximab and adalimumab have shown themselves highly effective in treating recalcitrant disease, which has led some to argue that these should be considered as first-line agents for treating PG.[71–75] Regardless of response to individual therapies, PG has a tendency to recur and may require maintenance therapy to ensure continued remission.

Peristomal pyoderma gangrenosum

Peristomal PG (PPG) is an uncommon, and likely underrecognized, occurrence near the site of stoma formation after bowel resection procedures for IBD (**Fig. 6**). Risk factors for development of PPG seem to be female gender, presence of other autoimmune disorders, and increased body mass index.[76] The differential for skin lesions in this area includes irritant and allergic contact dermatitis from stool and ostomy adhesives/pastes, respectively, as well as pressure ulceration from use of convex ostomy wafers. Infectious ulcerations can

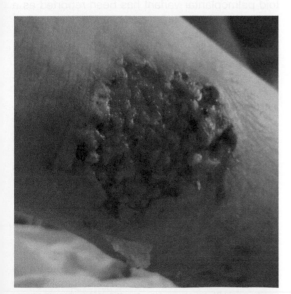

Fig. 5. PG on the lower leg of a patient with IBD. Note the violaceous border.

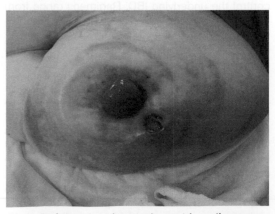

Fig. 6. Peristomal PG in a patient with an ileostomy.

also appear in this location. The timing for appearance of peristomal PG varies from 2 months to several decades after initial stoma creation.[77] Successful treatment has been reported with potent topical steroids (eg, clobetasol), tacrolimus, or intralesional corticosteroids and should be initiated as early as possible to avoid potential complications.[77,78] Topical application of crushed dapsone has also reportedly been effective for PPG.[79] Anecdotal off-label use of commercially available dapsone 5% gel has shown improvement in early disease (L.M.G., personal observation). However, topical therapy poses a challenge, because it may interfere with adhesion of the ostomy appliances. An intriguing alternative to topical cream and ointment formulations is the use of corticosteroid inhalers in the treatment of PPG, which may minimize complications with ostomy appliance adhesives.[80] Alternative vehicles, such as corticosteroid sprays and gels are also useful. As with lesions of classic PG, recalcitrant PPG has been shown to respond to biological therapy with variety of agents such as adalimumab, infliximab, etanercept, and ustekinumab.[81–84] Although it represents an extreme solution for most patients, successful resolution of PPG can be achieved in most cases with stoma closure, whereas revision or relocation are usually unsuccessful.[85,86]

Pyostomatitis Vegetans

Pustules, miliary abscesses, ulcerations, and vegetative plaques on the lips and buccal mucosa are the presenting symptoms of pyostomatitis vegetans, a rare reactive manifestation seen in the setting of IBD. Immune dysregulation is believed to underlie the development of the skin lesions, although the pathophysiology is still unclear.[87] Lesions of pyostomatitis vegetans tend to appear after the diagnosis of IBD and mirror the underlying disease activity. Treatment should initially be focused on symptomatic relief and simultaneously control the underlying IBD. Regimens range from topical corticosteroids and antiseptic mouthwashes to systemic infliximab, azathioprine, dapsone, or prednisolone.[88–90] Even with treatment, recrudescence is not uncommon.

Oral Aphthous Ulcers

Although certainly not a feature unique to CD, oral aphthae are frequently encountered in patients with CD and represent the most common oral mucosal finding in patients with IBD. Aphthae consist of single to multiple shallow, erythematous ulcers often accompanied by a fibrinous exudate and halo of erythema. The reported incidence of oral aphthae ranges widely depending on the source but may be present up to one-third of patients.[91] A variety of triggers and pathogenetic mechanisms have been proposed, including increased IBD activity, stress, food/medication allergies, local trauma, autoimmune disorders, a variety of nutritional deficiencies that are commonly seen in CD, and aberrant T-cell response to oral keratinocyte-associated antigens.[92,93] Although the diagnosis rarely requires a biopsy and is most often made clinically, a high degree of suspicion should be directed toward recalcitrant ulcers, especially in smokers, because these may represent oral squamous cell carcinoma. Treatment centers on addressing the underlying cause, whether it be untreated intestinal inflammation, infections, or nutritional deficiencies. Symptomatic therapy with viscous lidocaine or topical corticosteroid gels/pastes/mouthwashes should be instituted, with realization that corticosteroid preparations may increase the risk of oral candidiasis.

Sweet Syndrome

Sweet syndrome, also known as acute febrile neutrophilic dermatosis, has been infrequently associated with IBD.[94] Fever, myalgias, arthralgias, and malaise present with cutaneous erythematous to violaceous papules, nodules, and plaques, which may even progress to vesicles in some cases. Skin lesions are most commonly seen on the head, neck, and upper extremities. Episcleritis is a frequent ocular finding. Like many of the reactive conditions discussed, Sweet syndrome occurs in the setting of IBD with colonic involvement and is usually an indicator of active disease.[95,96] A targetoid palmoplantar variant has been reported as a presenting sign of severe underlying CD.[97] Although the pathogenesis of Sweet syndrome remains a subject of debate, various investigators implicate altered neutrophil activity, T-cell dysfunction, cytokine dysregulation, and hypersensitivity reactions as potential causes.[96]

If Sweet syndrome is suspected, a biopsy should be performed to confirm the presence of papillary dermal edema with a dense neutrophilic infiltrate and leukocytoclasia, typically without vasculitis, unless the inflammatory reaction is severe. Patients with Sweet syndrome may show the pathergy phenomenon at sites of tissue manipulation. Treatment centers on systemic corticosteroids, which should lead to rapid resolution of the lesions. Colchicine, dapsone, cyclosporine, cyclophosphamide, indomethacin, and clofazimine have also reportedly been effective, with more recent successes achieved with biological agents such as infliximab.[98–102] Azathioprine, a medication sometimes used in the setting of IBD, has been reported to induce Sweet syndrome in some patients.[103,104]

Cutaneous Polyarteritis Nodosa

In a few patients with CD, a chronic and recurrent small to medium-sized vasculitis known as cutaneous polyarteritis nodosa (CPN) has been observed, often with granulomatous inflammation reminiscent of the underlying CD. This finding, like many others discussed in this section, can precede development of IBD.[105,106] It differs from polyarteritis nodosa in that the disease spares the viscera and is limited to the reticular dermis and subcutaneous tissues, presenting clinically as a tender nodule, usually on the lower extremity. Reports estimate that approximately 10% of CPN is associated with underlying IBD, either ulcerative colitis or CD.[107,108] Treatment relies on low-dose corticosteroids and NSAIDs, but the disease does not run parallel to GI symptoms. However, use of NSAIDs carries well-known risks for patients with IBD.

Granulomatous Vasculitis

A superficial and deep granulomatous vasculitis characterized by neutrophils and histiocytes has also been described rarely in patients with CD.[109] There have also been cases in which extrapulmonary manifestations of Wegener granulomatosis are seen in association with CD.[110,111] This should prompt rapid therapy directed at the Wegener granulomatosis to prevent further morbidity and mortality.

Leukocytoclastic Vasculitis

Although reports in the literature are comparatively rare, there is evidence of an association between findings of leukocytoclastic vasculitis and CD (**Fig. 7**).[112–116] Biopsy findings show the classic angiocentric neutrophilic infiltrate without epidermal change, granuloma formation, or fibrinoid necrosis. Systemic corticosteroid therapy seems successful in treating the lesions.[113,114]

DISEASE-ASSOCIATED AND THERAPY-RELATED CONDITIONS

Some investigators further subdivide the conditions included in the following section into both disease-associated conditions and therapy-related conditions. Although there are certainly cases in which this distinction is possible, we have decided for the purpose of this article to include them together and highlight those entities in which the distinction is perhaps more clear.

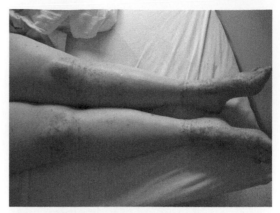

Fig. 7. Leukocytoclastic vasculitis on the lower legs.

Psoriasis

Along with EN, psoriasis is one of the most common cutaneous diseases seen in patients with CD.[66] A large study of 51,800 Taiwanese patients with psoriasis did not find an increased prevalence ratio for CD, suggesting perhaps that geographically variable genetic factors influence the development of this associated finding or that the reverse association of CD with underlying psoriasis is not present.[117] With regards to therapy-related conditions, paradoxic psoriasiform skin lesions are not uncommon in patients with CD undergoing anti-TNF therapy (**Fig. 8**).[118–120] These lesions are characterized by increased populations of Th17 and Th1 cells secreting IL-17A/IL-22 and interferon γ and seem to be more prevalent in patients who are smokers. The lesions respond well to anti-IL12/IL-23 therapy (eg, ustekinumab) in some cases.[120] There has been a case of CD induced in a patient receiving anti-TNF-α therapy for primary psoriasis.[121]

Vitiligo

Vitiligo is one of the more rare associated skin findings in patients with CD.[122–124] Although many believe that vitiligo risk is increased as a consequence of the ongoing autoimmune phenomenon active in patients with CD, some clinicians hypothesize that pigment loss can be a consequence of specific CD treatment regimens such as the anti-TNF-α agents.[125] Recent genetic studies have identified BACH2 as a key regulatory protein of Treg cells, with polymorphisms in the responsible gene leading to susceptibility to a wide range of immune-mediated diseases, including CD, vitiligo, celiac disease, multiple sclerosis, and type 1 diabetes.[126] Whether this situation, at least in part, underlies the phenomenon of coincident CD and vitiligo remains an unanswered question.

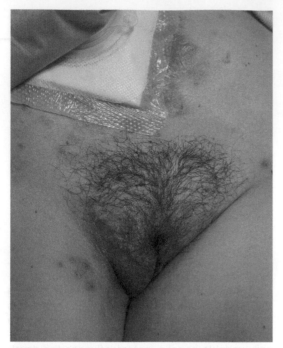

Fig. 8. TNF-α-induced psoriasis in a patient with IBD on adalimumab.

Epidermolysis Bullosa Acquisita

Patients with CD can rarely develop blistering of the skin in a phenotype consistent with epidermolysis bullosa acquisita (EBA).[127,128] EBA antigen (Col VII) is present in the human colon, and IgG autoantibodies have been shown in the sera of patients with CD.[129] In 1 report,[130] 25% of EBA cases were associated with underlying CD. Just as there have been instances of peristomal PG, peristomal EBA has also been reported in patients with CD.[131] A variety of treatments have been attempted for EBA, including dapsone, sulfapyridine, and colchicine in milder forms, and cyclosporine, mycophenolate mofetil, rituximab, intravenous immunoglobulins, and extracorporeal photochemotherapy in resistant and severe forms.[132,133]

Eczema

Eczematous eruptions have been reported with increased frequency in patients with IBD.[134–136] Early investigation for a genetic link between eczema and CD has led to findings of a shared susceptibility locus on chromosome 11q13.5.[137] It seems that, like psoriasis, eczema may also be a consequence of anti-TNF therapy in some patients.[138]

Alopecia Areata

Alopecia has been described in the setting of CD, both alopecia areata and alopecia universalis.[124,139,140] Similar to psoriasis, alopecia areata–like hair loss is a phenomenon that can be induced by treatment in patients receiving anti-TNF therapy. Reportedly, this form of alopecia can be distinguished from true alopecia areata by the presence of epidermal psoriasiform change and dermal plasma cells on biopsy.[141]

Nail Clubbing

Although it represents a subtle skin finding that is easily overlooked on examination, nail clubbing has been reported as a finding in patients with CD, with a likelihood ratio of 2.8 for underlying active disease.[142,143] Even if noted in the context of CD, nail clubbing should also prompt appropriate clinical workup to rule out pulmonary causes.

Acquired Zinc Deficiency

Acquired nutritional deficiencies can sometimes be seen in patients with CD, including findings that mimic acrodermatitis enteropathica but which are more appropriately termed acquired zinc deficiency.[140,144–146] Skin findings include alopecia, perlèche (angular cheilitis), glossitis, and genital skin erosions, as well as eczematous, psoriasiform, and bullous lesions.

SUMMARY

Mucocutaneous manifestations of CD encompass a broad array of clinical findings, some of which are common and can often be the presenting sign of underlying GI disease. These EIMs are traditionally divided into 3 categories: (1) disease-specific lesions that show the same histopathologic findings as the underlying GI disease, (2) reactive lesions that are inflammatory lesions that do not share the GI pathology, and (3) associated conditions believed to be caused by HLA linkage phenomenon, and most recently, (4) therapy-related sequelae. These conditions can be challenging to treat, because the skin disease does not always mirror the GI disease course. Health care providers should recognize these conditions and have a low threshold to initiate evaluation/consultation with gastroenterology. As the pathogenic mechanisms behind these conditions are not well understood, further research is needed to better define the connection between the gut and the skin.

DEDICATION

Dedicated to the memory of a consummate dermatologist and selfless colleague and educator who brought a wealth of knowledge, enthusiasm, and compassion to her patients and the residents she trained. This manuscript serves as a lasting testament to her passion for expanding the practice of dermatology to emerging and underserved diseases.

Lisa M. Grandinetti, MD, August 1976 – February 2015

REFERENCES

1. Loftus EV Jr. Clinical epidemiology of inflammatory bowel disease: incidence, prevalence, and environmental influences. Gastroenterology 2004; 126(6):1504–17.

2. Lichtenstein GR, Hanauer SB, Sandborn WJ. Management of Crohn's disease in adults. Am J Gastroenterol 2009;104(2):465–83 [quiz: 464, 484].

3. Farmer RG, Hawk WA, Turnbull RB Jr. Clinical patterns in Crohn's disease: a statistical study of 615 cases. Gastroenterology 1975;68(4 Pt 1):627–35.

4. Abraham C, Cho JH. Inflammatory bowel disease. N Engl J Med 2009;361(21):2066–78.

5. Thoreson R, Cullen JJ. Pathophysiology of inflammatory bowel disease: an overview. Surg Clin North Am 2007;87(3):575–85.

6. Ananthakrishnan AN, Higuchi LM, Huang ES, et al. Aspirin, nonsteroidal anti-inflammatory drug use, and risk for Crohn disease and ulcerative colitis: a cohort study. Ann Intern Med 2012;156(5):350–9.

7. Bernstein CN, Singh S, Graff LA, et al. A prospective population-based study of triggers of symptomatic flares in IBD. Am J Gastroenterol 2010;105(9):1994–2002.

8. Cosnes J, Carbonnel F, Carrat F, et al. Oral contraceptive use and the clinical course of Crohn's disease: a prospective cohort study. Gut 1999;45(2):218–22.

9. Brand S. Crohn's disease: Th1, Th17 or both? The change of a paradigm: new immunological and genetic insights implicate Th17 cells in the pathogenesis of Crohn's disease. Gut 2009;58(8):1152–67.

10. Vind I, Riis L, Jess T, et al. Increasing incidences of inflammatory bowel disease and decreasing surgery rates in Copenhagen City and County, 2003-2005: a population-based study from the Danish Crohn colitis database. Am J Gastroenterol 2006;101(6):1274–82.

11. Bernell O, Lapidus A, Hellers G. Recurrence after colectomy in Crohn's colitis. Dis Colon Rectum 2001;44(5):647–54 [discussion: 654].

12. Bernstein CN, Blanchard JF, Rawsthorne P, et al. The prevalence of extraintestinal diseases in inflammatory bowel disease: a population-based study. Am J Gastroenterol 2001;96(4):1116–22.

13. Isaacs KL. How prevalent are extraintestinal manifestations at the initial diagnosis of IBD? Inflamm Bowel Dis 2008;14(Suppl 2):S198–9.

14. Petrelli EA, McKinley M, Troncale FJ. Ocular manifestations of inflammatory bowel disease. Ann Ophthalmol 1982;14(4):356–60.

15. Gisbert JP, Luna M, Gonzalez-Lama Y, et al. Liver injury in inflammatory bowel disease: long-term follow-up study of 786 patients. Inflamm Bowel Dis 2007;13(9):1106–14.

16. Raj V, Lichtenstein DR. Hepatobiliary manifestations of inflammatory bowel disease. Gastroenterol Clin North Am 1999;28(2):491–513.

17. Kappelman MD, Horvath-Puho E, Sandler RS, et al. Thromboembolic risk among Danish children and adults with inflammatory bowel diseases: a population-based nationwide study. Gut 2011; 60(7):937–43.

18. Nguyen GC, Sam J. Rising prevalence of venous thromboembolism and its impact on mortality among hospitalized inflammatory bowel disease patients. Am J Gastroenterol 2008;103(9):2272–80.

19. Vavricka SR, Brun L, Ballabeni P, et al. Frequency and risk factors for extraintestinal manifestations in the Swiss inflammatory bowel disease cohort. Am J Gastroenterol 2011;106(1):110–9.

20. Thrash B, Patel M, Shah KR, et al. Cutaneous manifestations of gastrointestinal disease: part II. J Am Acad Dermatol 2013;68(2):211.e1–33 [quiz: 244–6].

21. Peltz S, Vestey JP, Ferguson A, et al. Disseminated metastatic cutaneous Crohn's disease. Clin Exp Dermatol 1993;18(1):55–9.

22. Palamaras I, El-Jabbour J, Pietropaolo N, et al. Metastatic Crohn's disease: a review. J Eur Acad Dermatol Venereol 2008;22(9):1033–43.

23. Tavarela Veloso F. Review article: skin complications associated with inflammatory bowel disease. Aliment Pharmacol Ther 2004;20(Suppl 4):50–3.

24. Hoffmann RM, Kruis W. Rare extraintestinal manifestations of inflammatory bowel disease. Inflamm Bowel Dis 2004;10(2):140–7.

25. Leu S, Sun PK, Collyer J, et al. Clinical spectrum of vulva metastatic Crohn's disease. Dig Dis Sci 2009; 54(7):1565–71.

26. Porzionato A, Alaggio R, Aprile A. Perianal and vulvar Crohn's disease presenting as suspected abuse. Forensic Sci Int 2005;155(1):24–7.

27. Figg RE, Church JM. Perineal Crohn's disease: an indicator of poor prognosis and potential proctectomy. Dis Colon Rectum 2009;52(4):646–50.

28. Rosmaninho A, Sanches M, Salgado M, et al. Vulvoperineal Crohn's disease responsive to metronidazole. An Bras Dermatol 2013;88(6 Suppl 1):71–4.

29. Khaled A, Ezzine-Sebai N, Fazaa B, et al. Vulvoperineal Crohn's disease: response to metronidazole. Skinmed 2010;8(4):240–1.

30. Kuloglu Z, Kansu A, Demirceken F, et al. Crohn's disease of the vulva in a 10-year-old girl. Turk J Pediatr 2008;50(2):197–9.

31. Girszyn N, Leport J, Arnaud L, et al. Crohn's disease affecting only vulvoperineal area. Presse Med 2007;36(12 Pt 1):1762–5 [in French].

32. Wickramasinghe N, Gunasekara CN, Fernando WS, et al. Vulvitis granulomatosa, Melkersson-Rosenthal syndrome, and Crohn's disease: dramatic response to infliximab therapy. Int J Dermatol 2012;51(8):966–8.

33. Bedioui H, Makni A, Magherbi H, et al. Hyperbaric oxygen in the treatment of perineal Crohn's disease era of infliximab: a renewal interest? Tunis Med 2012;90(6):427–30 [in French].

34. Bel Pla S, Garcia-Patos Briones V, Garcia Fernandez D, et al. Vulvar lymphedema: unusual manifestation of metastatic Crohn's disease. Gastroenterol Hepatol 2001;24(6):297–9 [in Spanish].

35. Reitsma W, Wiegman MJ, Damstra RJ. Penile and scrotal lymphedema as an unusual presentation of Crohn's disease: case report and review of the literature. Lymphology 2012;45(1):37–41.

36. Sackett DD, Meshekow JS, Figueroa TE, et al. Isolated penile lymphedema in an adolescent male: a case of metastatic Crohn's disease. J Pediatr Urol 2012;8(5):e55–8.

37. Murphy MJ, Kogan B, Carlson JA. Granulomatous lymphangitis of the scrotum and penis. Report of a case and review of the literature of genital swelling with sarcoidal granulomatous inflammation. J Cutan Pathol 2001;28(8):419–24.

38. Macaya A, Marcoval J, Bordas X, et al. Crohn's disease presenting as prepuce and scrotal edema. J Am Acad Dermatol 2003;49(2 Suppl Case Reports):S182–3.

39. Reinders MG, Kukutsch NA. Genital edema in childhood: harbinger of Crohn's disease? J Am Acad Dermatol 2011;65(2):449–50.

40. Patel M, Menter A. Reply: genital edema in Crohn's disease. J Am Acad Dermatol 2014;70(2):385.

41. Bunker CB, Shim TN. Male genital edema in Crohn's disease. J Am Acad Dermatol 2014;70(2):385.

42. Nunez EC, Penaranda JM, Alonso MS, et al. Acquired vulvar lymphangioma: a case series with emphasis on expanding clinical contexts. Int J Gynecol Pathol 2014;33(3):235–40.

43. Papalas JA, Robboy SJ, Burchette JL, et al. Acquired vulvar lymphangioma circumscriptum: a comparison of 12 cases with Crohn's associated lesions or radiation therapy induced tumors. J Cutan Pathol 2010;37(9):958–65.

44. Mu XC, Tran TA, Dupree M, et al. Acquired vulvar lymphangioma mimicking genital warts. A case report and review of the literature. J Cutan Pathol 1999;26(3):150–4.

45. van de Scheur MR, van der Waal RI, van der Waal I, et al. Ano-genital granulomatosis: the counterpart of oro-facial granulomatosis. J Eur Acad Dermatol Venereol 2003;17(2):184–9.

46. Williams AJ, Wray D, Ferguson A. The clinical entity of orofacial Crohn's disease. Q J Med 1991; 79(289):451–8.

47. Basu MK, Asquith P. Oral manifestations of inflammatory bowel disease. Clin Gastroenterol 1980; 9(2):307–21.

48. Bogenrieder T, Rogler G, Vogt T, et al. Orofacial granulomatosis as the initial presentation of Crohn's disease in an adolescent. Dermatology 2003; 206(3):273–8.

49. Gale G, Ostman S, Rekabdar E, et al. Characterisation of a Swedish cohort with orofacial granulomatosis with or without Crohn's disease. Oral Dis 2015;21(1):e98–104.

50. Campbell H, Escudier M, Patel P, et al. Distinguishing orofacial granulomatosis from Crohn's disease: 2 separate disease entities? Inflamm Bowel Dis 2011;17(10):2109–15.

51. Sanderson J, Nunes C, Escudier M, et al. Orofacial granulomatosis: Crohn's disease or a new inflammatory bowel disease? Inflamm Bowel Dis 2005;11(9):840–6.

52. Patel P, Brostoff J, Campbell H, et al. Clinical evidence for allergy in orofacial granulomatosis and inflammatory bowel disease. Clin Transl Allergy 2013;3(1):26.

53. White A, Nunes C, Escudier M, et al. Improvement in orofacial granulomatosis on a cinnamon- and benzoate-free diet. Inflamm Bowel Dis 2006;12(6): 508–14.

54. Elliott T, Campbell H, Escudier M, et al. Experience with anti-TNF-alpha therapy for orofacial granulomatosis. J Oral Pathol Med 2011;40(1):14–9.

55. Trost LB, McDonnell JK. Important cutaneous manifestations of inflammatory bowel disease. Postgrad Med J 2005;81(959):580–5.

56. Freeman HJ. Erythema nodosum and pyoderma gangrenosum in 50 patients with Crohn's disease. Can J Gastroenterol 2005;19(10):603–6.

57. Farhi D, Cosnes J, Zizi N, et al. Significance of erythema nodosum and pyoderma gangrenosum in inflammatory bowel diseases: a cohort study of 2402 patients. Medicine (Baltimore) 2008;87(5): 281–93.

58. Agrawal D, Rukkannagari S, Kethu S. Pathogenesis and clinical approach to extraintestinal manifestations of inflammatory bowel disease. Minerva Gastroenterol Dietol 2007;53(3):233–48.

59. Gilchrist H, Patterson JW. Erythema nodosum and erythema induratum (nodular vasculitis): diagnosis and management. Dermatol Ther 2010;23(4):320–7.

60. Biedermann L, Kerl K, Rogler G, et al. Drug-induced erythema nodosum after the administration of certolizumab in Crohn's disease. Inflamm Bowel Dis 2013;19(1):E4–6.

61. Lebwohl M, Lebwohl O. Cutaneous manifestations of inflammatory bowel disease. Inflamm Bowel Dis 1998;4(2):142–8.

62. Huang W, McNeely MC. Neutrophilic tissue reactions. Adv Dermatol 1997;13:33–64.

63. Jorizzo JL, Solomon AR, Zanolli MD, et al. Neutrophilic vascular reactions. J Am Acad Dermatol 1988;19(6):983–1005.

64. Prat L, Bouaziz JD, Wallach D, et al. Neutrophilic dermatoses as systemic diseases. Clin Dermatol 2014;32(3):376–88.

65. Boh EE, al-Smadi RM. Cutaneous manifestations of gastrointestinal diseases. Dermatol Clin 2002; 20(3):533–46.

66. Marzano AV, Borghi A, Stadnicki A, et al. Cutaneous manifestations in patients with inflammatory bowel diseases: pathophysiology, clinical features, and therapy. Inflamm Bowel Dis 2014;20(1):213–27.

67. Timani S, Mutasim DF. Skin manifestations of inflammatory bowel disease. Clin Dermatol 2008; 26(3):265–73.

68. Huang BL, Chandra S, Shih DQ. Skin manifestations of inflammatory bowel disease. Front Physiol 2012;3:13.

69. Su CG, Judge TA, Lichtenstein GR. Extraintestinal manifestations of inflammatory bowel disease. Gastroenterol Clin North Am 2002;31(1): 307–27.

70. Matis WL, Ellis CN, Griffiths CE, et al. Treatment of pyoderma gangrenosum with cyclosporine. Arch Dermatol 1992;128(8):1060–4.

71. Barrie A, Regueiro M. Biologic therapy in the management of extraintestinal manifestations of inflammatory bowel disease. Inflamm Bowel Dis 2007; 13(11):1424–9.

72. Regueiro M, Valentine J, Plevy S, et al. Infliximab for treatment of pyoderma gangrenosum associated with inflammatory bowel disease. Am J Gastroenterol 2003;98(8):1821–6.

73. Agarwal A, Andrews JM. Systematic review: IBD-associated pyoderma gangrenosum in the biologic era, the response to therapy. Aliment Pharmacol Ther 2013;38(6):563–72.

74. Arguelles-Arias F, Castro-Laria L, Lobaton T, et al. Characteristics and treatment of pyoderma gangrenosum in inflammatory bowel disease. Dig Dis Sci 2013;58(10):2949–54.

75. Fonder MA, Cummins DL, Ehst BD, et al. Adalimumab therapy for recalcitrant pyoderma gangrenosum. J Burns Wounds 2006;5:e8.

76. Wu XR, Mukewar S, Kiran RP, et al. Risk factors for peristomal pyoderma gangrenosum complicating inflammatory bowel disease. J Crohns Colitis 2013;7(5):e171–7.

77. Hughes AP, Jackson JM, Callen JP. Clinical features and treatment of peristomal pyoderma gangrenosum. JAMA 2000;284(12):1546–8.

78. Reichrath J, Bens G, Bonowitz A, et al. Treatment recommendations for pyoderma gangrenosum: an evidence-based review of the literature based on more than 350 patients. J Am Acad Dermatol 2005;53(2):273–83.

79. Handler MZ, Hamilton H, Aires D. Treatment of peristomal pyoderma gangrenosum with topical crushed dapsone. J Drugs Dermatol 2011;10(9): 1059–61.

80. Chriba M, Skellett AM, Levell NJ. Beclometasone inhaler used to treat pyoderma gangrenosum. Clin Exp Dermatol 2010;35(3):337–8.

81. Alkhouri N, Hupertz V, Mahajan L. Adalimumab treatment for peristomal pyoderma gangrenosum associated with Crohn's disease. Inflamm Bowel Dis 2009;15(6):803–6.

82. Fahmy M, Ramamoorthy S, Hata T, et al. Ustekinumab for peristomal pyoderma gangrenosum. Am J Gastroenterol 2012;107(5):794–5.

83. Kim FS, Pandya AG. The use of etanercept in the treatment of peristomal pyoderma gangrenosum. Clin Exp Dermatol 2012;37(4):442–3.

84. Mimouni D, Anhalt GJ, Kouba DJ, et al. Infliximab for peristomal pyoderma gangrenosum. Br J Dermatol 2003;148(4):813–6.

85. Poritz LS, Lebo MA, Bobb AD, et al. Management of peristomal pyoderma gangrenosum. J Am Coll Surg 2008;206(2):311–5.

86. Kiran RP, O'Brien-Ermlich B, Achkar JP, et al. Management of peristomal pyoderma gangrenosum. Dis Colon Rectum 2005;48(7):1397–403.

87. Femiano F, Lanza A, Buonaiuto C, et al. Pyostomatitis vegetans: a review of the literature. Med Oral Patol Oral Cir Bucal 2009;14(3):E114–7.

88. Brinkmeier T, Frosch PJ. Pyodermatitis-pyostomatitis vegetans: a clinical course of two decades with response to cyclosporine and low-dose prednisolone. Acta Derm Venereol 2001;81(2): 134–6.

89. Werchniak AE, Storm CA, Plunkett RW, et al. Treatment of pyostomatitis vegetans with topical tacrolimus. J Am Acad Dermatol 2005;52(4):722–3.

90. Bens G, Laharie D, Beylot-Barry M, et al. Successful treatment with infliximab and methotrexate of pyostomatitis vegetans associated with Crohn's disease. Br J Dermatol 2003;149(1):181–4.

91. Trikudanathan G, Venkatesh PG, Navaneethan U. Diagnosis and therapeutic management of extraintestinal manifestations of inflammatory bowel disease. Drugs 2012;72(18):2333–49.

92. Lourenco SV, Hussein TP, Bologna SB, et al. Oral manifestations of inflammatory bowel disease: a review based on the observation of six cases. J Eur Acad Dermatol Venereol 2010;24(2):204–7.

93. Slebioda Z, Szponar E, Kowalska A. Etiopathogenesis of recurrent aphthous stomatitis and the role of immunologic aspects: literature review. Arch Immunol Ther Exp (Warsz) 2014;62(3):205–15.

94. Larsen S, Bendtzen K, Nielsen OH. Extraintestinal manifestations of inflammatory bowel disease: epidemiology, diagnosis, and management. Ann Med 2010;42(2):97–114.

95. Ytting H, Vind I, Bang D, et al. Sweet's syndrome–an extraintestinal manifestation in inflammatory bowel disease. Digestion 2005;72(2–3): 195–200.

96. Catalan-Serra I, Martin-Moraleda L, Navarro-Lopez L, et al. Crohn's disease and Sweet's syndrome: an uncommon association. Rev Esp Enferm Dig 2010;102(5):331–7.

97. Smith SE, Gillon JT, Ferguson SB. Targetoid palmoplantar Sweet syndrome as presenting sign of severe Crohn's disease. J Am Acad Dermatol 2013; 69(4):e199–200.

98. Cohen PR. Neutrophilic dermatoses: a review of current treatment options. Am J Clin Dermatol 2009;10(5):301–12.

99. Spencer B, Nanavati A, Greene J, et al. Dapsone-responsive histiocytoid Sweet's syndrome associated with Crohn's disease. J Am Acad Dermatol 2008;59(2 Suppl 1):S58–60.

100. Meinhardt C, Buning J, Fellermann K, et al. Cyclophosphamide therapy in Sweet's syndrome complicating refractory Crohn's disease–efficacy and mechanism of action. J Crohns Colitis 2011;5(6): 633–7.

101. Rahier JF, Lion L, Dewit O, et al. Regression of Sweet's syndrome associated with Crohn's disease after anti-tumour necrosis factor therapy. Acta Gastroenterol Belg 2005;68(3):376–9.

102. Vanbiervliet G, Anty R, Schneider S, et al. Sweet's syndrome and erythema nodosum associated with Crohn's disease treated by infliximab. Gastroenterol Clin Biol 2002;26(3):295–7 [in French].

103. El-Azhary RA, Brunner KL, Gibson LE. Sweet syndrome as a manifestation of azathioprine hypersensitivity. Mayo Clin Proc 2008;83(9):1026–30.

104. Choonhakarn C, Chaowattanapanit S. Azathioprine-induced Sweet's syndrome and published work review. J Dermatol 2013;40(4):267–71.

105. Morgan AJ, Schwartz RA. Cutaneous polyarteritis nodosa: a comprehensive review. Int J Dermatol 2010;49(7):750–6.

106. Solley GO, Winklemann RK, Rovelstad RA. Correlation between regional enterocolitis and cutaneous polyarteritis nodosa. Two case reports and review of the literature. Gastroenterology 1975;69(1):235–9.

107. Khoo BP, Ng SK. Cutaneous polyarteritis nodosa: a case report and literature review. Ann Acad Med Singapore 1998;27(6):868–72.

108. Daoud MS, Hutton KP, Gibson LE. Cutaneous periarteritis nodosa: a clinicopathological study of 79 cases. Br J Dermatol 1997;136(5):706–13.

109. Burns AM, Walsh N, Green PJ. Granulomatous vasculitis in Crohn's disease: a clinicopathologic correlate of two unusual cases. J Cutan Pathol 2010;37(10):1077–83.

110. Vaszar LT, Orzechowski NM, Specks U, et al. Coexistent pulmonary granulomatosis with polyangiitis (Wegener granulomatosis) and Crohn disease. Am J Surg Pathol 2014;38(3):354–9.

111. Jacob SE, Martin LK, Kerdel FA. Cutaneous Wegener's granulomatosis (malignant pyoderma) in a patient with Crohn's disease. Int J Dermatol 2003; 42(11):896–8.

112. Zlatanic J, Fleisher M, Sasson M, et al. Crohn's disease and acute leukocytoclastic vasculitis of skin. Am J Gastroenterol 1996;91(11):2410–3.

113. Plaza Santos R, Jaquotot Herranz M, Froilan Torres C, et al. Leukocytoclastic vasculitis associated with Crohn's disease. Gastroenterol Hepatol 2010;33(6):433–5 [in Spanish].

114. Limdi JK, Doran HM, Crampton JR. Cutaneous vasculitis in Crohn's disease. J Crohns Colitis 2010;4(3):351–2.

115. Carlson JA, Chen KR. Cutaneous vasculitis update: neutrophilic muscular vessel and eosinophilic, granulomatous, and lymphocytic vasculitis syndromes. Am J Dermatopathol 2007;29(1):32–43.

116. Tsiamoulos Z, Karamanolis G, Polymeros D, et al. Leukocytoclastic vasculitis as an onset symptom of Crohn's disease. Case Rep Gastroenterol 2008; 2(3):410–4.

117. Tsai TF, Wang TS, Hung ST, et al. Epidemiology and comorbidities of psoriasis patients in a national database in Taiwan. J Dermatol Sci 2011;63(1): 40–6.

118. Ko JM, Gottlieb AB, Kerbleski JF. Induction and exacerbation of psoriasis with TNF-blockade therapy: a review and analysis of 127 cases. J Dermatolog Treat 2009;20(2):100–8.

119. Famenini S, Wu JJ. Infliximab-induced psoriasis in treatment of Crohn's disease-associated ankylosing spondylitis: case report and review of 142 cases. J Drugs Dermatol 2013;12(8): 939–43.

120. Tillack C, Ehmann LM, Friedrich M, et al. Anti-TNF antibody-induced psoriasiform skin lesions in patients with inflammatory bowel disease are characterised by interferon-gamma-expressing Th1 cells and IL-17A/IL-22-expressing Th17 cells and respond to anti-IL-12/IL-23 antibody treatment. Gut 2014;63(4):567–77.

121. Tichy M, Hercogova J. Manifestation of Crohn's disease in a young woman during the course of treatment for severe form of chronic plaque psoriasis with etanercept. Dermatol Ther 2014;27: 211–4.

122. Monroe EW. Vitiligo associated with regional enteritis. Arch Dermatol 1976;112(6):833–4.

123. McPoland PR, Moss RL. Cutaneous Crohn's disease and progressive vitiligo. J Am Acad Dermatol 1988;19(2 Pt 2):421–5.

124. Mebazaa A, Aounallah A, Naija N, et al. Dermatologic manifestations in inflammatory bowel disease in Tunisia. Tunis Med 2012;90(3):252–7.

125. Posada C, Florez A, Batalla A, et al. Vitiligo during treatment of Crohn's disease with adalimumab: adverse effect or co-occurrence? Case Rep Dermatol 2011;3(1):28–31.

126. Roychoudhuri R, Hirahara K, Mousavi K, et al. BACH2 represses effector programs to stabilize T(reg)-mediated immune homeostasis. Nature 2013;498(7455):506–10.

127. Reddy H, Shipman AR, Wojnarowska F. Epidermolysis bullosa acquisita and inflammatory bowel disease: a review of the literature. Clin Exp Dermatol 2013;38(3):225–9 [quiz: 229–30].

128. Caux F. Diagnosis and clinical features of epidermolysis bullosa acquisita. Dermatol Clin 2011; 29(3):485–91, x.

129. Chen M, O'Toole EA, Sanghavi J, et al. The epidermolysis bullosa acquisita antigen (type VII collagen) is present in human colon and patients with Crohn's disease have autoantibodies to type VII collagen. J Invest Dermatol 2002;118(6):1059–64.

130. Le Roux-Villet C, Prost-Squarcioni C. Epidermolysis bullosa acquisita: literature review. Ann Dermatol Venereol 2011;138(3):228–46 [in French].

131. Ormaechea-Perez N, Tuneu-Valls A, Borja-Consigliere HA, et al. Peristomal epidermolysis bullosa acquisita in a patient with Crohn's disease. Acta Derm Venereol 2014;94:489–90.

132. Gupta R, Woodley DT, Chen M. Epidermolysis bullosa acquisita. Clin Dermatol 2012;30(1):60–9.

133. Pellicer Z, Santiago JM, Rodriguez A, et al. Management of cutaneous disorders related to inflammatory bowel disease. Ann Gastroenterol 2012;25(1):21–6.

134. Pugh SM, Rhodes J, Mayberry JF, et al. Atopic disease in ulcerative colitis and Crohn's disease. Clin Allergy 1979;9(3):221–3.

135. Myrelid P, Dufmats M, Lilja I, et al. Atopic manifestations are more common in patients with Crohn disease than in the general population. Scand J Gastroenterol 2004;39(8):731–6.

136. Kappelman MD, Galanko JA, Porter CQ, et al. Association of paediatric inflammatory bowel disease with other immune-mediated diseases. Arch Dis Child 2011;96(11):1042–6.

137. Esparza-Gordillo J, Marenholz I, Lee YA. Genome-wide approaches to the etiology of eczema. Curr Opin Allergy Clin Immunol 2010;10(5):418–26.

138. Baumgart DC, Grittner U, Steingraber A, et al. Frequency, phenotype, outcome, and therapeutic impact of skin reactions following initiation of adalimumab therapy: experience from a consecutive cohort of inflammatory bowel disease patients. Inflamm Bowel Dis 2011;17(12):2512–20.

139. Santos G, Sousa L. Syndrome in question. An Bras Dermatol 2014;89(2):361–2.

140. Krasovec M, Frenk E. Acrodermatitis enteropathica secondary to Crohn's disease. Dermatology 1996; 193(4):361–3.

141. Doyle LA, Sperling LC, Baksh S, et al. Psoriatic alopecia/alopecia areata-like reactions secondary to anti-tumor necrosis factor-alpha therapy: a novel cause of noncicatricial alopecia. Am J Dermatopathol 2011;33(2):161–6.

142. Fawcett RS, Linford S, Stulberg DL. Nail abnormalities: clues to systemic disease. Am Fam Physician 2004;69(6):1417–24.

143. Myers KA, Farquhar DR. The rational clinical examination. Does this patient have clubbing? JAMA 2001;286(3):341–7.

144. Myung SJ, Yang SK, Jung HY, et al. Zinc deficiency manifested by dermatitis and visual dysfunction in a patient with Crohn's disease. J Gastroenterol 1998;33(6):876–9.

145. Gehrig KA, Dinulos JG. Acrodermatitis due to nutritional deficiency. Curr Opin Pediatr 2010;22(1): 107–12.

146. von Felbert V, Hunziker T. Acrodermatitis enteropathica-like skin lesions due to Crohn's disease-associated zinc deficiency. Hautarzt 2010;61(11):927–9 [in German].

Orofacial Granulomatosis

Arwa Al-Hamad, PhD[a,b],
Stephen Porter, BSc, MD, PhD, FDSRCS (Edin), FDSRCS (Eng), FHEA[a],
Stefano Fedele, DDS, PhD[a,c,d],*

KEYWORDS

- Orofacial granulomatosis • Melkersson-Rosenthal syndrome • Granulomatous cheilitis
- Granulomas • Crohn's disease

KEY POINTS

- Orofacial granulomatosis (OFG) is an uncommon granulomatous disorder of the orofacial tissues.
- Disease hallmarks include development of disfiguring labial or facial enlargement and intra-oral mucosal swelling and ulceration.
- Crohn's disease, sarcoidosis, and a range of other systemic disorders can present orofacial features similar to those of OFG; however, a strict case definition of OFG requires the exclusion of concomitant systemic granulomatous disease.
- A small subgroup of OFG patients, especially those with disease onset during childhood, will eventually develop intestinal Crohn's disease or, more rarely, sarcoidosis.
- Prolonged anti-inflammatory and immune-modulatory systemic therapy is usually needed to obtain long-term control of severe orofacial swelling and inflammation; however, intralesional corticosteroid therapy may provide notable long-term remission with no need of prolonged treatment.

INTRODUCTION

Orofacial granulomatosis (OFG) is an uncommon chronic inflammatory disorder that typically affects the soft tissues of the orofacial region.[1] It is histopathologically characterized by subepithelial noncaseating granulomas and has a spectrum of possible clinical manifestations ranging from subtle oral mucosal swelling to permanent disfiguring fibrous swelling of the lips and face.[2–6] Painful oral ulceration and neurologic manifestations to the head and neck region can also occur.[3–5] The first cases of a disorder causing recurrent/chronic orofacial swelling were initially reported in the nineteenth century[7,8]; eventually Melkersson[9] and Rosenthal[10] described the association between recurrent/chronic orofacial edema, facial palsy, and fissured tongue (lingua plicata). The term Melkersson-Rosenthal syndrome (MRS) was

---

Part of this work was undertaken at University College London/University College London Hospital, which received a proportion of funding from the Department of Health's National Institute for Health Research Biomedical Research Centre funding scheme.

Conflicts of Interest: The authors declare that they have no affiliation with any organization with a financial interest, direct or indirect, in the subject matter or materials discussed in the article that may affect the conduct or reporting of the work submitted.

Authorship: All authors named above meet the following criteria of the International Committee of Medical Journal Editors: Substantial contributions to conception and design, or acquisition of data, or analysis and interpretation of data; drafting the article or revising it critically for important intellectual content; final approval of the version to be published.

[a] Oral Medicine Unit, UCL Eastman Dental Institute, University College London, 256 Gray's Inn Road, London WC1X 8LD, UK; [b] Dental Services, Ministry of National Guard, King Abdulaziz Medical City-Riyadh, Riyadh, Saudi Arabia; [c] NIHR University College London Hospitals Biomedical Research Centre, Maple House, Suite A, 1st floor, 149 Tottenham Court Road, London W1T 7DN, UK; [d] Oral Medicine Unit, Eastman Dental Hospital, University College London Hospitals Trust, 256 Gray's Inn Road, London WC1X 8LD, UK
* Corresponding author. Oral Medicine Unit, Eastman Dental Institute and Hospital, University College London and University College London Hospitals Trust, 256 Gray's Inn Road, London WC1X 8LD, UK.
E-mail address: s.fedele@ucl.ac.uk

Dermatol Clin 33 (2015) 433–446
http://dx.doi.org/10.1016/j.det.2015.03.008

derm.theclinics.com

therefore introduced to describe individuals with the full triad of manifestations, whereas those with only labial swelling were referred to as having cheilitis granulomatosa (Miescher's cheilitis). In 1985, Wiesenfeld and colleagues[7] introduced the term OFG to encompass both MRS and Miescher's cheilitis. Over the years, many systemic granulomatous disorders (including Crohn's disease, sarcoidosis, leprosy, tuberculosis, chronic granulomatous disease, and possibly deep fungal infections) have been reported to cause orofacial manifestations[11] similar to those of OFG. It remains controversial whether it is appropriate to refer to them as OFG. The authors of the present article define OFG as an idiopathic granulomatous disease limited to the orofacial tissue, namely affecting individuals who do not show any evidence of previous or concomitant systemic granulomatous disease as per clinical, radiological, endoscopic, or serologic investigations; diagnosis of idiopathic OFG remains therefore one of exclusion.[3,5,6,12] Because it is well established that some of these patients would eventually develop additional extraoral/facial manifestations of a systemic granulomatous disease (eg, colonic Crohn's disease), the authors suggest that their diagnosis should be at that point revised and retermed (eg, from OFG to oral and colonic Crohn's disease). This classification has a pragmatic clinical relevance, because individuals with OFG limited to orofacial tissues would benefit from therapeutic interventions and monitoring that are significantly different from those with a systemic granulomatous disease. OFG is an uncommon disease. No reliable epidemiologic data are available because most cases series report small single-center groups of patients.[1] There remain few studies describing case series of 100 or more OFG patients, which, however, represent retrospective analysis of cohorts that are often heterogeneous (including patients with Crohn's disease) and observed for 2 or more decades.[1,13]

OFG seems to have no specific ethnic predilection, and most authors report that both genders are equally affected.[1,14] The disease occurs by the end of the third decade of life in the vast majority of reported patients.[1]

OFG can cause adverse effects on the quality of life of patients because of the disfiguring chronic orofacial swelling, painful oral ulceration, and occasional neurologic involvement.[15] Treatment of OFG has proven difficult and unsatisfactory, with no single predictable therapeutic model showing consistent efficacy in reducing orofacial swelling and mucosal inflammation.[16]

The aim of the present article is to present a comprehensive review of available literature about etiopathogenesis, clinical manifestations, prognosis, and management of OFG.

ETIOPATHOGENESIS

Although several possible causative factors have been associated with OFG,[12] the exact etiopathogenesis remains unknown. Existing literature has typically focused on the role of (1) delayed hypersensitivity to food substances, food preservatives, or dental materials; (2) microbial infections; and (3) inflammatory/immunologic factors.[12] Recent findings regarding the immunopathogenesis of granulomas in Crohn's disease[17] and other rare granulomatous disorders[18,19] could indicate that similar defects of the innate immunity may also play a part in the cause of granulomas of OFG.[12,20,21] Relevant studies are ongoing.[22]

Hereditary and Genetic Predisposition

There are no adequate data in the literature that support that OFG has a definite genetic background.[12,23] Reports of hereditary cases remain scarce, and studies have not found any convincing robust HLA association[24,25] in OFG patients versus population controls.

Inflammatory/Immunologic Factors

Characterization of granulomatous inflammation of OFG has led to conflicting and inconsistent results. It remains unclear whether lesional T cells of OFG represent clonal expansion as a result of chronic antigen stimulation.[12,26,27] Studies on the expression of cytokines and chemokines in OFG lesions have found a predominant Th1-mediated immune response.[12,28]

Hypersensitivity Reactions

A wide range of hypersensitivities have been reported in OFG patients, including dental restorative materials,[29,30] toothpastes and other dental hygiene products,[31,32] cocoa and chocolate,[31,32] cinnamon compounds, carvone, carbone piperitone, aspartate,[31,33–37] carmosine and sun yellow dye,[33] monosodium glutamate,[33,38] benzoates,[33,35–37,39,40] and tartrazine.[39] Cinnamon and benzoate compounds have been suggested to be the most common triggers.[31–33,36,39,40] A potential role of hypersensitivity in OFG pathogenesis seems to be supported and confirmed by the patient's history of symptoms aggravation associated with contact or ingestion of one or more of the above-mentioned triggering factors, positive response to elimination diet, and in some cases positive patch testing.[12,30] Furthermore, a recent article has reported OFG patients to have a higher prevalence of allergy than the general population as demonstrated by their medical history, skin prick test, and serum immunoglobulin E (IgE).[41] Nevertheless, other studies have failed to find convincing evidence of sensitization to foods, additives, or contactants in OFG patients.[42] Also, outcomes of avoidance diet remain controversial because they vary from 14%[13,43] to 70%[44] and seem not to correlate with patch testing results.[44] It is possible that delayed hypersensitivity mechanisms may have a pathogenetic role in a small subgroup of OFG patients.

Microbial Factors

Several investigators have investigated the potential role of microbial agents in triggering the immune response of OFG, including *Mycobacterium tuberculosis*, *Mycobacterium paratuberculosis*, *Saccharomyces cerevisiae*, *Borrelia burgdorferi*, *Candida albicans*, and *Streptococcus mutans*. Although some studies have reported the presence of *M tuberculosis* RNA in OFG samples[45] and raised IgG antibody titers to the mycobacterial stress protein 65[46] in OFG patients' serum, there remains little credible evidence to support a role of any of these agents in the etiopathogenesis of OFG.[25,47-50]

CLINICAL PRESENTATION

Disfiguring lip swelling remains the clinical hallmark of OFG and the most common reason for which OFG patients seek medical attention.[51] Other possible clinical manifestations include swelling and ulceration of the oral mucosa, swelling of facial (other than labial) tissues, and neurologic manifestations.[3,4] It is probable that OFG represents a disease with a spectrum of severity that ranges from localized granulomatous inflammation of the lips, through orofacial swelling with mucosal ulceration to a disease with additional neurologic deficit.[3,52-54] Available literature indicates that clinical manifestations at disease onset can be highly variable and multiform, although permanent disfiguring labial or facial swelling eventually develops in nearly all affected individuals.

Labial Swelling

Available literature clearly shows that labial enlargement is the most common feature of OFG, affecting more than 90% of patients.[5] Lip enlargement is typically recurrent and edematous in the early stages of the disease (**Fig. 1**), with each episode lasting a few days or weeks.[1,13,55] During the course of the disease and after several recurrent episodes, the swelling of the lips typically

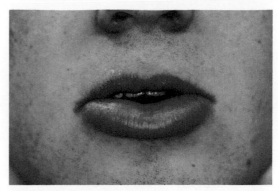

Fig. 1. Early stages of OFG showing recurrent mild-to-moderate edematous swelling of the lower lip.

becomes persistent, firm, and indurated (**Fig. 2**), assuming the characteristics of a granulomatous disorder.[5] Lip fissuring, exfoliation, and impetiginization can be associated, especially in severe cases, and intraoral labial mucosa may become erythematous and granular.[5,13] The peri-oral skin may become erythematous and exfoliated and some patients may develop angular cheilitis.[56] There is no site predisposition for the labial swelling, although it may be slightly more common on the lower lip.[3,5,7,57] The swelling rarely causes difficulties in speech or drooling.[4]

Facial Swelling

Swelling of nonlabial facial tissues has been described in OFG patients, sometimes in the absence of lip enlargement or other clinical manifestations, and can vary in severity. Patients can develop recurrent or persistent enlargement of the zygomatic, frontal, peri-orbital, or chin/submental region,[3,58] as well as the cheek and eyelids, which represent a diagnostic challenge because these are not favorable areas to obtain a biopsy specimen.[3] Indeed, blepharitis granulomatosa (or granulomatous blepharitis) it is likely to represent

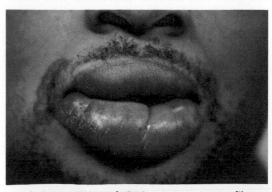

Fig. 2. Late stages of OFG causing severe fibrous swelling of both lips with desquamation and fissuring.

OFG-like disease.[59,60] Swelling of submandibular or cervical areas due to persistent lymph node enlargement can arise in about 25% of OFG individuals.[4,5]

Intra-oral Manifestations

Generalized swelling of the buccal and or labial mucosa gives rise to a cobblestone-like appearance,[4] a common intra-oral feature of OFG,[61] particularly in the posterior buccal mucosa.[4,52] Localized mucosal swelling manifests as discreet painless tags typically affecting the vestibular buccal and labial mucosa or floor of the mouth ("stag-horning").[5] Deep chronic linear ulcers with raised margins can arise in the buccal or labial sulcus and are often associated with significant pain.[5] Less commonly, flat and circular aphthous-like ulcers can arise on any oral mucosal surface. Pyostomatitis vegetans, which manifests with yellowish, linear pustules on the background of mucosal erythematous "snail track ulcerations," has also been described, although the vast majority of reports refer to individuals with evidence of inflammatory bowel disease (Crohn's disease).[4,62–65] Painless gingival swelling independent of plaque and calculus deposits may occur in up to one-third of patients with OFG.[2,6,66,67] The swelling can affect the attached or free gingivae, be localized or generalized, and is often associated with erythema and superficial "granular" appearance.[2,3] Generalized erythema/inflammation of the oral mucosa is uncommonly described as a separate intra-oral feature of OFG[68] possibly because it usually develops in association with either manifestation, including cobblestoning and ulceration. The tongue may have superficial fissures that are most pronounced on the lateral aspects of the dorsum.[4] The fissuring may rarely cause food accumulation leading to alteration in taste, oral malodor, and a local burning sensation.[66,69] Fissuring of the tongue has been inconsistently associated with neurologic manifestations.[69]

Neurologic Manifestations

A subgroup of patients with OFG may have lower motor nerve facial palsy at some point in the disease course.[66,70] Granuloma formation or inflammation within the course of the mainstem of the facial nerve is the most probable cause for the palsy.[4] The exact prevalence of facial palsy in OFG is unclear, but studies report a very wide range of 8% to 57%.[3,7,40,71] The palsy can be complete or partial but is typically unilateral. The palsy can occur before, with, or after (sometimes months to years) the facial swelling.[72] It also may be accompanied by otalgia or changes in hearing and taste.[60] Complete recovery of nerve function is usual but some residual weakness can occur.[70,73,74] Facial palsy can be considered a feature of MRS syndrome when associated with lip swelling and fissured tongue, although most clinicians now categorize MRS as a subtype of OFG. Many less common neurologic manifestations have been reported to develop in up to 30% of OFG patients.[2,3,7,71,74] These manifestations include blepharospasm, migraine-like headache, hypogeusia, glossodynia, hyperacusis, lacrimation, and sweating.[75,76] Relevant pathogenetic mechanisms remain unknown.

Clinical Manifestations of Early and Advanced Disease

Labial swelling is traditionally indicated as the most common clinical feature of OFG and was previously reported as being the most frequent manifestation at disease presentation. However, several investigators have more recently suggested that OFG can in fact present with multiple, temporary, and variable clinical features affecting oral mucosa, gingivae, facial tissues, and the craniofacial nervous system,[3] and that different clinical manifestations can develop at different time points during the course of the disease.[2,3] Zimmer and colleagues[2] reported that labial swelling was the initial disease manifestation in only 43% of their 42 patients, but this percentage increased to 74% during the course of the disease. Moreover, the overall number of clinical manifestations increased during the years as the percentage of patients with facial swelling increased from 26% to 50% and those with facial palsy increased from 19% to 33%. Mignogna and colleagues[3] reported that about half of their 19 OFG patients (9/19) had an "atypical" disease onset characterized by the absence of labial swelling, which, however, developed in 7 of these 9 patients at a later stage. Al Johani and colleagues[5] studied a cohort of 49 OFG patients and confirmed that OFG presents with lip swelling in only 50% of cases, whereas the remaining individuals had intra-oral or neurologic manifestations in the absence of labial or facial swelling. They also reported that most patients eventually developed a variety of additional features of OFG, with nearly all affected individuals (>90%) ultimately developing lip/facial swelling.[5]

SYSTEMIC ASSOCIATION

Considering the strict definition and nomenclature that the authors of the present review have adopted, the concomitant presence of orofacial and other systemic manifestations of a specific and well-characterized generalized granulomatous disorder (eg, Crohn's disease or sarcoidosis) should exclude the diagnosis of idiopathic OFG. Indeed, as mentioned above, a diagnosis of "true" idiopathic OFG would require that detailed medical history, clinical assessment, and comprehensive investigations are performed so to rule out the presence of these disorders and confirm that disease is limited to the orofacial tissues.[1,12,23] Nevertheless, potential associations with systemic disease can still exist in patients with idiopathic OFG.

Subsequent Development of Systemic Granulomatous Disease

It is well described that a subgroup of OFG individuals would eventually develop manifestations of systemic disease, typically intestinal Crohn's disease or respiratory/multiorgan sarcoidosis, even if at the moment of initial assessment there was no clinical, serologic, or radiological evidence of any relevant extra-oral abnormality.[13,68,77,78] As discussed, it would be sensible at that stage to re-label these cases as, for example, having oral and intestinal Crohn's disease or oral and respiratory sarcoidosis rather than maintaining the nomenclature of OFG in association with Crohn's disease or sarcoidosis. It is difficult to predict which OFG patients will eventually develop extra-oral manifestations of a granulomatous systemic disease, although the vast majority of them are thought to have disease that will remain limited to the orofacial tissues. Campbell and colleagues[13] reported that only 20% of OFG patients followed up in their cohort subsequently developed "true" symptomatic Crohn's disease. They also confirmed previous observations that childhood onset of OFG carries a higher risk of subsequent Crohn's disease development.[56,79] There is no convincing evidence that any particular clinical manifestation or hematological/histologic feature in OFG patients might be predictive of future Crohn's disease development, including early asymptomatic intestinal inflammation (see later discussion).

Several cases of multisystemic sarcoidosis developing in individuals with disease onset limited to the orofacial region have been reported.[80] Similarly to Crohn's disease, there remains no reliable clinical feature or test to predict development of systemic sarcoidosis in individuals with OFG-like disease, with the possible exception of raised serum angiotensin converting enzyme levels.[80]

Concomitant Intestinal Inflammation of Unclear Clinical Significance

A variable portion of OFG individuals have been reported to show concomitant endoscopic and histologic features of intestinal inflammation in the absence of specific gastrointestinal symptoms and of unclear clinical significance. Both Scully and colleagues[72] in 1982 and Sanderson and colleagues in 2005[68] reported evidence of intestinal inflammation in subgroups of OFG patients with no notable history of gastrointestinal symptoms.[32,37,40,43,81,82] The former study used rigid sigmoidoscopy and barium radiology on 19 patients and reported evidence of likely intestinal Crohn's disease in 37% of cases,[77] whereas the latter used flexible endoscopy and biopsies and found discrete granulomatous intestinal inflammation (but no convincing evidence of Crohn's disease) in 54% of the 35 patients studied.[68] Clinical significance of asymptomatic gut inflammation in these subgroups of OFG patients is unclear. Unfortunately, these studies were not followed by a long-term observation and it is unknown whether the presence of discrete intestinal inflammation in OFG patients might be predictive of subsequent development of symptomatic full-blown Crohn's disease.

Allergy

It has been found that a history of IgE-mediated clinical allergy in the form of hay fever, eczema, asthma, or oral allergy syndrome can be observed in up to 80% of OFG patients compared with 15% to 20% of the general population.[32,37,40,41,81,82] The most frequent skin prick testing-confirmed sensitizations were to grass, silver birch, ragweed, mugwort, latex, and pollens.[41,43] The clinical significance of IgE-mediated atopy in OFG patients is unclear because dietary avoidance of cross-reactive foods failed to demonstrate significant improvements in the majority patients.[43] Patients with OFG have also been described to have patch test–confirmed delayed-type hypersensitivity to several food substances and additives, including wheat, dairy products, chocolate, eggs, peanuts, cinnamaldehyde, carbone piperitone, cocoa, carvone, carmosine, sun yellow dye, monosodium glutamate, benzoate, and cow's milk.[12] Delayed hypersensitivity to some dental materials, including amalgam, mercury, gold, and cobalt, has also been reported.[12] Elimination diets and replacement of the relevant dental material have been reported to improve clinical manifestations by some, albeit not all, authors.[12,42] Significant limitations of available studies about dietary manipulation include concomitant use of immunosuppressive agents, open-label design with no controls, and surprising lack of correlation between patch testing results and dietary outcome.[13,37]

EVALUATION AND MANAGEMENT

Diagnosis and Assessment

Diagnosis of OFG requires (1) the presence of relevant orofacial clinical features, and (2) the exclusion of systemic disorders causing similar manifestations through detailed medical history and serologic, radiological, or endoscopic investigations (where clinically justified). Histopathological confirmation of noncaseating granulomas is not a required criterion, although it may provide useful information contributing to exclude other causes of granulomatous inflammation (**Table 1**). There is no consensus with respect to the most appropriate measure or instrument to assess OFG disease severity/activity and monitor response to treatment. Most authors have adopted a pragmatic, although highly subjective, patient- or clinician-centered assessment of swelling and inflammation, and some have used standardized clinical photographs to support patients' and clinicians' judgment.[6] Disease severity/activity scores have been suggested by different groups[51,68] but are limited by a lack of adequate validation. A newly developed quality-of-life questionnaire known as Chronic Oral Mucosal Diseases Questionnaire (COMDQ) was demonstrated to be a valid and reliable measure to assess quality of life in patients with chronic oral mucosal diseases, including OFG.[83] However, the number of OFG patients included in COMDQ validation study was very small, and further confirmatory evidence is needed. Chiandussi and colleagues[84] have proposed an objective method for assessing lip size and treatment-related morphologic changes based on lip impressions and measurement of related plaster models.

Management

The principal goal of OFG therapy is to lessen cosmetically undesirable orofacial swelling and control painful mucosal ulceration; however, treatment may not be always needed if symptoms or signs of OFG are mild. Many treatment strategies have been reported during the last 3 decades, but relevant outcomes remain variable and often unpredictable. The overall evidence regarding the effectiveness of available therapeutic options is not robust because of the lack of randomized controlled trials and the use of inconsistent, often subjective, outcome measures. Lack of multicenter collaborations recruiting large groups of OFG patients adds further limitations to the available data.

Table 1
Diagnostic investigations and criteria of orofacial granulomatosis

Results	Investigations
Should be normal	Full blood cell count
Should be normal	Hemoglobin
Should be normal	Serum angiotensin converting enzyme levels[a]
Should be normal	C-1 esterase inhibitor levels[b]
Should be normal	Serum iron and transferrin
Should be negative	Tuberculin skin test (when clinically justified)
Should be normal	Chest radiography (when clinically justified)
Should be normal; if inflammatory changes are present, Crohn's disease should be excluded	GI endoscopy/histopathology[c]
Should be present[d]	Histopathology I: dilated lymphatics, edema of corium, slight fibrosis, with/without multiple noncaseating granulomas with Langerhans giant cell and lymphocytes
Should be negative	Histopathology II: PAS reaction and Ziehl-Neelsen stain (when clinically justified)
Should be negative	Polarized light microscopy: identification of birefringent foreign-body material (when clinically justified)

Abbreviations: GI, gastrointestinal; PAS, periodic acid-Schiff.
[a] To be performed when there are clinical features compatible with potential diagnosis of sarcoidosis.
[b] To be performed when orofacial swelling is recurrent and edematous without signs of persistent tissue fibrosis.
[c] To be performed when clinical or laboratory features increase suggestion of GI inflammatory disease.
[d] Absence of histopathological features does not exclude OFG diagnosis if clinical features are compatible.

Available literature suggests that the treatment of the disfiguring orofacial swelling of OFG has proven exceedingly difficult and remains unsatisfactory.[16,51] Immunosuppressants, tumor necrosis factor-α (TNF-α) inhibitors, and other agents, as well as surgical cheiloplasty, have been used as single or combined therapy with some positive, although overall inconsistent, results in a variety of cases reports and small case series.[16] Similarly, the encouraging results of a benzoate- and cinnamon-free diet reported by White and colleagues[37] have never been replicated by other groups and need further research. Recently, a 3-week regimen of intralesional triamcinolone acetonide was reported to provide long-term reduction of disfiguring orofacial swelling of OFG.

Topical Corticosteroid and Immunosuppressants

Topical corticosteroids and tacrolimus applied directly onto the lips and oral mucosa have been reported to induce reduction of the labial swelling and oral ulceration in small numbers of patients,[85,86] although benefits are often temporary and disease can quickly recur.[4,5] Topical application of corticosteroid and tacrolimus is reported as generally safe with a low incidence of adverse side effects, including oral candidosis, mucosal burning sensation, sore throat, transient taste disturbance, mucosal staining, and headache.[87–92]

Intralesional Corticosteroids

Intralesional injections of corticosteroids in the treatment of orofacial swelling of OFG were originally introduced in 1971.[93] Initially, low-concentration triamcinolone acetonide (10 mg/mL) was used, requiring multiple sessions[11–19] of injections at approximately 2-week intervals to obtain a favorable, although transient, clinical response. Local block anesthesia at each session was required because of significant pain associated with injecting 1 to 2 mL of triamcinolone into affected tissues.[94,95] In 1992, Sakuntabhai and colleagues[96] suggested using a higher volume of triamcinolone to increase efficacy, reduce the number of treatment sessions, and attempt long-term swelling remission.[97] Under mental or infraorbital nerve blocks with 2% lidocaine, they injected a high volume of triamcinolone acetonide (mean, 6 mL) into the affected lip. Even if swelling increased immediately after the injections, their regimen was shown to be effective and led to nearly complete clinical remission and a long-term swelling-free period (10–12 months). Intralesional therapy was further modified in subsequent years with the introduction of highly concentrated triamcinolone acetonide (40 mg/mL).[98] This formulation allows injection of a high dose of triamcinolone within a reduced drug volume, thereby increasing efficacy, reducing associated pain, and avoiding the need for anesthetic block.[98,99]

The largest cohort of OFG patients managed with triamcinolone injections was reported by Fedele and colleagues.[51] They described the long-term outcomes of a homogeneous group of 22 OFG patients who had been managed with a standardized therapeutic regimen of triamcinolone injections.[51] The treatment led to a significant reduction in orofacial swelling, with most patients showing no disease recurrence after a single course of therapy for up to 4 years. Those who experienced swelling recurrence responded well to a second course of therapy. Of note, the vast majority of patients reached swelling-free status at a 2-week time point after the first course of therapy; all patients did so at the 1-month time point. Adverse side effects of intralesional therapy are uncommon and include local hematoma,[93,97] skin atrophy, mild transient swelling of the lip,[96] hypo-/hyperpigmentation,[98] and rarely, candidiasis.[53]

Systemic Corticosteroids and Immunosuppressants

Short courses of moderate dosage prednisolone (25–50 mg/d; 0.3–0.7 mg/kg/d) or deflazacort (30–60 mg/d; 1.2:1 therapeutic dosage ratio to prednisolone)[100] can quickly reduce orofacial swelling of OFG,[52–54] but benefits are typically short-lived and followed by disease recurrences. Long-term corticosteroid therapy is characterized by several adverse side effects, and therefore, systemic immunosuppressants are likely to represent a safer option in the long-term management of OFG. A recent report demonstrated a significant improvement in lip swelling and erythema after 1 month of mycophenolate mofetil 500 mg twice daily, with sustained benefits and no notable toxicity after 1 year of therapy.[101] Although azathioprine is commonly used by many clinicians to achieve long-term immunosuppression and swelling reduction in OFG patients, there are no articles reporting in detail the use of relevant therapeutic regimens and their outcomes.[102,103]

Antitumor Necrosis Factor Agents

Thalidomide, infliximab, and adalimumab have been occasionally used in the therapy of OFG in small groups of patients with variable outcomes. Low-dose thalidomide (20–100 mg daily) has been reported to induce notable reduction in OFG-related facial swelling,[85,104–107] even after previous failure of other topical and systemic immunosuppressant therapy.[85] The main limiting factor of thalidomide therapy is represented by its toxicity: in addition to its teratogenicity, thalidomide can cause sensory and motor neuropathies, and skin rash.[85,105,108,109] Infliximab and adalimumab have been used in small groups of patients with OFG and with oral manifestations of intestinal Crohn's disease.[110,111] Available evidence suggests that infliximab can provide good short-term response in most OFG patients (up to 70%); however, recurrences are common with only one-third of patients being still responsive after 2 years.[110,111] It has been suggested that patients failing infliximab therapy may benefit from adalimumab.[110,111] Because of the association with potentially serious adverse effects, which include infusion reactions, infection, and increased risk of malignancy,[110] use of infliximab and adalimumab in OFG should mirror that for intestinal Crohn's disease , that is, severe disease and intolerant or resistant to standard systemic therapy.

Diet Modification

Several studies have attempted treatment of OFG via elimination of potential allergens from the diet of affected patients. In addition to multiple case reports of patch test–proven hypersensitivity to a single antigen and relevant dietary avoidance,[12] a UK group has developed 3 separate dietary interventions aimed at reducing orofacial swelling and other intra-oral manifestations of OFG: a cinnamon- and benzoate-free diet,[37] a dietary avoidance of cross-reacting foods in OFG individuals with positive skin prick test to silver birch, grass, mugwort, ragweed, and latex,[43] and a low phenolic acid diet.[112] Although the investigators claim that some of these interventions can reduce orofacial inflammation of OFG in up to 70% of cases, there remains little robust evidence regarding their actual effectiveness due to methodological limitations of available studies.

Antileprotic Agents

Dapsone and clofazimine have been occasionally reported to reduce the orofacial swelling of OFG.[52,113–116] In one study, long-term treatment with low-dosage clofazimine (400–700 mg weekly for 3–11 months) led to complete remission in 5 of 10 treated patients and partial improvement in a further 3 patients.[117] There are only a few published cases of dapsone therapy in OFG, with relevant results ranging from complete relief to ineffectiveness.[58] It seems that antileprotic agents may be more effective during the early stages of the disease.[113]

Miscellaneous Drugs

There have been reports of a small number of patients with OFG having clinical benefits with methotrexate,[118] sulfasalazine,[119] lymecycline,[120] minocycline,[121] 5-aminosalicylic acid,[122] metronidazole[107,123–125] hydroxychloroquine,[114] and various combinations of these agents with systemic, topical, or intralesional corticosteroids.

Surgery and Low-Level Laser Therapy

OFG patients with long-standing and disfiguring fibrotic swelling that has proven to be unresponsive to treatment may benefit from surgical correction. Relevant plastic surgery procedures include cheiloplasty, commissuroplasty, facial liposuction, and tangential resection of labial mucosa, submucosa, and muscles.[126] It has been recommended that surgical correction of OFG should be undertaken during inactive phases of the disease,[23,114] and possibly in association with perioperative oral or intralesional corticosteroid therapy.[127–129] The long-term benefits of surgery are largely unknown, although recurrence of the labial swelling following surgery has been reported.[130,131]

Merigo and colleagues[132] reported complete remission of labial swelling with the use of low-level laser therapy in one OFG patient who had previuosly failed to respond to topical and systemic corticosteroid and immunosuppressive therapy. Low-level laser therapy is thought to have anti-inflammatory and wound-healing properties.[132] Of note, clinical remission was maintained for 2 years after treatment.[132]

Psychological Support

When orofacial enlargement of OFG becomes persistent and esthetically unacceptable, typically in cases of absent or partial response to therapy, psychological support and counseling may be beneficial in developing coping mechanisms and improving quality of life.[119] However, there are no studies investigating potential benefits of psychological interventions in OFG individuals.

CLINICAL OUTCOMES

Although variable and multiform in its early stages, the natural history of OFG is ultimately progressive, and permanent disfiguring labial or facial swelling eventually develops in nearly all affected individuals.[51] Spontaneous resolution is exceptionally rare and most patients would eventually require medical treatment. The long-term prognosis of OFG individuals is largely unknown. Al Johani and colleagues studied the long-term clinical outcomes of 49 patients with OFG who received a wide variety of treatments and reported that facial swelling of OFG tends to improve over time in those who are on therapy, with approximately 78% of patients showing some reduction in their clinical manifestations. However, only 46.8% eventually experienced complete resolution of orofacial swelling.[6] Historically, a variety of different topical or systemic agents have been used during the long-term management of OFG patients with a variable incidence of development of new manifestations, lack of response, and adverse side effects.[6] However, more recent and better designed studies seem to suggest that some single-treatment modalities could effectively provide long-term control of the disease, as in the case of intralesional corticosteroid injections.[51] A summary of clinical outcomes of available interventions is provided in **Table 2**.

Table 2
Clinical outcomes of orofacial granulomatosis therapy

Therapy	Clinical Outcome	Level of Evidence
Topical agents		
Corticosteroids[3,52,133]	Effective in managing moderate intra-oral lesions and mild labial swelling	D
Tacrolimus[86]	Marked improvement in lip swelling. Benefits can be transient	
Intralesional Corticosteroids		
Low-volume triamcinolone acetonide (10 mg/mL)[96,133,134]	Long-term effective in reducing lip swelling. It requires multiple injection sessions and local block anesthesia. Adverse effects: acute pain and transient worsening of swelling	D
High-volume triamcinolone acetonide (40 mg/mL)[51,99]	Effective in long-term reduction of orofacial swelling. Requires one single 3-week course and no block anesthesia. Adverse effects: mild discomfort, skin pigmentations	
Systemic Corticosteroids and Immunosuppressants		
Prednisolone[52,54]	Short-term courses effective in reducing facial swelling and oral ulcers. Side effects from chronic therapy: osteoporosis, diabetes, cataract, Cushing syndrome	D
Mycophenolate mofetil[101]	Long-term effectiveness in reducing orofacial swelling and ulceration. It requires monitoring of toxicity	
Anti-TNF Strategies		
Thalidomide[85,105,109]	Effective in the short-term management of OFG. Side effect: neuropathy and teratogenesis	D
Infliximab[109,111,135–138]	Short-term reduction in orofacial swelling and oral ulceration. It requires multiple infusions. Adverse effects: possible infusion reaction, infection, increased risk of cancer	
Adalimumab[139]	Satisfactory results for oral ulceration. Adverse effects: possible infusion reaction, infection, increased risk of cancer	
Diet Modification		
Cinnamon- and benzoate-free[37]	Improvement in swelling and inflammation. Compliance can be a limitation. Patch tests not predictive of response	D
Avoid cross-reacting food in patients with positive skin-prick testing[43]	Failed to show significant improvement	
Low phenolic acid diet[112]	Improvement in swelling and inflammation. The diet was nutritionally inadequate	

D, case series or case reports.

SUMMARY

OFG is an uncommon inflammatory disorder that typically affects children and young adults and causes disfiguring facial swelling and painful oral ulceration. Although a strict case definition of OFG requires the absence of any systemic granulomatous disease, an unpredictable subgroup of individuals with OFG limited to the orofacial tissues would eventually develop intestinal Crohn's disease or, more rarely, sarcoidosis. A significant number of OFG patients show evidence of concomitant IgE-mediated allergy and delayed-type hypersensitivity to many food and other antigens, although the relevant role in etiopathogenesis and therapy remains unclear. Management of OFG is often difficult and not evidence-based. Mild cases would benefit from topical immunosuppression, whereas long-term anti-inflammatory and immunosuppressive agents are needed to control more severe facial swelling and painful oral ulceration. Intralesional corticosteroid therapy may provide notable long-term remission with no need of prolonged treatment. It seems that the vast majority of OFG patients on therapy would eventually experience a variable degree of reduction in orofacial swelling.

REFERENCES

1. McCartan BE, Healy CM, McCreary CE, et al. Characteristics of patients with orofacial granulomatosis. Oral Dis 2011;17(7):696–704.

2. Zimmer WM, Rogers RS 3rd, Reeve CM, et al. Orofacial manifestations of Melkersson-Rosenthal syndrome. A study of 42 patients and review of 220 cases from the literature. Oral Surg Oral Med Oral Pathol 1992;74(5):610–9.

3. Mignogna MD, Fedele S, Lo Russo L, et al. The multiform and variable patterns of onset of orofacial granulomatosis. J Oral Pathol Med 2003;32(4):200–5.

4. Leão JC, Hodgson T, Scully C, et al. Review article: orofacial granulomatosis. Aliment Pharmacol Ther 2004;20(10):1019–27.

5. Al Johani K, Moles DR, Hodgson T, et al. Onset and progression of clinical manifestations of orofacial granulomatosis. Oral Dis 2009;15(3):214–9.

6. Al Johani KA, Moles DR, Hodgson TA, et al. Orofacial granulomatosis: clinical features and long-term outcome of therapy. J Am Acad Dermatol 2010; 62(4):611–20.

7. Wiesenfeld D, Ferguson MM, Mitchell DN, et al. Oro-facial granulomatosis–a clinical and pathological analysis. Q J Med 1985;54(213):101–13.

8. James J, Patton DW, Lewis CJ, et al. Oro-facial granulomatosis and clinical atopy. J Oral Med 1986;41(1):29–30.

9. Melkersson E. Case of recurrent facial paralysis with angioneurotic oedema. Hugiea 1928;90:737.

10. Rosenthal C. Klinisch-erbbiologischer Beitrag zur Konstitutions-pathologie. Z Gesampte Neurologie Psychiatrie 1931;131:475.

11. Dusi S, Poli G, Berton G, et al. Chronic granulomatous disease in an adult female with granulomatous cheilitis. Evidence for an X-linked pattern of inheritance with extreme lyonization. Acta Haematol 1990;84(1):49–56.

12. Tilakaratne WM, Freysdottir J, Fortune F. Orofacial granulomatosis: review on aetiology and pathogenesis. J Oral Pathol Med 2008;37(4):191–5.

13. Campbell H, Escudier M, Patel P, et al. Distinguishing orofacial granulomatosis from crohn's disease: two separate disease entities? Inflamm Bowel Dis 2011;17(10):2109–15.

14. Alawi F. Granulomatous diseases of the oral tissues: differential diagnosis and update. Dent Clin North Am 2005;49(1):203–21, x.

15. Somech R, Harel A, Rotshtein MS, et al. Granulomatosis cheilitis and Crohn disease. J Pediatr Gastroenterol Nutr 2001;32(3):339–41. Available at: http://journals.lww.com/jpgn/Fulltext/2001/03000/Granulomatosis_Cheilitis_and_Crohn_Disease.24.aspx.

16. Banks T, Gada S. A comprehensive review of current treatments for granulomatous cheilitis. Br J Dermatol 2012;166(5):934–7.

17. Somasundaram R, Nuij VJ, van der Woude CJ, et al. Peripheral neutrophil functions and cell signalling in Crohn's disease. PLoS One 2013;8(12):e84521.

18. Korzenik JR, Dieckgraefe BK. Is Crohn's disease an immunodeficiency? Dig Dis Sci 2000;45(6):1121–9.

19. Petersen HJ, Smith AM. The role of the innate immune system in granulomatous disorders. Front Immunol 2013;4:120. Available at: http://www.ncbi.nlm.nih.gov/pmc/articles/PMC3662972/. Accessed July 14, 2014.

20. Levy FS, Bircher AJ, Büchner SA. Delayed-type hypersensitivity to cow's milk protein in Melkersson-Rosenthal syndrome: coincidence or pathogenetic role? Dermatology 1996;192(2):99–102.

21. Taibjee SM, Prais L, Foulds IS. Orofacial granulomatosis worsened by chocolate: results of patch testing to ingredients of Cadbury's chocolate. Br J Dermatol 2004;150(3):595.

22. Petersen H, Hodgson T, Porter S, et al. Defects of the innate immune system in patients with orofacial franulomatosis. Oral Surg Oral Med Oral Pathol Oral Radiol 2014;117(5):e353.

23. Grave B, McCullough M, Wiesenfeld D. Orofacial granulomatosis–a 20-year review. Oral Dis 2009;15(1):46–51.

24. Satsangi J, Jewell DP, Rosenberg WM, et al. Genetics of inflammatory bowel disease. Gut 1994; 35(5):696–700.

25. Gibson J, Wray D. Human leucocyte antigen typing in orofacial granulomatosis. Br J Dermatol 2000; 143(5):1119–21.

26. Lim SH, Stephens P, Cao QX, et al. Molecular analysis of T cell receptor beta variability in a patient with orofacial granulomatosis. Gut 1997;40(5): 683–6.

27. De Quatrebarbes J, Cordel N, Bravard P, et al. Miescher's cheilitis and lymphocytic clonal expansion: 2 cases. Ann Dermatol Venereol 2004;131(1 Pt 1):55–7 [in French].

28. Freysdottir J, Zhang S, Tilakaratne WM, et al. Oral biopsies from patients with orofacial granulomatosis with histology resembling Crohn's disease have a prominent Th1 environment. Inflamm Bowel Dis 2007;13(4):439–45.

29. Pryce DW, King CM. Orofacial granulomatosis associated with delayed hypersensitivity to cobalt. Clin Exp Dermatol 1990;15(5):384–6.

30. Lazarov A, Kidron D, Tulchinsky Z, et al. Contact orofacial granulomatosis caused by delayed hypersensitivity to gold and mercury. J Am Acad Dermatol 2003;49(6):1117–20.

31. Patton DW, Ferguson MM, Forsyth A, et al. Orofacial granulomatosis: a possible allergic basis. Br J Oral Maxillofac Surg 1985;23(4):235–42.

32. Haworth RJ, MacFadyen EE, Ferguson MM. Food intolerance in patients with oro-facial granulomatosis. Hum Nutr Appl Nutr 1986;40(6):447–56.

33. Sweatman MC, Tasker R, Warner JO, et al. Orofacial granulomatosis. Response to elemental diet and provocation by food additives. Clin Allergy 1986;16(4):331–8.

34. Reed BE, Barrett AP, Katelaris C, et al. Orofacial sensitivity reactions and the role of dietary components. Case reports. Aust Dent J 1993;38(4):287–91.

35. McKenna KE, Walsh MY, Burrows D. The Melkersson-Rosenthal syndrome and food additive hypersensitivity. Br J Dermatol 1994;131(6):921–2.

36. Wray D, Rees SR, Gibson J, et al. The role of allergy in oral mucosal diseases. QJM 2000;93(8): 507–11.

37. White A, Nunes C, Escudier M, et al. Improvement in orofacial granulomatosis on a cinnamon- and benzoate-free diet. Inflamm Bowel Dis 2006;12(6): 508–14.

38. Oliver AJ, Rich AM, Reade PC, et al. Monosodium glutamate-related orofacial granulomatosis. Review and case report. Oral Surg Oral Med Oral Pathol 1991;71(5):560–4.

39. Pachor ML, Urbani G, Cortina P, et al. Is the Melkersson-Rosenthal syndrome related to the exposure to food additives? A case report. Oral Surg Oral Med Oral Pathol 1989;67(4):393–5.

40. Armstrong DK, Biagioni P, Lamey PJ, et al. Contact hypersensitivity in patients with orofacial granulomatosis. Am J Contact Dermatitis 1997;8(1):35–8.

41. Patel P, Brostoff J, Campbell H, et al. Clinical evidence for allergy in orofacial granulomatosis and inflammatory bowel disease. Clin Transl Allergy 2013;3(1):26.

42. Morales C, Peñarrocha M, Bagán JV, et al. Immunological study of Melkersson-Rosenthal syndrome. Lack of response to food additive challenge. Clin Exp Allergy 1995;25(3):260–4.

43. Campbell H, Escudier MP, Brostoff J, et al. Dietary intervention for oral allergy syndrome as a treatment in orofacial granulomatosis: a new approach? J Oral Pathol Med 2013;42(7):517–22.

44. Campbell HE, Escudier MP, Patel P, et al. Review article: cinnamon- and benzoate-free diet as a primary treatment for orofacial granulomatosis. Aliment Pharmacol Ther 2011;34(7):687–701.

45. Apaydin R, Bahadir S, Kaklikkaya N, et al. Possible role of Mycobacterium tuberculosis complex in Melkersson-Rosenthal syndrome demonstrated with Gen-Probe amplified Mycobacterium tuberculosis direct test. Australas J Dermatol 2004;45(2): 94–9.

46. Ivanyi L, Kirby A, Zakrzewska JM. Antibodies to mycobacterial stress protein in patients with orofacial granulomatosis. J Oral Pathol Med 1993;22(7): 320–2.

47. Riggio MP, Gibson J, Lennon A, et al. Search for Mycobacterium paratuberculosis DNA in orofacial granulomatosis and oral Crohn's disease tissue by polymerase chain reaction. Gut 1997;41(5): 646–50.

48. Muellegger RR, Weger W, Zoechling N, et al. Granulomatous cheilitis and Borrelia burgdorferi: polymerase chain reaction and serologic studies in a retrospective case series of 12 patients. Arch Dermatol 2000;136(12):1502–6.

49. Handa S, Saraswat A, Radotra BD, et al. Chronic macrocheilia: a clinico-pathological study of 28 patients. Clin Exp Dermatol 2003;28(3):245–50.

50. Savage NW, Barnard K, Shirlaw PJ, et al. Serum and salivary IgA antibody responses to Saccharomyces cerevisiae, Candida albicans and Streptococcus mutans in orofacial granulomatosis and Crohn's disease. Clin Exp Immunol 2004;135(3): 483–9.

51. Fedele S, Fung PP, Bamashmous N, et al. Long-term effectiveness of intralesional triamcinolone acetonide therapy in orofacial granulomatosis: an observational cohort study. Br J Dermatol 2014; 170:794–801.

52. Sciubba JJ, Said-Al-Naief N. Orofacial granulomatosis: presentation, pathology and management of 13 cases. J Oral Pathol Med 2003;32(10): 576–85.

53. El-Hakim M, Chauvin P. Orofacial granulomatosis presenting as persistent lip swelling: review of 6 new cases. J Oral Maxillofac Surg 2004;62(9): 1114–7.

54. Kauzman A, Quesnel-Mercier A, Lalonde B. Orofacial granulomatosis: 2 case reports and literature review. J Can Dent Assoc 2006;72:325–9.

55. Rogers RS 3rd. Melkersson-Rosenthal syndrome and orofacial granulomatosis. Dermatol Clin 1996; 14(2):371–9.

56. Sainsbury CP, Dodge JA, Walker DM, et al. Orofacial granulomatosis in childhood. Br Dent J 1987; 163(5):154–7.

57. Odukoya O. Orofacial granulomatosis: report of two Nigerian cases. J Trop Med Hyg 1994;97(6): 362–6.

58. Ratzinger G, Sepp N, Vogetseder W, et al. Cheilitis granulomatosa and Melkersson-Rosenthal syndrome: evaluation of gastrointestinal involvement and therapeutic regimens in a series of 14 patients. J Eur Acad Dermatol Venereol 2007;21(8):1065–70.

59. Yeatts RP, White WL. Granulomatous blepharitis as a sign of Melkersson-Rosenthal syndrome. Ophthalmology 1997;104(7):1185–9 [discussion: 1189–90].

60. Cocuroccia B, Gubinelli E, Annessi G, et al. Persistent unilateral orbital and eyelid oedema as a manifestation of Melkersson-Rosenthal syndrome. J Eur Acad Dermatol Venereol 2005;19(1):107–11.

61. Dupuy A, Cosnes J, Revuz J, et al. Oral Crohn disease: clinical characteristics and long-term follow-up of 9 cases. Arch Dermatol 1999;135(4):439–42.

62. Croft CB, Wilkinson AR. Ulceration of the mouth, pharynx, and larynx in Crohn's disease of the intestine. Br J Surg 1972;59(4):249–52.

63. Chan SW, Scully C, Prime SS, et al. Pyostomatitis vegetans: oral manifestation of ulcerative colitis. Oral Surg Oral Med Oral Pathol 1991;72(6):689–92.

64. Ruiz-Roca JA, Berini-Aytés L, Gay-Escoda C. Pyostomatitis vegetans. Report of two cases and review of the literature. Oral Surg Oral Med Oral Pathol Oral Radiol Endod 2005;99(4):447–54.

65. Kalman RS, Gjede JM, Farraye FA. Pyostomatitis vegetans in a patient with fistulizing Crohn's disease. Clin Gastroenterol Hepatol 2013;11(12):A24.

66. Worsaae N, Christensen KC, Schiødt M, et al. Melkersson-Rosenthal syndrome and cheilitis granulomatosa. A clinicopathological study of thirty-three patients with special reference to their oral lesions. Oral Surg Oral Med Oral Pathol 1982;54(4):404–13.

67. Levenson MJ, Ingerman M, Grimes C, et al. Melkersson-Rosenthal syndrome. Arch Otolaryngol 1984;110(8):540–2.

68. Sanderson J, Nunes C, Escudier M, et al. Orofacial granulomatosis: Crohn's disease or a new inflammatory bowel disease? Inflamm Bowel Dis 2005;11(9):840–6.

69. Greene RM, Rogers RS 3rd. Melkersson-Rosenthal syndrome: a review of 36 patients. J Am Acad Dermatol 1989;21(6):1263–70.

70. Alexander RW, James RB. Melkersson-Rosenthal syndrome: review of literature and report of case. J Oral Surg 1972;30(8):599–604.

71. Kanerva M, Moilanen K, Virolainen S, et al. Melkersson-Rosenthal syndrome. Otolaryngol Head Neck Surg 2008;138(2):246–51.

72. Vistnes LM, Kernahan DA. The Melkersson-Rosenthal syndrome. Plast Reconstr Surg 1971; 48(2):126–32.

73. Pino Rivero P, González Palomino A, Pantoja Hernández CG, et al. Melkersson-Rosenthal syndrome. Report of a case with bilateral facial palsy. An Otorrinolaringol Ibero Am 2005;32(5):437–43 [in Spanish].

74. Khandpur S, Malhotra AK, Khanna N. Melkersson-Rosenthal syndrome with diffuse facial swelling and multiple cranial nerve palsies. J Dermatol 2006;33(6):411–4.

75. Hornstein OP. Melkersson-Rosenthal syndrome. A neuro-muco-cutaneous disease of complex origin. Curr Probl Dermatol 1973;5:117–56.

76. Stosiek N, Birolleau S, Capesius C, et al. Chronicity and diagnostic doubts of Melkersson-Rosenthal syndrome. Analysis of developing ways in 5 cases. Ann Dermatol Venereol 1992;119(9):635–8 [in French].

77. Scully C, Cochran KM, Russell RI, et al. Crohn's disease of the mouth: an indicator of intestinal involvement. Gut 1982;23(3):198–201.

78. Zbar AP, Ben-Horin S, Beer-Gabel M, et al. Oral Crohn's disease: is it a separable disease from orofacial granulomatosis? A review. J Crohns Colitis 2012;6(2):135–42.

79. Saalman R, Mattsson U, Jontell M. Orofacial granulomatosis in childhood—a clinical entity that may indicate Crohn's disease as well as food allergy. Acta Paediatr 2009;98(7):1162–7.

80. Al-Azri AR, Logan RM, Goss AN. Oral lesion as the first clinical presentation in sarcoidosis: a case report. Oman Med J 2012 May;27(3):243–5.

81. Armstrong DK, Burrows D. Orofacial granulomatosis. Int J Dermatol 1995;34(12):830–3.

82. Patel P, Campbell H, Brostoff J, et al. Allergy in orofacial granulomatosis and inflammatory bowel disease. Gut 2010;59:A99.

83. Riordain RN, Meaney S, McCreary C. Impact of chronic oral mucosal disease on daily life: preliminary observations from a qualitative study. Oral Dis 2011;17(3):265–9.

84. Chiandussi S, Tappuni AR, Watson TF, et al. Lip impressions: a new method for monitoring morphological changes in orofacial granulomatosis. Oral Dis 2007;13(1):93–8.

85. Hegarty A, Hodgson T, Porter S. Thalidomide for the treatment of recalcitrant oral Crohn's disease

and orofacial granulomatosis. Oral Surg Oral Med Oral Pathol Oral Radiol Endod 2003;95(5):576–85.

86. Casson DH, Eltumi M, Tomlin S, et al. Topical tacrolimus may be effective in the treatment of oral and perineal Crohn's disease. Gut 2000;47(3):436–40.

87. Olivier V, Lacour J-P, Mousnier A, et al. Treatment of chronic erosive oral lichen planus with low concentrations of topical tacrolimus: an open prospective study. Arch Dermatol 2002;138(10):1335–8.

88. Rozycki TW, Rogers RS 3rd, Pittelkow MR, et al. Topical tacrolimus in the treatment of symptomatic oral lichen planus: a series of 13 patients. J Am Acad Dermatol 2002;46(1):27–34.

89. Shen JT, Pedvis-Leftick A. Mucosal staining after using topical tacrolimus to treat erosive oral lichen planus. J Am Acad Dermatol 2004;50(2):326.

90. Lozada-Nur FI, Sroussi HY. Tacrolimus powder in Orabase 0.1% for the treatment of oral lichen planus and oral lichenoid lesions: an open clinical trial. Oral Surg Oral Med Oral Pathol Oral Radiol Endod 2006;102(6):744–9.

91. Albert MH, Becker B, Schuster FR, et al. Oral graft vs. host disease in children–treatment with topical tacrolimus ointment. Pediatr Transplant 2007; 11(3):306–11.

92. Hodgson TA, Sahni N, Kaliakatsou F, et al. Long-term efficacy and safety of topical tacrolimus in the management of ulcerative/erosive oral lichen planus. Eur J Dermatol 2003;13(5):466–70.

93. Eisenbud L, Hymowitz SS, Shapiro R. Cheilitis granulomatosa. Report of case treated with injection of triamcinolone acetonide aqueous suspension. Oral Surg Oral Med Oral Pathol 1971;32(3): 384–9.

94. Krutchkoff D, James R. Cheilitis granulomatosa. Successful treatment with combined local triamcinolone injections and surgery. Arch Dermatol 1978; 114(8):1203–6.

95. Allen CM, Camisa C, Hamzeh S, et al. Cheilitis granulomatosa: report of six cases and review of the literature. J Am Acad Dermatol 1990;23(3 Pt 1):444–50.

96. Sakuntabhai A, MacLeod RI, Lawrence CM. Intralesional steroid injection after nerve-block in orofacial granulomatosis. Lancet 1992;340(8825):969.

97. Sakuntabhai A, MacLeod RI, Lawrence CM. Intralesional steroid injection after nerve block anesthesia in the treatment of orofacial granulomatosis. Arch Dermatol 1993;129(4):477–80.

98. Mignogna MD, Fedele S, Lo Russo L, et al. Effectiveness of small-volume, intralesional, delayed-release triamcinolone injections in orofacial granulomatosis: a pilot study. J Am Acad Dermatol 2004;51(2):265–8.

99. Mignogna MD, Pollio A, Leuci S, et al. Clinical behaviour and long-term therapeutic response in orofacial granulomatosis patients treated with intralesional triamcinolone acetonide injections alone or in combination with topical pimecrolimus 1%. J Oral Pathol Med 2013;42(1):73–81.

100. Van der Waal RI, Schulten EA, van de Scheur MR, et al. Cheilitis granulomatosa. J Eur Acad Dermatol Venereol 2001;15(6):519–23.

101. Antonyan AS, Pena-Robichaux V, McHargue CA. Orofacial granulomatosis successfully treated with mycophenolate mofetil. J Am Acad Dermatol 2014;70(6):e137–9.

102. Plauth M, Jenss H, Meyle J. Oral manifestations of Crohn's disease. J Clin Gastroenterol 1991;13: 9–37.

103. Mahadevan U, Sandborn WJ. Infliximab for the treatment of orofacial Crohn's disease. Inflamm Bowel Dis 2001;7(1):38–42.

104. Safa G, Joly P, Boullie MC, et al. Melkersson-Rosenthal syndrome treated by thalidomide. 2 cases. Ann Dermatol Venereol 1995;122(9): 609–11 [in French].

105. Odeka EB, Miller V. Thalidomide in oral Crohn's disease refractory to conventional medical treatment. J Pediatr Gastroenterol Nutr 1997;25(2):250–1.

106. Weinstein TA, Sciubba JJ, Levine J. Thalidomide for the treatment of oral aphthous ulcers in Crohn's disease. J Pediatr Gastroenterol Nutr 1999;28(2): 214–6.

107. Medeiros M Jr, Araujo MI, Guimarães NS, et al. Therapeutic response to thalidomide in Melkersson-Rosenthal syndrome: a case report. Ann Allergy Asthma Immunol 2002;88(4):421–4.

108. Thomas P, Walchner M, Ghoreschl K, et al. Successful treatment of granulomatous cheilitis with thalidomide. Arch Dermatol 2003;139(2):136–8.

109. Eustace K, Clowry J, Kirby B, et al. Thalidomide in the treatment of refractory orofacial granulomatosis. Br J Dermatol 2014;171(2):423–5.

110. O'Neill ID, Scully C. Biologics in oral medicine: oral Crohn's disease and orofacial granulomatosis. Oral Dis 2012;18(7):633–8.

111. Elliott T, Campbell H, Escudier M, et al. Experience with anti-TNF-α therapy for orofacial granulomatosis. J Oral Pathol Med 2011;40(1):14–9.

112. Campbell HE, Escudier MP, Milligan P, et al. Development of a low phenolic acid diet for the management of orofacial granulomatosis. J Hum Nutr Diet 2013;26:527–37.

113. Podmore P, Burrows D. Clofazimine–an effective treatment for Melkersson-Rosenthal syndrome or Miescher's cheilitis. Clin Exp Dermatol 1986;11(2): 173–8.

114. Van der Waal RI, Schulten EA, van der Meij EH, et al. Cheilitis granulomatosa: overview of 13 patients with long-term follow-up–results of management. Int J Dermatol 2002;41(4):225–9.

115. Camacho-Alonso F, Bermejo-Fenoll A, López-Jornet P. Miescher's cheilitis granulomatosa. A

presentation of five cases. Med Oral Patol Oral Cir Bucal 2004;9(5):427–9, 425–427.

116. Fdez-Freire LR, Serrano Gotarredona A, Bernabeu Wittel J, et al. Clofazimine as elective treatment for granulomatous cheilitis. J Drugs Dermatol 2005; 4(3):374–7.

117. Sussman GL, Yang WH, Steinberg S. Melkersson-Rosenthal syndrome: clinical, pathologic, and therapeutic considerations. Ann Allergy 1992;69(3): 187–94.

118. Tonkovic-Capin V, Galbraith SS, Rogers RS 3rd, et al. Cutaneous Crohn's disease mimicking Melkersson-Rosenthal syndrome: treatment with methotrexate. J Eur Acad Dermatol Venereol 2006;20(4):449–52.

119. Clayden AM, Bleys CM, Jones SF, et al. Orofacial granulomatosis: a diagnostic problem for the unwary and a management dilemma. Case reports. Aust Dent J 1997;42(4):228–32.

120. Pigozzi B, Fortina AB, Peserico A. Successful treatment of Melkersson-Rosenthal Syndrome with lymecycline. Eur J Dermatol 2004;14(3):166–7.

121. Stein SL, Mancini AJ. Melkersson-Rosenthal syndrome in childhood: successful management with combination steroid and minocycline therapy. J Am Acad Dermatol 1999;41(5 Pt 1):746–8.

122. Girlich C, Bogenrieder T, Palitzsch KD, et al. Orofacial granulomatosis as initial manifestation of Crohn's disease: a report of two cases. Eur J Gastroenterol Hepatol 2002;14(8):873–6.

123. Miralles J, Barnadas MA, de Moragas JM. Cheilitis granulomatosa treated with metronidazole. Dermatology 1995;191(3):252–3.

124. Dummer W, Lurz C, Jeschke R, et al. Granulomatous cheilitis and Crohn's disease in a 3-year-old boy. Pediatr Dermatol 1999;16(1):39–42.

125. Coskun B, Saral Y, Cicek D, et al. Treatment and follow-up of persistent granulomatous cheilitis with intralesional steroid and metronidazole. J Dermatolog Treat 2004;15(5):333–5.

126. Tan O, Atik B, Calka O. Plastic surgical solutions for Melkersson-Rosenthal syndrome: facial liposuction and cheiloplasty procedures. Ann Plast Surg 2006; 56(3):268–73.

127. Glickman LT, Gruss JS, Birt BD, et al. The surgical management of Melkersson-Rosenthal syndrome. Plast Reconstr Surg 1992;89(5):815–21.

128. Camacho F, García-Bravo B, Carrizosa A. Treatment of Miescher's cheilitis granulomatosa in Melkersson-Rosenthal syndrome. J Eur Acad Dermatol Venereol 2001;15(6):546–9.

129. Kruse-Lösler B, Presser D, Metze D, et al. Surgical treatment of persistent macrocheilia in patients with Melkersson-Rosenthal syndrome and cheilitis granulomatosa. Arch Dermatol 2005;141(9):1085–91.

130. Ellitsgaard N, Andersson AP, Worsaae N, et al. Long-term results after surgical reduction cheiloplasty in patients with Melkersson-Rosenthal syndrome and cheilitis granulomatosa. Ann Plast Surg 1993;31(5):413–20.

131. Oliver DW, Scott MJ. Lip reduction cheiloplasty for Miescher's granulomatous macrocheilitis (Cheilitis granulomatosa) in childhood. Clin Exp Dermatol 2002;27(2):129–31.

132. Merigo E, Fornaini C, Manfredi M, et al. Orofacial granulomatosis treated with low-level laser therapy: a case report. Oral Surg Oral Med Oral Pathol Oral Radiol 2012;113(6):e25–9.

133. Mignogna MD, Fedele S, Lo Russo L, et al. Orofacial granulomatosis with gingival onset. J Clin Periodontol 2001;28(7):692–6.

134. Kolokotronis A, Antoniades D, Trigonidis G, et al. Granulomatous cheilitis: a study of six cases. Oral Dis 1997;3(3):188–92.

135. Kaufman I, Caspi D, Yeshurun D, et al. The effect of infliximab on extraintestinal manifestations of Crohn's disease. Rheumatol Int 2005;25(6):406–10.

136. Ottaviani F, Schindler A, Capaccio P, et al. New therapy for orolaryngeal manifestations of Crohn's disease. Ann Otol Rhinol Laryngol 2003;112(1): 37–9.

137. Brunner B, Hirschi C, Weimann R, et al. Treatment-resistant lingual Crohn's disease disappears after infliximab. Scand J Gastroenterol 2005;40:1255–9.

138. Cardoso H, Nunes A, Carneiro F, et al. Successful infliximab therapy for oral Crohn's disease. Inflamm Bowel Dis 2006;12:337–8.

139. Sánchez AR, Rogers RS 3rd, Sheridan PJ. Oral ulcerations are associated with the loss of response to infliximab in Crohn's disease. J Oral Pathol Med 2005;34(1):53–5.

Granulomatous Rosacea and Periorificial Dermatitis
Controversies and Review of Management and Treatment

Grace L. Lee, MD, Matthew J. Zirwas, MD*

KEYWORDS

- Granulomatous rosacea • Perioral dermatitis • Periorificial dermatitis

KEY POINTS

- Granulomatous rosacea (GR) is a rare inflammatory skin condition characterized by reddish brown papules favoring the face.
- GR is thought to arise from various antigenic triggers causing granuloma formation.
- Treatment of GR is difficult and often requires a trial of various topical and systemic therapies.
- Periorificial dermatitis (PD) is a self-limiting inflammatory skin condition characterized by erythema, papules, pustules, and a distinct sparing around the vermillion border.
- Management of PD should include ending use of any triggering topical medication, especially topical steroids.

INTRODUCTION

Granulomatous rosacea (GR) and periorificial dermatitis (PD) are inflammatory skin conditions characterized by erythematous papules most commonly affecting the face (**Figs. 1** and **2**). These entities have been the topic of controversy because they are similar in clinical presentation, yet have variable causes and prognoses. They are both benign and self-limiting but GR tends to have a chronic course compared with PD. Some clinicians consider PD and its clinical variants on the same spectrum as rosacea because these entities have the same clinical response to similar therapies. Although acknowledging this controversy, for the sake of clarity this article describes them separate clinical entities. This article attempts to explain the origin of each disease and the different perspectives in terms of nomenclature and causes, as well as summarize existing literature on each entity.

In 2002, rosacea was classified and standardized by the National Rosacea Society Expert Committee into 4 recognized subtypes: erythematotelangiectatic, papulopustular, phymatous, and ocular.[1] Using this classification, epidemiologic studies show erythematotelangiectatic rosacea to be by far the most common type.[2] GR is not one of the subtypes of rosacea, but is thought to be a variant of rosacea based on unique clinical and histologic findings of granulomas.[1] At present, the Committee recognizes GR as a variant of

Disclosure statement: G.L. Lee has no relevant disclosure. M.J. Zirwas has been compensated for consulting work with Smart Practice and Sun Products.
The Ohio State University Wexner Medical Center, Columbus, OH, USA
* Corresponding author. Division of Dermatology, The Ohio State University Wexner Medical Center, 2012 Kenny Road, Columbus, OH 43221.
E-mail address: Matt.zirwas@osumc.edu

Dermatol Clin 33 (2015) 447–455
http://dx.doi.org/10.1016/j.det.2015.03.009
0733-8635/15/$ – see front matter © 2015 Elsevier Inc. All rights reserved.

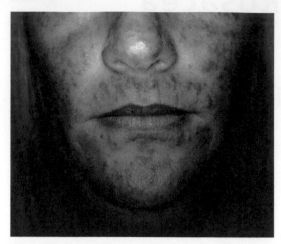

Fig. 1. GR. Firm papules involve the perioral, periocular, and perinasal regions.

rosacea and GR is diagnosed in the setting of histologically confirmed papular granulomas on the face after ruling out other entities, such as PD and sarcoidosis.

PD, which can involve the perinasal, perioral, and/or periorbital area, is an inflammatory skin eruption characterized by erythematous papules and pustules on the face. As such, PD has been erroneously referred to as perioral dermatitis even when lesions appear in locations other than the perioral area. In 1957, PD was first described by Frumess and Lewis[3] as a cyclic dermatitis called "light-sensitive seborrheid." In 1964 it became a distinct entity called "perioral dermatitis."[4] This condition is commonly found in young adult women between the ages of 16 and 45 years.[5] However, PD has also been reported

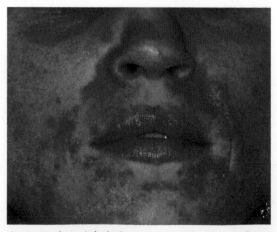

Fig. 2. PD from inhaled corticosteroids. The erythematous papules around the mouth spare the vermilion border of the lips.

in children between the ages of 6 months and 18 years.[6] Originally described in 1970by Gianotti and colleagues,[7] childhood granulomatous PD (CGPD) is a distinct subtype of PD typically seen in prepubertal children of darker skin color. Since then, several cases of children with a spectrum of skin colors with similar findings have been described.[8] In the literature, this entity has been given various names including childhood granulomatous perioral dermatitis, sarcoid-like granulomatous dermatitis, and facial Afro-Caribbean eruption (FACE). Currently, the most accepted term for this disease is CGPD, which the authors agree best describes the entity.[9] The granulomatous variant of PD can also be seen in adults and is clinically very similar to GR without the background erythema. The cause of this variant of PD is thought to be topical steroid use.[8]

GRANULOMATOUS ROSACEA
Etiopathogenesis

GR is a rare chronic inflammatory skin disease reported primarily in middle-aged women[10] that has been given various names in the literature. In 1896, Darier[11] first described the concept of tuberculids, which were defined as skin findings associated with a distant focus of active tuberculoid infection. In 1917, Lewandowsky[12] described a patient with a rosacea-like tuberculid granuloma that clinically mimicked the appearance of papular rosacea. Laymon[13] reported similar cases and called it "micropapular tuberculid." However, in 1949, Snapp[14] presented 20 patients with rosacea-like tuberculids; all except one displayed a low degree of tuberculin sensitivity. He concluded, therefore, that tuberculid rosacea does not exist and posited that it is a distinct form of rosacea.[14] Because the common features of rosacea (flushing, nontransient erythema, papules and pustules, and telangiectasia) are not necessary, or even typical, for the diagnosis of GR, it has been questioned whether the pathophysiology of GR is even related to that of rosacea.[15] For that reason, some investigators have even suggested the term granulomatous facial dermatitis for the condition.[15] Just as the nomenclature is controversial, the etiologic factors of both rosacea and GR are disputed. Several triggering and aggravating factors for rosacea have been described. These include systemic steroids, topical steroids, ultraviolet radiation (UVR), heat, spicy food, alcohol, and infectious organisms, including Demodex mites and GI bacteria.[16,17] Mullanax and Kierland[18] first reported cases of GR with the key pathologic finding of noncaseating epithelioid granulomas with a mixed inflammatory infiltrate. Because granulomas are thought to be a response to persistent antigen presence, researchers subsequently looked for antigens as the triggering factors.[17] *Demodex folliculorum* has been at the center of this discussion ever since histologic examination of a facial papule from a patient with GR showed foreign body granulomas along with *D folliculorum* species within enlarged hair follicles. Most recently, in 2008, a study reviewed pathologic specimens from 24 subjects with GR and *D folliculorum* was identified in only 7 out of these 24 specimens.[19] However, in those that were positive for *D folliculorum*, the mites were found within the granuloma suggesting their role in the pathogenesis of at least some cases.[19] Other researchers suggest it may not simply be the presence of the *D folliculorum* mites but the combination of location of the mites, density of the organisms, and host susceptibility that may play a role in the pathogenesis of GR.[17,20,21] Another recent study suggests the role of UVR in causing both sun damage and increased matrix metalloproteinase (MMP)-2 and MMP-9, contributing to tissue remodeling and, thereby, recruiting inflammatory cells that contribute to the formation of granuloma in the dermis.[22] Also of note is the historical but unsupported association between gastrointestinal disturbances caused by *Helicobacter pylori* and GR. There is a study showing improvement of GR after eradicating *H pylori*; however, there are no large trials supporting this data.[23] Currently, the consensus is that GR is a histologic variant of rosacea, not a distinct clinical subtype, and may have multifactorial causes that are distinct from rosacea.

Clinical Presentation

The lesions of GR consist of monomorphic, firm, yellow, red, brown, or flesh-colored papules or nodules localized around eyes, nose, and mouth on relatively normal appearing skin.[24] Specifically, the characteristic papules are on the lateral side of the face and on the neck below the mandible.[17] Other signs of rosacea, such as flushing, erythema, or telangiectasia, may be seen but are not needed for diagnosis.[24] However, if patients have overlap of GR and rosacea, they can have symptoms of burning or stinging, pruritus, facial swelling, or irritation.[15] In a review study of 53 patients with GR, 15% had extrafacial lesions in the ears, neck, axilla, shoulder, groin, thigh, and knees.[17] GR tends to be a chronic condition that is difficult to treat and has unpredictable responses to standard rosacea treatments. Based on case reports in the literature, the clinical course ranges from 6 months to 4 years.[23]

The differential diagnosis of GR includes PD, CGPD, lupus miliaris disseminatus faciei (LMDF), sarcoidosis, FACE, and cutaneous tuberculosis (**Table 1**). PD is a papulopustular facial dermatitis that typically spares the vermillion border. Clinically and histologically, PD can be similar to GR but typically has a less granulomatous histology, responds better to treatment, and has a shorter clinical course. CGPD is characterized by periorificial papules, pustules, and erythema and may be a subtype of GR. LMDF is a rare chronic skin condition characterized by papules distributed across the face symmetrically and can be differentiated by histologic findings of caseating granulomas.[26] LMDF tends to heal by leaving permanent scars.[26] Sarcoidosis can also cause granulomatous papules on the face but typically has other extracutaneous findings, such as granulomas, fatigue, fever, weight loss, pulmonary symptoms, and less mixed inflammation on histopathology.[27] FACE is similar to PD but is more commonly seen in children with dark skin. Some investigators think FACE is also a variant of GR.[5]

Systemic Associations

Involvement of other organ systems is not typically associated with GR. However, it is on the spectrum of rosacea. Ocular rosacea coexists in 50% of patients with cutaneous rosacea.[28] There is a case report of a patient with GR who developed lacrimal, parotid, and submandibular gland swelling after treatment with systemic steroids.[29] The scleritis, conjunctivitis, and parotiditis resolved after a month of minocycline therapy.[29] In fact, if patients have other systemic complaints, the clinician should seek out other possible diagnoses in the differential such as sarcoidosis.

Evaluation and Management

When approaching patients with facial papular dermatitis, differential diagnoses of GR, PD, CGPD, sarcoidosis, LMDF, FACE, and cutaneous tuberculosis should be considered. Diagnosis of these entities can be challenging and evaluation should include a thorough clinical history, physical examination, and skin biopsy. Depending on clinical suspicion of sarcoidosis or tuberculosis, evaluation can include routine complete blood cell count with differential, chemistry panel, purified protein-derived or QuantiFERON-TB Gold test (QTF-G, Cellestis Limited, Carnegie, Victoria, Australia), baseline pulmonary radiograph, and autoimmune panel.

Currently, there is no standard of treatment of GR and limited data on therapeutic effectiveness are reported in individual cases. With limited data

Table 1
Differential diagnosis of granulomatous papules on the face

	Patient Characteristics	Clinical Features	Histopathology
GR	Young adults, light skin	Periorificial, extrafacial papules	Noncaseating epithelioid cell granulomas with mixed infiltrate
PD	Children or young women	Periorificial erythema, papules and pustules	Perifollicular lymphocytic and perivascular infiltration
CGPD	Prepubertal	Periorificial, extrafacial papules	Perifollicular granulomatous infiltration on the upper half of body
LMDF	Adolescent or adult	Symmetric papules across central face	Perifollicular caseating granulomatous lymphohistiocytic infiltration with occasional neutrophils
Sarcoidosis	Any age	Noninflammatory facial papules and nodules May have systemic findings of fatigue, weight loss, joint pain, pulmonary symptoms	Naked, noncaseating granulomatous infiltration
FACE	Children, dark skin	Periorificial, favoring outer helix of the ear	Perifollicular granulomatous infiltration
Cutaneous tuberculosis	Any age	Systemic findings, weight loss, malaise, pulmonary symptoms	Caseating granuloma

Adapted from Refs.[5,18,25]

on treatment of GR, therapeutic efforts have been based on the use of medications that are effective for sarcoidosis and papulopustular rosacea, the 2 diseases with which it has the most in common. The tetracycline family of medications is the obvious first therapeutic choice. Use of tetracycline 250 mg daily to 500 mg 3 times a day, doxycycline 50 to 100 mg twice a day, or minocycline 50 to 100 mg twice a day has been reported in the literature.[10,18,30–32] Their mechanism of action against granuloma formation is thought to be due to inhibition of protein kinase C, a signaling enzyme in the inflammatory pathway.[33] Other therapeutic agents to consider include azelaic acid, benzoyl peroxide, topical metronidazole, topical corticosteroids, systemic corticosteroids, and oral erythromycin. There is a case report suggesting the role of H pylori in the pathogenesis of GR in which the patient's skin lesions resolved 2 months after taking clarithromycin 250 mg twice a day, oral metronidazole 500 mg twice a day, and pantoprazole 40 mg daily for 7 days.[23] There are 2 case reports of the use of pimecrolimus 1% cream applied to lesions twice a day with good efficacy.[34,35] One patient used pimecrolimus 1%

topical cream combined with sun block twice a day resulting in complete resolution of lesions after 4 months of therapy.[35] The other patient responded well to pimecrolimus 1% cream after failing a 45-day course of topical metronidazole and oral doxycyline.[34] There was no evidence of relapse after stopping the medication.

For recalcitrant GR, isotretinoin 0.7 mg/kg for 6 months as monotherapy showed some clinical resolution of disease without recurrence.[36] After failing systemic doxycycline, isotretinoin, and corticosteroid, 2 patients tried oral dapsone with clinical improvement.[37] Limited data on physical modalities as treatment options include laser and ablative laser therapy. One patient received 6 treatments at 2-week intervals of photodynamic therapy with aminolevulinic acid with improvement seen after the third treatment.[38] Another patient underwent 6 sessions of intense pulsed dye laser at 4-week interval with satisfactory improvement.[39]

Although unreported in the literature for specific use against GR, combination therapy with oral metronidazole and oral ivermectin has been shown to be the most effective regimen for eradication of *D folliculorum*. Given the role this organism is suspected to play in GR, a trial of this regimen would be reasonable in a case that does not respond to therapy with oral tetracyclines. The studied regimen for *D folliculorum* is metronidazole 250 mg 3 times a day for 14 days along with ivermectin 0.2 mg/kg of body weight on days 1 and 7 of the metronidazole course.[40] For current available treatments for GR, see **Table 2**.

PERIORIFICIAL DERMATITIS
Etiopathogenesis

Currently, the causes of PD and its clinical variants, granulomatous form and CGPD, are unknown. The most common known triggering factor for PD is prior exposure to topical steroids of any potency for treatment of other facial dermatitides and cutaneous exposure to steroids via exhaled steroid in patients using corticosteroid inhalers or nasal sprays.[6,44] However, not all patients have this clinical history. Several case reports also consider various historical etiologic factors, such as topical medications, cosmetic products, physical factors, and microorganisms, among others.[45] (**Table 3**) Another study compared the skin of subjects with rosacea and PD and found an association between PD and atopic dermatitis, suggesting either impaired skin barrier or incidental transfer of topical steroid to the face as the underlying pathologic condition.[61] A commonality among most of these factors is their irritant nature to the skin and alteration of microflora in the pilosebaceous unit.[5] Based on the current available evidence, the authors think that PD is induced by exogenous factors, such

as atopic dermatitis or hormonal disturbance, in a susceptible host.

Clinical Presentation

PD is an inflammatory disease limited to the face and characterized by erythema, papules, papulo-vesicles, papulopustules, and scaling with distinct sparing around the vermillion border. Most patients are women between ages of 20 and 45 years; however, PD can also affect children.[6,45] A variant of PD is CPGD, which occurs in prepubertal children typically presenting with monomorphic, yellow, reddish micronodular eruptions on the central face with predilection for the areas around the mouth, eyes, and nose.[62] Although rare, extra-facial involvement around the vaginal area has been described.[62] Adult patients commonly complain of an intense burning sensation accompanying skin erythema and scaling. Alternatively, a retrospective chart review from one institution of cases of children with PD showed 19% reporting pruritus with only 4% reporting burning.[6] The duration of disease ranged from 2 weeks to 4 years. Most of the cases resolved spontaneously with some patients reporting atrophic pinpoint scarring, likely from the inflammatory process.[9] The differential diagnoses for PD are similar to GR (see **Table 1**).

Systemic Associations

Both PD and CGPD are self-limiting conditions without associated systemic diseases.[62] However, some patients may develop emotional distress due to the disfiguring nature of the rash.[45] The lesions of PD may also run a chronic course and

Table 2
Therapeutic agents for granulomatous rosacea

Topical Agent	Level of Evidence[a]	Systemic Agent	Level of Evidence[a]
Azelaic acid	E	Clarithromycin, metronidazole, and pantoprazole combination[23]	D
Benzoyl peroxide	E	Dapsone[37]	D
Metronidazole[31,41]	D	Doxycycline[31]	D
Pimecrolimus[34,35]	D	Erythromycin[42]	D
Topical steroid	E	Isotretinoin[36,43]	D
—	—	Minocycline[10,32]	D
Other		Systemic steroid[43]	D
Intense pulsed dye laser[39]	D	Tetracycline[18,30]	D
Photodynamic therapy[38]	D	—	—

[a] D, case series or case reports; E, expert opinion.

Table 3
Causative factors of periorificial dermatitis

Medications	Topical steroids,[6] inhaled corticosteroids,[46,47] systemic corticosteroids[48]
Cosmetic products	Fluorinated toothpaste,[49] tartar control toothpaste,[50] moisturizers,[51] propolis,[52] sunscreens[53]
Physical factors	Ultraviolet light,[45] heat and cold[54]
Microorganisms	Fusobacteria,[55,56] *Candida* spp,[54] *Demodex folliculorum*[57]
Miscellaneous	Hormonal (oral contraceptives),[58] chewing gum,[59] amalgam dental filling[60]

evolve into lupoid form causing permanent scarring on the face.[44]

Evaluation and Management

Diagnosis of PD is made based on the typical clinical presentation and histologic examination is rarely necessary to exclude other diagnoses. Although the histology of CPGD is not diagnostic and can be very similar to GR, the age of the patient and the lack of pustules generally allow distinction.

A large armamentarium of treatment options is available based on the etiologic factors for PD. The first question the clinician should ask is whether the perioral skin has been exposed to steroids. If the patient cannot recall, the clinician should still maintain a high index of suspicion for exposure via any route, including topical application, inhaled steroids, or even "connubial" exposure from kissing another individual who uses topical steroids, and question the patient accordingly. If steroid use is ascertained, a frank discussion with the patient should ensue; there will be a direct correlation between reduction in steroid exposure and severity. In the authors' experience, a cold-turkey approach, with abrupt discontinuation of the steroid, leads to the worst flare but the most rapid resolution (1–3 months). When using this approach, we give the patient a class 1 topical steroid to use for 1 to 2 days up to twice a month for important social or work events. An alternative approach is to wean the patient off steroids, either by decreasing the potency, the frequency of application, or both. This approach generally leads to a significantly less severe flare but a much slower resolution (often greater than a year). The severity of the flare is directly proportional to how quickly the steroid is weaned, whereas the speed of resolution is inversely proportional.

All patients should be treated with topical and/or oral medications whether or not a steroid has been discontinued. Oral tetracycline is proven to be an effective agent for PD as seen in a randomized, multicenter clinical trial comparing it with topical metronidazole.[63] The recommended dosage varies from 250 mg 2 to 4 times a day to, in severe cases, up to 500 mg twice a day with treatment

Table 4
Therapeutic agents for periorificial dermatitis

Topical Agents	Level of Evidence[a]	Systemic Agents	Level of Evidence[a]
Metronidazole[63,70]	A	Tetracycline[63,71]	A
Erythromycin[71]	A	Erythromycin[62,68,69]	D
Pimecrolimus[72,73]	A	Doxycycline[66,74]	D
Sulfacetamide or sulfur[75]	B	Minocycline[67]	D
Azelaic acid[76,77]	B	Cefcapene pivoxil hydrochloride hydrate[55]	D
Clindamycin[66,78,79]	C	Isotretinoin[80]	D
Tacrolimus[67,81]	D	Other	—
Adapalene[82]	D	Zero therapy[71–73]	A
—	—	PDL[78]	C

[a] A, high-quality randomized controlled trial (RCT) or prospective study; B, lesser quality RCT or prospective study; C, case-control study or retrospective study; D, case series or case reports.

duration between 4 to 8 weeks.[5,64,65] Tetracycline also has been reported to help with CGPD, and can be considered in children older than age 9.[62] Doxycycline and minocycline, second-generation tetracyclines, in combination with other topical agents have also been used in CGPD with reasonable efficacy.[66,67] As a second-line agent especially for patients with contraindication to tetracycline, such as pregnant women or children younger than age 8, oral erythromycin can be considered; several reports show its efficacy for both PD and CGPD.[68] Dosages for oral erythromycin are generally in the range of 250 mg to 500 mg a day.[68,69] For patients who do not respond to conventional therapies as described above, the clinician can consider low-dose oral isotretinoin, initially 0.2 mg/kg/d, then lowering the dose to 0.1 mg/kg/d or to 0.05 mg/kg/d.[45] For PD in children, an effective treatment was reported with oral or topical metronidazole either alone, or in combination with erythromycin, that resulted in resolution of the primary and secondary lesions within 7 weeks.[6] Other topical agents that have shown effectiveness in case studies and series include pimecrolimus, tacrolimus, azelaic acid, sulfacetamide, topical adapalene, metronidazole, erythromycin, and clindamycin (**Table 4**).

SUMMARY

GR is a variant of rosacea that can occur with or without typical subtypes of rosacea. The cause of this entity is unknown but there are several reported antigenic factors triggering the granuloma formation. Clinically, the monomorphic papules favor periorificial areas on the face but can rarely occur in the extrafacial region. Treatment of this condition is difficult and the disease tends to be chronic but several modalities, including topical agents, oral antibiotics, oral retinoids, and laser, can be considered. PD shares similar clinical features with GR but is a common self-limiting inflammatory condition affecting young women. There are several triggering factors that may aggravate this condition. Management approach should include discontinuing any triggering factors, especially topical steroids. For children younger than 8 years of age, the first line agents to consider are topical metronidazole, erythromycin, and pimecrolimus. For patients older than 8 years of age, oral tetracycline is the first-line treatment.

REFERENCES

1. Wilkin J, Dahl M, Detmar M, et al. Standard classification of rosacea: report of the National Rosacea Society Expert Committee on the classification and staging of rosacea. J Am Acad Dermatol 2002; 46(4):584–7.

2. Tan J, Berg M. Rosacea: current state of epidemiology. J Am Acad Dermatol 2013;69(6 Suppl 1): S27–35.

3. Frumess GM, Lewis HM. Light-sensitive seborrheid. AMA Arch Derm 1957;75(2):245–8.

4. Mihan R, Ayress S. Perioral dermatitis. Arch Dermatol 1964;89:803–5.

5. Tempark T, Shwayder TA. Perioral dermatitis: a review of the condition with special attention to treatment options. Am J Clin Dermatol 2014;15(2):101–13.

6. Nguyen V, Eichenfield LF. Periorificial dermatitis in children and adolescents. J Am Acad Dermatol 2006;55(5):781–5.

7. Gianotti F, Ermacora E, Benelli MG, et al. "Perioral dermatitis" in children and adults. G Ital Dermatol Minerva Dermatol 1971;46(3):132 [in Italian].

8. Frieden IJ, Prose NS, Fletcher V, et al. Granulomatous perioral dermatitis in children. Arch Dermatol 1989;125(3):369–73.

9. Knautz MA, Lesher JL. Childhood granulomatous periorificial dermatitis. Pediatr Dermatol 1996; 13(2):131–4.

10. Khokhar O, Khachemoune A. A case of granulomatous rosacea: sorting granulomatous rosacea from other granulomatous diseases that affect the face. Dermatol Online J 2004;10(1):6.

11. Darier M. Des (tuberculides) cutanées. Ann Dermatol Syphiligr 1896;7:1431–6, 3rd series.

12. Lewandowsky F. Über Rosacea-ähnliche Tuberkulide des Geschiles. Corr Bl Schweiz Ärzte 1917;47: 1280–2.

13. Laymon CW, Schoch EP. Micropapular tuberculid and rosacea; a clinical and histologic comparison. Arch Derm Syphilol 1948;58(3):286–300.

14. Snapp RH. Lewandowsky's rosacea-like eruption; a clinical study. J Invest Dermatol 1949;13(4): 175–90.

15. Crawford GH, Pelle MT, James WD. Rosacea: I. Etiology, pathogenesis, and subtype classification. J Am Acad Dermatol 2004;51(3):327–41 [quiz: 342–4].

16. Steinhoff M, Schauber J, Leyden JJ. New insights into rosacea pathophysiology: a review of recent findings. J Am Acad Dermatol 2013;69(6 Suppl 1): S15–26.

17. Helm KF, Menz J, Gibson LE, et al. A clinical and histopathologic study of granulomatous rosacea. J Am Acad Dermatol 1991;25:1038–43.

18. Mullanax MG, Kierland RR. Granulomatous rosacea. Arch Dermatol 1970;101:206–11.

19. Sánchez JL, Berlingeri-Ramos AC, Dueño DV. Granulomatous rosacea. Am J Dermatopathol 2008; 30(1):6–9.

20. Ramelet AA, Perroulaz G. Rosacea: histopathologic study of 75 cases. Ann Dermatol Venereol 1988; 115(8):801–6 [in French].

21. Erbağci Z, Ozgöztaşi O. The significance of *Demodex folliculorum* density in rosacea. Int J Dermatol 1998;37(6):421–5.

22. Jang YH, Sim JH, Kang HY, et al. Immunohistochemical expression of matrix metalloproteinases in the granulomatous rosacea compared with the non-granulomatous rosacea. J Eur Acad Dermatol Venereol 2011;25(5):544–8.

23. Mayr-Kanhäuser S, Kränke B, Kaddu S, et al. Resolution of granulomatous rosacea after eradication of Helicobacter pylori with clarithromycin, metronidazole and pantoprazole. Eur J Gastroenterol Hepatol 2001;13(11):1379–83.

24. Wilkin J, Dahl M, Detmar M, et al. Standard grading system for rosacea: report of the National Rosacea Society Expert Committee on the classification and staging of rosacea. J Am Acad Dermatol 2002; 50(6):907–12.

25. Heinle R, Chang C. Diagnostic criteria for sarcoidosis. Autoimmun Rev 2014;13(4–5):383–7.

26. Rocas D, Kanitakis J. Lupus miliaris disseminatus faciei: report of a new case and brief literature review. Dermatol Online J 2013;19(3):4.

27. English JC, Patel PJ, Greer KE. Sarcoidosis. J Am Acad Dermatol 2001;44(5):725–43 [quiz: 744–6].

28. Del Rosso JQ, Thiboutot D, Gallo R, et al. Consensus recommendations from the American Acne & Rosacea Society on the management of rosacea, part 1: a status report on the disease state, general measures, and adjunctive skin care. Cutis 2013;92(5):234–40.

29. Ohata C, Saruban H, Ikegami R. Granulomatous rosacea affecting the lacrimal and salivary glands. Arch Dermatol 2004;140(2):240–2.

30. Patrinely JR, Font RL, Anderson RL. Granulomatous acne rosacea of the eyelids. Arch Ophthalmol 1990; 108(4):561–3.

31. Ajith C, Dogra S, Radotra BD, et al. Granulomatous rosacea mimicking eyelid dermatitis. Indian J Dermatol Venereol Leprol 2005;71(5):366.

32. Schewach-Millet M, Shpiro D, Trau H. Granulomatous rosacea. J Am Acad Dermatol 1988;18(6): 1362–3.

33. Webster G, Del Rosso JQ. Anti-inflammatory activity of tetracyclines. Dermatol Clin 2007;25(2):133–5, v.

34. Cunha PR, Rossi AB. Pimecrolimus cream 1% is effective in a case of granulomatous rosacea. Acta Derm Venereol 2006;86(1):71–2.

35. Gül U, Gönül M, Kiliç A, et al. A case of granulomatous rosacea successfully treated with pimecrolimus cream. J Dermatolog Treat 2008;19(5):313–5.

36. Rallis E, Korfitis C. Isotretinoin for the treatment of granulomatous rosacea: case report and review of the literature. J Cutan Med Surg 2012;16(6):438–41.

37. Ehmann LM, Meller S, Homey B. Successful treatment of granulomatous rosacea with dapsone. Hautarzt 2013;64(4):226–8 [in German].

38. Baglieri F, Scuderi G. Treatment of recalcitrant granulomatous rosacea with ALA-PDT: report of a case. Indian J Dermatol Venereol Leprol 2011; 77(4):536.

39. Lane JE, Khachemoune A. Use of intense pulsed light to treat refractory granulomatous rosacea. Dermatol Surg 2010;36(4):571–3.

40. Salem DA, El-Shazly A, Nabih N, et al. Evaluation of the efficacy of oral ivermectin in comparison with ivermectin-metronidazole combined therapy in the treatment of ocular and skin lesions of *Demodex folliculorum*. Int J Infect Dis 2013;17(5): e343–7.

41. Eghlileb AM, Finlay AY. Granulomatous rosacea in Cornelia de Lange syndrome. Indian J Dermatol Venereol Leprol 2009;75(1):74–5.

42. Sanchez-Viera M, Hernanz JM, Sampelayo T, et al. Granulomatous rosacea in a child infected with the human immunodeficiency virus. J Am Acad Dermatol 1992;27(6 Pt 1):1010–1.

43. Batra M, Bansal C, Tulsyan S. Granulomatous rosacea: unusual presentation as solitary plaque. Dermatol Online J 2011;17(2):9.

44. Lipozencic J, Ljubojevic S. Perioral dermatitis. Clin Dermatol 2011;29(2):157–61.

45. Lipozenčić J, Hadžavdić SL. Perioral dermatitis. Clin Dermatol 2014;32(1):125–30.

46. Dubus JC, Marguet C, Deschildre A, et al. Local side-effects of inhaled corticosteroids in asthmatic children: influence of drug, dose, age, and device. Allergy 2001;56(10):944–8.

47. Poulos GA, Brodell RT. Perioral dermatitis associated with an inhaled corticosteroid. Arch Dermatol 2007;143(11):1460.

48. Clementson B, Smidt AC. Periorificial dermatitis due to systemic corticosteroids in children: report of two cases. Pediatr Dermatol 2012;29(3):331–2.

49. Peters P, Drummond C. Perioral dermatitis from high fluoride dentifrice: a case report and review of literature. Aust Dent J 2013;58(3):371–2.

50. Beacham BE, Kurgansky D, Gould WM. Circumoral dermatitis and cheilitis caused by tartar control dentifrices. J Am Acad Dermatol 1990;22(6 Pt 1): 1029–32.

51. Abele DC. 'Moisturizers' and perioral dermatitis. Arch Dermatol 1977;113(1):110.

52. Budimir V, Brailo V, Alajbeg I, et al. Allergic contact cheilitis and perioral dermatitis caused by propolis: case report. Acta Dermatovenerol Croat 2012; 20(3):187–90.

53. Abeck D, Geisenfelder B, Brandt O. Physical sunscreens with high sun protection factor may cause perioral dermatitis in children. J Dtsch Dermatol Ges 2009;7(8):701–3.

54. Bradford LG, Montes LF. Perioral dermatitis and *Candida albicans*. Arch Dermatol 1972;105(6): 892–5.

55. Ishiguro N, Maeda A, Suzuki K, et al. Three cases of perioral dermatitis related to fusobacteria treated with β-lactam antibiotics. J Dermatolog Treat 2014; 25(6):507–9.

56. Takiwaki H, Tsuda H, Arase S, et al. Differences between intrafollicular microorganism profiles in perioral and seborrhoeic dermatitis. Clin Exp Dermatol 2003;28(5):531–4.

57. Hsu CK, Hsu MM, Lee JY. Demodicosis: a clinico-pathological study. J Am Acad Dermatol 2009; 60(3):453–62.

58. Hafeez ZH. Perioral dermatitis: an update. Int J Dermatol 2003;42(7):514–7.

59. Satyawan I, Oranje AP, van Joost T. Perioral dermatitis in a child due to rosin in chewing gum. Contact Dermatitis 1990;22(3):182–3.

60. Guarneri F, Marini H. Perioral dermatitis after dental filling in a 12-year-old girl: involvement of cholinergic system in skin neuroinflammation? ScientificWorldJournal 2008;8:157–63.

61. Dirschka T, Tronnier H, Fölster-Holst R. Epithelial barrier function and atopic diathesis in rosacea and perioral dermatitis. Br J Dermatol 2004;150(6): 1136–41.

62. Urbatsch AJ, Frieden I, Williams ML, et al. Extrafacial and generalized granulomatous periorificial dermatitis. Arch Dermatol 2002;138(10):1354–8.

63. Veien NK, Munkvad JM, Nielsen AO, et al. Topical metronidazole in the treatment of perioral dermatitis. J Am Acad Dermatol 1991;24(2 Pt 1):258–60.

64. Tarm K, Creel NB, Krivda SJ, et al. Granulomatous periorificial dermatitis. Cutis 2004;73(6):399–402.

65. Zalaudek I, Di Stefani A, Ferrara G, et al. Childhood granulomatous periorificial dermatitis: a controversial disease. J Dtsch Dermatol Ges 2005;3(4):252–5.

66. Kumar P, Parashette KR, Noronha P. Letter: Perioral dermatitis in a child associated with an inhalation steroid. Dermatol Online J 2010;16(4):13.

67. Misago N, Nakafusa J, Narisawa Y. Childhood granulomatous periorificial dermatitis: lupus miliaris disseminatus faciei in children? J Eur Acad Dermatol Venereol 2005;19(4):470–3.

68. Choi YL, Lee KJ, Cho HJ, et al. Case of childhood granulomatous periorificial dermatitis in a Korean boy treated by oral erythromycin. J Dermatol 2006; 33(11):806–8.

69. Ellis CN, Stawiski MA. The treatment of perioral dermatitis, acne rosacea, and seborrheic dermatitis. Med Clin North Am 1982;66(4):819–30.

70. Boeck K, Abeck D, Werfel S, et al. Perioral dermatitis in children–clinical presentation, pathogenesis-related factors and response to topical metronidazole. Dermatology 1997;195(3):235–8.

71. Weber K, Thurmayr R, Meisinger A. A topical erythromycin preparation and oral tetracycline for the treatment of perioral dermatitis: a placebo controlled trial. J Dermatol Treat 1993;4:57–9.

72. Oppel T, Pavicic T, Kamann S, et al. Pimecrolimus cream (1%) efficacy in perioral dermatitis - results of a randomized, double-blind, vehicle-controlled study in 40 patients. J Eur Acad Dermatol Venereol 2007;21(9):1175–80.

73. Schwarz T, Kreiselmaier I, Bieber T, et al. A randomized, double-blind, vehicle-controlled study of 1% pimecrolimus cream in adult patients with perioral dermatitis. J Am Acad Dermatol 2008; 59(1):34–40.

74. Adams SJ, Davison AM, Cunliffe WJ, et al. Perioral dermatitis in renal transplant recipients maintained on corticosteroids and immunosuppressive therapy. Br J Dermatol 1982;106(5):589–92.

75. Bendl BJ. Perioral dermatitis: etiology and treatment. Cutis 1976;17(5):903–8.

76. Jansen T. Azelaic acid as a new treatment for perioral dermatitis: results from an open study. Br J Dermatol 2004;151(4):933–4.

77. Jansen T, Melnik BC, Schadendorf D. Steroid-induced periorificial dermatitis in children–clinical features and response to azelaic acid. Podiatr Dermatol 2010;27(2):137–42.

78. Richey DF, Hopson B. Photodynamic therapy for perioral dermatitis. J Drugs Dermatol 2006;5(2 Suppl):12–6.

79. Coskey RJ. Perioral dermatitis. Cutis 1984;34(1): 55–6, 58.

80. Smith KW. Perioral dermatitis with histopathologic features of granulomatous rosacea: successful treatment with isotretinoin. Cutis 1990;46(5):413–5.

81. Hussain W, Daly BM. Granulomatous periorificial dermatitis in an 11-year-old boy: dramatic response to tacrolimus. J Eur Acad Dermatol Venereol 2007; 21(1):137–9.

82. Jansen T. Perioral dermatitis successfully treated with topical adapalene. J Eur Acad Dermatol Venereol 2002;16(2):175–7.

Adult Orbital Xanthogranulomatous Disease

A Review with Emphasis on Etiology, Systemic Associations, Diagnostic Tools, and Treatment

Justin Kerstetter, MD, Jun Wang, MD*

KEYWORDS

- Adult orbital xanthogranulomatous disease • Orbital inflammation • Erdheim-Chester disease
- Necrobiotic xanthogranuloma • Adult onset asthma with periorbital xanthogranuloma

KEY POINTS

- Taken as a whole, the adult orbital xanthogranulomatous disorders are rare.
- Recognition of these lesions are important owing to the occasionally clinically severe systemic associations seen in the different entities.
- Treatment options vary with no current consensus as to the most optimum therapeutic course.
- Prognosis of patients afflicted with these disorders depends primarily on the presence and severity of any accompanying systemic manifestations.

INTRODUCTION

Adult orbital xanthogranulomatous disease (AOXGD) comprises a heterogeneous group of rare orbital and ocular adnexal disorders that are classified as class II non-Langerhans histiocytic proliferations. Based primarily on the degree of systemic involvement, this disease can be classified into 4 subtypes: adult-onset xanthogranuloma, necrobiotic xanthogranuloma (NXG), Erdheim–Chester disease (ECD), and adult-onset asthma and periocular xanthogranuloma (AAPOX; **Table 1**).[1,2] Although some differences are present histologically, each of these entities is characterized by infiltration of foamy histiocytes and Touton-type giant cells, both of which are often negative for S100 protein and CD1a. Clinically, this infiltration, along with accompanying lymphocytes and varying degrees of fibrosis, can replace the normal lacrimal gland architecture, causing mass effects and loss of tear production.[1–4] This review discusses the etiopathogenesis of these lesions, along with clinicopathologic presentation and associated systemic manifestations. We conclude with a discussion about current evaluation and management in patients found to have this disease.

ETIOPATHOGENESIS

Orbital xanthogranulomatous disease is one of the non-Langerhans (type II) histiocytosis characterized by localized or systemic proliferation of histiocytes. Histiocytes are produced from bone

Department of Pathology and Laboratory Medicine, Loma Linda University Medical Center, 11234 Anderson Street, Room #2151, Loma Linda, CA 92354, USA
* Corresponding author.
E-mail address: jwang@llu.edu

Dermatol Clin 33 (2015) 457–463
http://dx.doi.org/10.1016/j.det.2015.03.010
0733-8635/15/$ – see front matter © 2015 Elsevier Inc. All rights reserved.

derm.theclinics.com

Table 1
Four adult types of orbital xanthogranuloma

Disease Type	Clinical Features and Systemic Associations	Prognosis	Therapeutic Modalities	Level of Evidence
Adult onset	Localized to the eye (anterior orbit)	Good; limited to eye	Surgical debulking	C
Adult onset with asthma	Anterior orbit; asthma and lymphadenopathy	Good; rarely associated with systemic findings	Surgery often successful; corticosteroids	C
Erdheim–Chester disease	Intraconal; long bone sclerolytic destruction; retroperitoneal fibrosis; cardiac involvement	Poor; mortality rate is increased (~66%)	Corticosteroids and immunosuppressive agents	C
Necrobiotic xanthogranuloma	Anterior orbit ulceration; multiple myeloma, lymphoma, paraproteinemia	Poor; systemic lymphoproliferative disorders	Combination of corticosteroid with immunosuppressive agent; surgical debulking is not recommended	C

C, case-control study or retrospective study.

marrow stem cells and mature into monocytes,[5] when they then enter into either the mononuclear–phagocytic system or the dendritic cell system.[6] These 2 groups are composed of unique cell types. The mononuclear–phagocytic system consists of phagocytic monocytes and free and fixed tissue macrophages.[5] The dendritic cell includes the follicular cells of the lymph nodes and the Langerhans cells of the skin, which both serve as antigen-presenting cells.[5] The current thinking is that xanthogranulomas develop secondary to a reactive proliferation of the free tissue macrophages. Although the etiopathogenesis of these proliferations is not known currently, a number of proposed mechanisms have been reported.

In 1971, Balfour and colleagues,[7] presented a case of an 11-week-old male infant with a xanthogranuloma of the salivary gland associated with cytomegalovirus infection. More recently, in 2001, Vasconcelos and colleagues[8] confirmed immunohistochemically the presence of immunolabeling for cytomegalovirus antigens in the histiocytes of an oral juvenile xanthogranuloma. These findings suggest the possibility that xanthogranulomatous diseases may be a virus-induced process. In addition, other patients with juvenile xanthogranulomas demonstrated chromosomal instability in lesional tissue and peripheral blood cells. It is theorized that chromosomal abnormalities constitute either a basic genetic defect or these aberrations may simply serve as evidence of a cellular response to an environmental agent (eg, virus), which would then initiate the proliferation of histiocytes.[9]

With regard to specific entities, the underlying mechanism for the pathogenesis of AAPOX is understood poorly, but recent research suggests a poorly understood systemic immunologic derangement with concurrent bronchiolar and ocular adnexal dysfunction.[1,3] In addition, because the association of NXG with paraproteinemia is well-known, this fact has led to a number of hypotheses regarding the pathogenesis of this variant of AOXGD. The paraproteinemia present is an immunoglobulin (Ig)G monoclonal gammopathy that is found in at least 80% of cases of NXG. The prevailing thought is that the paraprotein serves as either the primary inciting factor or it may act as a cofactor that facilitates in eliciting the characteristic giant cell granulomatous reaction.[10] To date, however, the precise pathogenesis of NXG and the other adult orbital xanthogranulomas is unknown.

CLINICAL PRESENTATION

Adult-onset xanthogranuloma is rare and as a group it affects patients from 17 to 85 years of age with no significant gender preference (73 male vs 64 female cases).[2] Adult-onset xanthogranuloma is an isolated xanthogranulomatous lesion without significant systemic involvement. It is the least common entity among AOXGDs, and affects patients ranging from 38 to 79 years with no significant gender preference. The significance of recognizing this entity is that it is often self-limited and does not require aggressive treatment, in contradistinction to the other subtypes of

AOXGDs, which can sometimes cause significant consequences.[2]

NXG is characterized by the presence of subcutaneous skin lesions that tend to ulcerate and become fibrotic. The most common clinical manifestation is an indurated papule, nodule, or plaque that can be violaceous, red-orange, or xanthomatous (yellow) in color.[11] Papules usually progressively enlarge to bulky nodules and plaques with scarring, atrophy, and telangiectasias. Ulcerations, which may be extensive, are seen in more than 40% of patients.[11] The size of the plaques can range from 0.3 to 25 cm. The most common site of involvement is the periorbital region (>80% of cases with other parts of the face, trunk, and extremities). Periorbital lesions may involve single or multiple eyelids and may be unilateral or bilateral. This entity often affects adults 20 to 85 years of age with no significant gender preference (32 for male and 40 for female).[11–13]

ECD is an idiopathic condition of lymphohistiocytic infiltration in the orbit as well as internal organs, including the heart, lungs, retroperitoneum, bones, and other tissues.[1,2,14] These patients typically present with bone pain and characteristic lesions are seen radiographically on further evaluation, which are ultimately what lead clinicians to arrive at the proper diagnosis. Other systemic symptoms leading to further workup include fever, weakness, weight loss, and night sweats.[15] Whereas skeletal manifestations are pathognomonic, cutaneous manifestations that may elevate the clinical suspicion include orbital disease with exophthalmos and xanthoma-like lesions of the eyelids.[16] Like AAPOX, it presents preferentially in male (male to female: 2:1) and affects patients ranging from 7 to 84 years of age.[17] This condition is often fatal, with death owing to cardiomyopathy, severe lung disease, or chronic renal failure. In addition, bone involvement is common, with frequent critical consequences despite aggressive therapies.[17] Because of its frequent and significant systemic involvement, bilateral diffuse orbital masses should alert the clinician to the possibility of this serious systemic disease.

AAPOX is rare, with fewer than 30 reported cases in the literature and a newly diagnosed case at our institution.[18] It often presents with bilateral yellow-orange, elevated, indurated, and nonulcerated xanthomatous eyelids and/or orbital masses. It typically extends into the anterior orbital fat, and sometimes involves the extraocular muscles and/or the lacrimal gland(s).[1–3] AAPOX is most often seen in adult patients ranging from 22 to 74 years old, with twice as many males being affected as females. Most patients experience adult-onset asthma within a few months to a few years of the onset of the orbital lesions. Interestingly, asthma has also been reported with some frequency in patients with sinus histiocytosis and massive lymphadenopathy. Even when asthmatic symptoms are severe enough to require systemic corticosteroids and inhalation therapy, a chest radiograph may be negative.

Because the eyelids usually remain intact and these xanthogranulomatous processes typically do not reach the deep orbital and perioptic nerve connective tissues, visual acuity may not be affected and ocular motility is generally well-preserved, unless the extraocular muscles are involved. Only rarely are the corneas exposed to the infiltrate, but in the rare cases where lacrimal gland involvement causes punctuate corneal epitheliopathy, the patient may suffer from a dry eye condition.[1] However, the eyelid and periocular infiltration can be very extensive and cause significant mass effect that prevents the patient from seeing properly (**Fig. 1**).

SYSTEMIC ASSOCIATIONS

The xanthogranulomatous disorders may be associated with a number of additional pathologic processes. Although AXO is seen commonly in the periorbital region, it may affect any part of the body. However, it is usually a self-limited process and is not associated typically with any other systemic abnormalities.

On the other hand, NXG is associated commonly with a paraproteinemia. As mentioned,

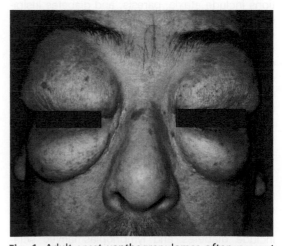

Fig. 1. Adult-onset xanthogranulomas often present with bilateral yellow-orange, elevated, indurated, and nonulcerated xanthomatous eyelids and/or orbital masses. It can be very extensive and causes significant mass effect that prevents the patient from seeing properly (shown here is a patient with adult-onset asthma and periocular xanthogranuloma).

this paraproteinemia is usually an IgG monoclonal gammopathy in up to 80% of the cases. Wood and colleagues,[13] in a review of 17 patients, showed that 12 (71%) had a monoclonal gammopathy, 8 of which showed kappa light chain restriction and 4 showing lambda light chain restriction. Three of their patients (18%) had multiple myeloma. Nine of 17 patients (53%) showed evidence of plasmacytosis or a plasma cell proliferative disorder on subsequent bone marrow examination. Of note, 1 patient had both multiple myeloma and type I cryoglobulinemia.[13] The mean time from the first appearance of NXG lesions to the development of hematologic disorders was 2.4 years. Recently, Balagula and colleagues[11] described the first reported case of a patient with NXG in a patient with Waldenstrom's macroglobulinemia. Given these features, close clinical monitoring of serum proteins is imperative in patients with confirmed NXG.

The histiocytic proliferations seen in ECD occur mainly in the long bones of the lower extremities, the central nervous system, retroperitoneum, lung, heart, liver, spleen, skin, and the orbit; they have been reported rarely in the testes, thyroid, and lymph nodes.[19] The associated bony lesions are essentially pathognomonic and are characterized by bilateral symmetric osteosclerosis involving metaphyseal and diaphyseal regions, with sparing of the epiphyses.[20] In addition, there are a number of extraskelatal and extraorbital manifestations. When the disease process extends to the retroperitoneum, obstructive renal impairment may occur.[21] Neurologic manifestations include ataxia, paresis, and diabetes insipidus.[22] Of significance, cardiac and pulmonary involvement by the histiocytic proliferation may lead to pericardial and pleural effusions, myocardial infiltration, and interstitial lung disease.[15] The extent of extraskeletal disease is what ultimately determines patient prognosis with more diffuse involvement portending a more ominous course.

Last, in addition to asthma, AAPOX is associated frequently with lymphadenopathy, paraproteinemia, and rarely with other lymphoproliferative disorders or internal organ dysfunction.[2,3] The most commonly reported hematologic malignancies included chronic lymphocytic leukemia/small lymphocytic lymphoma, multiple myeloma, and non-Hodgkin lymphoma. Other associations include diabetes and lymphoplasmacytic sclerosing pancreatitis.[23]

EVALUATION

All AOXGD subtypes share common histopathologic features characterized by sheets of mononucleated foamy histiocytes (xanthoma cells) infiltrating the orbicularis muscles and the orbital tissue, accompanied by variable numbers of dispersed and/or aggregates of lymphocytes, plasma cells and Touton giant cells (**Fig. 2**).[24] These infiltrating xanthoma cells often have small round nuclei and abundant clear or vacuolated cytoplasm (**Fig. 3**). Oil-red O staining of frozen sections confirms the lipid content of the xanthoma cells. Scattered among these xanthoma cells are Touton giant cells characterized by a ring of nuclei around a central eosinophilic zone that is surrounded by a zone of pallor extending to the periphery of the cell (see **Fig. 2**).[24] Lymphoid follicles are scattered commonly throughout with variable reactive germinal centers, especially seen in AAPOX.[24] Variable amounts of fibrosis is often present but without necrobiosis of collagen except for those patients with NXG.[24]

Immunohistochemically, the foamy histiocytes are strongly positive for CD68, CD163 (**Fig. 4**), and factor XIIIa, but are usually negative for CD21, CD35, S100, and CD1a (data not shown).[24] These foamy histiocytes, however, can be positive rarely for S100 and negative for factor XIIIa as in rare cases of juvenile xanthogranuloma. Therefore, neither a negative factor XIIIa nor a positive S100 result should preclude the diagnosis of AOXGDs.[12] The lymphoid infiltration has a reactive profile with germinal centers being positive for CD20 and negative for Bcl-2. The parafollicular T cells are CD3 positive and are often predominantly CD8 positive. There is often no influx of CD4-positive T cells.[1,2,4,25]

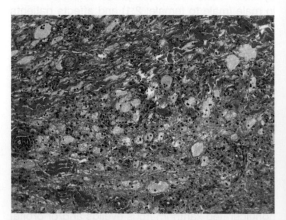

Fig. 2. Adult orbital xanthogranulomatous disease usually contains sheets of mononucleated foamy histiocytes (xanthoma cells) infiltrating the orbicularis muscles and the anteriorbital fibrous tissue, accompanied by variable numbers of dispersed and/or aggregates of lymphocytes, plasma cells (stain: hematoxylin and eosin; original magnification, ×200) and Touton giant cells.

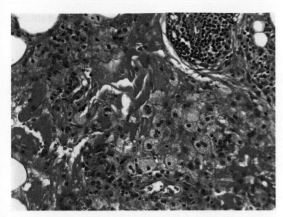

Fig. 3. These infiltrating xanthoma cells often have small round nuclei and abundant clear or vacuolated cytoplasm and lymphoid aggregates may be present (stain: hematoxylin and eosin; original magnification, ×400). Oil-red O staining of frozen sections confirms the lipid content of the xanthoma cells (not shown).

Immunophenotyping by flow cytometry, serum protein immunoelectrophoresis, or even bone marrow biopsy are sometimes performed and periodically repeated to evaluate the multiple myeloma, monoclonal gammopathy of undetermined significance or lymphoma that may be associated with AOXGDs. This evaluation is done much more commonly in patients with NXG, and occasionally in individuals with AAPOX. Because patients with xanthogranulomas can develop plasma cell dyscrasias and lymphoproliferative malignancies, especially in the presence of necrobiosis, a thorough baseline systemic evaluation and long-term follow-up is mandatory.[2,12] Although these extensive systemic evaluations are often unremarkable, the occurrence of

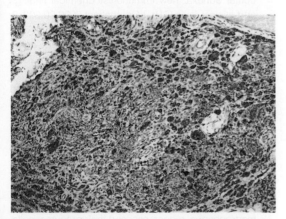

Fig. 4. These foamy histiocytes (xanthoma cells) are usually negative for CD21, CD35, CD1a, and S-100 (not shown), but are strongly positive for CD68 (stain: immunoperoxidase; original magnification, ×200) and CD163 (not shown).

paraproteinemia and/or a late onset of M-protein (IgG) on serum protein immunoelectrophoresis suggesting that the inflammatory infiltrates may have stimulated B-cell populations, as has been suggested in patients with AAPOX.[1–3]

Radiologic studies of patients with AOXGD may reveal evidence of proptosis with an abnormal infiltrative soft tissue mass and increased fat. Associated enlargement of extraocular muscles with possible lacrimal gland involvement is often present, whereas encasement of the optic nerve, bony destruction, and intracranial extension are not noted often. Particularly in patients with AAPOX, CT may reveal preseptal and anterior orbital involvement with occasional posterior tracking along or within the orbital muscles and fat, usually sparing the optic nerve and connective tissues. Facial bones are usually not involved.[1] MRI often discloses hypointense signals in the eyelids, extending into the anterior orbital fat.[1] Electron microscopic studies are sometimes used in difficult cases and often show cytoplasmic lipid vacuoles, mitochondria, and phagosomes, but no Birbeck granules within the xanthoma cells.[1]

TREATMENT

Because the mechanisms in the xanthogranulomatous disorders are understood poorly, to date there is no targeted therapy directed at the histiocytic proliferation and most therapies incorporate a strategy involving local and systemic control of the disease.[26] A myriad of therapies based primarily on anecdotal evidence has been used over the years: topical, intralesional, and systemic corticosteroid; alkylating agents, such as chlorambucil melphalan with or without systemic steroids; antimetabolites; interferon alpha-2b; radiation; plasmapheresis; and carbon dioxide have all been attempted.[11]

Intralesional corticosteroids have been successful in controlling the signs and symptoms of adult-onset xanthogranulomatous disease and, on occasion, have been shown effective in NXG with eyelid and orbital involvement.[24] Most commonly, however, these lesions are typically treated with systemic corticosteroids, typically starting at approximately 1 mg/kg per day with tapering once the lesions have abated, although numerous authors have reported recurrence of symptoms upon tapering.[1,23,27–30] In the largest series of patients with adult xanthogranulomatous disease, in the subset of patients with AAPOX, surgery was successful in 75% (6 of 8 patients), whereas corticosteroids were useful in both occasions they were administered.[2] However,

Jakobiec and colleagues[1] showed that patients who were treated with debulking surgery alone demonstrated recurrence within 6 to 12 months of their eyelid masses. It is their opinion that treatment with high-dose corticosteroids with low-dose radiotherapy is preferred over surgical debulking for AAPOX. It should be noted, in their series of 11 patients with orbital xanthogranulomas, Ebrahimi and colleagues[31] showed that of the 4 patients treated with orbital radiation owing to poor initial therapeutic response, at least 3 patients experienced exacerbation of their disease. Clearly, the role of radiotherapy in the treatment of orbital xanthogranulomatous disease is, for the time being, controversial at best.

More recently, the use of methotrexate has been proposed as a means to treat refractory cases of AOXGD or as a potential corticosteroid-sparing therapy. A dihydrofolate reductase inhibitor, the antiinflammatory mechanism in methotrexate is not well understood. It is hypothesized that it causes enhanced release of adenosine resulting in a decreased production of inflammatory cytokines.[32] Hayden and colleagues[33] reported a beneficial effect of methotrexate in their 3 patients with periocular xanthogranulomas. In Cavallazzi and colleague's series,[26] 3 patients responded with the use of methotrexate, 2 of whom had experienced treatment failure following initiation of corticosteroids. Both authors, however, reached the conclusion that it is unclear whether methotrexate should be a first-line therapy.

The eyelid lesions in NXG can be treated successfully with radiotherapy or systemic prednisolone and chlorambucil unless extensive destruction has occurred.[24] On the other hand, treatment modalities for ECD are broad, ranging from observation to systemic steroids, radiation therapy, and chemotherapy, including cyclophosphamide, doxorubicin, and vincristine.[15] Currently, interferon-α provides the best management strategy with sustainable stabilization of the disease in most cases. Interferon-α is administered in doses ranging from 3 million units 3 times per week to 9 million units 3 times per week. It should be noted that treatment with these therapies is long term and thus tolerance to the effects of the medication must be considered pivotal in management of these patients.[15] Additionally, Myra and colleagues[34] have shown that administering cladribine at 0.14 mg/kg per day for 5 days over the course of five weeks produced marked recovery in 1 patient with ECD. Corticosteroids once were considered promising given their immunosuppressive effects, but they have demonstrated little impact on the disease. Different chemotherapeutic regimens have been proposed, all only offering transient relief of symptoms. Retroorbital irradiation is often not effective. It should be noted that despite treatment ECD often follows an aggressive course.[15]

SUMMARY

AOXGDs are rare and pose challenges in daily clinical practice. They are discerned primarily by their associated systemic manifestations as well as the occasional distinctive histopathologic feature (ie, necrobiosis in cases of NXG). The mainstay of therapy remains immunosuppressive agents, primarily through the administration of systemic steroids, although a number of other modalities have been used, including chemotherapeutic agents. Having reviewed the literature, it is the authors' belief that debulking surgery should be used as a last resort. In addition, further study is necessary with regard to the use of radiation therapy, given the conflicted results reported in the literature. Further research is necessary given the rarity of these diseases, although a prospective, randomized controlled study remains unlikely. Ideally, this research would be tailored toward discerning the disease mechanisms with the goal of eventually developing more effective targeted therapy so that long-term effects of these disorders may be minimized, if not eliminated.

REFERENCES

1. Jakobiec FA, Mills MD, Hidayat AA, et al. Periocular xanthogranulomas associated with severe adult-onset asthma. Trans Am Ophthalmol Soc 1993;91: 99–125.
2. Sivak-Callcott JA, Rootman J, Rasmussen SL, et al. Adult xanthogranulomatous disease of the orbit and ocular adnexa: new immunohistochemical findings and clinical review. Br J Ophthalmol 2006;90:602–8.
3. Hammond MD, Niemi EW, Ward TP, et al. Adult orbital xanthogranuloma with associated adult-onset asthma. Ophthal Plast Reconstr Surg 2004; 20:329–32.
4. Vick VL, Wilson MW, Fleming JC, et al. Orbital and eyelid manifestations of xanthogranulomatous diseases. Orbit 2006;25:221–5.
5. Karcioglu ZA, Sharara N, Boles TL, et al. Orbital xanthogranuloma: clinical and morphologic features in eight patients. Ophthal Plast Reconstr Surg 2003; 19(5):372–81.
6. Van Furth R, Cohn ZA, Hirsch JG, et al. The mononuclear phagocytic system: a new classification of macrophages, monocytes, and their precursor cells. Bull World Health Organ 1972;46:845–55.
7. Balfour HH, Speicher CE, McReynolds DG, et al. Juvenile xanthogranuloma associated with cytomegalovirus infection. Am J Med 1971;50(3):380–4.

8. Vasconcelos FO, Oliveira LA, Naves MD, et al. Juvenile xanthogranuloma: case report with immunohistochemical identified of early and late cytomegalovirus antigens. J Oral Sci 2001;43:21–5.

9. Scappaticci S, Danesino C, Rossi E, et al. Cytogenetic abnormalities in PHA-stimulated lymphocytes from patients with Langerhans cell histiocytosis. Br J Haematol 2000;111:258–62.

10. Bolognia J, Jorizzo J, Rapini R. Dermatology. 1st edition. New York: Mosby; 2003.

11. Balagula Y, Straus DJ, Pulitzer MP, et al. Necrobiotic xanthogranuloma associated with immunoglobulin M paraproteinemia in a patient with Waldenstrom macroglobulinemia. J Clin Oncol 2011;29(11): e305–7.

12. Rayner SA, Duncombe AS, Keefe M, et al. Necrobiotic xanthogranuloma occurring in an eyelid scar. Orbit 2008;27:191–4.

13. Wood AJ, Wagner MV, Abbott JJ, et al. Necrobiotic xanthogranuloma: a review of 17 cases with emphasis on clinical and pathologic correlation. Arch Dermatol 2009;145(3):279–84.

14. Lau WW, Chan E, Chan CW. Orbital involvement in Erdheim-Chester disease. Hong Kong Med J 2007; 13:238–40.

15. Mazor R, Manevich-Mazor M, Shoenfeld Y. Erdheim-Chester disease: a comprehensive review of the literature. Orphanet J Rare Dis 2013;8:137.

16. Shields J, Karcioglu Z, Shields C, et al. Orbital and eyelid involvement with Erdheim-Chester disease: a report of two cases. Arch Ophthalmol 1991;109: 850–4.

17. Veyssier-Belot C, Cacour P, Caparros-Lefebvre D, et al. Erdheim-Chester disease: clinical and radiologic characteristics of 59 cases. Medicine (Baltimore) 1996;75(3):157–69.

18. Tokuhara KG, Agarwal MR, Rao NA. Adult-onset asthma and severe periocular xanthogranuloma: a case report. Ophthal Plast Reconstr Surg 2011; 27(3):e63–4.

19. Sheu SY, Wenzel RR, Kerstin C, et al. Erdheim-Chester disease: case report with multisystemic manifestations including testes, thyroid, and lymph nodes, and a review of literature. J Clin Pathol 2004;57: 1125–8.

20. Egan AJ, Boardman LA, Tazelaar HD, et al. Erdheim-Chester disease: clinical, radiologic, and histopathologic findings in five patients with interstitial lung disease. Am J Surg Pathol 1999;23(1):17–26.

21. Haroche J, Arnaud L, Amoura Z. Erdheim-Chester disease. Curr Opin Rheumatol 2012;117:2778–82.

22. Drier A, Haroche J, Savatovsky J, et al. Cerebral, facial, and orbital involvement in Erdheim-Chester disease: CT and MR imaging findings. Radiology 2010;255:586–94.

23. Roggin KK, Rudloff U, Kimstra DS, et al. Adult-onset asthma and periocular xanthogranulomas in a patient with lymphoplasmacytic sclerosing pancreatitis. Pancreas 2007;34:157–60.

24. Guo J, Wang J. Adult orbital xanthogranulomatous disease: review of the literature. Arch Pathol Lab Med 2009;133:1994–7.

25. Kraus MD, Haley JC, Ruiz R, et al. "Juvenile" xanthogranuloma: an immunophenotypic study with a reappraisal of histogenesis. Am J Dermatopathol 2001;23:104–11.

26. Cavallazzi R, Hirani A, Vasu TS, et al. Clinical manifestations and treatment of adult-onset asthma and periocular xanthogranuloma. Can Respir J 2009; 16(5):159–62.

27. Elner VM, Mintz R, Demirci H, et al. Local corticosteroid treatment of eyelid and orbital xanthogranuloma. Trans Am Ophthalmol Soc 2005;103:69–74 [discussion: 73–4].

28. Elner VM, Mintz R, Demirci H, et al. Local corticosteroid treatment of eyelid and orbital xanthogranuloma. Ophthal Plast Reconstr Surg 2006;22:36–40.

29. Zoumalan CI, Erb MH, Rao NA, et al. Periorbital xanthgranuloma after blephoroplasty. Br J Ophthalmol 2007;91:1088–9.

30. Nasr AM, Johnson T, Hidayat A, et al. Adult onset primary bilateral orbital xanthogranuloma: clinical. Diagnostic, and histopathologic correlations. Orbit 1991;10:13–22.

31. Ebrahimi KB, Miller NR, Sassani JW, et al. Failure of radiation therapy in orbital xanthogranuloma. Ophthal Plast Reconstr Surg 2010;26(4):259–64.

32. Krause D, Schleusser B, Herborn G, et al. Response to methotrexate treatment is associated with reduced mortality in patients with severe rheumatoid arthritis. Arthritis Rheum 2000;43:14–21.

33. Hayden A, Wilson DJ, Rosenbaum JT. Management of orbital xanthogranuloma with methotrexate. Br J Ophthalmol 2007;91:434–6.

34. Myra C, Sloper L, Tighe PJ. Treatment of Erdheim-Chester disease with cladribine: a rational approach. Br J Ophthalmol 2004;88:844–7.

Adult Xanthogranuloma, Reticulohistiocytosis, and Rosai-Dorfman Disease

Sarah S. Chisolm, MD[a], Joshua M. Schulman, MD[a,b],
Lindy P. Fox, MD[a,*]

KEYWORDS

- Xanthogranuloma • Histiocytosis • Reticulohistiocytosis • Self-healing reticulohistiocytosis
- Multicentric reticulohistiocytosis • Rosai-Dorfman disease

KEY POINTS

- In cases of adult xanthogranuloma, workup for lymphoproliferative disorders should be considered, but in general, treatment should be fairly conservative.
- Patients with solitary and multicentric reticulohistiocytosis should receive at minimum age-appropriate screening and thorough history and physical examination with aggressive pursuit of focal findings; the multicentric form is typically treated early and aggressively.
- Although the classic presentation of Rosai-Dorfman disease is cervical lymphadenopathy, many atypical cases are reported. Treatment must be tailored to the specific disease course.

ADULT XANTHOGRANULOMA
Overview

Adult xanthogranuloma is a disease in which lesions are indistinguishable clinically and histopathologically from the lesions of juvenile xanthogranuloma, tan to orange firm nodules (**Fig. 1**). The natural history of adult xanthogranulomas, however, may be quite different from that of xanthogranulomas in younger patients (see section titled Clinical Presentation below). Histopathologically, early xanthogranulomas consist of large collections of banal-appearing histiocytes in the dermis, sometimes extending into the subcutaneous fat and even the fascia.[1] Later, lesions may show foamy histiocytes, spindled mononuclear cells, Touton giant cells (classically), and also foreign body giant cells, with some eosinophils and lymphocytes also being present.[1] This process is characterized by non-Langerhans cell histiocytes (CD68[+], CD1a[−], usually S100[−], and factor XIIIa variable but often positive).[1]

Adult xanthogranuloma strictly defined is considered to be a separate form of histiocytosis that should be distinguished from necrobiotic xanthogranuloma and xanthoma disseminatum (XD).

Etiopathogenesis

The etiopathogenesis of adult xanthogranuloma is poorly understood. Various investigators have posited a role for physical trauma, infection, and malignancy (particularly bloodline tumors) in causing the disease.[2,3]

Clinical Presentation

Adult xanthogranuloma presents most commonly as a solitary lesion without systemic manifestations.[4,5] However, extracutaneous manifestations have been rarely reported (see section on Systemic Associations below). It is difficult to know for certain what the natural course of the disease is because many solitary lesions are excised for

No authors have relevant disclosures.
[a] Department of Dermatology, UCSF, 1701 Divisadero Street, San Francisco, CA 94115, USA; [b] Department of Pathology, UCSF, 1701 Divisadero Street, San Francisco, CA 94115, USA
* Corresponding author.
E-mail address: FoxLi@derm.ucsf.edu

Dermatol Clin 33 (2015) 465–473
http://dx.doi.org/10.1016/j.det.2015.03.011

derm.theclinics.com

Fig. 1. Xanthogranuloma. Orange to red-tan firm nodule.

cosmetic reasons, but in adults with multiple lesions, spontaneous resolution has been noted in about half of the patients.[4] Cases that present with many lesions are perhaps more concerning for association with lymphoproliferative disease; this is discussed further below.

Systemic Associations

Adult xanthogranuloma is primarily a disease of the skin without systemic manifestations. Associations with trauma (because of a few cases in which lesions arose shortly postoperatively), infection, and malignancy have been postulated, but with little to no understanding of a causal mechanism other than perhaps an inflammatory milieu leading to activation of the histiocytes.[1]

Recently, multiple cases of adult xanthogranuloma have been reported in association with lymphoproliferative disorders, including essential thrombocytosis, chronic lymphocytic leukemia, large B cell lymphoma, and monoclonal gammopathy.[3,6–8] In all these cases, the presentation was described as multiple xanthogranulomas, disseminated xanthogranulomas, or eruptive xanthogranulomas. In other reports, multiple xanthogranulomas have been described as possibly being associated with a benign course.[4,5] Although it is not yet entirely clear whether a more acute and widespread presentation is more worrisome for lymphoproliferative disease or whether there is simply variation in terminology, these reports do suggest that an underlying lymphoproliferative disease be considered in patients with eruptive or multiple lesions.

Extracutaneous manifestations of the disease itself, including cervical spine, intracardiac, and periocular lesion location (with the last being possibly associated with adult-onset asthma), have been rarely reported.[9–14] Although rare, when periocular xanthogranulomas are associated with adult-onset asthma, they are more likely to be associated with lymphadenopathy and/or lymphoproliferative disease.[15]

Evaluation and Management

As the differential diagnosis for adult xanthogranuloma is large, all patients with this suspected diagnosis should receive a thorough history including full review of systems, a full physical examination, and skin biopsy. Eruptive xanthogranulomas in an adult should prompt workup for lymphoproliferative disorder. Periocular xanthogranulomas require an ophthalmologic evaluation in addition to evaluation for asthma, lymphadenopathy, and lymphoproliferative disease. Other workup can likely be pursued as indicated based on any focal examination findings or symptoms.

Periorbital lesions should be followed up and treated locally (eg, topical corticosteroid or surgery) if appropriate, because they may have ophthalmologic complications.[12] Otherwise, use of chemotherapeutic agents, radiation, systemic corticosteroid, and cyclosporine have been reported, but data on efficacy are minimal.[2] As many cases may be indolent and/or self-resolving, management should not be overly aggressive such that harm outweighs benefit.

RETICULOHISTIOCYTOSIS
Overview

For the purposes of this article, the definition of reticulohistiocytosis is limited to 2 specific disease manifestations, solitary reticulohistiocytosis or giant cell reticulohistiocytosis (also known as reticulohistiocytoma), and multicentric reticulohistiocytosis. Both these diseases are non-Langerhans histiocytoses limited primarily to adults; this excludes congenital self-healing reticulohistiocytosis (Hashimoto-Pritzker disease), which is a congenital Langerhans-cell-type histiocytosis.

The histopathologies of solitary reticulohistiocytosis and multicentric reticulohistiocytosis are identical: a dermal collection of lymphocytes and histiocytes as well as scattered plasma cells and eosinophils. Histiocytes characteristically demonstrate a ground glass appearance, that is, copious eosinophilic granular cytoplasm.

Etiopathogenesis

The etiopathogenesis of reticulohistiocytoses, both solitary and multicentric, is not well understood. Associations with other systemic processes is more common in multicentric reticulohistiocytosis and includes autoimmune disease, malignancy, and trauma. Whether these associated conditions are pathophysiologically related to the development of reticulohistiocytomas or are a nonspecific reactive phenomenon is not known.

Clinical Presentation

Solitary reticulohistiocytoma is sometimes said to be a disease of young adults, although the age of onset in one of the larger case series ranged from 2.5 to 74 years.[16] Lesions are classically raised, fairly well-circumscribed, red or yellow-red dermal nodules, ranging from a few millimeters to about 2 cm.[17] Lesions may also be pink, brown, or gray.[17]

Multicentric reticulohistiocytosis is primarily a disease of middle-aged white women, with mean age of diagnosis of 40 to 50 years,[17–21] although some investigators question whether the disease may be overreported in this group and underreported in others.[22]

Multicentric reticulohistiocytosis is characterized by widespread papulonodular skin lesions, with a predilection for the hands and elbows, and a characteristic coral bead appearance of periungual lesions (**Figs. 2** and **3**). This condition is often associated with a symmetric erosive arthritis, particularly of the hands and wrists, and may have other systemic manifestations.

Joint symptoms occur first in nearly 40% of cases, sometimes accompanied by fever, fatigue, and weight loss.[17,23,24] Skin symptoms occur first in 30% of cases, and joint and skin symptoms occur simultaneously in the remaining 30% of cases.[17] Dysphagia may also rarely be a presenting symptom because of esophageal involvement.[25]

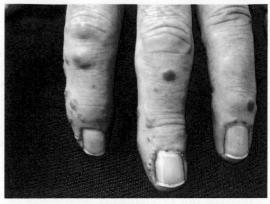

Fig. 3. Multicentric reticulohistiocytosis. Note predilection for periungual accentuation (coral bead sign). (*Courtesy of* Jeffrey P. Callen, MD, Louisville, KY.)

In one review, hands were most commonly affected by nodules, with the face, arms, trunk, legs, ears, mucosa, and neck also being affected.[17] The classic coral beads sign was present in 27%, palpebral xanthelasmas were present in 17%, and lesions described as vermicular, at the edge of nares, were present in 15%.[17] The course is often relapsing and remitting, with some cases resolving after around 7 years, and 11% to 45% of cases progressing to severe debilitating arthritis.[26]

Other associated signs and symptoms include weight loss (15%), anorexia (4%), dysphagia (3%), pruritus (10%), weakness (10%), cardiac symptoms (9%), myalgia (6%), fever (5%), malaise (5%), and lymphadenopathy (3%).[17]

Systemic Associations

Multicentric reticulohistiocytosis has been reported with a wide array of systemic diseases (**Table 1**). These diseases include disorders classically defined as autoimmune (primary biliary cirrhosis, systemic sclerosis, systemic lupus erythematosus, dermatomyositis, and Sjögren disease), as well as diabetes, celiac disease, hyperlipidemia, systemic vasculitis, and thyroid disease.[27,28] This condition has also been associated with many solid organ and lymphoproliferative malignancies, with no particular type of malignancy overrepresented.[22] The efficacy of control of multicentric reticulohistiocytosis via successful treatment of the underlying malignancy is a subject of debate. Finally, multicentric reticulohistiocytosis has been associated with pregnancy, along with a possible increased risk of preeclampsia.[29–31]

Solitary reticulohistiocytoma is generally thought to have few systemic manifestations or associations, although it has also been reported during pregnancy.[32]

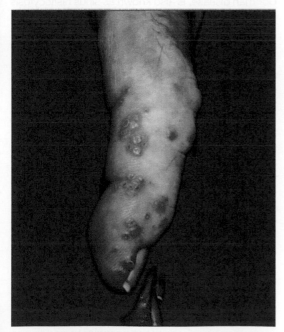

Fig. 2. Multicentric reticulohistiocytosis. Red to yellow-red dermal papules and nodules with a predilection for the hands and elbows. (*Courtesy of* Jeffrey P. Callen, MD, Louisville, KY.)

Table 1
Systemic conditions associated with multicentric reticulohistiocytosis

Autoimmune diseases	Primary biliary cirrhosis, systemic sclerosis, systemic lupus erythematosus, dermatomyositis, Sjögren disease
Malignancy	Breast, ovarian, cervical, endometrial, and penile cancers; pleural mesothelioma; sarcoma; lymphoma; leukemia; melanoma; and stomach, colon, and pancreatic cancers (no particular type overrepresented)
Pregnancy	Possible increased risk of preeclampsia
Other	Diabetes mellitus, celiac disease, hyperlipidemia, systemic vasculitis, thyroid disease

Adapted from Refs.[22,27–31]

Evaluation and Management

Although solitary reticulohistiocytomas may self-resolve, they are often treated surgically with excision, which typically is curative. There are no consensus guidelines for workup, but it is important to ensure that age-appropriate malignancy screening has been done, as well as a thorough history, review of systems, and physical examination with further exploration of any focal findings.

In multicentric reticulohistiocytosis, on the other hand, the workup is necessarily broad because of the frequency and wide range of associated systemic diseases. A thorough history and physical examination including complete skin and joint examination should be performed. One should consider radiographs of the hands, even in asymptomatic patients. Radiographs reveal erosive joint lesions, typically without osteoporosis, osteopenia, or periosteal new bone formation.[33,34] Referral to otolaryngology and/or gastroenterology to evaluate for mucosal involvement may be indicated. There are no serologic laboratory findings specific to the disease, but an elevated erythrocyte sedimentation rate (ESR) (about 50% of cases),[33] anemia, and hypercholesterolemia may be found. Tests for cold agglutinins and cryoglobulins may also occasionally yield positive results.[33] Very rarely, tests for rheumatoid factor and cyclic citrullinated peptide may yield positive result, which is important mainly because it may cause confusion between this condition and rheumatoid arthritis.[35]

No established guidelines exist for treatment of multicentric reticulohistiocytosis, although the consensus argues for early and aggressive treatment to prevent debilitating joint involvement.[33] Many consider nonsteroidal antiinflammatory drugs and corticosteroids (systemic or intralesional) to be the mainstays of treatment. According to a recent review article, treatments have included hydroxychloroquine, methotrexate, leflunomide, mycophenolate mofetil, azathioprine, cyclophosphamide, cyclosporine, chlorambucil, and dapsone.[22] According to the same review,

there is a current movement toward treatment with tumor necrosis factor-α (TNF-α) inhibitors (etanercept, infliximab, and adalimumab). Failure to respond to one TNF-α inhibitor does not predict failure to respond to another TNF-α inhibitor.[22,36] Another promising area of treatment is with bisphosphonates to mitigate bone destruction, because some studies have shown that inhibiting osteoclast formation and thus bone resorption may be helpful.[22,37,38] Often, combination treatments are used, but the risk of the underlying malignancy must be taken into advisement.

ROSAI-DORFMAN DISEASE
Overview

Rosai-Dorfman disease, or Destombes-Rosai-Dorfman disease, is also known as sinus histiocytosis with massive lymphadenopathy. The eponym is preferred, because several cases have been documented that are histopathologically classic for the disease but with extranodal clinical presentations and sometimes without lymphadenopathy. The clinical course is varied: in isolation, it can be self-limited and fairly benign, but it can also be persistent and cyclic.

The classic histopathologic findings involve lymph nodes with sinuses infiltrated by inflammatory cells, lymphocytes, plasma cells, and histiocytes.[39] These enlarged lymph node sinuses form the basis for the name sinus histiocytosis, although, somewhat confusingly, the disease can also have prominent nasal sinus involvement. Cutaneous lesions are also characterized by nodular inflammatory infiltrates containing many S100-positive histiocytes. Some histiocytes in Rosai-Dorfman disease exhibit emperipolesis, or uptake of entire, intact inflammatory cells within their cytoplasm, although this finding is neither pathognomonic for the disease nor necessary for diagnosis.

Etiopathogenesis

The etiopathogenesis of Rosai-Dorfman disease is unknown. Many suspect a viral cause, but this has not been shown conclusively. Involved lymphoid tissue has tested negative for the presence of human herpesvirus 8 (HHV-8), and although evidence of HHV-6 in involved tissue has been seen, it is unclear whether this is pathologic because HHV-6 has also been found coincidentally in nondiseased lymphoid tissue.[40]

Mutations in SLC29A3, the gene that encodes the equilibrative nucleoside transporter hENT3, have been found in 2 families with familial Rosai-Dorfman disease.[41] In addition, mutations in SLC29A3 have been described in both Faisalabad histiocytosis, an autosomal recessive histiocytosis with similarities to Rosai-Dorfman disease[41] and H syndrome, a genodermatosis that manifests with lymphadenopathy that mimics Rosai-Dorfman disease, insulin-dependent diabetes mellitus, hyperpigmentation, hearing loss, short stature, and flexion contractures of the fingers and toes.[42] How these diseases are related to classic Rosai-Dorfman disease discussed herein is still to be determined.

Clinical Presentation

The classic presentation is extensive, painless, bilateral cervical lymphadenopathy, but some cases have been entirely extranodal. Fever, elevated ESR, leukocytosis, anemia, and hypergammaglobulinemia are often seen.[43] Extranodal sites of involvement may include kidney, adrenal gland, and testes,[44] as well as bone, and rarely intracranial or meningeal lesions.[45–48] The condition has also been reported to involve upper airway and orbital/periorbital sites.[49] Some disagreement exists in the literature as to the average age of onset, but most commonly it is referred to as a disease of young adults. Cutaneous lesions, when present, are classically red to red-brown papules or nodules, although macules or plaques may also occur (**Figs. 4 and 5**).

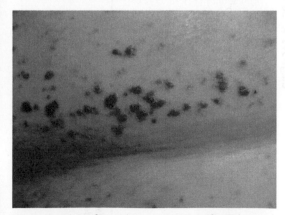

Fig. 4. Rosai-Dorfman disease. Nonspecific red to red-brown papules. (*Courtesy of* Kristen Losicco, MD, Arthur Huen, MD, Jonhan Ho, MD, Pittsburgh, PA.)

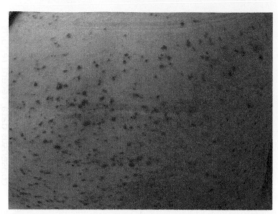

Fig. 5. Rosai-Dorfman disease. Nonspecific red to red-brown papules. (*Courtesy of* Kristen Losicco, Arthur Huen, Jonhan Ho, Pittsburgh, PA.)

Systemic Associations

Rosai-Dorfman disease has been recently linked with Crohn disease in a case series.[50] Other reported associations include bloodline malignancies.[44] Finally, histologic changes compatible with Rosai-Dortman disease have been found in children with autoimmune lymphoproliferative syndrome, an inherited disorder associated with defects in Fas-mediated apoptosis[51] as well as the genetic syndromes mentioned above.

Evaluation and Management

There is no recognized protocol for evaluation and management of Rosai-Dorfman disease, given the extreme rarity of the disease. However, a reasonable approach might include the following: thorough history and physical examination, complete blood cell count with differential (because anemia is a common finding and the disease has also been associated with bloodline malignancies), ESR, and imaging including computed tomography, MRI, ultrasonography, and/or radionuclide bone scan, as well as biopsy of any amenable lesions to confirm tissue diagnosis.[52]

Treatment plan may vary widely depending on the disease course. As many as half of the patients may have spontaneous resolution, making aggressive therapy undesirable.[43] Surgical intervention may be necessary if the airway or other vital structures are threatened.[53,54] Corticosteroids have been helpful in some cases, but benefit wanes after cessation of treatment.[52] Other modalities including radiotherapy, chemotherapy, and interferon are of unclear benefit.[55,56] Methotrexate alone or in combination with other therapies has been helpful in some cases.[57]

SUMMARY

Table 2

Table 2
Summary: adult xanthogranuloma, reticulohistiocytosis, and Rosai-Dorfman disease

	Epidemiology	Common Associations	Prognosis	Treatment
Adult xanthogranuloma[a]	No specific overrepresented subgroups	(Possibly) trauma, infection, malignancy.[1] Lymphoproliferative disorders[3,6–8]	Spontaneous resolution in about half of the patients with multiple lesions[4]	Periorbital lesions should be followed up, treated locally (eg, intralesional steroid or surgery) if appropriate; may have ophthalmologic complications.[12] Systemic agents reported, minimal data on efficacy[2]
Multicentric reticulohistiocytoma[a]	Middle-aged white females; mean age of diagnosis 40–50 y[17–21]	Autoimmune disease, diabetes, celiac disease, hyperlipidemia, systemic vasculitis, thyroid disease, lymphoproliferative disorders, pregnancy (see table 1)[22,27–31]	Relapsing and remitting—some cases resolve after about 7 y; 11%–45% progress to severe arthritis[26]	Many agents reported with no consensus data; recent reports on use of anti-TNF agents,[22,36] bisphosphonates[22,37,38]
Rosai-Dorfman disease[a]	Young age group[39]	Crohn disease, lymphoproliferative disorders (particularly non-Hodgkin lymphoma), and autoimmune lymphoproliferative syndrome[44,50,51]	Varied: self-limited in some, persistent in others	Aggressive therapy undesirable, because up to half may have spontaneous resolution. Surgical intervention if vital structures threatened.[53,54] Methotrexate may be helpful[57]; corticosteroid helpful but only while treatment continued[52]

Abbreviation: TNF, tumor necrosis factor.
[a] Evidence level D: case series or case reports.

REFERENCES

1. Asarch A, Thiele JJ, Ashby-Richardson H, et al. Cutaneous disseminated xanthogranuloma in an adult: case report and review of the literature. Cutis 2009;83:243–9.
2. Hernandez-Martin A, Baselga E, Drolet BA, et al. Juvenile xanthogranuloma. J Am Acad Dermatol 1997; 36:355–69.
3. Chiou CC, Wang PN, Yang LC, et al. Disseminated xanthogranulomas associated with adult T-cell leukaemia/lymphoma: a case report and review the association of haematologic malignancies. J Eur Acad Dermatol Venereol 2007;21:532–5.
4. Saad N, Skowron F, Dalle S, et al. Multiple adult xanthogranuloma: case report and literature review. Dermatology 2006;212:73–6.
5. Whitmore SE. Multiple xanthogranulomas in an adult: case report and literature review. Br J Dermatol 1992;127:177–81.
6. Shoo BA, Shinkai K, McCalmont TH, et al. Xanthogranulomas associated with hematologic malignancy in adulthood. J Am Acad Dermatol 2008;59:488–93.
7. Larson MJ, Bandel C, Eichhorn PJ, et al. Concurrent development of eruptive xanthogranulomas and hematologic malignancy: two case reports. J Am Acad Dermatol 2004;50:976–8.
8. Pino GM, Miquel FJ, Velasco M, et al. Multiple xanthogranulomas in an adult, associated with essential thrombocytosis. Br J Dermatol 1995;132:1018–21.
9. Inoue H, Seichi A, Yamamuro K, et al. Dumbbell-type juvenile xanthogranuloma in the cervical spine of an adult. Eur Spine J 2011;20(Suppl 2):S343–7.
10. Moreau E, Lefrancq T, Saint-Martin P. Incidental bilateral xanthogranuloma of the lateral ventricles at autopsy–a case report. J Forensic Leg Med 2013;20:647.
11. Lee SJ, Jo DJ, Lee SH, et al. Solitary xanthogranuloma of the upper cervical spine in a male adult. J Korean Neurosurg Soc 2012;51:54–8.
12. Minami-Hori M, Takahashi I, Honma M, et al. Adult orbital xanthogranulomatous disease: adult-onset xanthogranuloma of periorbital location. Am J Surg Pathol 2006;30:521–8.
13. Lehrke HD, Johnson CK, Zapolanski A, et al. Intracardiac juvenile xanthogranuloma with presentation in adulthood. Cardiovasc Pathol 2014;23:54–6.
14. Adam Z, Veselý K, Motyčková I, et al. Eyelids with yellow granulomas and cough - periocular xanthogranuloma associated with adult-onset asthma. A case study and an overview of clinical forms of juvenile xanthogranuloma and its therapy. Vnitr Lek 2012;58:365–77 [in Czech].
15. Sivak-Callcott JA, Rootman J, Rasmussen SL, et al. Adult xanthogranulomatous disease of the orbit and ocular adnexa: new immunohistochemical findings and clinical review. Br J Ophthalmol 2006;90:602–8.
16. Miettinen M, Fetsch JF. Reticulohistiocytoma (solitary epithelioid histiocytoma): a clinicopathologic and immunohistochemical study of 44 cases. Am J Surg Pathol 2006;30:521–8.
17. Luz FB, Gaspar TA, Kalil-Gaspar N, et al. Multicentric reticulohistiocytosis. J Eur Acad Dermatol Venereol 2001;15:524–31.
18. Tajirian AL, Malik MK, Robinson-Bostom L, et al. Multicentric reticulohistiocytosis. Clin Dermatol 2006;24: 486–92.
19. Goltz RW, Laymon CW. Multicentric reticulohistiocytosis of the skin and synovia; reticulohistiocytoma or ganglioneuroma. AMA Arch Derm Syphilol 1954;69: 717–31.
20. Lesher JL Jr, Allen BS. Multicentric reticulohistiocytosis. J Am Acad Dermatol 1984;11(4 Pt 2):713–23.
21. Rapini RP. Multicentric reticulohistiocytosis. Clin Dermatol 1993;11:107–11.
22. Islam AD, Naguwa SM, Cheema GS, et al. Multicentric reticulohistiocytosis: a rare yet challenging disease. Clin Rev Allergy Immunol 2013;45:281–9.
23. Outland JD, Keiran SJ, Schikler KN, et al. Multicentric reticulohistiocytosis in a 14-year-old girl. Pediatr Dermatol 2002;19:527–31.
24. Levine D, Miller S, Al-Dawsari N, et al. Paraneoplastic dermatoses associated with gynecologic and breast malignancies. Obstet Gynecol Surv 2010;65:455–61.
25. Zeale PJ, Miner D, Honig S, et al. Multicentric reticulohistiocytosis: a cause of dysphagia with response to corticosteroids. Arthritis Rheum 1985;28:231–4.
26. Barrow MV, Holubar K. Multicentric reticulohistiocytosis – a review of 33 Patients. Medicine 1969;48: 287–305.
27. Shiokawa S, Shingu M, Nishimura M, et al. Multicentric reticulohistiocytosis associated with subclinical Sjogren's syndrome. Clin Rheumatol 1991;10:201–5.
28. Ben Abdelghani K, Mahmoud I, Chatelus E, et al. Multicentric reticulohistiocytosis: an autoimmune systemic disease? Case report of an association with erosive rheumatoid arthritis and systemic Sjogren syndrome. Joint Bone Spine 2010;77:274–6.
29. Brackenridge A, Bashir T, Wheatley T. Multicentric reticulohistiocytosis and pregnancy. BJOG 2005; 112:672–3.
30. Tsubamoto H, Horinosono H, Horie M. Multicentric reticulohistiocytosis in a patient with severe preeclampsia. Arch Gynecol Obstet 2000;264:35–6.
31. Conaghan P, Miller M, Dowling JP, et al. A unique presentation of multicentric reticulohistiocytosis in pregnancy. Arthritis Rheum 1993;36:269–72.
32. Hunt SJ, Shin SS. Solitary reticulohistiocytoma in pregnancy: immunohistochemical and ultrastructural study of a case with unusual immunophenotype. J Cutan Pathol 1995;22:177–81.
33. Trotta F, Castellino G, Lo MA. Multicentric reticulohistiocytosis. Best Pract Res Clin Rheumatol 2004;18: 759–72.

34. Uhl M, Gutfleisch J, Rother E, et al. Multicentric reticulohistiocytosis. A report of 3 cases and review of literature. Bildgebung 1996;63:126–9.

35. Chauhan A, Mikulik Z, Hackshaw KV. Multicentric reticulohistiocytosis with positive anticyclic citrullinated antibodies. J Natl Med Assoc 2007;99:678–80.

36. Kalajian AH, Callen JP. Multicentric reticulohistiocytosis successfully treated with infliximab: an illustrative case and evaluation of cytokine expression supporting anti-tumor necrosis factor therapy. Arch Dermatol 2009;144:1360–6.

37. Adamopoulos IE, Wordsworth PB, Edwards JR, et al. Osteoclast differentiation and bone resorption in multicentric reticulohistiocytosis. Hum Pathol 2006; 37:1176–85.

38. Goto H, Inaba M, Kobayashi K, et al. Successful treatment of multicentric reticulohistiocytosis with alendronate: evidence for a direct effect of bisphosphonate on histiocytes. Arthritis Rheum 2003; 48:3538–41.

39. Warpe BM, More SV. Rosai-Dorfman disease: a rare clinico-pathological presentation. Australas Med J 2014;7:68–72.

40. Ortonne N, Fillet AM, Kosuge H, et al. Cutaneous Destombes-Rosai-Dorfman disease: absence of detection of HHV-6 and HHV-8 in skin. J Cutan Pathol 2002;29:113–8.

41. Morgan NV, Morris MR, Cangul H, et al. Mutations in SLC29A3, encoding an equilibrative nucleoside transporter ENT3, cause a familial histiocytosis syndrome (Faisalabad histiocytosis) and familial Rosai-Dorfman disease. PLoS Genet 2010;6:e1000833.

42. Molho-Pessach V, Ramot Y, Camille F, et al. H syndrome: the first 79 patients. J Am Acad Dermatol 2014;70:80–8.

43. Rosai J, Dorfman RF. Sinus histiocytosis with massive lymphadenopathy. A newly recognized benign clinicopathological entity. Arch Pathol 1969; 87:63–70.

44. Del Gobbo A, Moltrasio F, Young RH, et al. Involvement of the testis and related structures by Rosai-Dorfman disease: report of 2 new cases and review of the literature. Am J Surg Pathol 2013;37:1871–5.

45. Hashimoto K, Kariya S, Onoda T, et al. Rosai-Dorfman disease with extranodal involvement. Laryngoscope 2014;124:701–4.

46. Forest F, N'guyen AT, Fesselet J, et al. Meningeal Rosai-Dorfman disease mimicking meningioma. Ann Hematol 2014;93:937–40.

47. Molina-Carrión LE, Mendoza-Álvarez SA, Vera-Lastra OL, et al. Enfermedad de Rosai-Dorfman y lesiones espinales y craneales Informe de un caso clínico. Rev Med Inst Mex Seguro Soc 2014;52:218–23.

48. El Molla M, Mahasneh T, Holmes SE, et al. Rare presentation of Rosai-Dorfman disease mimicking a cervical intramedullary spinal cord tumor. World Neurosurg 2014;81:442.e7–9.

49. Kutlubay Z, Bairamov O, Sevim A, et al. Rosai-Dorfman disease: a case report with nodal and cutaneous involvement and review of the literature. Am J Dermatopathol 2014;36:353–7.

50. Salva KA, Stenstrom M, Breadon JY, et al. Possible association of cutaneous Rosai-Dorfman disease and chronic Crohn disease: a case series report. JAMA Dermatol 2014;150:177–81.

51. Maric I, Pittaluga S, Dale JK, et al. Histologic features of sinus histiocytosis with massive lymphadenopathy in patients with autoimmune lymphoproliferative syndrome. Am J Surg Pathol 2005;29:903–11.

52. Lai KL, Abdullah V, Ng KS, et al. Rosai-Dorfman disease: presentation, diagnosis, and treatment. Head Neck 2013;35:E85–8.

53. Ku PK, Tong MC, Leung CY, et al. Nasal manifestation of extranodal Rosai–Dorfman disease—diagnosis and management. J Laryngol Otol 1999;113:275–80.

54. Aluffi P, Prestinari A, Ramponi A, et al. Rosai–Dorfman disease of the larynx. J Laryngol Otol 2000;114:565–7.

55. Bernácer–Borja M, Blanco–Rodríguez M, Sanchez–Granados JM, et al. Sinus histiocytosis with massive lymphadenopathy (Rosai–Dorfman disease): clinico-pathological study of three cases. Eur J Pediatr 2006;165:536–9.

56. Komp DM. The treatment of sinus histiocytosis with massive lymphadenopathy (Rosai–Dorfman disease). Semin Diagn Pathol 1990;7:83–6.

57. Nasseri E, Belisle A, Funaro D. Rosai-Dorfman disease treated with methotrexate and low-dose prednisone: case report and review of the literature. J Cutan Med Surg 2012;16:281–5.

EDITOR'S ADDENDUM

XD is a rare non-Langerhans cell histiocytosis disorder of unknown cause. XD has been reported to have variable clinical presentations (self-healing, persistent, progressive) in young adults (with males being affected more than females). XD skin lesions present as reddish brown to yellow confluent papulonodular lesions that prefer the axilla, inguinal creases, buttock, as well as antecubital and popliteal fossa. Histologically, dense histiocytic infiltrates that are CD68+, S100−, and CD1a^s occur early with scalloped magrophages followed by the later development of Touton and multinucleated giant cells. Cutaneous lesions are benign in nature; however, in the more progressive variants, organ infiltration may occur causing significant systemic disease. Ocular disease can lead to blindness, and central nervous system lesions lead most commonly to diabetes insipidus; however, epilepsy and hydrocephalus can develop. Laryngeal lesions can cause dysphagia, dysphonia, and airway obstruction. Additionally, osteolytic bone lesions, plasma cell dyscrasia/monoclonal gammopathy, and hyperlipidemia have been described. Progressive disease requires therapeutic intervention with systemic steroids, immunosuppressants (cyclophosphamide, cyclosporine, azathioprine), statins, and vasopressin (if diabetes insipidus is present).

Atti AM, Bakry OA, Mohamed EE. Xanthoma disseminatum: a progressive case with multisystem involvement. J Postgrad Med 2014;60:69–71.

James WD, Berger TG, Elston DM. Andrews' diseases of the skin: clinical dermatology. 11th edition. Elsevier; 2011. p. 711.

Park M, Boone B, Devos S. Xanthoma disseminatum: case report and mini-review of the literature. Acta Dermatovenerol Croat 2014;22:150–4.

Seaton ED, Pillai GJ, Chu AC. Treatment of xanthoma disseminatum with cyclophosphamide. Br J Dermatol 2004;150:346–9.

Zinoun M, Hali F, Marnissi F, et al. Xanthoma disseminatum with asymptomatic multisystem involvement. Ann Dermatol Venereol 2015;142:276–80.

EDITOR'S ADDENDUM

XD is a rare non-Langerhans cell histiocytosis disorder of unknown cause. XD has been reported to have variable clinical presentations (self-healing, persistent, progressive) in young adults (with males being affected more than females). XD skin lesions present as reddish brown to yellow confluent papulonodular lesions that enter the axilla, inguinal creases, buttock, as well as antecubital and popliteal fossa. Histologically, dense histiocytic infiltrates that are CD68+, S100- and CD1a- occur early with scalloped macrophages followed by the later development of Touton and multinucleated giant cells. Cutaneous lesions are benign in nature, however, in the more progressive variants, organ infiltration may occur causing significant systemic disease. Ocular disease can lead to blindness, and central nervous system lesions lead most commonly to diabetes insipidus, however, epilepsy and hydrocephalus can develop. Laryngeal lesions can cause dysphagia, dysphonia, and airway obstruction. Additionally, osteolytic bone lesions, elevated cell dyscrasia/monoclonal gammopathy, and hyperlipidemia have been described. Prognosis for disease requires therapeutic intervention with systemic steroids, immunosuppressants (cyclophosphamide, cyclosporine, azathioprine), statins, and vasopressin (if diabetes insipidus is present).

Attia AM, Bakry OA, Mohamed EE. Xanthoma disseminatum: a progressive case with multisystem involvement. J Postgrad Med 2014;60:69-71.

James WD, Berger TG, Elston DM. Andrews' diseases of the skin: clinical dermatology. 11th edition. Elsevier; 2011. p. 711.

Park M, Boone B, Devos S. Xanthoma disseminatum: case report and mini-review of the literature. Acta Dermatovenereol Croat 2014;22:150-4.

Seaton ED, Pillai GJ, Chu AC. Treatment of xanthoma disseminatum with cyclophosphamide. Br J Dermatol 2004;150:346-9.

Zhou H, Hua P, Mennai F, et al. Xanthoma disseminatum with asymptomatic multisystem involvement. Ann Dermatol Venereol 2015;142:276-80.

Granulomatous Vasculitis

Aman Sharma, MD, MAMS, FICP, FACR, FRCP(London)[a],*,
Sunil Dogra, MD, MAMS, FRCP(London)[b], Kusum Sharma, MD, MAMS[c]

KEYWORDS

- Granulomatosis with polyangiitis • Eosinophilic granulomatosis with polyangiitis
- Microscopic polyangiitis • Polyarteritis nodosa • Cutaneous polyarteritis nodosa

KEY POINTS

- Systemic vasculitides are a group of disorders characterized by inflammation of the blood vessels.
- Granulomatosis with polyangiitis (GPA) is characterized by granulomatous inflammation of upper and lower airways, and by vasculitis of small and medium vessels, of which glomerulonephritis is common.
- Glomerulonephritis and lung hemorrhage are common manifestations of microscopic polyangiitis (MPA).
- The common presentations of polyarteritis nodosa (PAN) are in form of constitutional symptoms, with gastrointestinal (GI), nervous system, and cardiac involvement.
- Treatment is in form of immunosuppression and depends on the type of clinical presentation.

INTRODUCTION

Vasculitic disorders are characterized by inflammation of the blood vessels, which can either result in ischemia/infarction due to partial or total occlusion of the involved blood vessels, or cause hemorrhage due to the rupture of weakened vessel wall. The clinical manifestations depend on the size, type, and site of the blood vessels involved. These disorders may be primary, which in most cases are idiopathic, or secondary to other causes such as infections, connective tissue diseases, drugs, or hypersensitive disorders.

NOMENCLATURE AND CLASSIFICATION SYSTEM OF VASCULITIS

There have been various classification and nomenclature systems of vasculitis. Although it was Kussumaul and Maier who gave the first detailed clinical and pathologic report of systemic arteritis involving the medium and small vessels in 1866, it was Parla Zeek who made the first attempt to classify vasculitis, when she described 5 distinct vasculitides from the literature review.[1] In 1990, criteria for 7 types of systemic vasculitis were published by the American College of Rheumatology (ACR). These criteria were based on patient data from 48 centers, and the basis of diagnosis of each type was expert opinion.[2–8] These criteria had their limitations in the form of failure to include/identify MPA as a separate entity, lack of application of antinuclear cytoplasmic antibodies (ANCA), and the use of physician opinion as diagnostic gold standard.[9] The most widely cited nomenclature system is the Chapel Hill Consensus Conference (CHCC) system, which proposed the names and definitions of common systemic vasculitides in 1994.[10] This

Conflict of interest: None.
Disclosures: None.
[a] Rheumatology Division, Department of Internal Medicine, Postgraduate Institute of Medical Education and Research, Chandigarh 160012, India; [b] Department of Dermatology, Venereology and Leperology, Postgraduate Institute of Medical Education and Research, Chandigarh 160012, India; [c] Department of Medical Microbiology, Postgraduate Institute of Medical Education and Research, Chandigarh 160012, India
* Corresponding author.
E-mail address: amansharma74@yahoo.com

Dermatol Clin 33 (2015) 475–487
http://dx.doi.org/10.1016/j.det.2015.03.012
0733-8635/15/$ – see front matter © 2015 Elsevier Inc. All rights reserved.

nomenclature system was revised in 2012.[11] Among the changes that have been incorporated in the revised nomenclature include division of small-vessel vasculitis into categories of ANCA-associated vasculitis (AAV) and immune complex vasculitis, replacing Wegener granulomatosis with GPA, and replacing Churg-Strauss syndrome with eosinophilic granulomatosis with polyangiitis (EGPA). There have been attempts to classify the vasculitides based on their histopathologic manifestations, especially the division into granulomatous and nongranulomatous vasculitis among small-, medium- and large-vessel vasculitis. Savage and colleagues[12] tried to simplify it by incorporating the histopathologic element of granuloma formation (Table 1).

This review discusses the etiopathogenesis, clinical manifestations, and treatment of AAVs, namely, GPA; EGPA; MPA, which is a nongranulomatous small-vessel AAV, which shares clinical manifestation with GPA and EGPA; classic PAN, a nongranulomatous medium-vessel vasculitis and Cutaneous PAN.

ANTINEUTROPHIL CYTOPLASMIC ANTIBODY–ASSOCIATED VASCULITIDES

AAVs comprise 3 conditions, namely, GPA, EGPA, and MPA. They share a common feature in the form of ANCA positivity and have been clubbed together in the revised CHCC 2012. ANCA comprise a heterogeneous group of antibodies. These antibodies are usually detected by indirect immunofluorescence (IIF) or enzyme-linked immunosorbent assay (ELISA). Three patterns are observed on IIF, namely, cytoplasmic ANCA or cANCA, perinuclear ANCA or pANCA, and atypical ANCA or aANCA. It is recommended to use both the techniques for detection of ANCA.

ETIOPATHOGENESIS

The environmental factors may have a role in the disease pathogenesis. This is supported by variation in geographical distribution, relationship with exposure to silica, hydrocarbons and various drugs.[13] Infections such as *Staphylococcus aureus* have often been noted to precede the onset or flares of AAV, with decreased relapse rates reported after use of cotrimoxazole. Discovery of anti–lysosomal associated membrane protein 2 (LAMP2) antibodies in sera of patients with focal necrotizing glomerulonephritis defined the link between infection and AAV more clearly. Similar disease could be induced in animal models after immunizing with LAMP2.[14] Genetic associations, both human leukocyte antigen (HLA) and non-HLA, have been studied in various populations; these include, but are not restricted to, association of HLA-DRB1*04, DPB1*0401, PRTN3 (A546G poly), AAT polymorphisms (SERPINA1) with GPA, HLA-DRB4 with EGPA, and HLA-DRB1*0901 with MPA. There is unconfirmed or conflicting association with IL2RA, IL-10, LILRA2, CD226, and FCRIIIb.[15–23]

Distinct genetic association of HLA-DP, SERPINA1, and PRTN3 with anti-proteinase 3 (PR3) and HLA-DQ with anti-myeloperoxidase (MPO) ANCA has been shown in the genome wide association study (GVAS) study.[24] These results suggest that the future classification of AAV may be

Table 1
Classification of vasculitis based on histopathologic feature of granuloma formation

	Large-Vessel Vasculitis	Medium-Vessel Vasculitis	Small-Vessel Vasculitis
Granulomatous inflammation	Temporal arteritis Takayasu arteritis		Granulomatosis with polyangiitis[a] Eosinophilic granulomatosis with polyangiitis[b]
Nongranulomatous inflammation		Classic polyarteritis nodosa Kawasaki disease	Microscopic polyangiitis IgA vasculitis[c] Essential cryoglobulinemic vasculitis Cutaneous leucocytoclastic vasculitis

[a] Previously known as Wegener granulomatosis.
[b] Previously known as Churg-Strauss syndrome.
[c] Previously known as Henoch-Schönlein purpura.
Adapted from Savage CO, Harper L, Adu D. Primary systemic vasculitis. Lancet 1997;349:553–8; with permission.

based on antigen specificity and not phenotypic presentation.

This result is supported by the publication showing TLR 9 polymorphisms with PR3-ANCA vasculitis as opposed to MPO-ANCA vasculitis.[25] There is a role of epigenetic influences resulting in decreased histone demethylation at PR3 and MPO loci described in patients with AAV and alternate complement pathways. Amelioration of disease in mouse models when neutrophil depletion is done before antibody transfer proves the key role of neutrophils in AAV. Abnormal neutrophil extracellular traps containing PR3 and MPO have been demonstrated on activating neutrophils with ANCA derived from human sera. Activated neutrophils and macrophages have a role in propagation of AAV. Predominant effector cells implicated in EGPA are eosinophils. Activated neutrophils recruit and activate eosinophils, which further secrete IL-1, IL-3, IL-5, transforming growth factor (TGF)-α, and TGF-β. These proteins recruit helper T 2 cells and perpetuate granuloma formation and fibrosis.[26] Reduction in the number of circulating endothelial progenitor cells, responsible for endothelial repair, has been found to predict relapse in ANCA vasculitis. Robust animal models have been described for MPO-ANCA vasculitis but are yet to be described for anti-PR3–mediated vasculitis. Circulating levels of B-lymphocyte stimulator are elevated in AAV. Abnormalities of helper T cell–like Th1 skewing in localized GPA, Th2 skewing and Th17 expansion in systemic GPA and EGPA, and effector T cells have been demonstrated.[27,28]

CLINICAL FEATURES INCLUDING SYSTEMIC ASSOCIATIONS
Granulomatosis with Polyangiitis

The range of clinical presentations is wide and is characterized by granulomatous inflammation of upper and lower airways and vasculitis of small and medium vessels, of which glomerulonephritis is common. Upper or lower airway involvement occurs alone or in combination in about 90% of patients.[29]

Nasal symptoms include nasal obstruction, bloody nasal discharge, epistaxis, and saddle nose deformity (**Fig. 1**) due to nasal involvement. Chronic sinusitis is common. Nasal examination may show congested mucosa, superficial ulcerations of nasal mucosa, nasal crusting and septal perforation, and sinus tenderness. There may be ulcerative stomatitis, hyperplastic gingivitis, and subglottic stenosis. GPA can present with unique manifestation of strawberry gingival enlargement. There may also be mucosal ulcers on the tongue (**Fig. 2**), buccal mucosa, gums, or palate;

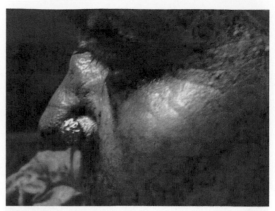

Fig. 1. Collapse of bridge of nose in a patient with GPA.

cobblestone-like lesion over the palate; nonhealing extraction socket; and oroantral fistula. Mastoiditis, otitis media, and orbital pseudotumor may be the other manifestations. Systemic features like fever, arthralgias, malaise, and signs of systemic vasculitis may not be present in the beginning, which is then known as localized form of vasculitis.

Arthralgias, fever, weight loss, and fatigue may occur in the generalized phase of GPA. Pulmonary involvement occurs in up to 85% of patients and may be asymptomatic in patients with pulmonary nodules or present in the form of cough, hemoptysis, and breathlessness. Radiologic features include pulmonary nodular infiltrates (**Fig. 3**), single or multiple cavities, and bilateral ground glass opacities, as seen in pulmonary hemorrhage. Renal involvement in the form of rapidly progressive glomerulonephritis is seen as presenting manifestation in 20% patients but occurs in up to 80% patients during the disease course. There is proteinuria, dysmorphic red blood cells and casts on urine examination, and renal dysfunction. Eye

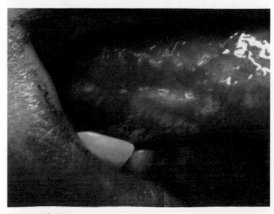

Fig. 2. Ulcer over the lateral margin of the tongue in a patient with GPA.

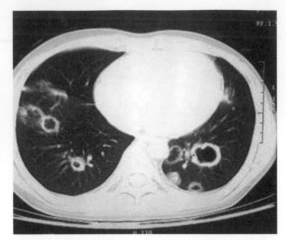

Fig. 3. Multiple cavitating lung nodules in a patient with GPA.

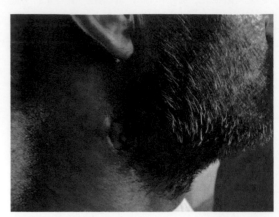

Fig. 5. Well-defined ulcer with a regular border sloping inward toward the base in a patient with GPA.

involvement occurs in half of these patients and may involve any structure. Common manifestations are in the form of episcleritis, scleritis (**Fig. 4**), and orbital disease. Cutaneous manifestations are seen in up to 46% patients and are in the form of verrucous lesions, skin ulcers (**Figs. 5** and **6**), nodules (**Fig. 7**), and nailfold infarcts. Sometimes there may be rare manifestations, such as tumefactive subcutaneous mass in the thigh, prostatomegaly with obstructive uropathy and advanced renal failure, and predominant GI vasculitis.[30]

Eosinophilic Granulomatosis with Polyangiitis

This condition was previously named Churg-Strauss syndrome after the initial description by

Churg and Strauss in 1951. This syndrome is characterized by eosinophil-rich granulomatous inflammations of the airways along with small- and medium-vessel vasculitis. There is asthma and eosinophilia. Three different disease phases are usually described, namely, prodromal, eosinophilic, and vasculitic. The main clinical feature in the prodromal stage is asthma and allergic rhinitis with or without polyposis. Asthma may occur many years before vasculitis. Faster progression from

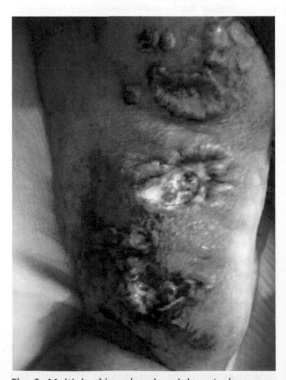

Fig. 6. Multiple skin colored nodules, at places coalescing together to form plaques. Some plaques show ulceration. Ulcers have an irregular margin and a base formed of granulation tissue with some purulent discharge.

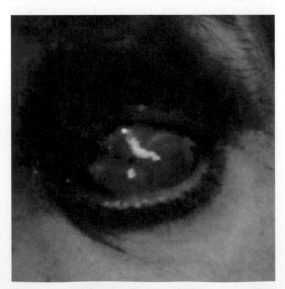

Fig. 4. Necrotizing perilimbal scleritis in a patient with GPA.

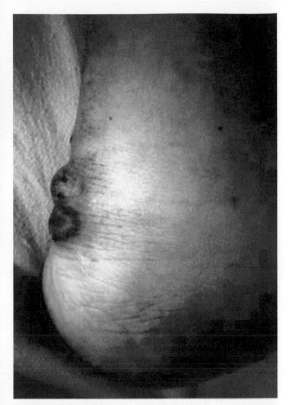

Fig. 7. Well-defined, erythematous to viloaceous bullae grouped over the ankle in a patient with GPA.

asthma to vasculitis portends poor prognosis. Although both upper and lower airways are involved, upper airway involvement is much milder than GPA. The second phase is of peripheral and tissue eosinophilia; this may be difficult to diagnose because of masking of eosinophilia by steroid use for asthma. Vasculitic manifestations are in the form of multisystem involvement of nerves, heart, lungs, GI tract, and kidneys.

Skin involvement is a dominant feature seen in one-third to two-thirds of patients and present in the form of nodules; urticaria and ulceration are less common. Neurologic involvement is seen in 60% to −70% patients and is commonly in the form of multiple mononeuropathies or symmetric polyneuropathy. Ischemic optic neuropathy, cranial neuropathies, and stroke are less common.

Cardiac involvement seen in up to 20% of patients contributes to half of deaths. Cardiac involvement may be in the form of myocarditis, pericarditis, endocarditis, valvulitis, and coronary vasculitis. Renal involvement in form of small-vessel vasculitis is less common than other AAVs. Migratory arthralgias and myalgias are common. There may be nonerosive arthritis in some patients. Positive rheumatoid factor can also be detected in these patients.[31,32]

Microscopic Polyangiitis

MPA is a nongranulomatous small-vessel AAV. It was initially thought to be a part of PAN and was recognized as a distinct entity in CHCC in 1994. The main manifestations are in the form of pauci-immune glomerulonephritis and pulmonary capillaritis. Granulomatous inflammation is absent. The dominant presenting manifestation in most patients is renal involvement in the form of rapidly progressive glomerulonephritis. There may be oliguria/anuria at the time of presentation, necessitating dialysis. Lung hemorrhage is the most catastrophic manifestation seen in about 10% of patients and is mostly associated with renal involvement. Most of these patients have constitutional symptoms, fever (temperature greater than 38°C), weight loss greater than 2 kg, arthralgias, and myalgias at the time of presentation. Neurologic involvement is common and is in the form of mononeuritis multiplex, axonal sensorimotor neuropathy, and cranial nerve involvement. Skin manifestations include purpura, ulcers, and digital gangrene. Ocular involvement is in the form of scleritis, episcleritis, blepharitis, conjunctivitis, keratitis, uveitis, and retinal vasculitis. The rare manifestations are involvement of heart and mesenteric ischemia.

EVALUATION AND MANAGEMENT OF ANTINEUTROPHIL CYTOPLASMIC ANTIBODY–ASSOCIATED VASCULITIS

There are no validated diagnostic criteria. There has to be a high index of suspicion, especially in the presence of multisystem involvement. Diagnosis is usually based on clinical features highlighted earlier, supported by positive ANCA and biopsy of the involved organ wherever feasible. It is recommended that ANCA testing should be carried out by both IIF and ELISA.[33] The main target antigens of ANCA are located in the cytoplasmic space of neutrophils and monocytes.[34] Two main targets, both part of azurophilic granules of neutrophils, are identified as enzymes, namely, PR3 and MPO.[35,36] The cANCA pattern of immunofluorescence is mainly associated with the reactivity to PR3. Although pANCA fluorescence pattern can be associated with various antigens, the clinically significant association is with MPO. The important clinical associations of types of ANCA are those of GPA with PR3 and cANCA, and MPA with MPO and pANCA. EGPA is associated with MPO-ANCA in approximately 50% of cases.[37] Biopsy of the involved organs must be pursued, wherever possible, unless it is contraindicated. The presence of fibrinoid necrosis or crescentic glomerulonephritis is highly suggestive of AAV.

A stepwise algorithm has been proposed by Watts and colleagues[38] for classification of vasculitis. It takes into account the ACR and Lanham criteria for Churg-Strauss syndrome and ACR criteria for Wegener granulomatosis. Various soft pointers considered suggestive of GPA are in the form of radiographic evidence of fixed pulmonary infiltrates; nodules or cavitations present for more than 1 month; bronchial stenosis; bloody nasal discharge and crusting for more than 1 month; nasal ulceration; chronic sinusitis, otitis media, or mastoiditis for more than 3 months; retro-orbital mass or inflammation (pseudotumor); subglottic stenosis; and saddle nose deformity/destructive sinonasal disease. The soft pointers for renal vasculitis are hematuria associated with red cell casts or greater than 10% dysmorphic erythrocytes or 2+ hematuria and 2+ proteinuria on urinalysis. These pointers help in reliably classifying patients into a single category. This algorithm has been validated in various population cohorts[39,40] and is valid even when the older CHCC nomenclature system is replaced with CHCC 2012.[41]

Once a diagnosis has been made, it is important to assess disease activity. Birmingham vasculitis activity score (BVAS) is the most widely used validated tool for assessing the disease activity. The first version was developed in 1994 by expert opinion, and at present, version 3 [BVAS (v3)] is being used. It has been validated in various population cohorts.[42,43] A simplified GPA-specific version of BVAS has also been developed. BVAS (v3) calculator can be accessed online at http://www.epsnetwork.co.uk/BVAS/bvas_flow.html. The other disease activity assessment tools such as Groningen index, which takes into account clinical and histologic features, and disease extent index are specific for GPA.[44,45]

Because there can be permanent, irreversible damage due to healed disease or drug toxicity, it is important to differentiate this damage from disease activity in these patients to prevent unnecessary or harmful immunosuppressive therapy. The most comprehensive and widely used validated damage index available is the vasculitis damage index.[46]

MANAGEMENT

Corticosteroids and cytotoxic drugs used in combination are the mainstay of treatment. Introduction of these cytotoxic therapies have drastically changed the outcomes of these diseases, which previously had a mortality rate of 90% at 2 years.[47] The current treatment recommendations are based on the disease severity. The European Vasculitis Study Group (EUVAS) recommends 5 grades of disease severity of AAV as follows: (1) localized—upper or lower airway disease without other systemic involvement or constitutional symptoms; (2) early systemic disease—systemic disease without organ or life-threatening disease; (3) generalized—renal or other organ-threatening disease, serum creatinine level less than 5.6 mg/dL; (4) severe—renal or other organ failure, serum creatinine level more than 5.6 mg/dL; (5) refractory—progressive disease unresponsive to glucocorticoids and cyclophosphamide.[48] The EUVAS has also given evidence-based recommendation for management of primary small- and medium-vessel vasculitis. The highlights are given in **Table 2**.

Remission Induction

Combination of methotrexate, and prednisolone may be used in patients with mild localized disease.[49] In patients with systemic non–life-threatening disease, cyclophosphamide may be used with corticosteroids. Intravenous pulse cyclophosphamide is preferred over oral daily cyclophosphamide because of lower rates of adverse events, although there may be an increased risk of relapse.[50,51] Rituximab can be used as a remission induction agent in patients in whom cyclophosphamide is contraindicated.[52,53] Plasmapheresis has an adjunct role to cyclophosphamide and rituximab in patients with rapidly progressive renal failure (serum creatinine level >5.6 mg/dL or oliguria or need for dialysis) or lung hemorrhage; this may prevent organ damage, although the survival advantage may not be there.[54,55]

Remission Maintenance

The choice of therapy depends on the initial agent used for remission induction. When methotrexate has been used in induction, it can be used as maintenance agent also. However, emerging evidence suggests that patients treated with methotrexate may have a higher relapse rate than the group in which cyclophosphamide is used.[56] When cyclophosphamide is used as the remission induction agent, azathioprine is the remission maintenance agent of choice.[57] Leflunomide or methotrexates are alternative choices when azathioprine cannot be used.[48] Mycophenolate mofetil can also be used but has a higher relapse rate than azathioprine.[58] In patients in whom rituximab has been used for induction, it can be used as a maintenance agent every 4 to 6 months.[59,60] 15-Deoxyspergualin has been used in patients with refractory GPA.[61]

POLYARTERITIS NODOSA
Introduction

PAN or classic PAN is a nongranulomatous medium-vessel vasculitis. It was first described by Kussumaul and Maier in 1866, who named it periarteritis nodosa.[1] It is an uncommon disease. The initial descriptions included patients with MPA, and it was only after CHCC that MPA was identified as a separate entity.

Etiopathogenesis

The exact etiopathogenesis is not known. There are no well-characterized animal models of PAN. A disease closely mimicking human PAN develops in *Cynomolgus macaques* monkeys.[62] The rarity of PAN makes genomewide association studies unlikely. A recent publication has reported mutations in CECR1, a gene encoding ADA2, causing a familial PAN in Jewish and German families.[63]

PAN is associated with hepatitis B virus (HBV) infection. The incidence of HBV-associated PAN has decreased with increased screening of blood products before transfusion and increasing vaccination.[64,65] The most probable mechanism of HBV PAN is type III or immune complex reaction. The immune complexes precipitate and are trapped in the vessel walls, thus resulting in vessel injury.[66–70] The primary role of immune complexes in the pathogenesis is suggested by the presence of large masses of HBsAg immune complexes in the recent vascular lesions, lesser amount of these complexes in healing lesions, and their absence in healed lesions.[71]

Clinical Features Including Systemic Associations

The spectrum of clinical manifestations varies from mild to progressive disease. The classic presentation is in the form of constitutional symptoms of fever, myalgias, and weight loss along with manifestations of multisystem involvement. The multisystem involvement may be in the form of skin rash, peripheral neuropathy, asymmetrical arthritis, and kidney, gut, and GI involvement. Skin manifestations include palpable purpura, livedo reticularis, infarctions, nodules, and peripheral gangrene. Arthralgias and myalgias are common, seen in half of these patients. Neurologic manifestations are in the form of peripheral neuropathy and mononeuritis multiplex with rare manifestations in form of central nervous system involvement, which carries poor prognosis. Renal manifestations are in the form of renal artery stenosis, renal artery microaneurysms, and renal infarcts. The glomerulus is classically spared. GI involvement manifesting as pain abdomen, diarrhea, hemorrhage, and abnormal liver enzyme levels, and cardiac involvement are the other major manifestations of PAN. The clinical manifestations of HBV-associated PAN are largely similar to non–HBV-associated PAN. PAN occurs early in the course of HBV infection. In a study of 348 patients, patients with HBV-associated PAN had higher weight loss, peripheral neuropathy, mononeuritis multiplex, mesenteric artery microaneurysms, abdominal pain, GI manifestations requiring surgery, cardiomyopathy, orchitis, hypertension, and/or elevated transaminase levels. Renal artery microaneurysms (**Fig. 8**) and skin manifestations, however, were less common.[72]

Associations

PAN can be associated with other diseases such as hairy cell leukemia, Sjögren syndrome, rheumatoid arthritis, mixed cryoglobulinemia, myelodysplastic syndrome, and other hematologic malignancies.

Diagnosis

There are no diagnostic criteria. The ACR criteria did not differentiate between PAN and MPA. It was only after CHCC that MPA was differentiated from PAN. In the CHCC 2014, HBV-associated PAN has been grouped separately as vasculitis associated with probable etiology.[11]

The presence of ANCA, glomerulonephritis, or histologic involvement of arterioles, capillaries, or venules is against the diagnosis of PAN and more in favor of small-vessel vasculitis. Five factor score (FFS) given by the French Vasculitis Group has been used to evaluate prognosis in patients with PAN, EGPA, and MPA.[73] A score of 1 is given for each of the following factors while calculating FFS: proteinuria greater than 1 g/24 hours, creatinine greater than 140 µmol/L, specific GI involvement, specific cardiomyopathy, and specific central nervous system involvement. Five-year survival rate and relative risk of death with FFS of 0 were 88.1% and 0.62; with FFS of 1 were 74.1% and 1.35; and FFS of greater than 2 were 54.1% and 2.40, respectively.[74]

Wherever possible, diagnosis should be confirmed with histopathology and angiography. The most accessible tissues for biopsy include sural nerve, testes, and skeletal muscles. The pathology consists of focal necrotizing lesions extending through the walls of small and medium-sized vessels. There may be granulomatous inflammation rarely.[75] Typical angiographic findings include arterial stenosis, occlusions, and

Table 2
European League against Rheumatism recommendations on management of primary small- and medium-vessel vasculitis

	Recommendation	Level of Evidence	Strength of Recommendation
1	Patients with primary small- and medium-vessel vasculitis be managed in collaboration with or at centers of expertise	3	D
2	Antineutrophilic cytoplasmic antibody (ANCA) testing (including indirect immunofluorescence and ELISA) should be performed in the appropriate clinical context	1A	A
3	A positive biopsy result is strongly supportive of vasculitis and we recommend the procedure to assist diagnosis and further evaluation for patients suspected of having vasculitis	3	C
4	Use of a structured clinical assessment, urine analysis, and other basic laboratory tests at each clinical visit for patients with vasculitis	3	C
5	Patients with ANCA-associated vasculitis be categorized according to different levels of severity to assist treatment decisions	2B	B
6	Combination of cyclophosphamide (intravenous or oral) and glucocorticoids for remission induction of generalized primary small- and medium-vessel vasculitis	1A for GPA and MPA, 1B for PAN and EGPA	A
7	A combination of methotrexate (oral or parenteral) and glucocorticoid as a less toxic alternative to cyclophosphamide for the induction of remission in non–organ-threatening or non–life-threatening ANCA-associated vasculitis	1B	B
8	Use of high-dose glucocorticoids as an important part of remission induction therapy	3	C
9	Plasma exchange for selected patients with rapidly progressive severe renal disease to improve renal survival	1B	A

#	Recommendation	1B for azathioprine, leflunomide, 2B for methotrexate	A for azathioprine and B for methotrexate, leflunomide
10	Remission-maintenance therapy with a combination of low-dose glucocorticoid therapy and azathioprine, leflunomide, or methotrexate	1B for azathioprine, leflunomide, 2B for methotrexate	A for azathioprine and B for methotrexate, leflunomide
11	Alternative immunomodulatory therapy choices should be considered for patients who do not achieve remission or relapse on maximal doses of standard therapy: these patients should be referred to an expert center for further management and enrollment in clinical trials	3	C
12	Immunosuppressive therapy for patients with mixed essential cryoglobulinemic vasculitis (nonviral)	4	D
13	Use of antiviral therapy for the treatment of hepatitis C-associated cryoglobulinemic vasculitis	1B	B
14	Combination of antiviral therapy, plasma exchange, and glucocorticoids for hepatitis B-associated PAN	3	C
15	Investigation of persistent unexplained hematuria in patients with prior exposure to cyclophosphamide	2B	C

1A, from meta-analysis of randomized controlled trials; 1B, from at least 1 randomized controlled trial; 2B, from at least 1 type of quasi-experimental study; 3, from descriptive studies, such as comparative studies, correlation studies, or case–control studies; 4, from expert committee reports or opinions and/or clinical experience of respected authorities. Strength of recommendation: A, category 1 evidence; B, category 2 evidence or extrapolated recommendations from category 1 evidence; C, category 3 evidence or extrapolated recommendations from category 1 or 2 evidence; D, category 4 evidence or extrapolated recommendations from category 2 or 3 evidence.

Adapted from Mukhtyar C, Guillevin L, Cid MC, et al. EULAR recommendations for the management of primary small and medium vessel vasculitis. Ann Rheum Dis 2009;68:310–7; with permission.

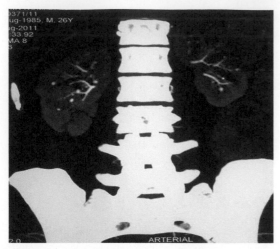

Fig. 8. Computed tomographic angiogram in a patient with polyarteritis nodosa showing renal microaneurysms.

saccular and fusiform aneurysms without significant atherosclerosis.

Treatment

Corticosteroids are the cornerstone of therapy. Cyclophosphamide can be used in patients with disease refractory to steroids or with major organ-threatening manifestations. The treatment of HBV-associated PAN is different from that of non–HBV-associated PAN, targeting clearance of immune complexes with plasma exchange (PE) along with use of antiviral drugs for suppression of HBV replication. Corticosteroids are given only for 2 weeks; their abrupt stoppage results in enhanced immunologic clearance of HBV-infected hepatocytes and favors seroconversion from HBsAg to anti-HBe antibody. PE and antivirals become the cornerstone of therapy subsequently.[64]

Summary

The vasculitides generally present with multisystem involvement. The presentations depend on the site and size of vessel involved. There are no diagnostic criteria, and diagnosis is usually based on clinical manifestations, supported by ANCA serology for AAV and angiographic findings for PAN and tissue biopsy wherever feasible. Immunosuppressive drugs are the cornerstone of therapy. The differences in characteristics of various vasculitides are shown in **Table 3**.

CUTANEOUS POLYARTERITIS NODOSA
Introduction

Cutaneous PAN is a vasculitis involving small and medium-sized vessels of subcutaneous and deep dermal parts of the skin. This condition has been proposed as an entity that is different from classic PAN.[76]

Etiopathogenesis

The exact etiopathogenesis is not known. Among the proposed hypotheses are hypersensitivity due to its development after administration of various drugs and transfer of antigens from mother to fetus due to development of disease in newborn infants of mother with the disease.

Clinical Features

This condition is slightly more common in the female population. Depending on the severity, 3 different classes have been described (mild cutaneous, severe cutaneous, and progressive systemic). In the mild cutaneous form, skin manifestations are in the form of nodular skin lesions and livedo reticularis. The skin nodules are tender and, numbers may vary from single to multiple. The most commonly involved sites are the lower

Table 3
Comparison of different features of various vasculitides

Disease	ANCA	ENT	Lungs	Kidneys	Heart	Nerves	Skin
GPA	PR3 80%–95% MPO 5%–20% ANCA-Neg	+++	Nodules Infiltrates	++++	+	++	++
EGPA	MPO 40% PR3 35%	+	Asthma Infiltrates	++++	+	+++	+++
MPA	MPO 40%–80% PR3 35%	−	Infiltrates	+++	++	++++	+++
PAN	−	−	−	−	++	++++	+++
Cut PAN	−	−	−	−	−	+	++++

Abbreviations: ANCA-Neg, ANCA negative; Cut PAN, cutaneous polyarteritis nodosa; ENT, ear, nose, and throat.

limbs. Mild polyneuropathy may be present. In the severe cutaneous form, besides nodular skin lesions, there can be ulceration and more prominent livedo reticularis. Mild polyneuropathy is frequent. These patients can have constitutional symptoms such as fever malaise and arthralgias in the acute stage. Patients with progressive systemic disease have necrotizing livedo reticularis along with digital gangrene. There is progressive musculoskeletal involvement in the form of arthralgias/arthritis. The peripheral neuropathy can be severe and is commonly in form of mononeuritis multiplex.

Diagnosis

There is no serologic test. Diagnosis is based on clinical examination and histopathologic findings. The lesions are similar to those of systemic PAN on microscopic examination.[77] There is necrotizing inflammation of small to medium-sized vessels. Cellular infiltrate depends on the stage of illness, with neutrophilic infiltration in and around the vessel wall in the early stage and the healing stage characterized by infiltration of mononuclear cells. In patients with systemic symptoms, careful search should be done to exclude systemic PAN.

Treatment

Although nonsteroidal anti-inflammatory drugs may be effective in some of these patients, most require glucocorticoids for induction of remission. Patients with refractory skin disease may require other drugs, such as dapsone. Drugs such as methotrexate, azathioprine, and cyclophosphamide are used in patients with severe manifestations like mononeuritis multiplex. There are reports of successful use of anti-TNF agents and rituximab in patients with refractory skin disease.

REFERENCES

1. Zeek PM. Periarteritis nodosa; a critical review. Am J Clin Pathol 1952;22:777–90.
2. Hunder GG, Bloch DA, Michel BA, et al. The American College of Rheumatology 1990 criteria for the classification of giant cell arteritis. Arthritis Rheum 1990;33:1122–8.
3. Arend WP, Michel BA, Bloch DA, et al. The American College of Rheumatology 1990 criteria for the classification of Takayasu arteritis. Arthritis Rheum 1990;33:1129–34.
4. Leavitt RY, Fauci AS, Bloch DA, et al. The American College of Rheumatology 1990 criteria for the classification of Wegener's granulomatosis. Arthritis Rheum 1990;33:1101–7.
5. Masi AT, Hunder GG, Lie JT, et al. The American College of Rheumatology 1990 criteria for the classification of Churg-Strauss syndrome (allergic granulomatosis and angiitis). Arthritis Rheum 1990;33:1094–100.
6. Lightfoot RW Jr, Michel BA, Bloch DA, et al. The American College of Rheumatology 1990 criteria for the classification of polyarteritis nodosa. Arthritis Rheum 1990;33:1088–93.
7. Mills JA, Michel BA, Bloch DA, et al. The American College of Rheumatology 1990 criteria for the classification of Henoch-Schonlein purpura. Arthritis Rheum 1990;33:1114–21.
8. Calabrese LH, Michel BA, Bloch DA, et al. The American College of Rheumatology 1990 criteria for the classification of hypersensitivity vasculitis. Arthritis Rheum 1990;33:1108–13.
9. Waller R, Ahmed A, Patel I, et al. Update on the classification of vasculitis. Best Pract Res Clin Rheumatol 2013;27:3–17.
10. Jennette JC, Falk RJ, Andrassy K, et al. Nomenclature of systemic vasculitides. Proposal of an international consensus conference. Arthritis Rheum 1994;37:187–92.
11. Jennette JC, Falk RJ, Bacon PA, et al. 2012 Revised International Chapel Hill Consensus Conference nomenclature of vasculitides. Arthritis Rheum 2013;65:1–11.
12. Savage CO, Harper L, Adu D. Primary systemic vasculitis. Lancet 1997;349:553–8.
13. Mahr AD, Neogi T, Merkel PA. Epidemiology of Wegener's granulomatosis: lessons from descriptive studies and analyses of genetic and environmental risk determinants. Clin Exp Rheumatol 2006;24:S82–91.
14. Kain R, Exner M, Brandes R, et al. Molecular mimicry in pauci-immune focal necrotizing glomerulonephritis. Nat Med 2008;14:1088–96.
15. Gencik M, Borgmann S, Zahn R, et al. Immunogenetic risk factors for anti-neutrophil cytoplasmic antibody (ANCA)-associated systemic vasculitis. Clin Exp Immunol 1999;117:412–7.
16. Morris H, Morgan MD, Wood AM, et al. ANCA-associated vasculitis is linked to carriage of the Z allele of alpha(1) antitrypsin and its polymers. Ann Rheum Dis 2011;70:1851–6.
17. Tsuchiya N, Kobayashi S, Hashimoto H, et al. Association of HLA-DRB1*0901-DQB1*0303 haplotype with microscopic polyangiitis in Japanese. Genes Immun 2006;7:81–4.
18. Vaglio A, Martorana D, Maggiore U, et al. HLA-DRB4 as a genetic risk factor for Churg-Strauss syndrome. Arthritis Rheum 2007;56:3159–66.
19. Cao Y, Schmitz JL, Yang J, et al. DRB1*15 allele is a risk factor for PR3-ANCA disease in African Americans. J Am Soc Nephrol 2011;22:1161–7.
20. Carr EJ, Niederer HA, Williams J, et al. Confirmation of the genetic association of CTLA4 and PTPN22 with ANCA-associated vasculitis. BMC Med Genet 2009;10:121.

21. Gencik M, Meller S, Borgmann S, et al. Proteinase 3 gene polymorphisms and Wegener's granulomatosis. Kidney Int 2000;58:2473–7.

22. Mahr AD, Edberg JC, Stone JH, et al. Alpha(1)-antitrypsin deficiency-related alleles Z and S and the risk of Wegener's granulomatosis. Arthritis Rheum 2010;62:3760–7.

23. Tsuchiya N, Kobayashi S, Kawasaki A, et al. Genetic background of Japanese patients with antineutrophil cytoplasmic antibody-associated vasculitis: association of HLA-DRB1*0901 with microscopic polyangiitis. J Rheumatol 2003;30:1534–40.

24. Lyons PA, Rayner TF, Trivedi S, et al. Genetically distinct subsets within ANCA-associated vasculitis. N Engl J Med 2012;367:214–23.

25. Husmann CA, Holle JU, Moosig F, et al. Genetics of toll like receptor 9 in ANCA associated vasculitides. Ann Rheum Dis 2014;73:890–6.

26. Jennette JC, Falk RJ, Hu P, et al. Pathogenesis of antineutrophil cytoplasmic autoantibody-associated small-vessel vasculitis. Annu Rev Pathol 2013;8: 139–60.

27. Wilde B, Thewissen M, Damoiseaux J, et al. T cells in ANCA-associated vasculitis: what can we learn from lesional versus circulating T cells? Arthritis Res Ther 2010;12:204.

28. Free ME, Bunch DO, McGregor JA, et al. Patients with antineutrophil cytoplasmic antibody-associated vasculitis have defective Treg cell function exacerbated by the presence of a suppression-resistant effector cell population. Arthritis Rheum 2013;65: 1922–33.

29. Hoffman GS, Kerr GS, Leavitt RY, et al. Wegener granulomatosis: an analysis of 158 patients. Ann Intern Med 1992;116:488–98.

30. Sharma A, Gopalakrishan D, Nada R, et al. Uncommon presentations of primary systemic necrotizing vasculitides: the Great Masquerades. Int J Rheum Dis 2014;17(5):562–72.

31. Churg J, Strauss L. Allergic granulomatosis, allergic angiitis, and periarteritis nodosa. Am J Pathol 1951; 27:277–301.

32. Guillevin L, Cohen P, Gayraud M, et al. Churg-Strauss syndrome. Clinical study and long-term follow-up of 96 patients. Medicine (Baltimore) 1999;78:26–37.

33. Savige J, Gillis D, Benson E, et al. International consensus statement on testing and reporting of antineutrophil cytoplasmic antibodies (ANCA). Am J Clin Pathol 1999;111:507–13.

34. Bartunkova J, Tesar V, Sediva A. Diagnostic and pathogenetic role of antineutrophil cytoplasmic autoantibodies. Clin Immunol 2003;106:73–82.

35. Jenne DE, Tschopp J, Ludemann J, et al. Wegener's autoantigen decoded. Nature 1990;346:520.

36. Falk RJ, Jennette JC. Anti-neutrophil cytoplasmic autoantibodies with specificity for myeloperoxidase in patients with systemic vasculitis and idiopathic necrotizing and crescentic glomerulonephritis. N Engl J Med 1988;318:1651–7.

37. Gayraud M, Guillevin L, le Toumelin P, et al. Long-term follow-up of polyarteritis nodosa, microscopic polyangiitis, and Churg-Strauss syndrome: analysis of four prospective trials including 278 patients. Arthritis Rheum 2001;44:666–75.

38. Watts R, Lane S, Hanslik T, et al. Development and validation of a consensus methodology for the classification of the ANCA-associated vasculitides and polyarteritis nodosa for epidemiological studies. Ann Rheum Dis 2007;66:222–7.

39. Kamali S, Artim-Esen B, Erer B, et al. Re-evaluation of 129 patients with systemic necrotizing vasculitides by using classification algorithm according to consensus methodology. Clin Rheumatol 2012;31:325–8.

40. Sharma A, Mittal T, Rajan R, et al. Validation of the consensus methodology algorithm for the classification of systemic necrotizing vasculitis in Indian patients. Int J Rheum Dis 2014;17:408–11.

41. Abdulkader R, Lane SE, Scott DG, et al. Classification of vasculitis: EMA classification using CHCC 2012 definitions. Ann Rheum Dis 1888;2013:72.

42. Luqmani RA, Bacon PA, Moots RJ. Birmingham vasculitis activity score (BVAS) in systemic necrotizing vasculitis. QJM 1994;87:671–8.

43. Suppiah R, Mukhtyar C, Flossmann O, et al. A cross-sectional study of the Birmingham vasculitis activity score version 3 in systemic vasculitis. Rheumatology (Oxford) 2011;50:899–905.

44. Kallenberg CG, Tervaert JW, Stegeman CA. Criteria for disease activity in Wegener's granulomatosis: a requirement for longitudinal clinical studies. APMIS Suppl 1990;19:37–9.

45. de Groot K, Gross WL, Herlyn K, et al. Development and validation of a disease extent index for Wegener's granulomatosis. Clin Nephrol 2001;55:31–8.

46. Exley A, Carruthers DM, Luqmani RA. Damage occurs early in systemic vasculitis and is an index of outcome. QJM 1997;90:391–9.

47. Phillip R, Luqmani R. Mortality in systemic vasculitis: a systematic review. Clin Exp Rheumatol 2008;26: S94–104.

48. Mukhtyar C, Guillevin L, Cid MC, et al. EULAR recommendations for the management of primary small and medium vessel vasculitis. Ann Rheum Dis 2009; 68:310–7.

49. De Groot K, Rasmussen N, Bacon PA, et al. Randomized trial of cyclophosphamide versus methotrexate for induction of remission in early systemic antineutrophil cytoplasmic antibody-associated vasculitis. Arthritis Rheum 2005;52:2461–9.

50. de Groot K, Harper L, Jayne DR, et al. Pulse versus daily oral cyclophosphamide for induction of remission in antineutrophil cytoplasmic antibody-associated vasculitis: a randomized trial. Ann Intern Med 2009; 150:670–80.

51. Harper L, Morgan MD, Walsh M, et al. Pulse versus daily oral cyclophosphamide for induction of remission in ANCA-associated vasculitis: long-term follow-up. Ann Rheum Dis 2012;71:955–60.

52. Jones RB, Tervaert JW, Hauser T, et al. Rituximab versus cyclophosphamide in ANCA-associated renal vasculitis. N Engl J Med 2010;363:211–20.

53. Stone JH, Merkel PA, Spiera R, et al. Rituximab versus cyclophosphamide for ANCA-associated vasculitis. N Engl J Med 2010;363:221–32.

54. Guillevin L, Cevallos R, Durand-Gasselin B, et al. Treatment of glomerulonephritis in microscopic polyangiitis and Churg-Strauss syndrome. Indications of plasma exchanges, meta-analysis of 2 randomized studies on 140 patients, 32 with glomerulonephritis. Ann Med Interne (Paris) 1997;148:198–204.

55. Jayne DR, Gaskin G, Rasmussen N, et al. Randomized trial of plasma exchange or high-dosage methylprednisolone as adjunctive therapy for severe renal vasculitis. J Am Soc Nephrol 2007;18:2180–8.

56. Faurschou M, Westman K, Rasmussen N, et al. Brief report: long-term outcome of a randomized clinical trial comparing methotrexate to cyclophosphamide for remission induction in early systemic antineutrophil cytoplasmic antibody-associated vasculitis. Arthritis Rheum 2012;64:3472–7.

57. Jayne D, Rasmussen N, Andrassy K, et al. A randomized trial of maintenance therapy for vasculitis associated with antineutrophil cytoplasmic autoantibodies. N Engl J Med 2003;349:36–44.

58. Hiemstra TF, Walsh M, Mahr A, et al. Mycophenolate mofetil vs azathioprine for remission maintenance in antineutrophil cytoplasmic antibody-associated vasculitis: a randomized controlled trial. JAMA 2010;304:2381–8.

59. Smith RM, Jones RB, Guerry MJ, et al. Rituximab for remission maintenance in relapsing antineutrophil cytoplasmic antibody-associated vasculitis. Arthritis Rheum 2012;64:3760–9.

60. Rhee EP, Laliberte KA, Niles JL. Rituximab as maintenance therapy for anti-neutrophil cytoplasmic antibody-associated vasculitis. Clin J Am Soc Nephrol 2010;5:1394–400.

61. Flossmann O, Baslund B, Bruchfeld A, et al. Deoxyspergualin in relapsing and refractory Wegener's granulomatosis. Ann Rheum Dis 2009;68:1125–30.

62. Colmegna I, Maldonado-Cocco JA. Polyarteritis nodosa revisited. Curr Rheumatol Rep 2005;7:288–96.

63. Navon Elkan P, Pierce SB, Segel R, et al. Mutant adenosine deaminase 2 in a polyarteritis nodosa vasculopathy. N Engl J Med 2014;370:921–31.

64. Guillevin L, Mahr A, Callard P, et al. Hepatitis B virus-associated polyarteritis nodosa: clinical characteristics, outcome, and impact of treatment in 115 patients. Medicine (Baltimore) 2005;84:313–22.

65. Lane SE, Watts R, Scott DG. Epidemiology of systemic vasculitis. Curr Rheumatol Rep 2005;7:270–5.

66. Belizna CC, Hamidou MA, Levesque H, et al. Infection and vasculitis. Rheumatology (Oxford) 2009;48:475–82.

67. Mahr A, Guillevin L, Poissonnet M, et al. Prevalences of polyarteritis nodosa, microscopic polyangiitis, Wegener's granulomatosis, and Churg-Strauss syndrome in a French urban multiethnic population in 2000: a capture-recapture estimate. Arthritis Rheum 2004;51:92–9.

68. Pernice W, Sodomann CP, Luben G, et al. Antigen-specific detection of HBsAg-containing immune complexes in the course of hepatitis B virus infection. Clin Exp Immunol 1979;37:376–80.

69. Zuckerman AJ. Proceedings: hepatitis B, immune complexes, and the pathogenesis of polyarteritis nodosa. J Clin Pathol 1976;29:84–5.

70. Trepo CG, Zucherman AJ, Bird RC, et al. The role of circulating hepatitis B antigen/antibody immune complexes in the pathogenesis of vascular and hepatic manifestations in polyarteritis nodosa. J Clin Pathol 1974;27:863–8.

71. Michalak T. Immune complexes of hepatitis B surface antigen in the pathogenesis of periarteritis nodosa. A study of seven necropsy cases. Am J Pathol 1978;90:619–32.

72. Pagnoux C, Seror R, Henegar C, et al. Clinical features and outcomes in 348 patients with polyarteritis nodosa: a systematic retrospective study of patients diagnosed between 1963 and 2005 and entered into the French Vasculitis Study Group database. Arthritis Rheum 2010;62:616–26.

73. Guillevin L, Lhote F, Gayraud M, et al. Prognostic factors in polyarteritis nodosa and Churg-Strauss syndrome. A prospective study in 342 patients. Medicine (Baltimore) 1996;75:17–28.

74. Pagnoux C, Cohen P, Guillevin L. Vasculitides secondary to infections. Clin Exp Rheumatol 2006;24:S71–81.

75. Lie JT. Histopathologic specificity of systemic vasculitis. Rheum Dis Clin North Am 1995;21:883–909.

76. Daoud MS, Hutton KP, Gibson LE. Cutaneous polyarteritis nodosa: a clinicopathological study of 79 cases. Br J Dermatol 1997;136:706–13.

77. Kleeman D, Kempf W, Burg G, et al. Cutaneous polyarteritis nodosa. Vasa 1998;27:54–7.

Granulomatous Lymphoproliferative Disorders
Granulomatous Slack Skin and Lymphomatoid Granulomatosis

Pamela Gangar, MD, Sangeetha Venkatarajan, MD, MBA*

KEYWORDS

- Lymphomatoid granulomatosis • Granulomatous cutaneous T-cell lymphoma
- Granulomatous mycosis fungoides • Granulomatous slack skin
- EBV-positive lymphoproliferative disorder

KEY POINTS

- Granulomatous cutaneous T-cell lymphomas (CTCL) are rare and present a diagnostic challenge.
- Granulomatous mycosis fungoides and granulomatous slack skin, the 2 most common types of granulomatous CTCL, display overlapping histologic findings, but differ clinically by circumscribed areas of pendulous lax skin seen in granulomatous slack skin.
- Recent studies have suggested that the prognosis of granulomatous mycosis fungoides is worse than that of classic mycosis fungoides.
- Lymphomatoid granulomatosis is a rare Epstein-Barr virus driven lymphoproliferative disease.
- Therapeutic options include oral corticosteroids, rituximab, interferon-α, and combined chemoimmunotherapy, and are based on the histologic grading of the lesion.

GRANULOMATOUS CUTANEOUS T-CELL LYMPHOMA
Introduction

Granulomatous cutaneous T-cell lymphoma (CTCL) is a rare entity. Approximately 2% of all cutaneous lymphomas involve granulomatous infiltrates.[1–3] The most common types of granulomatous CTCL are granulomatous mycosis fungoides (GMF) and granulomatous slack skin (GSS) **(Table 1)**.[4]

GMF is an entity distinct from GSS. GMF is a rare histopathologic variant of mycosis fungoides (MF) characterized by a prominent granulomatous infiltrate.[5] The term GMF was coined by Ackerman and Flaxman in 1970.[6] GSS is recognized by the World Health Organization and European Organization for Research and Treatment of Cancer classification for cutaneous lymphomas as 1 of 3 subtypes of mycosis fungoides.[7] GMF and GSS display overlapping histologic findings, but differ clinically by circumscribed areas of pendulous lax skin seen in GSS.[8]

Etiopathogenesis

The pathogenesis of granulomatous CTCLs is unknown. Histologically, GMF and GSS show

Disclosures: The authors do not have any financial disclosures or conflicts of interest.
MD Anderson Cancer Center, Department of Dermatology, 1400 Pressler Street FCT11.6074, Houston, TX 77030, USA
* Corresponding author.
E-mail address: Sangeetha.venkatarajan@gmail.com

Dermatol Clin 33 (2015) 489–496
http://dx.doi.org/10.1016/j.det.2015.03.013
0733-8635/15/$ – see front matter © 2015 Elsevier Inc. All rights reserved.

Table 1
Clinical results and outcomes in the literature: granulomatous mycosis fungoides and granulomatous slack skin

Clinical and Therapeutic Data from a Series of 19 Patients with Granulomatous Cutaneous T-Cell Lymphoma

Patient No.	Stage	Therapy	Treatment Response	Outcome/Follow-Up (years)
Granulomatous Mycosis Fungoides				
1	IB	IFN, PUVA	PR	AWD/8
2	III	IFN, chemo	SD	DOD/1
3	IA	CS, MC, RT, IFN	CR	ACR/20
4	IB	CS, MC	PR	AWD/6
5	IIB	RT, chemo	PR	DOD/2
6	IB	PUVA, RT	PD	DOD/1
7	IA	Imiq, IFN, PUVA, RT	CR	ACR/6
8	IA	Chemo	SD	AWD/1
9	IVA	Chemo	CR	AWD/4
10	IIA	Pred	PD	AWD/5
11	IA	PUVA, IFN	PR	AWD/4
12	IA	PUVA, RT, IFN	PD	DOD/9
13	IA	CS, PUVA, IFN, ret	SD	AWD/7
14	IB	PUVA, IFN, RT, chemo	PD	DOD/1
15	IA	CS, IFN, ret, RT	PD	DOD/5
Granulomatous Slack Skin				
16	IA	PUVA, ret, IFN	PR	AWD/10
17	IA	NA	NA	AWD/16
18	IA	Excision, CS, MC, PUVA, IFN	PD	AWD/15
19	IA	Excision, carmustine	PR	AWD/28

Abbreviations: ACR, alive with complete remission; AWD, alive with disease; chemo, chemotherapy; CR, complete tumor regression; CS, topical corticosteroids; DOD, died of disease; IFN, interferon-α; imiq, imiquimod; MC, mechlorethamine hydrochloride; NA, not available; PD, progressive disease; PR, partial tumor regression; pred, oral prednisone; PUVA, psoralen/UV-A light therapy; ret, retinoids; RT, radiotherapy; SD, stable disease.

Adapted from Kempf W, Ostheeren-Michaelis S, Paulli M, et al. Granulomatous mycosis fungoides and granulomatous slack skin: a multicenter study of the Cutaneous Lymphoma Histopathology Task Force Group of the European Organization for Research and Treatment of Cancer (EORTC). Arch Dermatol 2008;144(12):1610.

overlapping findings and cannot be discriminated by histologic examination alone. Typically, GMF has an atypical lichenoid CD4+CD8− lymphocytic infiltrate with interstitial histiocytes and/or perivascular granulomas with concomitant eosinophils and multinucleated giant cells.[9] Sarcoidal granulomas are also commonly encountered.[8] Tuberculoid, periadnexal, and granuloma annulare–like patterns are occasionally seen.[9]

Classic histologic features of GSS include dense diffuse dermal infiltrate of atypical, irregular, and convoluted lymphocytes that may extend to the subcutaneous tissue.[10] In the dermis, diffuse multinucleate giant cells and numerous histiocytes, which exhibit prominent elastophagocytosis and lymphophagocytosis, are observed.[10] The multinucleated giant cells show 20 to 30 nuclei in the periphery of the cytoplasm.[11] Loss of elastic

fibers usually correlates with the extent of the granulomatous infiltrate, and is a universal finding in GSS.[10] In the past, elastolysis involving the full thickness of the dermis was thought to be pathognomonic for GSS.[5] However, a more recent study showed loss of elastic fibers in both patients with GSS and patients with GMF.[8]

Clinical Presentation

The clinical presentation and skin manifestations of GMF are similar to those of classic MF, and patients may present with patches, plaques, tumors, erythroderma, poikilodermatous patches, and granuloma annulare–like lesions.[9] GMF may coexist with classic MF lesions.[11] Unlike GSS, patients with GMF present without pendulous skin folds, and extracutaneous spread is common.[8]

GSS is an extremely rare type of CTCL. GSS usually presents initially as asymptomatic, erythematous papules and plaques that progress, with elastic tissue loss, to bulky pendulous skin folds with a predilection for the axillae and groin of Caucasian men in their third to fifth decades of life.[5,8,11] Unlike granulomatous MF, extracutaneous spread is rare.[8] Most patients have a very slow progressive course.[11]

Systemic Associations

Patients with GMF and GSS are at risk for the development of second lymphoid neoplasias. Hodgkin lymphoma is the most common second neoplasia in patients with granulomatous CTCL and occurs in approximately 50% of cases.[8,11] Granulomatous CTCL may also be associated with MF, CD30+ anaplastic large-cell lymphoma, follicular lymphoma, chronic lymphocytic leukemia, diffuse large B-cell lymphoma, and lymphomatoid papulosis.[9,11]

Patients with CD8+ granulomatous CTCL appear to have an associated immunodeficiency. In a retrospective study of 4 patients with CD8+ granulomatous CTCL, nodal involvement was not seen but lung granulomas were found in all cases. All 4 patients had a history of immunodeficiency, either primary or iatrogenic, in addition to slowly progressive disease. Evaluation for an underlying immunodeficiency may be considered in patients with CD8+ granulomatous CTCL.[4]

Evaluation and Management

Granulomatous CTCLs are a diagnostic challenge. Predominant granuloma formation may obscure the atypical lymphoid infiltrate, delaying diagnosis and treatment.[1] Epidermotropism may or may not be present.[8–11] Detection of a monoclonal T-cell receptor (TCR) gene rearrangement can be a useful diagnostic adjunct in granulomatous CTCLs. However, a monoclonal T-cell population may also be found in reactive granulomatous disorders. In a recent study, rearrangement of TCRγ genes had sensitivity of 94% and specificity of 96% for granulomatous CTCL over reactive granulomatous disorders.[12] Diagnosis of GSS should be made on clinical findings and be restricted to patients presenting with lax skin folds.[1]

Granulomatous CTCLs show a therapy-resistant, slowly progressive course.[8] Treatment options for patients with GMF are similar to those recommended for patients with classic MF.[9] To date, there is no standard treatment for GSS.[11] Multiple treatment modalities, both individually and in combination, have been tried with some success. Partial remissions have been reported with psoralen in combination with ultraviolet A light (PUVA), radiotherapy, (poly)chemotherapy, systemic steroids, azathioprine, immunomodulating drugs such as interferon-α and interferon-γ, surgery, and some combination therapies.[13] Rapid recurrences of GSS after surgical excision have been reported.[14]

Clinical Results and Outcomes in the Literature

In a study of 15 patients with GMF and 4 with GSS, the disease showed a slowly progressive course. The most common treatment modalities were PUVA and interferon-α in addition to radiotherapy. Extracutaneous disease was observed in one-third of patients with GMF, and 6 of 15 patients with GMF died of the disease. By contrast, all patients with GSS were alive after a median follow-up of 17 years. GSS was therapy resistant, and complete remission was not achieved in any patient.[8]

In a recent retrospective case-control study of 27 patients with GMF and age-matched and stage-matched patients with classic MF, patients with GMF had poorer response to skin-directed therapies and progressed more frequently. Compared with patients with classic MF, patients with GMF achieved fewer partial or complete responses with topical (57% vs 83%) or ultraviolet light (62% vs 90%) therapy. Patients with GMF also required a longer time to achieve best response (median 35 vs 9 months) compared with patients with classic MF. The 5- and 10-year progression-free survival rates were significantly lower in the GMF group (59% and 33%) compared with the classic MF group (84% and 56%). However, this significant difference did not translate into worse overall survival. The 5- and 10-year overall survival rates were similar in patients with GMF (86% and 72%) and those with classic MF (85% and 85%) (**Table 2**).[9]

In a recent case report, a 35-year-old Caucasian man with GSS was successfully treated with ultraviolet A1 phototherapy. He was treated 3 times a week with 20 J/cm^2 and increasing in increments of 5 J/cm^2 to a dose of 50 J/cm^2 per session. He underwent a total of 45 sessions with a cumulative dose of 1495 J/cm^2, without any adverse events. A decrease in erythema and skin thickness was noted at the conclusion of the phototherapy, with continued treatment benefit at a 12-month follow-up.[15]

Summary

GMF and GSS are the most common types of granulomatous CTCL. GMF and GSS display

Table 2
Therapies and therapeutic responses in patients with granulomatous mycosis fungoides

Treatments	No. of Patients	No. of Patients Achieving PR or CR
	N = 25	
Skin directed		
Topical therapy[a]	23	13 (57%)
PUVA or NB-UVB	13	8 (62%)
TSEBT	4	4 (100%)
Systemic		
Oral bexarotene	9	5 (56%)
Interferon	1	1 (100%)
Romidepsin/vorinostat	5	1 (20%)
Alemtuzumab/zanolimumab	3	1 (33%)
Denileukin diftitox	2	1 (50%)
Pralatrexate	4	2 (50%)
Methotrexate	4	3 (75%)
Chemotherapy[b]	9	7 (78%)
Allogeneic SCT	2	2 (50%)
No treatment	1	1 (100%)
Treatments (median)		
Topical	2	
Systemic	1	
Total	4	
Systemic therapy		
Yes	16 (67%)	
No	8 (33%)	
Time to best response, mo		
Median	35	
Mean	56	
Best response		
CR	9 (38%)	
PR	13 (54%)	
Stable disease	2 (8%)	

Abbreviations: CR, complete response; NB, narrowband; PR, partial response; PUVA, psoralen plus ultraviolet A; SCT, stem cell transplantation; TSEBT, total skin electron beam therapy; UV, ultraviolet.
[a] Topical corticosteroids, nitrogen mustard, and bexarotene.
[b] Cladribine, liposomal doxorubicin, gemcitabine, vinorelbine, and combination chemotherapy with cyclophosphamide, doxorubicin, vincristine, prednisone (CHOP) or CHOP-based.
Adapted from Li JY, Pulitzer MP, Myskowski PL, et al. A case-control study of clinicopathologic features, prognosis, and therapeutic responses in patients with granulomatous mycosis fungoides. J Am Acad Dermatol 2013;69(3):371.e4; with permission.

overlapping histologic findings, but differ clinically by circumscribed areas of pendulous lax skin seen in GSS. Patients with GMF and GSS are at risk for the development of second lymphoid neoplasias, and require life-long observation.[8]

Granulomatous CTCLs show a therapy-resistant, slowly progressive course.[8] To date there is no standard treatment for granulomatous CTCL, and treatment options are similar to those recommended for patients with classic MF. In the past there has been controversy as to whether patients with GMF have a different prognosis than patients with classic MF. However, more recent studies have suggested that the prognosis of GMF is worse than that of classic MF.[8,9] Thus, patients with GMF may require a more aggressive treatment approach, and earlier systemic therapy may be warranted.[9]

LYMPHOMATOID GRANULOMATOSIS
Introduction

Lymphomatoid granulomatosis (LYG), a rare Epstein-Barr virus (EBV)-driven lymphoproliferative disorder, was first described in 1972 by Minars and colleagues.[16] It was initially considered to be a peripheral T-cell lymphoma because of the predominance of T lymphocytes, primarily helper T cells on histology.[17] However, TCR gene rearrangement clonality was not identified. LYG was reclassified as a T-cell–rich, large B-cell lymphoma, based on the presence of EBV-positive large B cells.[18]

Etiopathogenesis

The pathogenesis of this disease is unknown. Histologically, LYG is a pleomorphic angiocentric and angiodestructive infiltrate with atypical lymphohistiocytic cells.[19] Liebow and colleagues[20] discussed possible causes, including an oncogenic viral infection caused by EBV, chronic autoimmune disease, or immunodeficiency. There has been considerable debate in the past regarding the presence of B-cell populations in these T-cell infiltrates. Katzenstein and Peiper[21] evaluated 29 patients with lymphomatoid granulomatosis for EBV infection, and found 72% (21 of 29 patients) of patients to be positive for EBV DNA via polymerase chain reaction. McNiff and colleagues[22] evaluated 4 patients with LYG of the skin and lung. Biopsies revealed EBV RNA restricted to B lymphocytes in the skin of 1 patient and lung of 3 patients, suggesting that EBV may be associated with LYG (**Table 3**).

Clinical Presentation

LYG predominantly involves the lungs but can also present in the skin, kidneys (32%), central and peripheral nervous systems (33%), and, less commonly, the upper respiratory tract.[16,19,23,24] Lymph nodes and spleen are typically spared at initial diagnosis.[25] LYG occurs more commonly in men than in women and presents between the fourth and sixth decades.[25] Clinically, patients with pulmonary involvement present with cough, shortness of breath, and chest pain.[25,26] Systemic symptoms such as fever, malaise, weight loss, and myalgias commonly occur. Other common symptoms include peripheral neuropathy and arthralgias.[17,25,26] Although pulmonary involvement occurs in more than 90% of patients with LYG, it is not necessary for the diagnosis of LYG.

Cutaneous lesions, which occur in 20% to 60% of cases of LYG, can develop 2 weeks to 9 years before the development of pulmonary nodules, or develop simultaneously or after pulmonary involvement.[17,24] James and colleagues,[26] reporting on 44 patients with LYG, noted that skin manifestations can be painful and include subcutaneous nodules, dermal nodules, maculopapular eruptions, macular erythema, and ulcerations. These lesions are caused by arteritis of the small vessels of dermal and subcutaneous tissue. Cutaneous lesions can be transient and resolve spontaneously. Carlson and Gibson[17] presented 47 patients with LYG, of whom 24 had skin involvement. The most common cutaneous lesions they noted were red nodules ranging in size from 0.5 to 4 cm, the second most common being ulcerations.

Systemic Associations

LYG has been associated with lymphoma, which usually involves the central nervous system.[26] Lymphoma can develop in patients during the course of LYG, and has been reported to occur in 12% to 46% of patients.[24,26] Case reports also disclose an association with immunodeficiency states such as acquired immunodeficiency syndrome, common variable immunodeficiency, X-linked agammaglobulinemia, and hypogammaglobulinemia. Katzenstein and colleagues[27] reported patients with LYG to have a history of lymphoma, leukemia, biliary cirrhosis, chronic hepatitis, ulcerative colitis, sarcoidosis, and retroperitoneal fibrosis.

Evaluation and Management

There are no laboratory tests that can confirm the diagnosis of LYG, and they are usually nonspecific.[17] EBV serology is usually positive and immunoglobulin heavy-chain gene rearrangements may show monoclonality, oligoclonality, or polyclonality.[25] Chest radiographs commonly show bilateral nodular densities.[17] Skin biopsy is useful in the diagnosis of LYG, and helps differentiate LYG from other diseases in the differential including Wegener granulomatosis, lymphomatoid papulosis, malignant lymphoma, and other granulomatous disease.[17,22] Classically, pathology shows a pleomorphic, angiocentric, and angiodestructive granulomatous vasculitis, but histologic findings can be nonspecific. Typically these lesions show a small number of atypical EBV-positive B cells with a background of mononuclear cells made up of T cells, plasma cells, and histiocytes.[25] Neutrophils or eosinophils are not seen in biopsy specimens.

LYG can be divided into 3 grades based on histopathology, specifically the proportion of large B cells and the number of EBV-positive cells per

Table 3
Clinical results and outcomes in the literature: lymphomatoid granulomatosis (LYG)

Author, Year	No. of Patients	Treatment	Response	Duration of Remission (y)	Median Survival (mo)	Mortality Rate	Level of Evidence
Fauci et al,[29] 1982	15	13: cyclophosphamide 2 mg/kg/d and prednisone 1 mg/kg/d, dosing adjusted to maintain remission	7 complete responses (no relapse of LYG or lymphoma), 1 partial response	Median 5.2		53% (8 of 15 patients); 7 of these 8 patients developed malignant lymphoma	C
Katzenstein et al,[30] 1979	152	67: corticosteroids 42: corticosteroids and chemotherapy 13: chemotherapy 21: antibiotics 2: radiotherapy	38 patients with CR	Median 4.5	14	63.5% (94 of 148 patients)	C

C, case-control study or retrospective study.

Data from Fauci AS, Haynes BF, Costa J, et al. Lymphomatoid granulomatosis: prospective clinical and therapeutic experience over 10 years. N Engl J Med 1982;306(2):68–74; and Katzenstein AA, Carrington CB, Liebow AA. Lymphomatoid granulomatosis. A clinicopathologic study of 152 cases. Cancer 1979;43(1):360–73.

high-power field.[27] Lesions of grades 1 and 2 are considered low grade while grade 3 lesions are considered high grade.[25] Grade 1 lesions have rare large lymphoid cells and less than 5 EBV-positive cells per high-power field.[27] Grade 2 lesions have occasional large lymphoid cells and 5 to 50 EBV-positive cells per high-power field. Grade 3 lesions have "readily identified" large atypical B cells and more than 50 EBV-positive cells per high-power field.

Therapies that have been used include systemic corticosteroids, chemotherapy, and radiation therapy.[28] Corticosteroids improve neurologic and pulmonary symptoms transiently but are not effective as maintenance therapy. Patients with low-grade lesions can be observed, as a small percentage of these patients will have spontaneous remissions or no progression of their disease.[25] Low-grade lesions are typically treated with interferon, which enhances the host's immune system. It is given as interferon-α2b, 7.5 million units subcutaneously 3 times weekly, and the dose is increased based on the response and toxicities. Patients with high-grade lesions should be treated as for those with diffuse large B-cell lymphoma, and require immediate treatment. Rituximab is an anti-CD20 monoclonal antibody that has been used as a single agent in the treatment of LYG, with only limited data in the literature. Patients with high-grade LYG should be treated with a combination chemoimmunotherapy regimen, including rituximab, prednisone, etoposide, vincristine, cyclophosphamide, and adriamycin, for a total of 6 cycles. Another regimen includes rituximab, cyclophosphamide, vincristine, and prednisone. When disease recurrence is suspected, a repeat biopsy must be taken to determine recurrence and establish the grade, as management differs based on grading. Prognostic factors that indicate a poor outcome include the development of lymphoma and bilateral pulmonary involvement.[17]

Summary

LYG is a rare EBV-positive lymphoproliferative disorder with a male predominance, which typically presents between the fourth and sixth decades. The lungs are almost always affected. Therapy depends on the grade of the LYG lesion and can include oral corticosteroids, rituximab, and combined chemoimmunotherapy. In LYG patients with EBV-positive biopsies that show clonal B-cell proliferation, therapeutic options including antiviral therapy may be beneficial.[22]

REFERENCES

1. Scarabello A, Leinweber B, Ardigó M, et al. Cutaneous lymphomas with prominent granulomatous reaction: a potential pitfall in the histopathologic diagnosis of cutaneous T-and B-cell lymphomas. Am J Surg Pathol 2002;26(10):1259–68.

2. Shapiro PE, Pinto FJ. The histologic spectrum of mycosis fungoides/sezary syndrome (cutaneous T-cell lymphoma): a review of 222 biopsies, including newly described patterns and the earliest pathologic changes. Am J Surg Pathol 1994;18(7): 645–67.

3. Gallardo F, García-Muret M, Servitje O, et al. Cutaneous lymphomas showing prominent granulomatous component: clinicopathological features in a series of 16 cases. J Eur Acad Dermatol Venereol 2009;23(6):639–47.

4. Gammon B, Robson A, Deonizio J, et al. CD8(+) granulomatous cutaneous T-cell lymphoma: a potential association with immunodeficiency. J Am Acad Dermatol 2014;71:555–60.

5. LeBoit PE, Zackheim HS, White CR Jr. Granulomatous variants of cutaneous T-cell lymphoma: The histopathology of granulomatous mycosis fungoides and granulomatous slack skin. Am J Surg Pathol 1988;12(2):83–95.

6. Ackerman AB, Flaxman BA. Granulomatous mycosis fungoides. Br J Dermatol 1970;82(4):397–401.

7. Willemze R, Jaffe ES, Burg G, et al. WHO-EORTC classification for cutaneous lymphomas. Blood 2005;105(10):3768–85.

8. Kempf W, Ostheeren-Michaelis S, Paulli M, et al. Granulomatous mycosis fungoides and granulomatous slack skin: a multicenter study of the Cutaneous Lymphoma Histopathology Task Force Group of the European Organization for Research and Treatment of Cancer (EORTC). Arch Dermatol 2008;144(12): 1609–17.

9. Li JY, Pulitzer MP, Myskowski PL, et al. A case-control study of clinicopathologic features, prognosis, and therapeutic responses in patients with granulomatous mycosis fungoides. J Am Acad Dermatol 2013;69(3):366–74.

10. El-Khoury J, Kurban M, Abbas O. Elastophagocytosis: underlying mechanisms and associated cutaneous entities. J Am Acad Dermatol 2014;70(5): 934–44.

11. Shah A, Safaya A. Granulomatous slack skin disease: a review, in comparison with mycosis fungoides. J Eur Acad Dermatol Venereol 2012; 26(12):1472–8.

12. Pfaltz K, Kerl K, Palmedo G, et al. Clonality in sarcoidosis, granuloma annulare, and granulomatous mycosis fungoides. Am J Dermatopathol 2011;33(7):659–62.

13. Teixeira M, Alves R, Lima M, et al. Granulomatous slack skin. Eur J Dermatol 2007;17(5):435–8.

14. Clarijs M, Poot F, Laka A, et al. Granulomatous slack skin: treatment with extensive surgery and review of the literature. Dermatology 2003;206(4):393–7.

15. Oberholzer PA, Cozzio A, Dummer R, et al. Granulomatous slack skin responds to UVA1 phototherapy. Dermatology 2009;219(3):268–71.

16. Minars N, Kay S, Escobar MR. Lymphomatoid granulomatosis of the skin: a new clinicopathologic entity. Arch Dermatol 1975;111(4):493–6.

17. Carlson KC, Gibson LE. Cutaneous signs of lymphomatoid granulomatosis. Arch Dermatol 1991; 127(11):1693–8.

18. Colby TV. Current histological diagnosis of lymphomatoid granulomatosis. Mod Pathol 2012;25:S39–42.

19. Whittaker S, Foroni L, Luzzatto L, et al. Lymphomatoid granulomatosis–evidence of a clonal T-cell origin and an association with lethal midline granuloma. QJM 1988;68(256):645–55.

20. Liebow AA, Carrington CR, Friedman PJ. Lymphomatoid granulomatosis. Hum Pathol 1972;3(4): 457–558.

21. Katzenstein AL, Peiper SC. Detection of Epstein-Barr virus genomes in lymphomatoid granulomatosis: analysis of 29 cases by the polymerase chain reaction technique. Mod Pathol 1990;3(4):435–41.

22. McNiff JM, Cooper D, Howe G, et al. Lymphomatoid granulomatosis of the skin and lung: an angiocentric T-cell-rich B-cell lymphoproliferative disorder. Arch Dermatol 1996;132(12):1464–72.

23. Kessler S, Lund HZ, Leonard DD. Cutaneous lesions of lymphomatoid granulomatosis comparison with lymphomatoid papulosis. Am J Dermatopathol 1981;3(2):115–28.

24. Brodell RT, Miller CW, Eisen AZ. Cutaneous lesions of lymphomatoid granulomatosis. Arch Dermatol 1986;122(3):303–6.

25. Roschewski M, Wilson WH. Lymphomatoid granulomatosis. Cancer J 2012;18(5):469–74.

26. James WD, Odom RB, Katzenstein AA. Cutaneous manifestations of lymphomatoid granulomatosis: report of 44 cases and a review of the literature. Arch Dermatol 1981;117(4):196–202.

27. Katzenstein AL, Doxtader E, Narendra S. Lymphomatoid granulomatosis: insights gained over 4 decades. Am J Surg Pathol 2010;34(12):e35–48.

28. Holden C, Wells R, MacDonald D. Cutaneous lymphomatoid granulomatosis. Clin Exp Dermatol 1982;7(4):449–54.

29. Fauci AS, Haynes BF, Costa J, et al. Lymphomatoid granulomatosis: prospective clinical and therapeutic experience over 10 years. N Engl J Med 1982; 306(2):68–74.

30. Katzenstein AA, Carrington CB, Liebow AA. Lymphomatoid granulomatosis. A clinicopathologic study of 152 cases. Cancer 1979;43(1):360–73.

Foreign Body Granulomas

Ana M. Molina-Ruiz, MD, PhD*, Luis Requena, MD, PhD

KEYWORDS

- Granuloma • Foreign body • Dermatopathology • Management • Tattoos • Cosmetic fillers
- Drugs • Minerals

KEY POINTS

- The essential feature of foreign body granulomas is the presence of either identifiable *exogenous* (foreign) material or of *endogenous* material that has become altered in some way so that it acts as a foreign body.
- Foreign substances may penetrate the skin because of voluntary reasons, such as materials used in tattoos and cosmetic implants, or involuntary reasons, such as accidental inclusion of external substances secondary to cutaneous trauma.
- Cosmetic fillers can induce adverse reactions that can be very difficult to treat. Each filler has specific histopathologic features that can clearly associate the filler with the subsequent skin reaction.
- Cutaneous granulomatous reactions to drugs and medication can occur with (1) systemic medications, such as polyvinylpyrrolidone; (2) topical application of several substances for hemostasis or cosmetic reasons; and (3) following the injection of different drugs and vaccines.
- The correct diagnosis of most cutaneous granulomatous reactions is usually established by histopathologic study; however, imaging techniques like sonography can sometimes be useful.
- Complications associated with foreign body granulomatous reactions in the skin include inflammation, infection, persistent nodule formation, and poor cosmetic result. A thorough understanding of these issues is essential to maximize a correct treatment.

INTRODUCTION

A large list of foreign substances may penetrate the skin because of both voluntary and involuntary reasons. The first group includes the particle materials used in tattoos and cosmetic fillers, whereas the second group is almost always caused by accidental inclusion of external substances secondary to cutaneous trauma.[1] **Box 1** summarizes the most common foreign body agents found in cutaneous biopsies.

Histopathologically, most of these substances induce a foreign body granuloma with histiocytes (including epithelioid histiocytes), multinucleate giant cells derived from histiocytes, and variable numbers of other inflammatory cells. Multinucleate giant cells are often of foreign body type, with nuclei scattered irregularly throughout the cytoplasm; but Langhans giant cells are also seen.[2] This foreign body granuloma involves the dermis and often extends to the subcutaneous tissue. The causative agent may or may not be birefringent when sections are examined under polarized light.[2] Sometimes, secondary infection occurs in the preexisting foreign body granuloma.

Cutaneous foreign body granulomas may also develop secondary to endogenous material that has become altered in such a way that it is recognized as a foreign substance, as is the case of calcium deposits, urate, oxalate, keratin, and hair

Disclosures: The authors do not have any conflicts of interest to declare. The authors do not have any financial support for this article.
Department of Dermatology, Fundación Jiménez Díaz, Universidad Autónoma, Avda. Reyes Católicos 2, Madrid 28040, Spain
* Corresponding author.
E-mail address: amolinar@fjd.es

Dermatol Clin 33 (2015) 497–523
http://dx.doi.org/10.1016/j.det.2015.03.014

Box 1
Foreign substances that may be found in the skin

Tattoo pigments

Cosmetic fillers

  Collagen

  Hyaluronic acid

  Purified polysaccharide alginate

  Hyaluronic acid + dextranomer microparticles

  Poly-L-lactic acid

  Calcium hydroxylapatite

  Paraffin

  Silicone

  Polyvinylpyrrolidone

  Polymethyl-methacrylate microspheres and bovine collagen

  Hydroxyethylmethacrylate/ethylmethacrylate + hyaluronic acid

  Polyacrylamide hydrogel

  Polyalkylimide gel

Drugs and medications

  Polyvinylpyrrolidone

  Monsel solution

  Hydroquinone

  Glatiramer acetate

  Phosphatidylcholine

  Copolymer pentazocine

  Vitamin K1

  Interferon beta-1b

  Interferon beta

  Interferon alfa-2a

  Hepatitis B vaccine

  Disodium clodronate

  Leuprorelin acetate

  Sodium bisulfite

  Anabolic corticosteroids

  Zinc-containing insulin

  Exenatide

Mineral, metallic, and other particles

  Aluminum

  Silica

  Beryllium

  Zirconium

  Titanium

  Mercury

  Nickel

  Other metals

Miscellaneous particles

  Glass

  Sutures

  Fibers

  Starch

  Plants

  Splinters

  Cactus bristles

  Arthropod fragments

  Sea urchin spines

  Food particles

  Artificial hair

shafts. These endogenous materials are not included in this article. Herein, the authors focus on the most recent etiopathogenesis, clinical presentations, systemic associations, evaluation, and evidence-based management concerning cutaneous reactions to exogenous agents, with special emphasis on the microscopic morphology of the external particles, in order to specifically recognize the involved substance, something that is becoming increasingly important in case of litigation.

Concerning the pathogenesis, like other inflammatory processes, foreign body reactions are dynamic processes. It seems to be that the initial response against a foreign substance in the skin involves a neutrophilic infiltrate, which usually fails to deal with the foreign body. This neutrophilic infiltrate is later replaced by histiocytes and macrophages that engulf the foreign material. Sometimes macrophages are successful digesting the foreign body, but more often the foreign material resists degradation and remains within the cytoplasm of macrophages. Macrophages containing foreign body material within their cytoplasm are activated; they secrete different cytokines, which attract additional macrophages to the inflammatory focus. The result is the formation of a granuloma around the foreign body, which attempts to isolate the rest of the body from the sequestered indigestible material. Individual macrophages coalesce to form multinucleated foreign body giant cells, and T lymphocytes and fibroblasts are also components of the inflammatory response.

TATTOO PIGMENTS

Tattoos are produced by the mechanical introduction of insoluble pigments into the dermis. Most tattoos have cosmetic purposes, but occasionally carbon or some other pigment is traumatically implanted in an industrial or firearm accident.[3,4] In recent years, cosmetic tattooing is also used as permanent makeup in adult women for lips, eyelids, and eyebrows.[5] Also, henna tattoos are becoming more popular, especially among teenagers[6]; allergic and irritant reactions have been reported, especially when henna is used in combination with other coloring agents.[7] **Box 2** summarizes the main components of the most commonly used substances for tattooing according to the wanted color.

Tattoo Complications

In recent years, the incidence of complications secondary to tattoos is becoming rarer because of better hygiene during the tattooing process and because of the declining use of strong irritant substances, such as mercury salts. However, complications of tattoos are still sporadically reported and may be grouped into several broad categories:

- Infections introduced at the time of tattooing
- Cutaneous diseases that localize in tattoos, often in a Koebner-type phenomenon
- Allergic reactions to the tattoo pigments
- Photosensitivity reactions
- Tumors developed on preexisting tattoos
- Miscellaneous reactions

Rare systemic complications described in patients with tattoos include uveitis[8] and systemic sarcoidosis.[9]

DIAGNOSTIC EVALUATION
Histopathology

Histopathologically, usually tattoo pigments are easily visualized in hematoxylin-eosin stained sections. The pigment is mostly localized around the blood vessels of the upper and mid dermis; most pigment is seen as extracellular deposits between collagen bundles, although small amounts of pigmented particles may also be visualized within the cytoplasm of macrophages.[1] In many instances, the pigment is seen lying free in the dermis without an apparent inflammatory response (**Fig. 1**). Often the pigment is slightly refractile but not doubly refractile. In general, traumatic implanted pigments during working or sport accidents are larger and more variable in size and shape when compared with the relative small and homogeneous size and shape of the pigment particles used in decorative tattoos. Histopathologic patterns vary according to the composition of the used pigment. Hypersensitivity reactions include the development of a diffuse lymphohistiocytic infiltrate involving the full thickness of the dermis,[10] lichenoid reactions (which seem to be more frequent with red pigments) (**Fig. 2**),[11] sarcoidal granulomas,[12] granuloma annulare–like reaction,[13] necrobiosis lipoidica,[14] perforating granulomatous dermatitis,[15] vasculitis,[16] a pseudolymphomatous pattern,[17] and a morphealike reaction.[18] The overlying epidermis is usually normal, although spongiosis and pseudoepitheliomatous hyperplasia have been described.

Imaging

Other methods, such as ultrasound scanning, optical coherence tomography (OCT), or confocal scanning laser microscopy (CLSM), can be used for diagnostic evaluation of tattoo reactions and pre-evaluation of tattoos before laser removal. Carlsen and colleagues[19] have recently demonstrated for the first time that ultrasound, with histopathology as the comparative method, can quantify the severity of tattoo reactions and noninvasively diagnose the depth of the inflammatory process in the dermis. They proposed preoperative 20-MHz ultrasound scanning as a potentially useful method to guide therapeutic interventions by surgery and lasers. Other investigators suggest that examination by OCT[20] and CLSM[21] has an important future potential predicting good or poor outcome of laser removal.

TREATMENT
Tattoo Removal

Although tattoos were once considered to be permanent, technical and scientific progress in recent years has made it possible to remove tattoos by various treatment modalities. Contemporary technology involves the use of nonablative quality-switched lasers, which are considered to be the

---

Box 2
Composition of the tattoo pigments according to the color

- Black: coal and graphite
- Red: mercury salts, ferric hydrate, cadmium selenide
- Blue: cobalt compounds
- Green: chromium compounds
- Yellow: cadmium sulfide
- Purple: manganese compounds

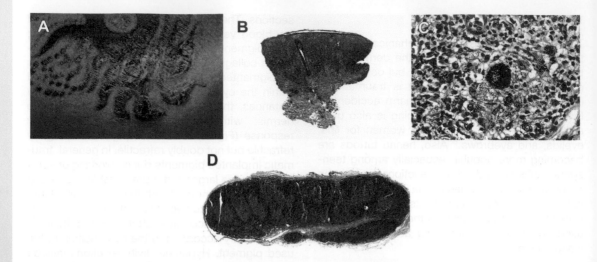

Fig. 1. Granulomatous reaction in a black tattoo. (*A*) Clinical features. (*B*) Scanning power showing a dense infiltrate involving the upper half of the dermis (H&E ×10). (*C*) Numerous black granules both inside the histiocytes and extracellularly (H&E ×400). (*D*) Abundant black pigment in the sentinel lymph node (H&E ×10).

gold standard treatment option for the removal of unwanted tattoo ink.[22] However, lasers may be invalidated in thick tattoo reactions and not curative as the power of the laser becomes diminutive already in the superficial dermis. In these cases, the culprit tattoo ink pigment deposited in the superficial dermis can be removed by surgery, including dermatome shaving. Topical tacrolimus has also been used successfully to treat a lichenoid tattoo reaction[23] and etanercept to treat a granulomatous reaction.[24] Current research in tattoo removal is focused on faster lasers and more effective targeting of tattoo pigment particles, including picosecond laser devices,[25]

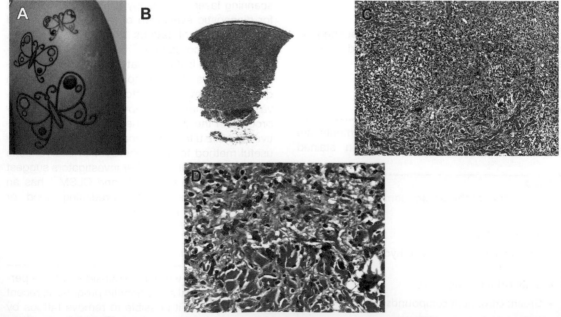

Fig. 2. Granulomatous reaction on the red areas of a tattoo. (*A*) Clinical features. (*B*) Scanning power showing a dense diffuse infiltrate involving the upper half of the dermis (H&E ×10). (*C*) The infiltrate is mostly composed of histiocytes (H&E ×200). (*D*) Numerous extracellular red granules of the tattoo material (H&E × 400).

multi-pass treatments, picosecond laser devices,[26] application of imiquimod,[27] and the use of microencapsulated tattoo ink.[22]

Cosmetic Implants

Injection techniques with filler agents are often used in cosmetic dermatology for wrinkle treatment, correction of atrophic scars, and soft tissue augmentation. Although fillers have low intrinsic toxicity,[28] all cosmetic implants can induce adverse reactions that have been recently reviewed.[29] Moreover, microneedle therapy, which includes skin puncture with multiple microsized needles to promote skin rejuvenation or increase transdermal delivery of topical medications, has been reported to introduce immunogenic particles into the dermis producing local or systemic hypersensitivity reactions.[30] **Table 1** summarizes the most common fillers currently used, and they appear classified into 2 main categories:

1. Transitory biodegradable or resorbable within months and years, respectively
2. Permanent or nonresorbable

Agents that are degraded within months, such as collagen, hyaluronic acid (HA), and agarose gel, may induce severe complications; but these will in general disappear spontaneously in a variable period of time. All other fillers can give rise to severe adverse reactions (**Fig. 3**), and these show little or no tendency to spontaneous improvement.

DIAGNOSTIC EVALUATION

Although the incidence of cosmetic filler injections is increasing worldwide, neither exact details of the procedure nor the agent used are always reported or remembered by patients. Thus, the availability of a precise diagnostic tool to detect cutaneous filler deposits could help clarify the association between the procedure and the underlying pathology. In litigation cases, dermatopathologic evaluation of skin specimens has been used as the most consistent proof of association between the filler and the subsequent skin reaction. The evaluation can be done because each filler has specific histopathologic features that are described in detail later. Unfortunately, patients who are subjects of cosmetic interventions try to avoid invasive procedures, such as biopsies in highly exposed areas (eg, in the face). For this reason, cutaneous sonography is also being used in the detection and identification of cosmetic filler deposits and to describe dermatologic abnormalities found associated with the presence of these agents. Wortsman and colleagues[31] have recently studied ultrasound to accurately identify in situ a filler agent, determine the location and size of cutaneous deposits, their presence in ectopic locations, and also measure local blood flow. They concluded that no other technology

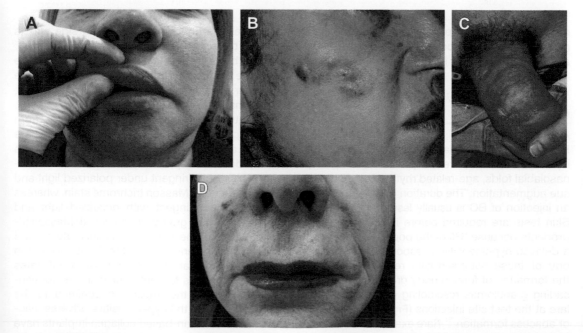

Fig. 3. Clinical features of granulomatous reactions to fillers. (A) Bovine collagen. (B) Silicone. (C) Paraffinoma. (D) Ethylmethacrylate and hydroxyethylmethacrylate particles (Dermalive).

Table 1
The most common fillers used for soft tissue augmentation

Category	Chemical Composition	Trademark
Resorbable within months	Bovine collagen	Zyderm, Zyplast
	Porcine collagen	Dermicol-P35
	Human-derived collagen	Autologen, Cosmoderm, Cosmoplast, Cymetra
	Hyaluronic acid	Hylaform, Restylane, Juvederm, Perlane, Macrolane
	Purified polysaccharide alginate	Novabel
Resorbable within years	Hyaluronic acid + dextranomer microparticles	Matridex, Reviderm Intra
	Poly-L-lactic acid microspheres + sodium carboxymethylcellulose, nonpyrogenic mannitol, sterile water	Sculptra, New Fill
	Calcium hydroxylapatite + carboxymethylcellulose and glycerin	Radiance, Radiesse
Permanent	Paraffin	—
	Silicone oil	Silikon 1000, Silskin
	Silicone gel	MDX 4-4011
	Silicone elastomer particles + polyvinylpyrrolidone	Bioplastique
	Polymethyl-methacrylate microspheres and bovine collagen	Artecoll, Arteplast, Artefill
	Hydroxyethylmethacrylate/ethylmethacrylate fragments and hyaluronic acid	DermaLive, DermaDeep
	Polyacrylamide hydrogel	Aquamid, Interfall, OutLine, Royamid, Formacryl, Argiform, Amazing gel, Bio-Formacryl, Kosmogel
	Polyalkylimide gel	Bio-Alcamid
	Polyvinylhydroxide microspheres + polyacrylamide gel	Evolution

currently available will provide all those parameters noninvasively and proposed ultrasound as a useful adjunct tool for further investigation into this field.

Transitory Biodegradable or Resorbable Implants

Animal collagen
Bovine collagen (BC) has been used as a transitory injectable filler to correct depressed scars, deep nasolabial folds, age-related rhytides, and soft tissue augmentation. The duration of the effect from an injection of BC is usually less than 6 months. Skin tests are required before injection of these products because 3% of the population develops a delayed hypersensitivity response. Histopathology of these hypersensitive reactions includes the formation of foreign body granulomas,[32] palisading granulomas resembling granuloma annulare at the test site injections (**Fig. 4**A),[33] and cyst or abscess formation.[34] Rare examples of disseminated and recurrent sarcoid like granulomatous panniculitis caused by BC injection have also

been described.[35] More uncommon side effects include bruising, reactivation of herpetic infection, verified bacterial infection, and local necrosis. The last one is mostly seen with BC injected at the glabellar area because of vascular interruption; injections should, thus, be avoided in this region. Histopathologically, BC appears different from human collagen (HC) because bundles of BC are thicker and show a homogeneous appearance nearly devoid of spaces between them. Furthermore, HC is birefringent under polarized light and stains green with Masson trichrome stain, whereas BC is not birefringent with polarized light and stains with a pale gray-violet color with Masson trichrome stain. The inflammatory infiltrate around the implant is denser when the BC is injected in the deep reticular dermis or partially infiltrates the subcutaneous fat, but panniculitis is not usually seen when the implant is confined to the dermis. To avoid the hypersensitive adverse reactions to BC, human-based collagen implants have been produced in recent years. No skin tests for hypersensitive reactions are required with

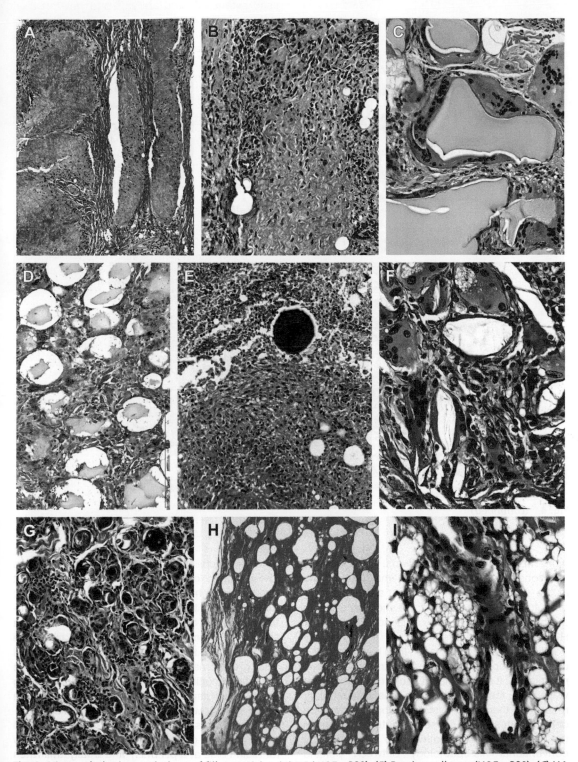

Fig. 4. Histopathologic morphology of filler particles. (*A*) BC (H&E ×200). (*B*) Porcine collagen (H&E ×200). (*C*) HA (H&E ×400). (*D*) Purified polysaccharide alginate (Novabel) (H&E ×400). (*E*) Dextranomer microparticles (Matridex) (H&E ×400). (*F*) Poly-ʟ-lactic acid (New-Fill) (H&E ×400). (*G*) Calcium hydroxylapatite + carboxymethylcellulose and glycerin (Radiance) (H&E ×400). (*H*) Paraffin (H&E ×400). (*I*) Silicone (H&E ×400). (*J*) Elastomer particles + polyvinylpyrrolidone (Bioplastique) (H&E ×400). (*K*) Polymethyl-methacrylate microspheres and BC (Artecoll) (H&E ×400). (*L*) Hydroxyethylmethacrylate/ethylmethacrylate fragments and HA (Dermalive) (H&E ×400). (*M*) Polyacrylamide hydrogel (Aquamid) (H&E ×200). (*N*) Polyalkylimide gel (Bio-Alcamid) (H&E ×400).

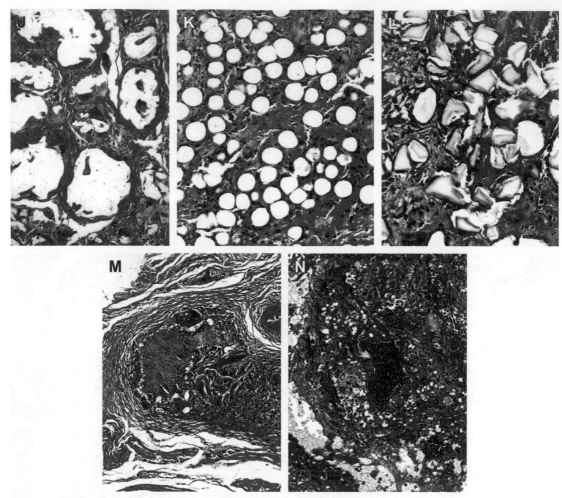

Fig. 4. (*continued*)

human-derived collagen products. Local adverse reactions include bruising, erythema, and swelling at the site of injection. However, a few cases of granulomatous reactions at the injection site[36] or at the skin test site after injection of acellular HC[37] have also been reported.

Fillers with porcine collagen (PC) have also been used with good cosmetic results and few adverse reactions.[38] It seems that PC does not require previous skin testing; it induces less inflammatory response than BC; histopathologic evaluation demonstrates that PC seems integrated within the host tissue, being difficult to distinguish by conventional histopathology between porcine and HC bundles (see **Fig. 4**B).[39]

Hyaluronic acid

Injections of HA gel are now used as resorbable filler for filling out wrinkles of the face, soft tissue augmentation, and correction of all types of

defects, such as scars and facial lipoatrophy. The longevity of the injected gel lasts for about 6 months. HA has no organ or species specificity; thus, in theory there is no risk of an allergic reaction. Very few adverse hypersensitivity reactions secondary to injections of HA used as filler have been reported. Histopathologically, they consisted of a granulomatous foreign body reaction, with abundant multinucleated giant cells surrounding an extracellular basophilic amorphous material (see **Fig. 4**C), which was the injected HA gel.[40,41] Scant amounts of HA may also be seen within multinucleated giant cells. The HA stains positively for alcian blue at a pH of 2.7 and is negative when examined under polarized light. Rarely described histopathologic findings at the injection sites of HA include a prominent eosinophilic granulomatous reaction[42] and a suppurative granuloma without evidence of infection.[43] Sonographically, pure HA appears as scattered anechoic round structures (pseudocysts), whereas the mixed formulation (HA and lidocaine) presents pseudocysts with inner echoes (debris) and septa.[31] The most serious complication of HA injections is the iatrogenic blindness as a direct consequence of filler embolization into the ophthalmic artery following cosmetic injections.[44,45]

Purified polysaccharide alginate

Five cases of granulomatous reactions to a new resorbable filler consisting of the purified polysaccharide alginate (Novabel) have been described when injected into tear troughs and/or the dorsa of hands.[46,47] No systemic complications have been described as secondary to the injections of this filler. Histopathologically, the granulomatous reaction was confined to the deep dermis and subcutaneous fat, which were involved by numerous multinucleated giant cells and histiocytes. Within this granulomatous reaction, a nonpolarizing exogenous material was identified consisting of slightly bluish deposits of variable size and shape, some of which were well delineated, others with a blurred or spiky perimeter, and frequently showed retraction in a clear vacuole (see **Fig. 4**D). These particles of Novabel reacted weakly with periodic acid-Schiff (PAS) and alcian blue but were intensely stained with toluidine blue.

Hyaluronic acid + dextranomer microparticles

A mixture of nonanimal-stabilized HA and dextranomer microspheres (Matridex, Reviderm Intra) has also been used as a resorbable filler. Only one case of a granulomatous reaction caused by this filler has been described in the literature. Histopathology of that case demonstrated a suppurative granuloma surrounding the HA and the spherical dark bluish particles that represented the dextranomer microparticles (see **Fig. 4**E).[48]

Poly-L-lactic acid

Poly-L-lactic acid (PLLA) is a resorbable filler that has been used to correct the signs of lipoatrophy in human immunodeficiency virus (HIV)–infected patients receiving antiprotease treatment as well as for facial cosmetic augmentation. It induces tissue augmentation that lasts up to at least 24 months. This filler frequently develops nodules at the site of injection, which are palpable but generally nonvisible. Histopathology of the nodules demonstrates a foreign-body granulomatous reaction, with numerous multinucleated giant cells surrounding translucent particles of different sizes, most of them showing a fusiform, oval, or spiky shape, which are birefringent under polarized light examination (see **Fig. 4**F).[49]

Calcium hydroxylapatite

Calcium hydroxylapatite (CH) is another resorbable filler composed of CH microspheres that stimulate the endogenous production of collagen. These microspheres induce almost no foreign body reaction and they show a bluish color and a round or oval shape. When this agent is injected in the lips, it tends to be associated with a high incidence of nodules. However, in some patients, CH microspheres may induce a foreign body granulomatous reaction, and blue-gray microspheres in the extracellular matrix or within multinucleated giant cells can be seen (**Fig. 4**G).[41] On ultrasound, CH appears as hyperechoic deposits with variable degrees of posterior acoustic shadowing.[31]

Nonresorbable or Permanent Implants

Paraffin

Paraffin is no longer used as filler because of its frequent adverse reactions; but because it is a nonresorbable material, it is still possible to see granulomatous reactions secondary to injections performed many years ago. These granulomatous reactions, also named paraffinomas, consist histopathologically of a mostly lobular panniculitis, in which the subcutaneous fat exhibits a Swiss-cheese appearance, with cystic spaces of variable size and shape, surrounded by foamy histiocytes and multinucleated giant cells. The surrounding dermis and the connective tissue of the subcutaneous septa show considerable sclerosis.[50] Sclerosing lipogranuloma is a specific form of paraffinoma, which results from injection of paraffin in the penis causing fibrosis and deformity of the penis body (see **Fig. 4**H).[51]

Silicone

Silicone is the most widely used filler material for soft tissue augmentation. Recently, it has also been injected as a filler to circumvent facial lipoatrophy in HIV infected patients receiving antiprotease treatment. Silicone gel is capable of migrating to distant sites, where it may give rise to an inflammatory reaction and hamper clinical diagnosis. Although in the past decade there has been considerable controversy in the literature about the relationship between systemic scleroderma and other connective tissue diseases and the use of breast implants containing silicone gel, there seems to be little scientific basis for any association between silicone breast implants and any well-defined connective tissue disease. Recently, 4 cases of a new type of adverse reaction to injected silicone simulating orofacial granulomatosis have been described.[52] The reaction consisted of recurrent episodes of unilateral, asymmetric facial edema of the cheek. Histopathology demonstrated a granulomatous reaction around silicone particles.[53] Histopathologic findings in local reactions to implants of silicone are variable depending mainly on the form of the injected silicone. Solid elastomer silicone induces an exuberant foreign body granulomatous reaction, whereas silicone oil and gel induce a sparser inflammatory response.[54] Silicone particles appear as groups of round empty vacuoles of different sizes between collagen bundles or within macrophages, and the particles are not birefringent under polarized light (see **Fig. 4**I). Sonographically, silicone oil appears as hyperechoic deposits snow storm with a high degree of sound scattering, similar to the pattern reported in patients with ruptured breast implants whereby the initially anechoic silicone is suddenly expelled and can freely mix and/or spread through the fat lobules of the subcutaneous tissue.[31] Pure silicone appears anechoic when injected without pressure in the porcine skin.[31]

Polyvinylpyrrolidone

A permanent filler, composed of particles of polymerized silicone elastomer dispersed in a carrier of polyvinylpyrrolidone (PVP) (Bioplastique), has been recently introduced for correction of facial rhytides and lip augmentation. Granulomas secondary to this filler are uncommon but when develop consist of irregularly shaped cystic spaces containing translucent, jagged pop corn, nonbirefringent particles of varying size dispersed in a sclerotic stroma, surrounded by abundant multinucleated foreign body giant cells (see **Fig. 4**J).[55] Although the material is nonbirefringent, crystalloid particles are better seen when lowering the microscope condenser.

Polymethyl-methacrylate microspheres and bovine collagen

Another permanent biphasic filler, composed of polymethylmethacrylate microspheres suspended in a degradable BC solution as a carrier (Artecoll), is used mostly in Europe as a cosmetic microimplant for correction of facial wrinkles and furrows, perioral lines, small scars, and other subdermal defects. Because this filler contains BC, it is mandatory to perform an intradermal test before the first use of this filler. Histopathologically, adverse reactions to this filler show a nodular or diffuse granulomatous infiltrate surrounding rounded vacuoles of similar shape and size, which mimic normal adipocytes and correspond to the implanted polymethylmethacrylate microspheres (see **Fig. 4**K).[56] The microspheres may be distinguished from normal adipocytes because they

are markedly homogeneous in size and shape. Recently, a study analyzed the biological behavior of Artecoll injected into the mouse ear.[57] Histopathologic analyses of the ear, liver, and kidney were performed revealing the development of an intense granulomatous reaction of the foreign body type in the right ear, periportal and intralobular infiltrates in the liver, and interstitial nephritis and chronic pyelonephritis in the kidney. Sonographically, polymethylmethacrylate deposits at early stages are generally small (<1 cm), appearing as multiple bright hyperechoic dots producing a mini comet-tail-shaped artifact (posterior reverberance); later on (more than 6 months after injection), some of the larger filler deposits acquire posterior acoustic shadowing artifacts.[31]

Hydroxyethylmethacrylate/ethylmethacrylate fragments and hyaluronic acid

Another permanent biphasic filler is composed of ethylmethacrylate and hydroxyethylmethacrylate particles suspended in an HA gel (Dermalive). Histopathologically, granulomatous reactions to this filler consist of nodular infiltrates of macrophages and multinucleated giant cells with numerous pseudocystic structures of different sizes and shapes containing polygonal, pink, translucent, nonbirefringent foreign bodies (see **Fig. 4**L).[58] Transepidermal elimination of the product may occur.

Polyacrylamide hydrogel

An injected hydrophilic gel of polyacrylamide (Aquamid) has been used in large quantities mostly in China, Ukraine, and the former Soviet Union for breast, buttock, and calf augmentation. More recently, it has been used in European countries for treatment of antiretroviral-related facial lipoatrophy in HIV-infected patients as well as for correction of acquired or congenital malformations with depressed skin. This permanent filler may cause nodules after the injections that frequently develop secondary localized bacterial infection.[59] Granulomas secondary to this filler are composed of macrophages, foreign body giant cells, lymphocytes, and red cells surrounding a basophilic multivacuolated nonbirefringent material, which corresponds to the polyacrylamide hydrogel (see **Fig. 4**M). This material shows some histopathologic similarity to HA, although granulomas secondary to HA usually show a less dense inflammatory infiltrate than those secondary to polyacrylamide hydrogel. Polyacrylamide hydrogel is positive with alcian blue stain, and it is not birefringent under polarizing microscopy.

Polyalkylimide gel

Bio-Alcamid is a permanent translucent gel filler made of a hydrophilic biopolymer composed of sterile water and polyalkylimide polymer. It has been used to increase volume in the cheeks in HIV-infected patients with facial lipoatrophy related to antiretroviral therapy as well as for buttock augmentation, correction of scar depressions, and posttraumatic subcutaneous atrophy. Few histopathologic studies describing the adverse reactions to this filler have been reported, and they described basophilic amorphous material corresponding to the implanted material, surrounded by epithelioid histiocytes, foreign body multinucleated giant cells, neutrophils, and red cells (see **Fig. 4**N).[60]

Granulomatous Reactions Associated with Microneedle Therapy

Microneedle therapy includes skin puncture with multiple microsized needles to promote skin rejuvenation or increase transdermal delivery of topical medications. In cosmetic practices, various nonapproved cosmeceuticals are applied before microneedling to enhance the therapeutic effects, introducing immunogenic particles into the dermis and potentiating local or systemic hypersensitivity reactions. Despite the increasing popularity of these cosmetic practices, there are few data about their safety; the use of products for intradermal injection in humans has not been regulated yet.

Soltani-Arabshahi and colleagues[30] recently described 3 cases of facial granulomas following microneedle therapy for skin rejuvenation. Two patients had undergone microinjection of the same branded topical moisturizer (Vita C Serum) during microneedle therapy and had a positive patch test reaction to this agent. Biopsy showed foreign body–type granulomas in all cases. Treatment with topical and oral corticosteroids as well as oral tetracyclines led to partial improvement in one case and resolution in another.

Granulomatous Reactions Associated with Mesotherapy

Mesotherapy is a procedure that involves the injection of substances into the dermis and subcutaneous tissue for medical or esthetic problems. Although mesotherapy is gaining popularity in most countries, there is limited knowledge about its efficacy and safety. The products used in mesotherapy are a combination of herbal and allopathic medicines, and their mechanism of action is unknown or doubtful. Previously, it was thought that side effects of mesotherapy were limited to minor bruising. Recently, many skin reactions to mesotherapy have been reported in the literature, including atypical mycobacterial infections, urticaria, lichenoid eruptions, exacerbation of psoriasis, sporotrichosis, pigmentation problems, skin

necrosis, ecchymoses, prolonged swelling and tenderness, ulceration, and hematoma formation. Cutaneous granulomatous reactions and panniculitis have also been noted.[61]

Treatment of Complications Associated with Filler Injections

Complications associated with filler injections can be categorized as immediate-, early, or late-onset events and subcategorized into mild, moderate, and severe. A thorough understanding of these issues is essential to ensure the safe use of these soft tissue fillers and to maximize the treatment of soft tissue filler complications.[62]

Immediate-onset complications

Immediate-onset complications include undercorrection and overcorrection, implant visibility, and vascular compromise. Venous obstruction is typically associated with shallower skin breakdown, whereas arterial occlusion may lead to sudden iatrogenic blindness and broad and deep skin loss.[63] In the case of HA injection, firm massage can be used to disperse excessive, superficial, or unaesthetic filler placement; in some cases, hyaluronidase can also be of help. Other filling agents may require reduction of the product using several methods, including simple unroofing with a needle tip or superficial dermabrasion. Treatment of vascular occlusion should be swift and aggressive.[64] Injection should be stopped and aspiration attempted; the area should be massaged and warm compresses applied to increase vasodilatation. Additionally, 2% nitroglycerine paste can be considered to cause further vasodilatation. The use of hyperbaric oxygen can also be considered in the case of dramatic vascular compromise and impending necrosis. Localized skin breakdown should be treated with topical or systemic antibiotics, and conservative debridement should also be performed when necessary.

Early onset complications

Early onset (3–14 days) complications include noninflammatory and inflammatory persistent nodules and angioedema. Noninflammatory nodules can be treated with observation, gentle massage, patient reassurance, and, sometimes, hyaluronidase. Inflammatory nodules can be treated with incision and drainage (with culture) and empiric treatment with a macrolide or tetracycline antibiotic (which also have antiinflammatory and immunomodulatory effects).[65] Antibiotic treatment should be continued for a total of 4 to 6 weeks; if the inflammatory nodule persists, intralesional corticosteroids may also be used. Angioedema can be related to the material or to host factors; true immune-mediated angioedema is rare, estimated as less than 1 to 5 in 10,000, and thought to be related to protein contaminants present in the material.[66,67] HA-related angioedema can be treated with hyaluronidase or removal of the HA derivative.

Delayed-onset complications

Delayed-onset (>14 days) complications include persistent erythema and telangiectasias at the site of injection that can be treated with hyaluronidase and a 532- or 1064-nm laser.[68] However, the more problematic delayed-onset complications are inflammatory nodules, granulomas, and sterile abscesses. These complications can be managed with multidrug oral antibiotic therapy and intralesional corticosteroid injection using ultradilute solutions and treating repeatedly. Sometimes, surgical excision or destruction of the injected agent is the only therapeutic possibility, resulting in worse cosmetic results than those that were attempted to correct by filler in the first place. Anecdotic reports have described improvement of the foreign body granulomas with colchicine,[53] laser therapy,[69] allopurinol,[70] cyclosporin, tacrolimus, ascomycin,[71] and isotretinoin.[72]

DRUGS AND MEDICATIONS

Numerous reports of cutaneous granulomatous reactions to different drugs and medications have been described in the literature. These reactions can occur with (1) systemic medications,

such as PVP, that may show dermal deposits as the cutaneous expression of the PVP storage disease; (2) topical application of several substances for hemostasis or cosmetic reasons; and (3) following injection of different drugs and vaccines.

Both tuberculoid or foreign body granulomatous reactions after topical applications of several substances as well as local panniculitis secondary to injections of different drugs and medications have been described. The exact mechanism of these reactions is not known, but probably they occur as consequence of a multifactorial etiopathogenesis whereby vasoconstriction with tissue ischemia, inflammatory response to precipitated drug in the tissues, trauma, and hypersensitivity reactions after repeated injections are implicated. Some of these reactions show specific histopathologic findings that allow the diagnosis of the applied or injected medication.[1]

Systemic Drugs

PVP was originally developed as a plasma expander but is currently widely used in skin care products, fruit juices, and as a retarding agent in some drugs. It has also been inappropriately used for intravenous injections as a "blood tonic."[73] Larger polymers of PVP are phagocytized by macrophages and permanently stored in the reticular endothelial system, leading to the so-called PVP storage disease (Fig. 5).[74] A variety of skin changes ranging from clinically normal skin to swelling, papules, granulomas, and

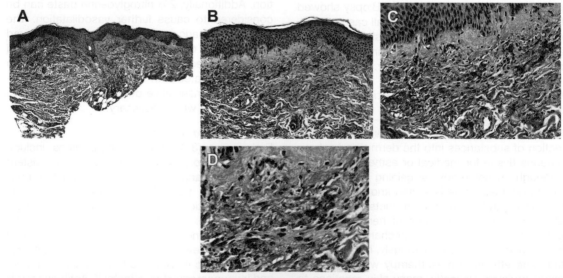

Fig. 5. Histopathologic findings in the skin of a patient with polyvinylpyrrolidone storage disease. (*A*) Low power showing a basophilic granular material in the superficial dermis (H&E ×20). (*B*) The basophilic granular material is arranged interstitially (H&E ×40). (*C*) Some of the histiocytes contain the same basophilic material within their cytoplasm(H&E ×200). (*D*) Still higher magnification showing both intra and extracellular basophilic granular material (H&E ×400).

pseudotumors may occur.[75] Clinically, it may be confused with connective tissue disease, pigmented purpura, storage disease, or osteomyelitis. Histopathologically, blue-gray vacuolated histiocytes are found around blood vessels and adnexal structures.[76] The cells are large and are positive with mucicarmine, colloidal iron, and alkaline Congo red stains. They are negative with PAS and alcian blue stains. By immunohistochemistry, these cells are CD68 positive. Usually, there is little if any accompanying inflammation; but occasionally, there may be foreign body reaction.

Many HIV-infected patients initiating antiretroviral therapy develop immune reconstitution inflammatory syndrome (IRIS). IRIS is defined as a paradoxic clinical worsening caused by a subclinical opportunistic pathogen (unmasking IRIS) or by a previously known treated, completed, or ongoing opportunistic infection (paradoxic IRIS). Several noninfective cutaneous diseases have also been described as an expression of IRIS. One of them consisted of multiple, linear nodular lesions that develop at cutaneous intravenous drug injection sites and that may mimic polyarteritis nodosa, false aneurysms, and lymphatic spread of infections.[77] Histopathologically, these lesions show a sarcoidal granulomatous reaction to extravasated suspended drug particles in which inert material has been identified.[77] An IRIS-associated foreign body granulomatous reaction has also been described in tattoos and in tribal scars containing long-standing burnt carbon.[78] It has been hypothesized that a highly active antiretroviral therapy–augmented T-helper response

with macrophage activation via interleukin 2 and interferon delta is responsible for these granulomatous reactions as an expression of IRIS.[78]

Topical Medications

Application of Monsel solution (20% aqueous ferric subsulfate) for hemostasis in minor surgical procedures causes ferrugination of dermal collagen, which appears coated with a slightly refractile, gray-brown substance, which is strongly positive with Perl's reaction for iron.[79] Some of the ferruginated collagen fibers may become calcified and eliminated through the epidermis. These ferruginated collagen fibers act as foreign bodies to elicit a granulomatous reaction (**Fig. 6**).[80]

Chronic application of certain topical agents containing hydroquinone, mercury, quinine, phenol, or picric acid can induce the development of the so-called exogenous ochronosis.[81] This disease affects mainly patients with high skin phototypes (IV, V, and VI) in the Fitzpatrick scale and manifests as pigmented papular lesions located on the areas of the face where the cream was applied, mostly the forehead, malar areas, neck, and sometimes the ears (**Fig. 7**A).[82] Skin atrophy, striae distensae, and acne also develop.[83] Ochronosis is histopathologically characterized by a striking discoloration (basophilia) of the collagen fibers in the upper dermis, followed by the appearance of characteristic yellow-brown or ochre-colored, banana-shaped fibers in the papillary dermis (banana bodies) (see **Fig. 7**B–D).[84] Sometimes a foreign body granuloma[85] develops

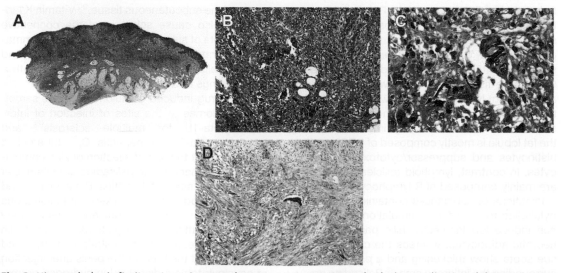

Fig. 6. Histopathologic findings in a pigmented area secondary to Monsel solution application. (*A*) Scanning power showing a diffuse infiltrate involving the upper half of the dermis (H&E ×10). (*B*) Ferruginated collagen bundles surrounded by a granulomatous reaction (H&E ×200). (*C*) Higher magnification of the ferrugination of the collagen bundles (H&E ×400). (*D*) Perls' prussian blue stain ×200 showing strong positivity for iron.

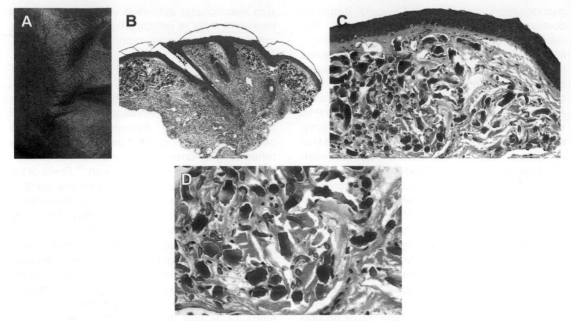

Fig. 7. Exogenous ochronosis. (*A*) An African American woman with hyperpigmentation around the eyes. (*B*) Scanning power showing yellow bodies in the upper dermis (H&E ×20). (*C*) Higher magnification shows a flattened epidermis and a thin band of spared superficial dermis with banana bodies beneath (H&E ×200). (*D*) Still higher magnification of the banana bodies (H&E ×400).

around these banana bodies; in rare instances, transepidermal elimination of these altered collagen bundles has been described.[86]

Injected Drugs

Subcutaneous glatiramer acetate injections for the treatment of multiple sclerosis have been reported to induce localized panniculitis (**Fig. 8**).[87] Histopathology can orientate the diagnosis in these cases showing a mostly lobular panniculitis with lipophagic granuloma, with scattered neutrophils and eosinophils both in the septa and the fat lobules. Connective tissue septa show widening, fibrosis, and frequent lymphoid follicles with germinal center formation. Immunohistochemistry demonstrates that the inflammatory infiltrate involving the fat lobule is mostly composed of CD68 positive histiocytes and suppressor/cytotoxic T lymphocytes. In contrast, lymphoid follicles at the septa are mainly composed of B lymphocytes.[87]

Injections of substances containing phosphatidylcholine to treat fat accumulation and lipomas can induce lobular neutrophilic panniculitis with necrotic adipocytes, whereas the connective tissue septa show thickening and a pseudocapsule surrounding the inflamed area.[88] Palisading granulomas with necrobiosis have been also described associated with the presence of foreign material introduced through the use of a lubricating agent

containing a copolymer (Carbopol 934) for liposuction.[89]

Pentazocine injections cause sclerodermoid plaques at the sites of injection secondary to thrombosis of small vessels and endoarteritis, with subsequent granulomatous inflammation, necrosis of adipocytes, lipophagic granuloma, and pronounced fibrosis of the dermis and connective septa of the subcutaneous tissue.[90] Vitamin K1 injections also cause sclerosis of the connective tissue septa of subcutaneous fat and an inflammatory infiltrate composed of lymphocytes and plasma cells, closely resembling the histopathologic findings of deep morphea.[91]

Other drug-induced granulomas include sarcoidal granulomas at the sites of injection of interferon beta-1b for multiple sclerosis[92] and interferon alfa-2a for hepatitis C,[93] tuberculoid granulomas at the site of injection of zinc containing insulin,[94] necrobiotic palisading granulomas at the injection sites of hepatitis B vaccine[95] and disodium clodronate,[96] mixed granulomatous reaction combining sarcoidal and foreign body granulomas after depot injections of leuprorelin acetate for treatment of prostatic cancer,[97] and granulomas at the base of the penis after injection of acyclovir tablets dissolved in hydrogen peroxidase as self-treatment for recurrent genital herpes.[98] Ophthalmologic drops containing sodium bisulfite may induce facial papules

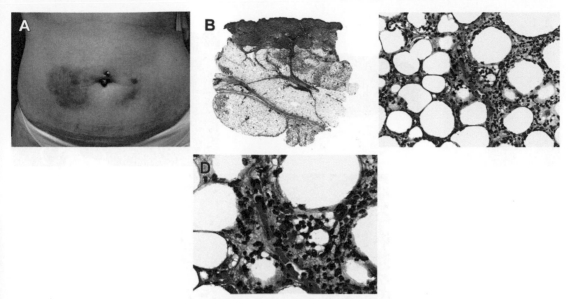

Fig. 8. Panniculitis at the injection sites of glatiramer acetate. (*A*) Erythematous plaque at the paraumbilical region. (*B*) Scanning power showing a mostly lobular panniculitis (H&E ×10). (*C*) Lipophagic granuloma with some scattered neutrophils and eosinophils (H&E ×200). (*D*) Higher magnification shows a polymorphous infiltrate composed of lymphocytes, histiocytes, neutrophils and eosinophils (H&E ×400).

histopathologically characterized by sarcoidal granulomas containing black-brown pigment within the cytoplasm of multinucleated giant cells.[99] Injected anabolic corticosteroids, which are often used for bodybuilders, have been reported to induce a cutaneous granulomatous reaction.[100] Foreign bodies typical of steroids can be found, together with areas of calcification and ossification with lamellar bone. Multi-vacuolated macrophages can be observed in the fibrous tissue close to these areas of calcification and ossification (**Fig. 9**).

Exenatide is a glucagonlike peptide-1 agonist medication, belonging to the group of incretin mimetics, approved in 2005 for the treatment of diabetes mellitus type 2. It is administered as a subcutaneous injection and may cause a nodular, eosinophilic-rich granulomatous panniculitis.[101,102] The authors have seen a case of granulomatous reaction at the site of injection of exenatide, probably elicited by the medisorb microspheres used for delayed release of exenatide (**Fig. 10**).

MINERAL AND METALLIC PARTICLES
Aluminum

Aluminum hydroxide is used as an effective adjuvant in a wide range of vaccines for enhancing the immune response to the antigen. Contact sensitivity,[103] inflammatory nodular reactions,[104] and cases of late-onset cutaneous lymphoid nodules (pseudolymphomatous reaction)[105,106] have been described in the skin after aluminum-adsorbed vaccination (**Fig. 11**). Aluminum chloride (Drysol) is used as a hemostatic agent for minor surgical procedures and often provokes an unusual histiocytic reaction in biopsies of skin previously treated with it. These lesions are usually not clinically apparent.[107] Aluminum salts used in tattooing rarely cause a granulomatous reaction in the skin; however, a delayed hypersensitivity granulomatous reaction has been reported on the eyelids following the use of aluminum-silicate in blepharopigmentation, a process that attempts to produce a permanent line along the eyelid margin, simulating a cosmetic eyeliner.[108]

Histopathologic examination of the nodular lesions after aluminum-adsorbed vaccines show deep dermal or subcutaneous nodules characterized by a central zone of degenerated collagen surrounded by a rim of histiocytes containing bluish granules in their cytoplasm and lymphoid aggregates, some of them with germinal center formation, and abundant eosinophils.[109] The aluminum can be confirmed by x-ray microanalysis or by the solochrome azurine stain, in which crystals of aluminum salts stain a deep gray-blue color.[110] Skin biopsies of aluminum tattoos after the topical application of aluminum chloride show individual and clusters of histiocytes containing round to slightly indented single nuclei with abundant basophilic or occasionally amphophilic granules. Granules vary slightly in size and shape and measure up to 1 to 2 mm in diameter

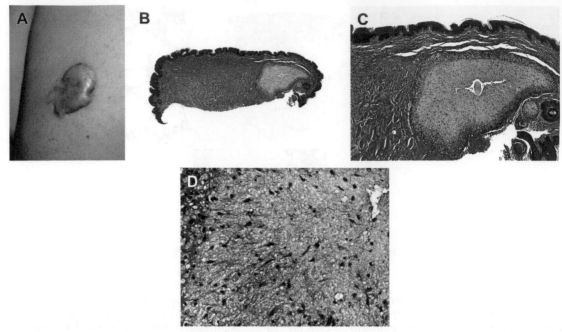

Fig. 9. Keloid scar treated with triamcinolone injections. (*A*) An indurated plaque on the lateral side of the left arm. (*B*) Scanning magnification showing a keloid on the left side of the picture and a rounded deposit of triamcinolone on the right side of the picture (H&E ×10). (*C*) At higher magnification, triamcinolone appears as a foamy material surrounded by a palisade of histiocytes (H&E ×40). (*D*) At still higher magnification, triamcinolone shows a basophilic granular appearance (H&E ×400).

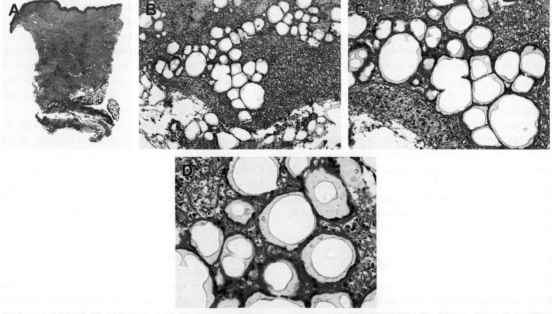

Fig. 10. Histopathologic findings at the site of exenatide injection. (*A*) Scanning power showing a normal dermis with an inflammatory process in the upper subcutaneous tissue (H&E ×10). (*B*) Higher magnification shows cystic spaces replacing the fat lobules (H&E ×100). (*C*) At higher magnification, a ring of foreign material can be observed at the periphery of these structures (H&E ×200). (*D*) Detailed view of the foreign material showing its amphophilic and slightly refractile appearance (H&E ×400).

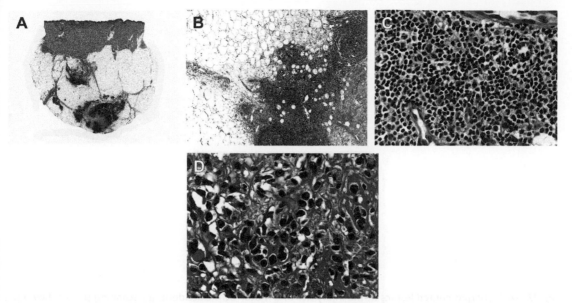

Fig. 11. Histopathologic findings of a hypersensitivity reaction at the site injection of an aluminum-containing vaccine. (*A*) Scanning power showing nodular infiltrates in the subcutaneous tissue (H&E ×10). (*B*) Dense nodular lymphocytic infiltrate at the interface between the septa and the fat lobule (H&E ×40). (*C*) Higher magnification showing that the infiltrate was mostly composed of lymphocytes with scattered plasma cells and eosinophils (H&E ×200). (*D*) Still higher magnification demonstrated that almost all histiocytes contained a basophilic granular material within their cytoplasm (H&E ×400).

and correspond to aluminum particles.[107] Histopathologic examination in the case of blepharopigmentation with aluminum salts revealed a delayed-hypersensitivity granulomatous reaction to aluminum with pigment granules in the lower dermis associated with epithelioid cells, giant cells, lymphohistiocytic infiltration, and tissue necrosis.[108]

Silica

Silica is a frequent contaminant of the skin wounds after sports or motor traffic accidents. Silica particles appear as dirt, sand, rock, or glass; they induce papules and nodules at the sites of trauma. Histopathologically, silica particles included in the skin induce sarcoidal granulomas, with abundant number of Langhans or foreign body multinucleated giant cells, whereby the causing particles are difficult to see with routine microscopy. However, silica particles are easily identified with polarized light microscopy because they are strongly birefringent (**Fig. 12**).[111] Histopathologic differential diagnosis with authentic cutaneous sarcoidosis may be difficult; moreover, it has been suggested that particles of foreign material may serve as a trigger for granuloma formation in true sarcoidosis.[112] Silica granulomas are interpreted as response to colloidal silica particles rather than as result of a hypersensitivity reaction.[113]

Beryllium

Beryllium is one of the lightest metals, and it is used as an alloy with other metals. Chronic beryllium disease is a granulomatous disorder characterized by a cell-mediated immune response to beryllium. Most reports of chronic beryllium disease describe pulmonary involvement. Cutaneous manifestations of beryllium exposure were first described in 1951[114]; since then, 5 classes of beryllium skin disease have been described: irritant contact dermatitis, allergic contact dermatitis, chemical ulcers, ulcerating granulomas, and allergic dermal granulomas.[115] These granulomas were histopathologically characterized by sarcoidal-like granulomas with areas of central fibrinoid necrosis.[115]

Zirconium

Zirconium compounds used as topical deodorants may induce granulomas identical to those of sarcoidosis at the sites of application; therefore, axillary folds are the most common location.[116,117] These granulomas seems to develop by allergic mechanism and, therefore, only appear in previously sensitized individuals.[116]

Titanium

Titanium alloys are often considered to be rather inert within the body; however, there exist several

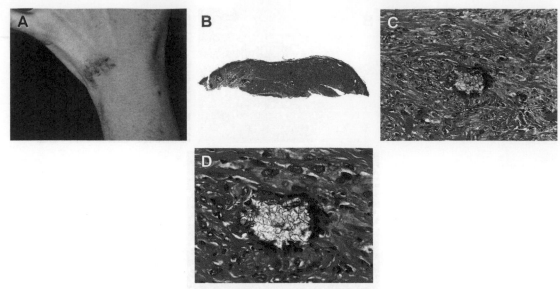

Fig. 12. (*A*) Hyperpigmented lesions at the injury site of a motor traffic accident. (*B*) Scanning power showing a diffuse infiltration of the dermis (H&E ×10). (*C*) Higher magnification demonstrated that the infiltrate was mostly composed of epithelioid histiocytes. Foreign body material with a crystalloid appearance can be seen at the center of the infiltrate (H&E ×200). (*D*) Histiocytes surrounding the silica particles (H&E ×400).

reports of granulomatous tissue reactions attributed to titanium alloy contained within pacemaker implants,[118,119] ear piercings,[120] and titanium screws used in a hip replacement.[121] On microscopic examination, a granulomatous response with minute, intracellular, brown-black particles within macrophages was observed. Titanium dioxide is a compound extensively used in industry as an ingredient in house paints and as a food additive.[122] The effects of titanium dioxide on human tissues are not clearly defined, but several reports of cutaneous lesions after exposure to titanium dioxide exist in the literature.[122,123] One patient developed small papules on the penis after the application of an ointment containing titanium dioxide for the treatment of herpetic lesions. Histopathologic examination showed numerous brown granules, confirmed as titanium by electron probe microanalysis, in the upper dermis, both free and in macrophages.[122]

Mercury

Mercury granulomas may develop after the accidental penetration of mercury through the skin from a broken thermometer or from deliberate intradermal or subcutaneous injections.[124] Clinically, these suppurative granulomas present as erythematous subcutaneous or cutaneous ulcerated nodules. Microscopic examination shows large black spheres of mercury within the neutrophilic aggregates at the center of the granulomas.[124]

Nickel and Other Metals

Sarcoidal granulomas have also been described as an uncommon complication of piercing in the ear lobule and other sites. These lesions are not caused by trauma or scarring, but they develop as consequence of contact allergy to nickel and other metals contained in the rings (**Fig. 13**). Histopathologically, they consist of sarcoidal granulomas involving the entire thickness of the dermis; but in contrast with true sarcoidosis, a dense lymphoid infiltrate surrounds the aggregates of epithelioid histiocytes.[125] Usually, no foreign material is identified with routine microscopy and polarized light. In one reported case, the granulomatous reaction developed against the titanium alloy used in the ear piercing.[120]

ATYPICAL FOREIGN SUBSTANCES

Finally, a large list of disparate foreign substances may induce different types of granulomas in the skin including

- Food particles (the so-called pulse granulomas)[126–129]
- Starch[130]
- Talc[131]
- Suture,[132,133] acrylic or nylon fibers[134]
- Glass[135]
- Cactus bristles[136,137]
- Plant,[138] wood, and steal splinters[139]
- Fragments of a chain saw blade[140]
- Sea urchin spines[141]

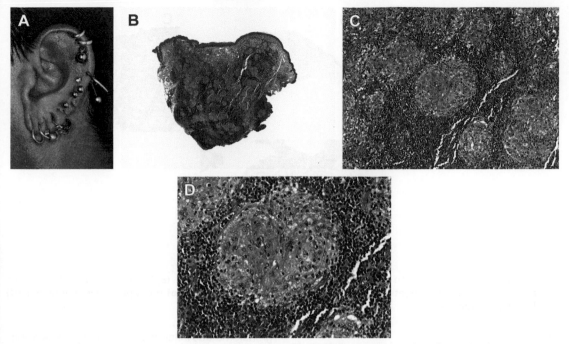

Fig. 13. Granulomatous reaction to piercing. (*A*) Patient with multiple piercings in the left ear. (*B*) Scanning power showing a diffuse involvement of the entire thickness of the dermis by multiple small granulomas (H&E ×10). (*C*) Rounded granulomas composed of epithelioid histiocytes with a peripheral rim of small lymphocytes (H&E ×200). (*D*) Detail of the granulomas (H&E ×400).

- Wheat stubble[142]
- Pencil lead[143,144]
- Artificial hair[145]
- Golf club graphite[146]
- Insect fragments after arthropod bites[147]
- At the points of entry of needles coated with silicone for acupuncture, catheters, and venepunctures[148–150]
- Retained epicardial pacing wires[151,152]
- Materials used to cut heroin and other addictive drugs[153]

The diagnosis of these foreign body reactions is usually establish histopathologically, but the elemental nature of the unknown inorganic material can be determined using energy-dispersive x-ray analysis techniques if necessary. It is also recommended to perform stains for bacteria and fungi to exclude contaminating organisms when foreign bodies, such as wood splinters or bone fragments, are found. Plant material may be readily identified by its characteristic structure and may be PAS positive.[139] Talc particles are birefringent, as are starch granules; the latter exhibit a characteristic Maltese cross birefringence in polarized light.[154]

Plant Splinters and Spines

Splinters and spines of plant matter are common foreign bodies in skin wounds of the extremities and often present embedded in the dermis or subcutaneous tissue. Vegetative foreign bodies are highly inflammatory and, if not completely removed, can cause infection, toxic reactions, or granuloma formation (**Fig. 14**). The most common error in plant splinter and spine management is failure to detect their presence.

Arthropod Bite

A granulomatous reaction at the site of an arthropod bite may be a reaction to insect fragments or introduced epidermal elements.[155] Local reactions to tick bites display a variety of histologic pictures, which are mostly considered nonspecific, and have been reviewed by Castelli and colleagues.[156] In the granulomatous reactions, the finding of recognizable remnants of the mouthparts and the presence of special vascular changes may provide a clue to the etiologic diagnosis (**Fig. 15**). A florid granulomatous reaction producing an exophytic tumor has been reported following multiple bee stings used as a folk remedy.[157] Histology of this case showed epidermal ulceration with granulomatous inflammatory cell infiltration of many eosinophils. No microorganisms or foreign bodies were identified. Intralesional triamcinolone acetonide was not effective, but an excellent outcome was obtained using carbon dioxide laser vaporization of the lesion.

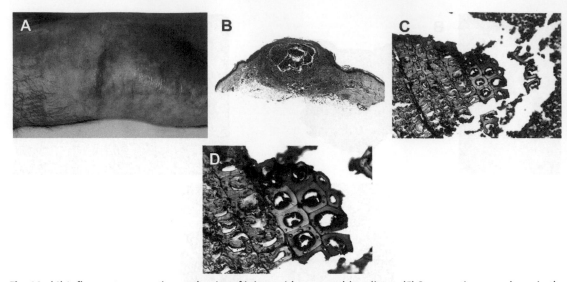

Fig. 14. (*A*) Inflammatory reaction at the site of injury with a vegetable splinter. (*B*) Suppurative granuloma in the upper dermis. (*C*) Parts of a vegetable splinter can be observed at the center of the suppurative granuloma. (*D*) Detail of the foreign body.

Sea Urchin Spine

Puncture with the spine of the rigid external skeleton of sea urchins may cause mechanical injury by skin penetration. It causes immediate local symptoms and, in some cases, a delayed reaction occurs in the site of injury, weeks to months later. In this case, persistent, firm, flesh-colored papules or nodules develop. Histopathologic examination of sea urchin granulomas shows a nonspecific granulomatous inflammation, in most cases of sarcoidal type. Being aware of the triggering event is necessary for the correct diagnosis.[158] Some polymerase chain reaction studies have found *Mycobacterium marinum* in sea urchin granulomas.[159]

Food Particles

Pulse granulomas, also named hyalin angiopathy, is a rare granulomatous reaction to particles of

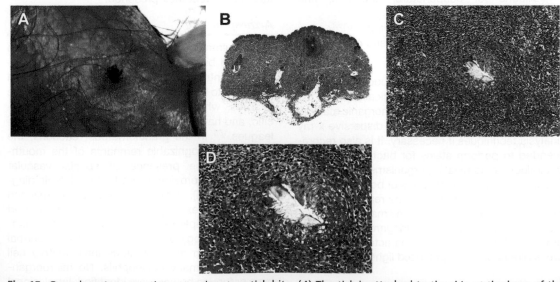

Fig. 15. Granulomatous reaction secondary to a tick bite. (*A*) The tick is attached to the skin at the base of the penis. (*B*) Scanning power showing a nodular infiltrate on the mid dermis (H&E ×10). (*C*) Granulomatous reaction surrounding parts of the tick mouth (H&E ×200). (*D*) Still higher magnification showing a palisade of histiocytes surrounding a fragment of the tick (H&E ×400).

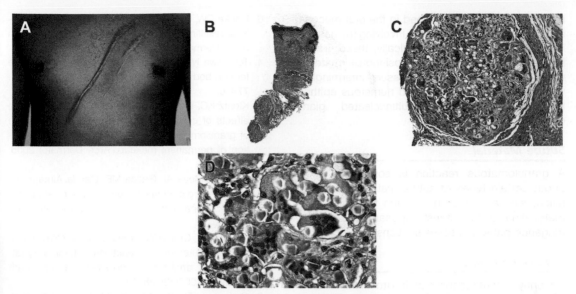

Fig. 16. (*A*) Linear hypertrophic scar on the chest. (*B*) Punch biopsy showing granulomatous aggregates in the deeper areas of the biopsy (H&E ×10). (*C*) The nodular aggregates are composed of histiocytes and multinucleated giant cells surrounding the suture filaments (H&E ×200). (*D*) Higher magnification showing histiocytes and multinucleated giant cells engulfing the suture material (H&E ×400).

Table 2
Treatment of the cutaneous foreign body reactions

Foreign Body	Treatment (Level of Evidence-Based Ratings)
Tattoos	Quality-switched lasers (D) Topical tacrolimus (D) Etanercept (D) Picosecond laser devices (D) Imiquimod (D) Microencapsulated tattoo ink (D)
BC	Wait and see (D)
HA	Wait and see (D), intralesional hyaluronidase (D)
Purified polysaccharide alginate	Wait and see (D)
HA + dextranomer microparticles	Surgery, cephalexin, and methylprednisolone (D)
PLLA	Intralesional injections of corticosteroids (D)
Calcium hydroxylapatite	Wait and see (D), intralesional injections of corticosteroids (D)
Paraffin	Surgery (D), intralesional injections of corticosteroids (D)
Silicone	Surgery (D), imiquimod (D), intralesional corticosteroids (D), oral minocycline (D)
Polymethyl-methacrylate microspheres and BC	Intralesional corticosteroids (D), allopurinol (D), intralesional 5-fluorouracil (D)
Granulomatous reactions associated with microneedle therapy	Topical and oral corticosteroids (D), oral tetracyclines (D)
Hydroxyethylmethacrylate/ethylmethacrylate	Intralesional corticosteroids (D), intralesional 5-fluorouracil (D)
Other foreign bodies	Surgical excision (D), colchicine (D), laser therapy (D), allopurinol (D), cyclosporine (D), tacrolimus (D), ascomycin (D), isotretinoin (D)

(A) High-quality randomized controlled trial or prospective study; (B) lesser-quality randomized controlled trial or prospective study; (C) case-control study or retrospective study; (D) case series or case report.

food that has been described in the oral mucosa and in the skin around fistulae involving the gastrointestinal tract. Histopathologically, these granulomas consist of amorphous eosinophilic material within and around blood vessels intermingled with chronic inflammation and numerous epithelioid histiocytes and multinucleated giant cells.[126–129]

Suture Material

A granulomatous reaction is sometimes seen about certain types of suture material, including nylon, silk, and dacron.[132] Each type of suture material has a characteristic appearance and birefringence pattern in tissue sections (**Fig. 16**).[133]

Lava Lamp Liquid

Recently, a cutaneous reaction to the unheated liquid contents of a broken lava lamp has been reported.[160] Small umbilicated erythematous papules containing central keratotic spines developed within the affected areas. Biopsy showed a granulomatous foreign body reaction with focal transepidermal elimination. Electron microscopy and energy-dispersive x-ray spectroscopy analysis of the tissue revealed carbon-based material, consistent with substances reported to be present in lava lamp liquid.

SUMMARY

Cutaneous foreign granulomatous reactions are a group of unrelated conditions caused by the penetration of exogenous substances through the skin. Cutaneous foreign body granulomas may also develop secondary to endogenous material, which has become altered in such a way that it is recognized as a foreign substance. The differential diagnosis of these disorders can be challenging. **Table 2** summarizes the different therapies that have been used for the treatment of the foreign body reactions described in this article. After reading this article, participants should be familiar with the clinical and histologic findings relevant to each disorder. Basic mechanisms of pathogenesis, diagnostic modalities, and treatment options are also described for several of these entities.

REFERENCES

1. Requena L, Cerroni L, Kutzner H. Histopathologic patterns associated with external agents. Dermatol Clin 2012;30:731–48.

2. Weedon D. The granulomatous reaction pattern. In: Weedon D, editor. Weedon's skin pathology. China: Beijing, Elsevier; 2010. p. 170–96.

3. Hanke CW, Conner AC, Probst EL, et al. Blast tattoos resulting from black powder firearms. J Am Acad Dermatol 1987;17:819–25.

4. Terasawa N, Kishimoto S, Kibe Y, et al. Graphite foreign body granuloma. Br J Dermatol 1999;141:774–6.

5. Klontz KC, Lambert LA, Jewell RE, et al. Adverse effects of cosmetic tattooing: an illustrative case of granulomatous dermatitis following the application of permanent makeup. Arch Dermatol 2005;141:918–9.

6. Sánchez Moya AI, Gatica ME, García Almagro D, et al. Allergic contact dermatitis for temporary "black henna" tattoos. Arch Argent Pediatr 2010;108:96–9.

7. Chung WH, Chang YC, Yang LJ, et al. Clinicopathologic features of skin reactions to temporary tattoos and analysis of possible causes. Arch Dermatol 2002;138:88–92.

8. Ostheimer TA, Burkholder BM, Leung TG, et al. Tattoo-associated uveitis. Am J Ophthalmol 2014;158(3):637–43.e1.

9. Papageorgiou PP, Hongcharu W, Chu AC. Systemic sarcoidosis presenting with multiple tattoo granulomas and an extra-tattoo cutaneous granuloma. J Eur Acad Dermatol Venereol 1999;12:51–3.

10. Goldstein AP. VII. Histologic reactions in tattoos. J Dermatol Surg Oncol 1979;5:896–900.

11. Mortimer NJ, Chave TA, Johnson GA. Red tattoo reactions. Clin Exp Dermatol 2003;28:508–10.

12. Morales-Callaghan AM Jr, Aguilar-Bernier M, Martínez-Garcia G, et al. Sarcoid granuloma on black tattoo. J Am Acad Dermatol 2006;55:S71–3.

13. Bagwan IN, Walker M, Theaker JM. Granuloma annulare-like tattoo reaction. J Cutan Pathol 2007;34:804–5.

14. Bethune GC, Miller RA, Murray SJ, et al. A novel inflammatory reaction in a tattoo: challenge. Am J Dermatopathol 2011;33:740–1, 749.

15. Sweeney SA, Hicks LD, Ranallo N, et al. Perforating granulomatous dermatitis reaction to exogenous tattoo pigment: a case report and review of the literature. Am J Dermatopathol 2013;35:754–6.

16. Kluger N, Jolly M, Guillot B. Tattoo-induced vasculitis. J Eur Acad Dermatol Venereol 2008;22:643–4.

17. Blumental G, Okun MR, Ponitch JA. Pseudolymphomatous reaction to tattoos. J Am Acad Dermatol 1982;6:485–8.

18. Mahalingman M, Kim E, Bhawan J. Morphea-like tattoo reaction. Am J Dermatopathol 2002;24:392–5.

19. Carlsen KH, Tolstrup J, Serup J. High-frequency ultrasound imaging of tattoo reactions with histopathology as a comparative method. Introduction of preoperative ultrasound diagnostics as a guide to therapeutic intervention. Skin Res Technol 2013;20(3):257–64.

20. Morsy H, Mogensen M, Thrane L, et al. Imaging of intradermal tattoos by optical coherence tomography. Skin Res Technol 2007;13:444–8.

21. O'goshi K, Suihko C, Serup J. In vivo imaging of intradermal tattoos by confocal scanning laser microscopy. Skin Res Technol 2006;12:94–8.

22. Luebberding S, Alexiades-Armenakas M. New tattoo approaches in dermatology. Dermatol Clin 2014;32:91–6.

23. Campbell FA, Gupta G. Lichenoid tattoo reaction responding to topical tacrolimus ointment. Clin Exp Dermatol 2006;31:293–4.

24. Bachmeyer C, Blum L, Petitjean B, et al. Granulomatous tattoo reaction in a patient treated with etanercept. J Eur Acad Dermatol Venereol 2007;21: 550–2.

25. Fabi SG, Metelitsa AI. Future directions in cutaneous laser surgery. Dermatol Clin 2014;32:61–9.

26. Fox MA, Diven DG, Sra K, et al. Dermal scatter reduction in human skin: a method using controlled application of glycerol. Lasers Surg Med 2009;41: 251–5.

27. Ricotti CA, Colaco SM, Shamma HN, et al. Laser-assisted tattoo removal with topical 5% imiquimod cream. Dermatol Surg 2007;33:1082–91.

28. Nel A, Xia T, Mädler L, et al. Toxic potential of materials at the nanolevel. Science 2006;311:622–7.

29. Requena L, Requena C, Christensen L, et al. Adverse reactions to injectable soft tissue fillers. J Am Acad Dermatol 2011;64:1–34.

30. Soltani-Arabshahi R, Wong JW, Duffy KL, et al. Facial allergic granulomatous reaction and systemic hypersensitivity associated with microneedle therapy for skin rejuvenation. JAMA Dermatol 2014; 150:68–72.

31. Wortsman X, Wortsman J, Orlandi C, et al. Ultrasound detection and identification of cosmetic fillers in the skin. J Eur Acad Dermatol Venereol 2012;26:292–301.

32. Barr RJ, Stegman SJ. Delayed skin test reaction to injectable collagen implant (Zyderm). J Am Acad Dermatol 1984;10:652–8.

33. Barr RJ, King DF, McDonald RM, et al. Necrobiotic granulomas associated with bovine collagen test site injections. J Am Acad Dermatol 1982;6:867–9.

34. McCoy JP Jr, Schade WJ, Siegle RJ, et al. Characterization of the humoral immune response to bovine collagen implants. Arch Dermatol 1985; 121:990–4.

35. Garcia-Domingo MI, Alijotas Rey J, Cistero-Bahima A, et al. Disseminated and recurrent sarcoid-like granulomatous panniculitis due to bovine collagen injection. J Invest Allergol Clin Immunol 2000;10:107–9.

36. Sclafani A, Romo T, Jacono AA, et al. Evaluation of acellular dermal graft in sheet (Alloderm) and injectable (micronized Alloderm) forms for soft tissue augmentation: clinical observations and histologic findings. Arch Facial Plast Surg 2000; 2:130–6.

37. Moody BR, Sengelmann RD. Self-limited adverse reaction to human-derived collagen injectable product. Dermatol Surg 2000;26:936–8.

38. Lorenc ZP, Nir E, Azachi M. Characterization of physical properties and histologic evaluation of injectable Dermicol-p35 porcin-collagen dermal filler. Plast Reconstr Surg 2010;125:1805–13.

39. Braun M, Braun S. Nodule formation following lip augmentation using porcine collagen-derived filler. J Drugs Dermatol 2008;7:579–81.

40. Ghislanzoni M, Bianchi F, Barbareschi M, et al. Cutaneous granulomatous reaction to injectable hyaluronic acid gel. Br J Dermatol 2006;154:755–8.

41. Dadzie OE, Mahalingam M, Parada M, et al. Adverse reactions to soft tissue fillers-a review of the histological features. J Cutan Pathol 2008;35: 536–48.

42. Okada S, Okuyama R, Tagami H, et al. Eosinophilic granulomatous reaction after intradermal injection of hyaluronic acid. Acta Derm Venereol 2008;88: 69–70.

43. Fernandez Aceñero MJ, Zamora E, Borbujo J. Granulomatous foreign body reaction against hyaluronic acid: report of a case after lip augmentation. Dermatol Surg 2003;29:1225–6.

44. Lazzeri D, Agostini T, Figus M, et al. Blindness following cosmetic injections of the face. Plast Reconstr Surg 2012;129:995–1012.

45. He MS, Sheu MM, Huang ZL, et al. Sudden bilateral vision loss and brain infarction following cosmetic hyaluronic acid injection. JAMA Ophthalmol 2013;131:1234–5.

46. Moulonguet I, de Goursac V, Plantier F. Granulomatous reaction after injection of a new resorbable filler Novabel. Am J Dermatopathol 2011; 33:710–1.

47. Schuller-Petrović S, Pavlović MD, Schuller SS, et al. Early granulomatous foreign body reactions to a novel alginate dermal filler: the system's failure? J Eur Acad Dermatol Venereol 2013;27:121–3.

48. Massone C, Horn M, Kerl H, et al. Foreign body granuloma due to Matridex injection for cosmetic purposes. Am J Dermatopathol 2009;31:197–9.

49. Dijkema SJ, van der Lei B, Kibbelaar RE. New-fill injections may induce late-onset foreign body granulomatous reaction. Plast Reconstr Surg 2005;115:76e–8e.

50. Darsow U, Bruckbauer H, Worret WI, et al. Subcutaneous oleomas induced by self-injection of sesame seed oil for muscle augmentation. J Am Acad Dermatol 2000;42:292–4.

51. Claudy A, Garcier F, Schmitt D. Sclerosing lipogranuloma of the male genitalia: ultrastructural study. Br J Dermatol 1981;105:451–5.

52. Requena C, Requena L, Alegre A, et al. Adverse reaction to silicone simulating orofacial granulomatosis. J Eur Acad Dermatol Venereol 2015;29: 998–1001.

53. Aivaliotis M, Kontochristopoulos G, Hatziolou E, et al. Successful colchicine administration in facial granulomas caused by cosmetic implants: report of a case. J Dermatolog Treat 2007;18:112–4.

54. Morgan AM. Localized reactions to injected therapeutic materials. Part 2. Surgical agents. J Cutan Pathol 1995;22:289–303.

55. Zimmermann US, Clerici TJ. The histological aspects of fillers complications. Semin Cutan Med Surg 2004;23:241–50.

56. Rudolph CM, Soyer HP, Schuller-Petrovic S, et al. Foreign body granulomas due to injectable aesthetic microimplants. Am J Surg Pathol 1999; 23:113–7.

57. Rosa SC, de Magalhães AV, de Macedo JL. An experimental study of tissue reaction to polymethyl methacrylate (PMMA) microspheres (Artecoll) and dimethylsiloxane (DMS) in the mouse. Am J Dermatopathol 2008;30:222–7.

58. Requena C, Izquierdo MJ, Navarro M, et al. Adverse reactions to injectable aesthetic microimplants. Am J Dermatopathol 2001;23:197–202.

59. Christensen L, Breiting V, Vuust J, et al. Adverse reactions following injection with a permanent facial filler polyacrylamide hydrogel (Aquamid): causes and treatment. Eur J Plast Surg 2006;28:464–71.

60. Gómez-de la Fuente E, Alvarez-Fernández JG, Pinedo F, et al. Reacción cutánea tras implante con Bio-Alcamid. Actas Dermosifiliogr 2007;98:271–5.

61. Gokdemir G, Küçükünal A, Sakiz D. Cutaneous granulomatous reaction from mesotherapy. Dermatol Surg 2009;35:291–3.

62. Sclafani AP, Fagien S. Treatment of injectable soft tissue filler complications. Dermatol Surg 2009; 35(Suppl 2):1672–80.

63. Glaich AS, Cohen JL, Goldberg LH. Injection necrosis of the glabella: protocol for prevention and treatment after use of dermal fillers. Dermatol Surg 2006;3:276–81.

64. Narins RS, Jewell M, Rubin M, et al. Clinical conference: management of rare events following dermal fillers–focal necrosis and angry red bumps. Dermatol Surg 2006;32:426–34.

65. Lowe NJ, Maxwell CA, Patnaik R. Adverse reactions to dermal fillers: review. Dermatol Surg 2005;31:1616–25.

66. Leonhardt JM, Lawrence N, Narins RS. Angioedema acute hypersensitivity reaction to injectable hyaluronic acid. Dermatol Surg 2005;31:577–9.

67. Brody HJ. Use of hyaluronidase in the treatment of granulomatous hyaluronic acid reactions or unwanted hyaluronic acid misplacement. Dermatol Surg 2005;31:893–7.

68. Lemperle G, Rullan PP, Gauthier-Hazan N. Avoiding and treating dermal filler complications. Plast Reconstr Surg 2006;118(Supp I):92–107.

69. Reddy KK, Brauer JA, Anolik R, et al. Calcium hydroxylapatite nodule resolution after fractional carbon dioxide laser therapy. Arch Dermatol 2012;148:634–6.

70. Wiest LG, Stolz W, Schroeder JA. Electron microscopic documentation of late changes in permanent fillers and clinical management of granulomas in affected patients. Dermatol Surg 2009;35(Suppl 2):1681–8.

71. De Boulle K. Management of complications after implantation of fillers. J Cosmet Dermatol 2004;3: 2–15.

72. Lloret P, España A, Leache A, et al. Successful treatment of granulomatous reactions secondary to injection of esthetic implants. Dermatol Surg 2005;31:486–90.

73. Kuo T, Hu S, Huang C, et al. Cutaneous involvement in polyvinylpyrrolidone disease. A clinicopathologic study of five patients including two patients with severe anemia. Am J Surg Pathol 1997;21:1361–7.

74. Chi C, Wang SH, Kuo TT. Localized cutaneous polyvinylpyrrolidone storage disease mimicking cheilitis granulomatosa. J Cutan Pathol 2006;33:454–7.

75. Mensing H, Koster W, Schaeg G, et al. Zur klinischen Varianz der Polyvinylpyrrolidon-Dermatose. Z Hautkr 1984;59:1027–37.

76. Kuo T, Hsueh S. Mucicarminophilic histiocytosis. A polyvinylpyrrolidone (PVP) storage disease simulating signet-ring cell carcinoma. Am J Surg Pathol 1984;8:419–28.

77. Fernández-Casado A, Martin-Ezquerra G, Yébenes M, et al. Progressive supravenous granulomatous nodular eruption in a human immunodeficiency virus-positive intravenous drug user treated with highly active antiretroviral therapy. Br J Dermatol 2008;158:145–9.

78. Farrant P, Higgins E. A granulomatous response to tribal medicine as a feature of the immune reconstitution syndrome. Clin Exp Dermatol 2004;29:366–8.

79. Amazon K, Robinson MJ, Rywlin AM. Ferrugination caused by Monsel's solution. Clinical observation and experimentations. Am J Dermatopathol 1980; 2:197–205.

80. Olmstead PM, Lund HZ, Leonard DD. Monsel's solution: a histologic nuisance. J Am Acad Dermatol 1980;3:492–8.

81. Katsambas AD, Stratigos AJ. Depigmenting and bleaching agents: coping with hyperpigmentation. Clin Dermatol 2001;19:483–8.

82. Hoshaw RA, Zimmerman KG, Menter A. Ochronosis-like pigmentation from hydroquinone bleaching creams in American blacks. Arch Dermatol 1985; 121:105–8.

83. Bongiorno MR, Aricò M. Exogenous ochronosis and striae atrophicae following the use of bleaching creams. Int J Dermatol 2005;44:112–5.

84. Snider RL, Thiers BH. Exogenous ochronosis. J Am Acad Dermatol 1993;28:662–4.

85. Jordaan HF, Mulligan RP. Actinic granuloma-like change in exogenous ochronosis: case report. J Cutan Pathol 1990;17:236–40.

86. Phillips JI, Isaacson C, Carman H. Ochronosis in black South Africans who used skin lighteners. Am J Dermatopathol 1986;8:14–21.

87. Soares-Almeida LM, Requena L, Kutzner H, et al. Localized panniculitis secondary to subcutaneous glatiramer acetate injections for the treatment of multiple sclerosis: a clinicopathologic and immunohistochemical study. J Am Acad Dermatol 2006;55:968–74.

88. Bechara F, Sand M, Hoffman K, et al. Fat tissue after lipolysis of lipomas: a histopathological and immunohistochemical study. J Cutan Pathol 2007;34:552–7.

89. Shanesmith RP, Vogiatzis PI, Binder SW, et al. Unusual palisading and necrotizing granulomas associated with a lubricating agent used in lipoplasty. Am J Dermatopathol 2010;32:448–52.

90. Palestine RF, Millns JL, Spigel GT, et al. Skin manifestations of pentazocine abuse. J Am Acad Dermatol 1980;2:47–55.

91. Pujol RM, Puig L, Moreno A, et al. Pseudoscleroderma secondary to phytonadione (vitamin K1) injections. Cutis 1989;43:365–8.

92. Mehta CL, Tyler RJ, Cripps DJ. Granulomatous dermatitis with focal sarcoidal features associated with recombinant Interferon β-1b injections. J Am Acad Dermatol 1988;39:1024–8.

93. Eberlein-Köning B, Hein R, Abeck D, et al. Cutaneous sarcoid foreign body granulomas developing at sites of previous skin injury after systemic interferon-alpha treatment for chronic hepatitis C. Br J Dermatol 1999;140:370–2.

94. Jordaan HF, Sandler M. Zinc-induced granuloma - a unique complication of insulin therapy. Clin Exp Dermatol 1989;14:227–9.

95. Ajithkumar K, Anand U, Pulimood S, et al. Vaccine-induced necrobiotic granulomas. Clin Exp Dermatol 1998;23:222–4.

96. Lalinga AV, Pellegrino M, Laurini L, et al. Necrobiotic palisading granuloma at injection site of disodium clodronate: a case report. Dermatology 1999;198:394–5.

97. Yasukawa K, Sawamura D, Sugawara H, et al. Leuprorelin acetate granulomas: case reports and review of the literature. Br J Dermatol 2005;152:1045–7.

98. Porter WM, Grabczynska S, Francis N, et al. The perils and pitfalls of penile injections. Br J Dermatol 1999;141:736–8.

99. Carlson JA, Schutzer P, Pattison T, et al. Sarcoidal foreign-body granulomatous dermatitis associated with ophthalmic drops. Am J Dermatopathol 1998;20:175–8.

100. Fernandez-Flores A, Valerdiz S, Crespo LG, et al. Granulomatous response due to anabolic steroid injections. Acta Dermatovenerol Croat 2011;19:103–6.

101. Boysen NC, Stone MS. Eosinophil-rich granulomatous panniculitis caused by exenatide injection. J Cutan Pathol 2014;41:63–5.

102. Shan SJ, Guo Y. Exenatide-induced eosinophilic sclerosing lipogranuloma at the injection site. Am J Dermatopathol 2013;36(6):510–2.

103. Akyol A, Boyvat A, Kundakçi N. Contact sensitivity to aluminum. Int J Dermatol 2004;43:942–3.

104. Cosnes A, Flechet ML, Revuz J. Inflammatory nodular reactions after hepatitis B vaccination due to aluminium sensitization. Contact Dermatitis 1990;23:65–7.

105. Maubec E, Pinquier L, Viguier M, et al. Vaccination-induced cutaneous pseudolymphoma. J Am Acad Dermatol 2005;52:623–9.

106. Hernández I, Sanmartín O, Cardá C, et al. B-cell pseudolymphoma caused by aluminium hydroxide following hyposensitization therapy. Actas Dermosifiliogr 2008;99:213–6.

107. Del Rosario RN, Barr RJ, Graham BS, et al. Exogenous and endogenous cutaneous anomalies and curiosities. Am J Dermatopathol 2005;27:259–67.

108. Schwarze HP, Giordano-Labadie F, Loche F, et al. Delayed-hypersensitivity granulomatous reaction induced by blepharopigmentation with aluminum-silicate. J Am Acad Dermatol 2000;42:888–91.

109. Fawcett HA, Smith NP. Injection-site granuloma due to aluminium. Arch Dermatol 1984;120:1318–22.

110. Slater DN, Underwood JC, Durrant TE, et al. Aluminium hydroxide granulomas: light and electron microscopic studies and X-ray microanalysis. Br J Dermatol 1982;107:103–8.

111. Mowry RG, Sams WM Jr, Caufield JB. Cutaneous silica granuloma. Arch Dermatol 1991;127:692–4.

112. Walsh NM, Hanly JG, Tremaine R, et al. Cutaneous sarcoidosis and foreign bodies. Am J Dermatopathol 1993;15:203–7.

113. Shelley WB, Hurley HJ. The pathogenesis of silica granulomas in man: a non-allergic colloidal phenomenon. J Invest Dermatol 1960;34:107–23.

114. Curtis GH. Cutaneous hypersensitivity due to beryllium: a study of thirteen cases. AMA Arch Derm Syphilol 1951;54:470–82.

115. Berlin JM, Taylor JS, Sigel JE, et al. Beryllium dermatitis. J Am Acad Dermatol 2003;49:939–41.

116. Shelley WB, Hurley HJ. Allergic origin of zirconium deodorant granuloma. Br J Dermatol 1958;70:75–101.

117. Skelton HG III, Smith KJ, Johnson FB, et al. Zirconium granuloma resulting from an aluminum zirconium complex: a previously unrecognized agent in development of hypersensitivity granulomas. J Am Acad Dermatol 1993;28:874–6.

118. Viraben R, Boulinguez S, Alba C. Granulomatous dermatitis after implantation of a titanium containing pacemaker. Contact Dermatitis 1995;33:437.

119. Abdallah HI, Balsara RK, O'Riordan AC. Pacemaker contact sensitivity: clinical recognition and management. Ann Thorac Surg 1994;57:1017–8.

120. High WA, Ayers RA, Adams JR, et al. Granulomatous reaction to titanium alloy: an unusual reaction to ear piercing. J Am Acad Dermatol 2006;55:716–20.

121. Akimoto M, Hara H, Suzuki H. Metallosis of the skin mimicking malignant skin tumour. Br J Dermatol 2003;149:653.

122. Dupre A, Touron P, Daste J, et al. Titanium pigmentation. An electron probe microanalysis study. Arch Dermatol 1985;121:656–8.

123. Moran CA, Mullick FG, Ishak KG, et al. Identification of titanium in human tissues: probable role in pathologic processes. Hum Pathol 1991;22:450–4.

124. Rachman R. Soft-tissue injury by mercury from a broken thermometer. A case report and review of the literature. Am J Clin Pathol 1974;61:296–300.

125. Casper C, Groth W, Hunzelmann N. Sarcoidal-type allergic contact granuloma. A rare complication of ear piercing. Am J Dermatopathol 2004;26:59–62.

126. Martin RW III, Lumadue JA, Corio RL, et al. Cutaneous giant cell hyalin angiopathy. J Cutan Pathol 1993;20:356–8.

127. Rhee DD, Wu ML. Pulse granulomas detected in gallbladder, fallopian tube, and skin. Arch Pathol Lab Med 2006;130:1839–42.

128. Beer TW, Cole JM. Cutaneous pulse granulomas. Arch Pathol Lab Med 2007;131:1513–4.

129. Tschen JA, Tschen JA. Pulse granuloma in a rectocutaneous fistula. J Cutan Pathol 2008;35:343–5.

130. Leonard DD. Starch granulomas. Arch Dermatol 1973;107:101–3.

131. Tye MJ, Hashimoto K, Fox F. Talc granulomas of the skin. JAMA 1966;198:1370–2.

132. Postlethwait RW, Willigan DA, Ulin AW. Human tissue reaction to sutures. Ann Surg 1975;181:144–50.

133. Holzheimer RG. Adverse events of sutures: possible interactions of biomaterials? Eur J Med Res 2005;10:521–6.

134. Pimentel JC. Sarcoidal granulomas of the skin produced by acrylic and nylon fibers. Br J Dermatol 1977;96:673–7.

135. Pimentel JC, Alves MC. Clinical course, particularities, and possibility of etiologic characterization of sarcoid-type granulomas of the skin. Acta Med Port 1994;7:237–41.

136. Gutiérrez MC, Martín L, Arias PD, et al. Granulomas faciales por espinas de cactus. Med Cutan Ibero Lat Am 1990;18:197–200.

137. Madkan VK, Abraham T, Lesher JL Jr. Cactus spine granuloma. Cutis 2007;79:208–10.

138. Vizzini GM. A case of granuloma caused by a plant foreign body retained in the perineal subcutaneous tissue. Minerva Med 1975;66:4603–10.

139. Snyder RA, Schwartz RA. Cactus bristle implantation. Report of an unusual case initially seen with rows of yellow hairs. Arch Dermatol 1983;119:152–4.

140. Osawa R, Abe R, Inokuma D, et al. Chain saw blade granuloma: reaction to deeply embedded metal fragment. Arch Dermatol 2006;142:1079–80.

141. De La Torre C, Toribio J. Sea-urchin granuloma: histologic profile. A pathologic study of 50 biopsies. J Cutan Pathol 2001;28:223–8.

142. Pimentel JC. The "wheat-stubble sarcoid granuloma": a new epithelioid granuloma of the skin. Br J Dermatol 1972;87:444–9.

143. Hatano Y, Asada Y, Komada S, et al. A case of pencil core granuloma with unusual temporal profile. Dermatology 2000;201:151–3.

144. Gormley RH, Kovach SJ 3rd, Zhang PJ. Role for trauma in inducing pencil "lead" granuloma in the skin. J Am Acad Dermatol 2010;62:1074–5.

145. Peluso AM, Fanti PA, Monti M, et al. Cutaneous complications of artificial hair implantation: a pathological study. Dermatology 1992;184:129–32.

146. Young PC, Smack DP, Sau P, et al. Golf club granuloma. J Am Acad Dermatol 1995;32:1047–8.

147. Allen AC. Persistent "insect bites" (dermal eosinophilic granulomas) simulating lymphoblastomas, histiocytes, and squamous cell carcinomas. Am J Pathol 1948;24:367–75.

148. Yanagihara M, Fujii T, Wakamatu N, et al. Silicone granuloma on the entry points of acupuncture, venepuncture and surgical needles. J Cutan Pathol 2000;27:301–5.

149. Kenmochi A, Satoh T, Igawa K, et al. Silica granuloma induced by indwelling catheter. J Am Acad Dermatol 2007;57:S54–5.

150. Alani RM, Busam K. Acupuncture granulomas. J Am Acad Dermatol 2001;45:S225–6.

151. Matwiyoff GN, McKinlay JR, Miller CH, et al. Transepidermal migration of external cardiac pacing wire presenting as a cutaneous nodule. J Am Acad Dermatol 2000;42:865–6.

152. Gilaberte M, Delclós J, Yebenés M, et al. Delayed foreign body granuloma secondary to an abandoned cardiac pacemaker wire. J Eur Acad Dermatol Venereol 2007;21:107–9.

153. Posner DI, Guill MA 3rd. Cutaneous foreign body granulomas associated with intravenous drug abuse. J Am Acad Dermatol 1985;13:869–72.

154. Lázaro C, Reichelt C, Lázaro J, et al. Foreign body post-varicella granulomas due to talc. J Eur Acad Dermatol Venereol 2006;20:75–8.

155. Lee NR, Lee SY, Lee WS. Granulomatous inflammation with chronic folliculitis as a complication of bee sting acupuncture. Indian J Dermatol Venereol Leprol 2013;79:554.

156. Castelli E, Caputo V, Morello V, et al. Local reactions to tick bites. Am J Dermatopathol 2008;30:241–8.

157. Park JH, Kim JG, Cha SH, et al. Eosinophilic foreign body granuloma after multiple self-administered bee stings. Br J Dermatol 1998;139:1102–5.

158. Suárez-Peñaranda JM, Vieites B, Del Río E, et al. Histopathologic and immunohistochemical features of sea urchin granulomas. J Cutan Pathol 2013;40:550–6.

159. De la Torre C, Vega A, Carracedo A, et al. Identification of Mycobacterium marinum in sea-urchin granulomas. Br J Dermatol 2001;145:114–6.

160. Thom GA, Cheah KC. Perforating foreign body reaction to unheated liquid contents of lava lamp. Pediatr Dermatol 2013;31(5):623–4.

Granulomatous Drug Eruptions

Roni P. Dodiuk-Gad, MD[a,b], Neil H. Shear, MD, FRCPC[a,c],*

KEYWORDS

- Granuloma • Drug • Granulomatous drug eruptions • Skin • Noninfectious granuloma

KEY POINTS

- Granulomatous drug eruptions (GDEs) , defined by a predominance of histiocytes in the inflammatory infiltrate, are rare and include 4 major types: interstitial granulomatous drug reaction, drug-induced accelerated rheumatoid nodulosis, drug-induced granuloma annulare, and drug-induced sarcoidosis.
- The diagnosis of GDEs is challenging because of the long time lapse between initiation and cessation of the drug, and the emergence and clearance of lesions that usually appear over periods ranging from several weeks to months.
- GDEs may be localized to the skin or may include major systemic involvement.
- It is reasonable to consider continuing the offending medication in disease limited to the skin if the drug has proved effective in treating a systemic disease, the risks and benefits have been assessed, and proper follow-up is conducted.
- GDEs should always be considered in the differential diagnosis of noninfectious granulomatous diseases of the skin.

INTRODUCTION

Granulomas represent a pattern of inflammation that develops during the body's attempt to enclose foreign bodies or inciting agents. The causative agent is walled off and sequestered by cells of the mononuclear phagocyte system, allowing it to be contained, if not destroyed altogether.[1] The mononuclear phagocyte system consists of macrophages, epithelioid cells, and multinucleated giant cells. In most instances these cells are aggregated into well-demarcated focal lesions called granulomas, although a looser, more diffuse arrangement may be found. There is usually an admixture of other cells, especially lymphocytes, plasma cells, and fibroblasts.[2] The characteristics of a granuloma depend not only on the properties of the causative irritant but also greatly on host factors.[2] The granulomatous inflammation is initiated by antigen-presenting cells, which activate T cells to secrete interleukin-2 and interferon (IFN)-γ, which then activate additional T cells and macrophages, respectively. The activated macrophages transform into epithelioid histiocytes and giant cells.[2] Noninfectious granulomatous diseases of the skin are a broad group of distinct reactive inflammatory conditions that share important similarities. As a group, they are relatively difficult to diagnose and distinguish both clinically and

Conflicts of Interest: The authors have no financial or other conflicts of interest, including financial interests and relationships and affiliations relevant to the subject of this submission.
^a Division of Dermatology, Department of Medicine, Sunnybrook Health Sciences Centre, 2075 Bayview Ave., Room M1-737, Toronto, ON M4N 3M5, Canada; ^b Department of Dermatology, Ha'emek Medical Center, Afula 18101, Israel; ^c Division of Clinical Pharmacology and Toxicology, Department of Medicine, Sunnybrook Health Sciences Centre, University of Toronto, 2075 Bayview Avenue, Room M1-737, Toronto, Ontario M4N 3M5, Canada
* Corresponding author. Dermatology Division, Sunnybrook Health Sciences Centre, 2075 Bayview Avenue, Room M1-737, Toronto, Ontario M4N 3M5, Canada.
E-mail address: neil.shear@sunnybrook.ca

Dermatol Clin 33 (2015) 525–539
http://dx.doi.org/10.1016/j.det.2015.03.015
0733-8635/15/$ – see front matter © 2015 Elsevier Inc. All rights reserved.

histologically.[3] These diseases include granuloma annulare, annular elastolytic giant cell granuloma, necrobiosis lipoidica, necrobiotic xanthogranuloma, interstitial granulomatous dermatitis, palisaded neutrophilic granulomatous dermatitis (PNGD), sarcoidosis, and metastatic Crohn disease.[4] Granulomatous drug eruptions are an additional rare subgroup of noninfectious granulomatous diseases of the skin.[4] This review summarizes current knowledge on the various types of granulomatous drug eruptions, which include the following types of reactions:

- Interstitial granulomatous drug reaction (IGDR), including the subtype drug-associated reversible granulomatous T-cell dyscrasia
- Drug-induced accelerated rheumatoid nodulosis
- Drug-induced granuloma annulare (GA)
- Drug-induced sarcoidosis.
- Other granulomatous drug eruptions: cutaneous granulomatous reaction to injectable drugs and vaccinations, photoinduced granulomatous eruption, and miscellaneous.

INTERSTITIAL GRANULOMATOUS DRUG REACTION

IGDR, described by Magro and colleagues[5] in 1998, is a rare entity of unknown prevalence, with a peculiar histopathology characterized by the dermal presence of histiocytes between fragmented collagen bundles, leading to the term IGDR.[5]

Etiopathogenesis

The list of drugs capable of inducing IGDR, which includes various groups, is increasing (**Box 1**). The pathogenesis is unknown. It has been proposed that the drug alters the antigenicity of dermal collagen and elicits an immune response.[6]

Clinical Presentation

The most common cutaneous features are symptomatic erythematous to violaceous annular plaques with a predilection for the flexures (intertriginous areas, medial thighs, and inner aspects of the arms),[5] and, occasionally, indurated borders and central clearing.[6,7] Other reported clinical presentations include generalized erythematous macules and papules[6,7]; erythroderma[8]; multiple tender, erythematous, violaceous, poorly demarcated, firm papules and plaques on both palms and soles[9,10]; and erythema nodosum–like lesions.[11]

> **Box 1**
> **Drugs that induce an interstitial granulomatous drug reaction**
>
> Calcium-channel blockers[a,5,8]
>
> Angiotensin-converting enzyme inhibitors[5]
>
> Lipid-lowering agents[5,13]
>
> Brompheniramine (antihistamine)[5]
>
> Histamine H2-receptor antagonists[5]
>
> Furosemide[5]
>
> Carbamazepine[5]
>
> Bupropion and tricyclic antidepressants[5]
>
> Anti–tumor necrosis factor (TNF) agents: infliximab, adalimumab, etanercept, and lenalidomide[16,70]
>
> Sennoside (laxative)[71]
>
> Herbal medications[11,72]
>
> β-Blockers[5]
>
> Ganciclovir[10]
>
> Sorafenib (kinase inhibitor)[9]
>
> Strontium ranelate[73]
>
> Febuxostat (selective xanthine oxidase inhibitor)[7]
>
> Anakinra (interleukin-1 inhibitor)[6]
>
> Trastuzumab (immunoglobulin-1 recombinant humanized monoclonal antibody)[74]
>
> Darifenacin (muscarinic receptor antagonist)[75]
>
> [a]The most common drug inducing the reaction.

Lag period

There may be a prolonged period between the initiation and cessation of the drug and the emergence and clearance of IGDR lesions, ranging from several weeks to months.[6] Twenty patients with IGDR in the study by Magro and colleagues[5] had ingested the offending drugs 4 weeks to 25 years (average, 5 years) before the onset of the eruption.

Differential diagnosis

The erythematous or violaceous plaques in the area of skin folds may mimic the scaly plaques of mycosis fungoides (cutaneous T-cell lymphoma). The differential diagnosis also includes erythema annulare centrifugum, lupus erythematosus, pigmented purpura, lichen planus, dermatomyositis, macular GA,[4] and interstitial granulomatous dermatitis with arthritis (Ackerman syndrome).[12]

Systemic Associations

Characteristically, there is no systemic association in IGDR.[5]

Evaluation and Management

The clinical and histologic findings must be correlated for the diagnosis of this entity.[5] A temporal association between the initiation of drug therapy and lesion onset and resolution after cessation of the implicated drug is characteristic. However, the diagnosis may be challenging because of the prolonged time course between initiation and cessation of the drug and emergence and clearance of IGDR lesions, ranging from several weeks to months.[13] In many cases, the lesions resolve on discontinuation of the drug and reappear on reintroduction of the drug-positive drug provocation test.[13]

Histology

IGDRs have variable histologic presentations. Microscopically they typically exhibit a diffuse interstitial infiltrate of lymphocytes and histiocytes with elastic and collagen fiber fragmentation, vacuolar interface dermatitis, and scant to absent mucin deposition.[14] Tissue eosinophilia is present in most cases.[5] Of note, some 50% of cases exhibit atypical lymphocytes with hyperchromatic convoluted nuclei, found either in the interstitium or along the dermoepidermal junction, with variable epidermotropism.[5] The clinical and histopathologic appearances of IGDR and the granulomatous slack skin variant of cutaneous T-cell lymphoma are strikingly similar: both present as violaceous plaques on intertriginous areas and show elastolysis, tissue eosinophilia, and granulomatous infiltrates with atypical lymphocytes. In IGDR, however, typical intraepidermal cells do not include Sézary cells and do not exceed the atypia of the dermal component, findings typical of granulomatous slack skin. Other features supporting the diagnosis of IGDR are hypersensitivity reactions, such as papillary dermal edema, vesiculation, basilar vacuolopathy, and dyskeratosis.[5] Differentiation between IGDR and Ackerman syndrome is based on the appearance of vacuolar interface dermatitis with an interstitial histiocytic infiltrate in IGDR.[12]

Treatment

The condition is treated by identifying and discontinuing the drug causing the reaction.[5] Complete resolution of the lesions usually follows the withdrawal of the causative medication.[5] Awareness of this will avoid prolonged disease and unnecessary treatments. In cases where IGDR does not resolve in several months, repeat biopsy is recommended to exclude granulomatous slack skin, and should include gene rearrangement studies.[4] Histopathology suggesting malignancy will require further investigation.[15] The frequent time lapse between the initial ingestion of the offending agent and the onset of cutaneous findings and polypharmacy may further complicate the identification of the culprit.[15] Fifteen of 20 patients with IGDR in the study by Magro and colleagues[5] had 1 or more of the implicated drugs discontinue, and the eruption resolved within 1 to 40 weeks (mean, 8 weeks) in 14 patients with improvement, although not complete resolution, in 1 patient. No recurrences developed at a 12-month follow-up. In the cases of IGDR induced by anti–tumor necrosis factor (TNF) medications, it is recommended that all patients undergo a careful workup to rule out an infectious process.[16]

A distinct subset of the IGDR is drug-associated reversible granulomatous T-cell dyscrasia, a novel reaction pattern characterized by atypical T-lymphocytic infiltrates that manifest a light microscopic, phenotypic, and molecular profile that closely parallels cutaneous T-cell lymphoma but regresses when the causal drug is withdrawn. Margo and colleagues[17] labeled this distinct subset in 2010 based on a series of 10 patients with atypical cutaneous T-cell lymphocytic infiltration associated with granulomatous features, and combined light microscopic, phenotypic, and molecular profile resembling a subtype of mycosis fungoides, which they designated granulomatous mycosis fungoides. The cutaneous findings included persistent eczematous papules, plaques, or patches, or infiltrative plaque-like lesions, often in fold areas of the skin, which resolved or mostly resolved following discontinuation of the offending drug in 2 weeks to 10 months. In all cases the biopsies showed a diffuse interstitial lymphocytic and histiocytic infiltrate. Other histologic findings in these cases included epidermotropism, and angiocentric infiltrates containing large transformed cells and cells with an atypical cerebriform morphology. All cases showed a dominance of CD4 cells over those of the CD8 subset. There was a reduction in the expression of CD7 in most cases and, in a few cases, CD62L expression of greater than or equal to 50%. The large transformed cells in an angiocentric array showed CD30 expression. Molecular studies demonstrated clonality at 2 different biopsy sites in one case, oligoclonality in another, and a polyclonal profile in the remainder. In one case where clonality was identified in the skin biopsies, the peripheral blood analysis showed an oligoclonal profile without any commonality between the dominant clones detected in the peripheral blood and those detected in the skin.[17] One patient continued to have a peripheral blood monoclonal T-cell population despite the absence of skin lesions, indicating the importance of drug modulation to prevent the conversion of what is initially a reversible T-cell dyscrasia to one that may become irreversible.[17]

DRUG-INDUCED ACCELERATED RHEUMATOID NODULOSIS
Etiopathogenesis

Kremer and Lee[18] first noted accelerated rheumatoid nodulosis in 1986 during a study of long-term methotrexate (MTX) therapy for rheumatoid arthritis (RA). In 2001, Ahmed and colleagues[19] termed this acceleration MTX-induced accelerated rheumatoid nodulosis (MIARN). Other medications have been implicated in accelerated rheumatoid nodulosis (Box 2). However, as MTX is the most common drug to be associated with this condition,[15,20] this section focuses on MIARN. A double-blind study that compared MTX and azathioprine in patients with refractory RA showed an 8% incidence of MIARN (with arthritic improvement) and none with azathioprine.[21] Other collagen vascular diseases besides RA were associated with accelerated rheumatoid nodulosis, including juvenile RA,[22] psoriatic arthritis,[23] and systemic lupus erythematosus.[24] Although the mechanism of accelerated nodulosis is unclear, studies have suggested a genetic etiology or, at least, predisposition.[19,25] In 2001, a retrospective study of 79 Caucasian patients with RA identified the HLA-DRB1*0401 allele as an HLA class II gene that associates with nodule formation.[19] A 2007 cross-sectional study identified a polymorphism of the methionine synthase reductase gene in RA patients that was increased in these patients in comparison with the general population and was associated with MIARN.[25] Of interest, accelerated rheumatoid nodulosis does not appear in patients receiving MTX therapy for disorders other than collagen vascular diseases (eg, patients with psoriasis). Therefore, it seems possible that there is a synergistic pathogenic effect between the underlying collagen vascular disease and the drug inducing the nodulosis.[20]

Box 2
Drugs that induce accelerated rheumatoid nodulosis

Methotrexate[a,19–22,26]

Anti-TNF agents: etanercept,[27] adalimumab,[28] infliximab[29]

Aromatase inhibitors[30]

Azathioprine[31]

Leflunomide[32]

[a]The most common drug inducing the reaction.

Clinical Presentation

Clinical presentation of MIARN includes multiple flesh-colored to erythematous indurated papules and nodules.[20] MIARN affects mainly the hands, usually the metacarpophalangeal and proximal interphalangeal joints,[12,19–21] although other locations have been reported including knees, heel pads, Achilles tendons, arms, elbows, thighs, shoulder girdle, buttocks, and feet.[22,26] The nodules are typically painful, but discomfort is minimal in most patients.[19] Regarding the clinical presentation of accelerated rheumatoid nodulosis induced by drugs other than MTX, Cunnane and colleagues[27] reported 3 patients with refractory seropositive erosive RA who, despite clinical improvement with etanercept, developed new nodulosis, 2 cases of cutaneous nodulosis, and 1 case of pulmonary nodulosis. Scrivo and colleagues[28] reported on a patient with RA who developed subcutaneous nodules in the extensor side of the elbows following treatment with adalimumab. Mackley and colleagues[29] reported a patient with seropositive RA who developed nodules on the fingers of both hands despite continued remission of her rheumatoid arthritis following treatment with infliximab. Chao and colleagues[30] described a patient with RA who developed subcutaneous nodules on the fingers of both hands following treatment with an aromatase inhibitor. Langevitz and colleagues[31] reported on a patient with seropositive, erosive RA who developed subcutaneous nodules on the elbows and extensor surfaces of the arms and hands during treatment with azathioprine. Three patients reported by Braun and colleagues[32] developed subcutaneous nodules on the extensor side of the hands and elbows following leflunomide therapy.

Lag period
Nodule formation is not related to cumulative MTX dosage. The duration of MTX therapy reported before MIARN ranges widely from hours to months.[19,20,22,26] In a retrospective study by Ahmed and colleagues,[19] of 30 cases with MIARN the mean duration of MTX therapy was 36.4 ± 27.2 months before developing MIARN.

The lag period reported with medications other than MTX that induce accelerated rheumatoid nodulosis is as follows. Anti-TNF agents: 2 to 3 months for etanercept,[27] 26 months for adalimumab,[28] and 12 months for infliximab[29]; aromatase inhibitors, 15 months[30]; azathioprine, 1 month[31]; and leflunomide, 6 months.[32]

Differential diagnosis
Rheumatoid nodules comprise 3 clinical types: classic rheumatoid nodules associated with RA,

rheumatoid nodulosis, considered a benign variant of RA, and MTX-induced rheumatoid nodulosis.[4] Differentiation between these types of nodules may be challenging. MIARN is characterized by multiple lesions that disappear with termination of MTX and do not recur in previously affected areas in the absence of MTX therapy. The differential diagnosis also includes pseudorheumatoid nodules,[15] cutaneous extravascular necrotizing granuloma of Churg-Strauss,[20] and rheumatoid neutrophilic dermatitis.[20]

Systemic Associations

One patient in the report by Ahmed and colleagues[19] developed lung disease with biopsy-proven intrapulmonary nodules that resolved completely after MTX withdrawal. Another patient developed extensive cutaneous nodulosis associated with new cardiac murmurs of aortic and tricuspid regurgitation. Other reported organ involvement includes the lungs,[33] heart,[34] and brain.[35]

Evaluation and Management

Histology
Nodules have a histology similar to that of rheumatoid nodules[19]: multinodular foci of massive necrobiosis with adjacent scarring in soft tissue or subcutaneous fat, surrounded by a histiocytic palisade, with fibrin deposition, often seen with rosettes of histiocytes surrounding collagen bundles in the reticular dermis.[3] In 4 cases with cutaneous lesions caused by methotrexate therapy[20] (2 with systemic lupus erythematosus, 1 with RA, and 1 with Sharp syndrome), histopathology of the papules showed an inflammatory infiltrate composed mainly of histiocytes interstitially arranged between collagen bundles of the dermis, intermingled with few neutrophils. Some foci of deeper reticular dermis contained small rosettes composed of clusters of histiocytes surrounding a thick central collagen bundle.

Treatment
MIARN often regresses with discontinuation of MTX and reappears once MTX is restarted.[19] In the report by Ahmed and colleagues,[19] nodules regressed within 6.1 ± 4.5 months when MTX was discontinued but persisted for 41.2 ± 14.9 months when MTX was continued.[19] It was suggested that unless the nodules are painful or interfere with the patient's usual activities, MTX therapy may be continued, especially if the arthritis has improved.[22] The addition of hydroxychloroquine,[19,22] etanercept,[19] D-penicillamine,[36] and colchicine[19] have been shown to accelerate

healing in cases where MTX was continued. Discontinuation of MTX and aggressive intervention may be warranted with development of symptoms, ulceration, infection, or mechanical issues.[15]

In the cases of accelerated rheumatoid nodulosis induced by drugs other than MTX, treatment included discontinuation of the offending drug,[30] changing the dosage of the offending drug,[28] adding an immunosuppressive drug,[27] and not changing or adding any treatment.[29]

DRUG-INDUCED GRANULOMA ANNULARE
Etiopathogenesis

GA is a benign, self-limited disorder of unknown etiology, first described by Colcott-Fox in 1895, and named granuloma annulare by Radcliffe-Crocker in 1902.[37] GA has various clinical variants, including localized, generalized (generalized annular GA, disseminated papular GA, and atypical generalized GA), subcutaneous, and perforating, providing for a wide spectrum of clinical lesions.[38] Several systemic associations have been proposed but not proven, including diabetes mellitus, malignancy, thyroid disease, and dyslipidemia.[38] The first association between GA and drugs was reported in 1980,[39] since then various drugs have been implicated in its etiology (**Box 3**). The pathogenesis of drug-induced GA is not known, although the possible role of immune dysregulation induced by immunosuppressive drugs has been suggested.[40] Several cases of TNF-α antagonists inducing GA were reported,[41] a curious finding given that TNF-α inhibitors can be used

---

Box 3
Drugs that induce granuloma annulare

Anti-TNF agents[a]: infliximab, adalimumab, etanercept, thalidomide[41,50]

Amlodipine[47]

Gold[39,49]

Allopurinol[44]

Diclofenac[76]

Intranasal calcitonin[77]

Immunizations (hepatitis B and antitetanus vaccination)[46,78]

Paroxetine: drug-induced photodistributed granuloma annulare[51]

Pegylated interferon-α[40,45]

Desensitization injections[79]

Topiramate (anticonvulsant)[48]

[a]The most common drug inducing the reaction.

for the treatment of refractory GA.[42,43] The pathogenesis of TNF-α antagonist–induced GA may be related to the autoimmune phenomena induced by anti-TNF-α therapy in genetically predisposed individuals.[41]

Clinical Presentation

Various clinical presentations of drug-induced GA have been reported with different drugs, with the generalized type being the most common.[41,44–47] Although the cutaneous manifestations and the lag period varied with each drug, the histologic findings were consistent with GA in all cases. Allopurinol-induced generalized interstitial GA presented as multiple, asymptomatic, red, raised lesions that appeared after 6 months of treatment with allopurinol.[44] Pegylated IFN-α for hepatitis C infection was reported to induce generalized GA in 2 different reports following 6 and 24 weeks of treatment.[45] Generalized GA was also reported following hepatitis B vaccine,[46] amlodipine,[47] and topiramate.[48] Gold was reported to induce papular GA.[39,49] Anti-TNF was reported also to induce GA.[41] A case series study assessed 199 patients with RA and 127 with spondyloarthropathies, treated with anti-TNF antagonists.[41] Nine cases of GA were identified (4.5%) in the group of patients with RA: 2 treated with infliximab, 6 with adalimumab, and 1 with etanercept. No patient with spondyloarthropathies developed such skin lesions. In 7 patients the skin eruptions developed during the first year of anti-TNF treatment, and in 2 patients during the second year. All 9 patients developed a generalized type of GA located mostly on the hands, forearms, and fingers.[41] Another type of medication in the anti-TNF group, thalidomide, was reported to induce GA[50]: a violaceous, ring-like, firm papular eruption localized on the dorsal aspect of both hands 15 days after starting the treatment of multiple myeloma with thalidomide. GA photoinduced by paroxetine following 1 year of treatment and confirmed by photobiological study was reported.[51]

Systemic Associations

There was no systemic involvement with any of the drugs except for the case of GA induced by amlodipine, whereby the patient developed a transient fever within 10 days of starting the drug. Three days after the febrile episode, the patient developed bilateral ankle edema with a rash on the lower legs.[47]

Evaluation and Management

The association between GA and a drug is considered when: (1) the GA appears only after the initiation of the drug; (2) the cutaneous lesion vanishes after the discontinuation of the drug; (3) the granulomatous lesion reappears with the resumption of the drug in the same area and with the same characteristics as the first lesion; and (4) the histology is characteristic of GA.[48]

The histologic findings of drug-induced GA are palisading granulomas, collagen degeneration, mucin, and a lymphohistiocytic infiltrate. The presence of mucin is the key histologic feature that distinguishes GA from other noninfectious granulomatous diseases.[52]

In most cases the lesions regress with discontinuation of the offending drug.[44,47–49] However, it may also be decided to continue the medication following explanation of the risks and benefits and obtaining the patient's consent. In a case series of 9 patients with RA who developed generalized granuloma attributable to anti-TNF treatment, only 2 had to stop the anti-TNF therapy because of the extent of skin lesions while the other 7 responded well to local corticosteroid therapy, with resolution of the lesions without discontinuing the treatment.[41]

DRUG-INDUCED SARCOIDOSIS
Etiopathogenesis

Sarcoidosis is an autoimmune disease of unknown origin characterized by the presence of noncaseating epithelioid cell granulomas in multiple organs (lymph nodes, lungs, spleen, liver, skin, salivary and lacrimal glands).[4] Proposed causes include infections, organisms, environmental agents, and autoantigens, but to date no specific etiologic agent has been identified. Genetic and immunologic factors are thought to play an important role in the development of the disease through increased susceptibility to antigenic stimulation.[4]

Sarcoidal granulomas have been described as a battle between an antigen and cell-mediated and humoral immunity whereby macrophages are stimulated by the attack of an antigen and converted into epithelioid and giant cells through the mediation of T-helper (Th) cells that also increase the activity of B lymphocytes.[15] The current understanding of disease pathogenesis involves an overactive Th-1 immune response in genetically susceptible individuals exposed to one of a variety of proposed exogenous antigens.[15] Sarcoidosis is a CD4 Th cell driven process, with presentation of unknown antigens by monocytes via major histocompatibility complex II receptors. Cytokine production in sarcoidosis is characterized by a Th-1 profile with the elaboration of IFN-γ and transforming growth factor β. The infiltrating monocytes are thought to present the inciting antigen to Th cells, and eventually develop into the multinucleated giant cell and epithelioid histiocytes characteristic of sarcoidal granulomas.[15]

Various drugs were reported to induce cutaneous sarcoidosis (Box 4), and several theories were suggested to explain the pathogenesis of this process.[4] In 1987, Abdi and colleagues[53] reported the first case of histologically proven sarcoidosis in a woman treated with IFN-α. The role of IFN-α in the induction of sarcoidosis is probably related to its capacity to induce a predominant Th-1 immune response, which is considered the main immunologic event in granuloma formation.[54] In the cases of IFN-α–induced sarcoidosis koebnerized along venous drainage lines in former intravenous drug users, it was suggested that repeated venipuncture over several years resulted in tissue injury, chronic subclinical inflammation, and scar formation, which koebnerized the cutaneous sarcoidosis.[55] Sarcoidosis has been effectively treated with TNF-α blockers, owing to the important role of TNF-α in granuloma formation and maintenance.[56] However, there have also been case reports of an unexpected, paradoxic effect of the development of sarcoidosis in patients on anti–TNF-α therapy.[57–60] Most cases of sarcoidosis developing on TNF-α therapy involved organs other than skin, although cases of only cutaneous sarcoidosis have been reported.[57] In a retrospective case review assessing 34 cases of sarcoidosis that developed during anti-TNF therapy,[58] cutaneous sarcoidosis was documented in 32% of cases. The association was seen with various TNF inhibitors, including etanercept in most cases but also with infliximab and adalimumab. Although the cause of sarcoidosis in these cases is not known, several mechanisms have been postulated: that the granulomatous reaction is part of an autoimmune phenomenon resulting from cytokine imbalance secondary to TNF-α suppression[57]; that blocking TNF-α modifies the pathways of p38 kinase and adenosine A2A and A3 receptors in CD4 cells—biochemical modifications that unbalance the activity of CD4 cells, in particular Th-17, which may contribute to the generation of granulomatous processes such as sarcoidosis[59]; and that genetic variation of the TNF-α gene is an important factor in determining sarcoidosis predisposition and course, while polymorphism of the genes that mediate cytokine production may be associated with distinct immune pathways.[60]

Clinical Presentation

Sarcoidosis is one of the "great mimickers," with polytypic morphology.[15] Cutaneous involvement in sarcoidosis may be either specific (noncaseating granulomas) or nonspecific (reactive processes), and both have been observed in patients with drug-induced sarcoidosis.[57,58,60] In a report of sarcoidal foreign body granulomatous dermatitis associated with ophthalmic drops,[61] multiple brown-black asymptomatic papules were described over the chin, involving nasal mucosa and columella. In a retrospective case review assessing 34 cases of sarcoidosis developing during anti-TNF therapy,[58] the most common clinical sign of cutaneous sarcoidosis was erythema nodosum–like lesions; the average amount of time between initiation of therapy and onset of symptoms in this study was 22 months. In a report on exacerbation of recalcitrant cutaneous sarcoidosis with adalimumab,[60] the cutaneous lesions of sarcoidosis became more erythematous, infiltrated, and ulcerated, and associated with retroauricular adenopathies following the third injection. The cutaneous manifestation of sarcoidosis-like reaction associated with ipilimumab[62] included grouped erythematous papules, some in linear array, in a patient with stage IIIC melanoma following the second dose of high-dose ipilimumab 10 mg/kg. In a review of the literature on cutaneous signs of IFN-α–induced sarcoidosis,[63] cutaneous lesions were found to be a frequent sign of IFN-induced sarcoidosis, with skin involvement documented in 56% of the reports. Cutaneous lesions were found to appear among the presenting and diagnostic signs of a sarcoid reaction in 51% of cases in this study. Symptoms appeared from 1 to 6 months after drug intake and skin lesions usually took the form of erythema nodosum, subcutaneous nodules, plaques, and scars. In an assessment of sarcoidosis among 68 patients with chronic hepatitis C virus (HCV) infection,[54] a temporal relationship between initiation of antiviral therapy and diagnosis of

---

Box 4
Drugs that induce cutaneous sarcoidosis

Interferon-α[a,54,55,63,65]

Anti-TNF agents: etanercept, infliximab, adalimumab[57,58,60]

Synthetic fillers used for cosmetic procedures (hyaluronic acid)[64]

Zinc[80]

Desensitization injections[81]

Ipilimumab (a monoclonal antibody directed against cytotoxic T-lymphocyte antigen-4)[62]

Ophthalmic drops containing sodium bisulfite[61]

[a]The most common drug inducing the reaction.

sarcoidosis was found in 47 cases. The sarcoidosis appeared during the first 6 months after commencing antiviral therapy in 31 of 47 (66%) patients, between 6 and 12 months in 9 (19%), and after 12 months in the remaining 7 (15%). In 8 cases, the initiation of antiviral therapy for HCV reactivated preexisting sarcoidosis. The clinical picture of sarcoidosis in these 47 cases included predominantly pulmonary and cutaneous features. Thirty patients (60%) presented with cutaneous involvement, including painful subcutaneous nodules in 16 cases, plaques in 8, erythema nodosum in 6, and exanthema in 1. The main sites of cutaneous sarcoidosis were the arms in 13 patients, legs in 9, knees in 7, head in 6, and neck in 3. In 4 patients, cutaneous lesions appeared adjacent to older scars or tattoos. In the 2 cases of IFN-α–induced sarcoidosis koebnerized along venous drainage lines,[55] painless, firm, erythematous skin papules developed in a linear distribution along the cephalic and median antebrachial veins of both forearms in former areas of drug injections. The cases were reported in 2 former intravenous drug users following 16 and 30 weeks of treatment with IFN-α and ribavirin for chronic hepatitis C.[55] In a case report of hyaluronic acid injections inducing cutaneous sarcoidosis, tender nodules in both nasolabial folds that had developed 4 months after the injection of hyaluronic acid for wrinkles were described.[64]

Systemic Associations

Drug-induced sarcoidosis may involve only the skin or present as a multisystem disease that includes cutaneous involvement.[58,59,62,63] In the case of sarcoidosis-like reaction associated with ipilimumab, shortness of breath and hypoxemia requiring supplemental oxygen were signs of pulmonary involvement in addition to the cutaneous manifestations.[62] In a review of the literature on cutaneous signs of IFN-α–induced sarcoidosis,[63] nonspecific respiratory symptoms were noted in 54% and mediastinal lymphadenopathy in 50% of the patients. It should be mentioned that many cases of sarcoidosis developing while on anti-TNF therapy involve organs other than the skin,[59] with lung and surrounding lymph nodes the most commonly affected.[58] Other organs include liver, eyes, salivary glands, central nervous system, joints, kidneys, and bone marrow.[58,65] In the case of IFN-α–induced sarcoidosis, because systemic symptoms of sarcoidosis (eg, fatigue, pulmonary dysfunction, arthromyalgias, adenopathies) match the side effects of the antiviral therapy, special attention to dermatologic signs may offer a clue to an early diagnosis of IFN-induced

sarcoidosis. In these cases, skin biopsy provides an easy route to rapid histologic confirmation and diagnosis of sarcoidosis.[63]

Evaluation and Management

The diagnosis of drug-induced sarcoidosis is established when clinical findings are supported by histologic evidence.[54] The histologic findings of drug-induced sarcoidosis are similar to those of sarcoidosis and include classically naked tubercles (granulomas), which are characterized by dermal, noncaseating, epithelioid, histiocytic granulomas; multinucleated giant cells; and lack of an additional extensive inflammatory infiltrate.[15] Most patients experience resolution, or at least improvement of symptoms, on discontinuing the medication,[58] a relatively mild course of disease in contrast to the natural history of sarcoidosis in general.[65] Few cases of persistent or relapsing course require immunosuppressive treatment.[58,62,64] In the cases of hyaluronic acid injections inducing cutaneous sarcoidosis,[64] and cutaneous and pulmonary sarcoidosis-like reaction associated with ipilimumab,[62] prednisone treatment improved the symptoms. In a retrospective case review assessing 34 cases of sarcoidosis developing during anti-TNF therapy,[58] the primary treatment for 33 of the 34 cases was discontinuation of the TNF-inhibitor therapy. A small number of patients were treated with systemic corticosteroids and antituberculosis medications. Complete clearance of disease was reported in 33 of the 34 cases, with a mean time of 5.2 months for clearance after the discontinuation of the TNF inhibitor. In a retrospective study of 60 cases of sarcoidosis induced by IFN-α,[65] management of the disease consisted of discontinuation of IFN-α either alone or in combination with corticosteroid administration. Most patients experienced resolution or, at least, improvement of symptoms. The few (11%) who had a persistent or relapsing course needed additional immunosuppressive treatment. In the case of IFN-α–induced cutaneous sarcoidosis koebnerized along venous drainage lines,[55] because there was no systemic involvement the IFN and ribavirin therapy was continued for a total of 48 weeks, after which the skin lesions spontaneously disappeared. The investigators designed a decision algorithm for the management of IFN-induced sarcoidosis in HCV infection (Fig. 1).[55] A few important points were highlighted: (1) IFN discontinuation should be based on the extent of sarcoidosis; (2) maintaining treatment to maximize hepatitis C remission must be evaluated jointly with hepatologists; (3) systemic steroids should be considered with caution in symptomatic

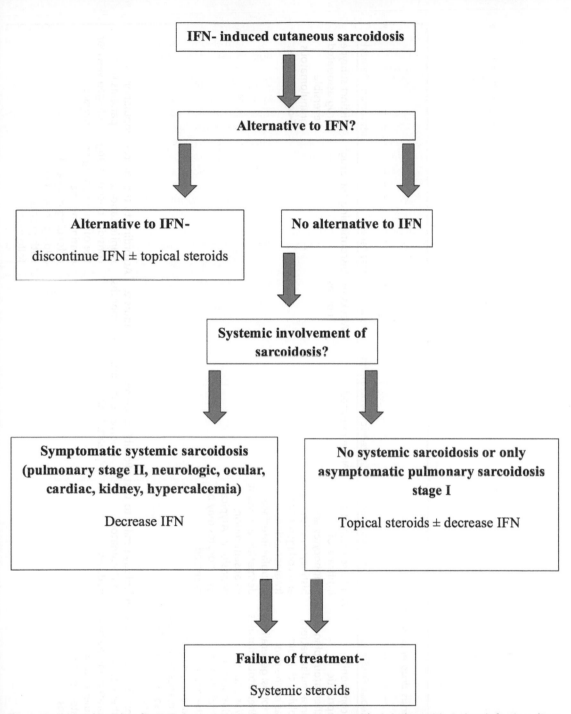

Fig. 1. Decision algorithm for interferon (IFN)-induced cutaneous sarcoidosis in hepatitis C virus infection. (*Data from* Buss G, Cattin V, Spring P, et al. Two cases of interferon-alpha-induced sarcoidosis Koebnerized along venous drainage lines: new pathogenic insights and review of the literature of interferon-induced sarcoidosis. Dermatology 2013;226(4):289–97.)

IFN-induced sarcoidosis, because it may increase the viral load; and (4) aggressive treatment of neurologic, ocular, cardiac, and renal sarcoidosis or hypercalcemia is recommended.

OTHER GRANULOMATOUS DRUG ERUPTIONS

Other granulomatous drug eruptions have been reported, including cutaneous granulomatous

Table 1
Summary of granulomatous drug eruptions

	Cutaneous Findings	Histologic Findings	Systemic Involvement	Lag Period	Treatment	Important Remarks
Interstitial granulomatous drug reaction (IGDR)	Most commonly nonpruritic erythematous plaques in an annular pattern involving the fold areas of the skin Other forms: generalized erythematous macules and/or papules, erythroderma, multiple tender erythematous-violaceous, papules and plaques on palms and soles, erythema nodosum-like lesions	A diffuse interstitial infiltrate of lymphocytes and histiocytes with elastic and collagen fiber fragmentation, vacuolar interface dermatitis, and scant to absent mucin deposition. Atypical lymphocytes may be observed	None reported	Weeks to months	Discontinuing the drug[c]	A distinct subtype: drug-associated reversible granulomatous T-cell dyscrasia
Drug-induced accelerated rheumatoid nodulosis	Multiple flesh-colored to erythematous indurated and painful papules and nodules located mainly on the hands	Histology similar to that of rheumatoid nodules	Possible systemic involvement: lung, heart, brain	Hours to months	According to the clinical manifestations, consider discontinuing the offending drug or continuing the offending drug and adding treatment[a] with proper follow-up[D]	Population of patients with collagen vascular disease

	Clinical presentation	Histology	Systemic involvement	Time course	Treatment	Notes
Drug-induced granuloma annulare (GA)	Various clinical presentations; mostly generalized type of GA	Histology similar to that of GA	No systemic involvement reported except in 1 case[b]	Weeks to months	According to the clinical manifestations, consider discontinuing the drug or continuing the drug and adding local corticosteroid if needed[D]	A distinct subtype: GA photoinduced by paroxetine
Drug-induced sarcoidosis	Polymorphic morphology Specific: papules, nodules, and plaques or Nonspecific: erythema nodosum	Histology similar to that of sarcoidosis	Possible systemic involvement: lung, lymph nodes, liver, eyes, salivary glands, central nervous system, bone marrow, kidney, heart, joints	Weeks to months	According to the clinical manifestations, consider discontinuing the drug or continuing the drug and adding local corticosteroid and systemic immunosuppressive treatment if needed[D]	A distinct subtype: sarcoidosis koebnerized along venous drainage lines in former intravenous drug users

Level of evidence for treatment: A, high-quality randomized controlled trial (RCT) or prospective study; B, lesser quality RCT or prospective study; C, case-control study or retrospective study; D, case series or case reports; E, expert opinion.

[a] Hydroxychloroquine,[19,22] etanercept,[19] D-penicillamine,[36] and colchicine[19] have been shown to accelerate healing in cases of methotrexate-induced accelerated rheumatoid nodulosis.

[b] Transient fever and bilateral ankle edema in a patient with amlodipine-associated GA.[47]

reaction to injectable drugs[66] and vaccinations,[67] photoinduced granulomatous eruption by hydroxyurea,[68] and a characteristic drug eruption secondary to granulocyte colony-stimulating factor (G-CSF) whereby patients presented with an eruption 1 day to 3 weeks after the administration of this medication. Histopathologic analyses of these cases revealed a dermal infiltrate composed primarily of CD68-positive enlarged histiocytes.[69] An interesting and previously unreported association was published recently on 2 patients with melanoma who developed cutaneous granulomatous eruptions during targeted BRAF inhibitor therapy.[1] In case 1, after 2 months of treatment with dabrafenib and trametinib (MEK inhibitor), a papular eruption appeared, and concern regarding the progression of the disease prompted cessation of treatment. After the histopathologic diagnosis of granulomas, the patient was treated with clobetasol ointment, with resolution within days and resumption of therapy. In case 2, after 5 months of vemurafenib treatment, the patient developed a granulomatous eruption that resolved 3 weeks after cessation of therapy. It is interesting that in case 1 the histology revealed melanoma cells central to the granulomatous reaction, suggesting that the reaction was incited by the melanoma cells. The authors propose that in this case, granuloma formation represents immune activation toward possible melanoma regression, and therefore it is unnecessary to discontinue the therapy.

SUMMARY

Granulomatous drug eruptions are rare and include 4 major types: IGDR, drug-induced accelerated rheumatoid nodulosis, drug-induced GA, and drug-induced sarcoidosis. A summary of these 4 types is presented in **Table 1**. IGDR and drug-induced GA are mostly localized to the skin, whereas both drug-induced accelerated rheumatoid nodulosis and drug-induced sarcoidosis may include major systemic involvement. In all 4 types, a temporal association between the initiation of drug therapy and lesion onset and resolution after cessation of the implicated drug is characteristic. A positive drug provocation test was reported in all of these subtypes, with lesions reappearing on reintroduction of the drug. Because a prolonged time course between initiation and cessation of the drug and the emergence and clearance of lesions is common, ranging from several weeks to months, the diagnosis of granulomatous drug eruptions and identification of the offending medication can be challenging. Among the various cutaneous and histologic presentations reported, all cases include predominance of histiocytes in the inflammatory infiltrate. Most patients experience resolution, or at least improvement of symptoms, on discontinuing the medication. In cases of persistent or relapsing course, immunosuppressive treatment is needed. It is also reasonable to consider continuing the offending medication in skin-limited disease, especially if the drug has been proved to be effective in treating a systemic disease, the risks and benefits have been assessed with the patient, and proper follow-up is conducted (eg, patients with RA who develop generalized GA due to anti-TNF treatment, and patients developing drug-induced cutaneous sarcoidosis resulting from IFN treatment of hepatitis C). Granulomatous drug eruptions should always be considered in the differential diagnosis of noninfectious granulomatous diseases of the skin, as awareness of this entity will avoid prolonged disease and unnecessary treatments.

REFERENCES

1. Park JJ, Hawryluk EB, Tahan SR, et al. Cutaneous granulomatous eruption and successful response to potent topical steroids in patients undergoing targeted BRAF inhibitor treatment for metastatic melanoma. JAMA Dermatol 2014;150(3):307–11.
2. Williams GT, Williams WJ. Granulomatous inflammation—a review. J Clin Pathol 1983;36(7):723–33.
3. Hawryluk EB, Izikson L, English JC III. Non-infectious granulomatous diseases of the skin and their associated systemic diseases. Am J Clin Dermatol 2010;11(3):171–81.
4. Izikson L, English JC. Noninfectious granulomatous diseases: an update. Adv Dermatol 2006;22:31–53.
5. Magro CM, Crowson AN, Schapiro BL. The interstitial granulomatous drug reaction: a distinctive clinical and pathological entity. J Cutan Pathol 1998;25(2):72–8.
6. Regula CG, Hennessy J, Clarke LE, et al. Interstitial granulomatous drug reaction to anakinra. J Am Acad Dermatol 2008;59(2 Suppl 1):S25–7.
7. Laura A, Luca P, Luisa PA. Interstitial granulomatous drug reaction due to febuxostat. Indian J Dermatol Venereol Leprol 2014;80(2):182–4.
8. Chen YC, Hsiao CH, Tsai TF. Interstitial granulomatous drug reaction presenting as erythroderma: remission after discontinuation of enalapril maleate. Br J Dermatol 2008;158(5):1143–5.
9. Martinez-Moran C, Nájera L, Ruiz-Casado AI, et al. Interstitial granulomatous drug reaction to sorafenib. Arch Dermatol 2011;147(9):1118–9.
10. Marcollo Pini A, Kerl K, Kamarachev J, et al. Interstitial granulomatous drug reaction following intravenous ganciclovir. Br J Dermatol 2008;158(6):1391–3.
11. Lee MW, Choi JH, Sung KJ, et al. Interstitial and granulomatous drug reaction presenting as

erythema nodosum-like lesions. Acta Derm Venereol 2002;82(6):473–4.

12. Sayah A, English JC 3rd. Rheumatoid arthritis: a review of the cutaneous manifestations. J Am Acad Dermatol 2005;53(2):191–209 [quiz: 210–2].

13. Hernandez N, Penate Y, Borrego L. Generalized erythematous-violaceous plaques in a patient with a history of dyslipidemia. Interstitial granulomatous drug reaction (IGDR). Int J Dermatol 2013;52(4): 393–4.

14. Justiniano H, Berlingeri-Ramos AC, Sánchez JL. Pattern analysis of drug-induced skin diseases. Am J Dermatopathol 2008;30(4):352–69.

15. Goldminz AM, Gottlieb AB. Noninfectious granulomatous dermatitides: a review of 8 disorders (Part 3 of 3). Semin Cutan Med Surg 2013;32:e7–11.

16. Hu S, Cohen D, Murphy G, et al. Interstitial granulomatous dermatitis in a patient with rheumatoid arthritis on etanercept. Cutis 2008;81(4):336.

17. Magro CM, Cruz-Inigo AE, Votava H, et al. Drug-associated reversible granulomatous T cell dyscrasia: a distinct subset of the interstitial granulomatous drug reaction. J Cutan Pathol 2010;37(Suppl 1):96–111.

18. Kremer JM, Lee JK. The safety and efficacy of the use of methotrexate in long-term therapy for rheumatoid arthritis. Arthritis Rheum 1986;29(7):822–31.

19. Ahmed SS, Arnett FC, Smith CA, et al. The HLA-DRB1*0401 allele and the development of methotrexate-induced accelerated rheumatoid nodulosis: a follow-up study of 79 Caucasian patients with rheumatoid arthritis. Medicine (Baltimore) 2001;80(4):271–8.

20. Goerttler E, Kutzner H, Peter HH, et al. Methotrexate-induced papular eruption in patients with rheumatic diseases: a distinctive adverse cutaneous reaction produced by methotrexate in patients with collagen vascular diseases. J Am Acad Dermatol 1999;40(5 Pt 1):702–7.

21. Kerstens PJ, Boerbooms AM, Jeurissen ME, et al. Accelerated nodulosis during low dose methotrexate therapy for rheumatoid arthritis. An analysis of ten cases. J Rheumatol 1992;19(6):867–71.

22. Muzaffer MA, Schneider R, Cameron BJ, et al. Accelerated nodulosis during methotrexate therapy for juvenile rheumatoid arthritis. J Pediatr 1996; 128(5 Pt 1):698–700.

23. Smith MD. Accelerated nodulosis in a patient with psoriasis and arthritis during treatment with methotrexate. J Rheumatol 1996;23(11):2004.

24. Rivero MG, Salvatore AJ, Gómez-Puerta JA, et al. Accelerated nodulosis during methotrexate therapy in a patient with systemic lupus erythematosus and Jaccoud's arthropathy. Rheumatology (Oxford) 2004;43(12):1587–8.

25. Berkun Y, Abou Atta I, Rubinow A, et al. 2756GG genotype of methionine synthase reductase gene is more prevalent in rheumatoid arthritis patients treated with

methotrexate and is associated with methotrexate-induced nodulosis. J Rheumatol 2007;34(8):1664–9.

26. Matsushita I, Uzuki M, Matsuno H, et al. Rheumatoid nodulosis during methotrexate therapy in a patient with rheumatoid arthritis. Mod Rheumatol 2006; 16(6):401–3.

27. Cunnane G, Warnock M, Fye KH, et al. Accelerated nodulosis and vasculitis following etanercept therapy for rheumatoid arthritis. Arthritis Rheum 2002; 47(4):445–9.

28. Scrivo R, Spadaro A, Iagnocco A, et al. Appearance of rheumatoid nodules following anti-tumor necrosis factor alpha treatment with adalimumab for rheumatoid arthritis. Clin Exp Rheumatol 2007;25(1):117.

29. Mackley CL, Ostrov BE, Ioffreda MD. Accelerated cutaneous nodulosis during infliximab therapy in a patient with rheumatoid arthritis. J Clin Rheumatol 2004;10(6):336–8.

30. Chao J, Parker BA, Zvaifler NJ. Accelerated cutaneous nodulosis associated with aromatase inhibitor therapy in a patient with rheumatoid arthritis. J Rheumatol 2009;36(5):1087–8.

31. Langevitz P, Maguire L, Urowitz M. Accelerated nodulosis during azathioprine therapy. Arthritis Rheum 1991;34(1):123–4.

32. Braun MG, Van Rhee R, Becker-Capeller D. Development and/or increase of rheumatoid nodules in RA patients following leflunomide therapy. Z Rheumatol 2004;63(1):84–7 [in German].

33. Alarcon GS, Koopman WJ, McCarty MJ. Nonperipheral accelerated nodulosis in a methotrexate-treated rheumatoid arthritis patient. Arthritis Rheum 1993; 36(1):132–3.

34. Bruyn GA, Essed CE, Houtman PM, et al. Fatal cardiac nodules in a patient with rheumatoid arthritis treated with low dose methotrexate. J Rheumatol 1993;20(5):912–4.

35. Karam NE, Roger L, Hankins LL, et al. Rheumatoid nodulosis of the meninges. J Rheumatol 1994; 21(10):1960–3.

36. Dash S, Seibold JR, Tiku ML. Successful treatment of methotrexate induced nodulosis with D-penicillamine. J Rheumatol 1999;26(6):1396–9.

37. Wolff KE. Fitzpatrick's dermatology in general medicine. New York: McGraw-Hill. J Am Acad Dermatol 2004;51(2):325–26.

38. Goldminz AM, Gottlieb AB. Noninfectious granulomatous dermatitides: a review of 8 disorders (Part 1 of 3). Semin Cutan Med Surg 2013;32(3):177–82.

39. Rothwell R, Schloss E. Granuloma annulare and gold therapy. Arch Dermatol 1980;116(8):863.

40. Kluger N, Moguelet P, Chaslin-Ferbus D, et al. Generalized interstitial granuloma annulare induced by pegylated interferon-alpha. Dermatology 2006; 213(3):248–9.

41. Voulgari PV, Markatseli TE, Exarchou SA, et al. Granuloma annulare induced by anti-tumour

necrosis factor therapy. Ann Rheum Dis 2008; 67(4):567–70.

42. Murdaca G, Colombo BM, Barabino G, et al. Anti-tumor necrosis factor-alpha treatment with infliximab for disseminated granuloma annulare. Am J Clin Dermatol 2010;11(6):437–9.

43. Torres T, Pinto Almeida T, Alves R, et al. Treatment of recalcitrant generalized granuloma annulare with adalimumab. J Drugs Dermatol 2011;10(12): 1466–8.

44. Singh SK, Manchanda K, Bhayana AA, et al. Allopurinol induced granuloma annulare in a patient of lepromatous leprosy. J Pharmacol Pharmacother 2013;4(2):152–4.

45. Ahmad U, Li X, Sodeman T, et al. Hepatitis C virus treatment with pegylated interferon-alfa therapy leading to generalized interstitial granuloma annulare and review of the literature. Am J Ther 2013; 20(5):585–7.

46. Wolf F, Grezard P, Berard F, et al. Generalized granuloma annulare and hepatitis B vaccination. Eur J Dermatol 1998;8(6):435–6.

47. Lim AC, Hart K, Murrell D. A granuloma annulare-like eruption associated with the use of amlodipine. Australas J Dermatol 2002;43(1):24–7.

48. Cassono G, Tumiati B. Granuloma annulare as a possible new adverse effect of topiramate. Int J Dermatol 2014;53(2):259–61.

49. Martin N, Belinchón I, Fuente C, et al. Granuloma annulare and gold therapy. Arch Dermatol 1990; 126(10):1370–1.

50. Ferreli C, Atzori L, Manunza F, et al. Thalidomide-induced granuloma annulare. G Ital Dermatol Venereol 2014;149(3):329.

51. Alvarez-Perez A, Gómez-Bernal S, Gutiérrez-González E, et al. Granuloma annulare photoinduced by paroxetine. Photodermatol Photoimmunol Photomed 2012;28(1):47–9.

52. Thornsberry LA, English JC 3rd. Etiology, diagnosis, and therapeutic management of granuloma annulare: an update. Am J Clin Dermatol 2013;14(4): 279–90.

53. Abdi EA, Nguyen GK, Ludwig RN, et al. Pulmonary sarcoidosis following interferon therapy for advanced renal cell carcinoma. Cancer 1987;59(5):896–900.

54. Ramos-Casals M, Mañá J, Nardi N, et al. Sarcoidosis in patients with chronic hepatitis C virus infection: analysis of 68 cases. Medicine (Baltimore) 2005;84(2):69–80.

55. Buss G, Cattin V, Spring P, et al. Two cases of interferon-alpha-induced sarcoidosis Koebnerized along venous drainage lines: new pathogenic insights and review of the literature of interferon-induced sarcoidosis. Dermatology 2013;226(4): 289–97.

56. Wanat KA, Rosenbach M. Case series demonstrating improvement in chronic cutaneous sarcoidosis following treatment with TNF inhibitors. Arch Dermatol 2012;148(9):1097–100.

57. Lamrock E, Brown P. Development of cutaneous sarcoidosis during treatment with tumour necrosis alpha factor antagonists. Australas J Dermatol 2012;53:e87–90.

58. Cathcart S, Sami N, Elewski B. Sarcoidosis as an adverse effect of tumor necrosis factor inhibitors. J Drugs Dermatol 2012;11(5):609–12.

59. Vigne C, Tebib JG, Pacheco Y, et al. Sarcoidosis: an underestimated and potentially severe side effect of anti-TNF-alpha therapy. Joint Bone Spine 2013; 80(1):104–7.

60. Santos G, Sousa LE, Joao AM. Exacerbation of recalcitrant cutaneous sarcoidosis with adalimumab—a paradoxical effect? A case report. An Bras Dermatol 2013;88(6 Suppl 1):26–8.

61. Carlson JA, Schutzer P, Pattison T, et al. Sarcoidal foreign-body granulomatous dermatitis associated with ophthalmic drops. Am J Dermatopathol 1998; 20(2):175–8.

62. Reule RB, North JP. Cutaneous and pulmonary sarcoidosis-like reaction associated with ipilimumab. J Am Acad Dermatol 2013;69:e272–3.

63. Fantini F, Padalino C, Gualdi G, et al. Cutaneous lesions as initial signs of interferon α-induced sarcoidosis: report of three new cases and review of the literature. Dermatol Ther 2009;22(s1):S1–7.

64. Bardazzi F, Ruffato A, Antonucci A, et al. Cutaneous granulomatous reaction to injectable hyaluronic acid gel: another case. J Dermatolog Treat 2007;18(1): 59–62.

65. Goldberg HJ, Fiedler D, Webb A, et al. Sarcoidosis after treatment with interferon-alpha: a case series and review of the literature. Respir Med 2006; 100(11):2063–8.

66. Ball RA, Kinchelow T, ISR Substudy Group. Injection site reactions with the HIV-1 fusion inhibitor enfuvirtide. J Am Acad Dermatol 2003;49(5):826–31.

67. Nikkels AF, Nikkels-Tassoudji N, Piérard GE. Cutaneous adverse reactions following anti-infective vaccinations. Am J Clin Dermatol 2005;6(2):79–87.

68. Leon-Mateos A, Zulaica A, Caeiro JL, et al. Photo-induced granulomatous eruption by hydroxyurea. J Eur Acad Dermatol Venereol 2007;21(10): 1428–9.

69. Scott GA. Report of three cases of cutaneous reactions to granulocyte macrophage-colony-stimulating factor and a review of the literature. Am J Dermatopathol 1995;17(2):107–14.

70. Deng A, Harvey V, Sina B, et al. Interstitial granulomatous dermatitis associated with the use of tumor necrosis factor α inhibitors. Arch Dermatol 2006; 142(2):198–202.

71. Fujita Y, Shimizu T, Shimizu H. A case of interstitial granulomatous drug reaction due to sennoside. Br J Dermatol 2004;150(5):1035–7.

72. Du XF, Yin XP, Zhang GL, et al. Interstitial granulomatous drug reaction to a Chinese herb extract. Eur J Dermatol 2012;22(3):419–20.

73. Groves C, McMenamin ME, Casey M, et al. Interstitial granulomatous reaction to strontium ranelate. Arch Dermatol 2008;144(2):268–9.

74. Martin G, Cañueto J, Santos-Briz A, et al. Interstitial granulomatous dermatitis with arthritis associated with trastuzumab. J Eur Acad Dermatol Venereol 2010;24(4):493–4.

75. Mason HR, Swanson JK, Ho J, et al. Interstitial granulomatous dermatitis associated with darifenacin. J Drugs Dermatol 2008;7(9):895–7.

76. Le Corre Y, Léonard F, Fertin C, et al. Granuloma-annulare type photosensitivity disorder caused by diclofenac. Ann Dermatol Venereol 1992;119(11): 932–3 [in French].

77. Goihman-Yahr M. Disseminated granuloma annulare and intranasal calcitonin. Int J Dermatol 1993;32(2): 150.

78. Baykal C, Ozkaya-Bayazit E, Kaymaz R. Granuloma annulare possibly triggered by antitetanus vaccination. J Eur Acad Dermatol Venereol 2002;16(5): 516–8.

79. Spring P, Vernez M, Maniu CM, et al. Localized interstitial granuloma annulare induced by subcutaneous injections for desensitization. Dermatol Online J 2013;19(6):18572.

80. Jordaan HF, Sandler M. Zinc-induced granuloma—a unique complication of insulin therapy. Clin Exp Dermatol 1989;14(3):227–9.

81. Healsmith MF, Hutchinson PE. The development of scar sarcoidosis at the site of desensitization injections. Clin Exp Dermatol 1992;17(5):369–70.

Tuberculosis and Leprosy
Classical Granulomatous Diseases in the Twenty-First Century

 CrossMark

David M. Scollard, MD, PhD[a],*, Mara M. Dacso, MD, MS[b,c],
Ma. Luisa Abad-Venida, MD, FPDS[d]

KEYWORDS

- Granuloma - Atypical mycobacteria - Tuberculosis - Lupus vulgaris - Leprosy - Hansen disease
- Leprosy reaction - Cell-mediated immunity

KEY POINTS

- Cutaneous lesions are rare in tuberculosis but are common in leprosy.
- *Mycobacterium tuberculosis* is cultivable; *Mycobacterium leprae* is not.
- Both infections are curable, but optimal multidrug regimens for them are different.
- Standard Ziehl-Neelsen staining may fail to stain many *M leprae,* because they are weakly acid-fast compared with *M tuberculosis.*
- A delay or failure to diagnose cutaneous tuberculosis may be associated with mortality if there is concomitant systemic disease; delay or failure to diagnose leprosy is associated with a high risk of peripheral neuropathy and disability.
- Hypoesthesia and intraneural or perineural localization of granulomas are helpful in distinguishing leprosy from tuberculosis clinically and histologically.

INTRODUCTION

Tuberculosis (TB) and leprosy, the 2 major mycobacterial infections of humans, are classic granulomatous diseases that still affect millions of people. Both infections are now curable, but no highly effective vaccine is yet available for either of them. Both are ancient scourges with a wide range of cutaneous manifestations, and both are infamous for their ability to mimic other diseases and sometimes fool even the most skilled diagnostician.

Etiopathogenesis

TB and leprosy are both chronic infections, but they are very different diseases (**Table 1**).

Mycobacterium tuberculosis Is cultivable; *Mycobacterium leprae* is not. *M leprae* infects peripheral nerves; *M tuberculosis* does not. Untreated tuberculosis has a high mortality; untreated leprosy has a high disability rate due to peripheral neuropathy. Cutaneous lesions are typical of leprosy, but rare in tuberculosis.

The cell-mediated immune response (CMI) to these agents is the critical determinant in individual susceptibility to these infections and in the range of clinical and histologic appearances of their cutaneous lesions (**Fig. 1**). The organisms express pathogen-associated molecular patterns on their surfaces, which are recognized by pattern recognition receptors of macrophages and

All authors declare that they have no conflicts of interest.

[a] National Hansen's Disease Programs, 1770 Physician Park Drive, Baton Rouge, LA 70816, USA; [b] Center for Dermatology and Cosmetic Laser Surgery, 5026 Tennyson Parkway, Plano, TX 75024, USA; [c] Department of Dermatology, University of Texas Southwestern Medical Center, 5323 Harry Hines Boulevard, Dallas, TX 75390-9069, USA; [d] Department of Dermatology, Jose R. Reyes Memorial Medical Center, Rizal Avenue, Manila 1008, Philippines

* Corresponding author.
E-mail address: dscollard@hrsa.gov

Table 1
A comparison of tuberculosis and leprosy

	TB	Leprosy
Etiologic agent	*M tuberculosis*	*M leprae*
Acid-fastness	Strong (Ziehl-Neelsen stain)	Weak (Fite stain preferred)
Growth in tissue	Extracellular or in macrophages	Obligate intracellular pathogen, in macrophages and Schwann cells
Cultivable	Yes	No
Growth temperature	37°C	33°C
Number of protein genes	3993	1614
Number of pseudogenes	6	1133
Transmission	Airborne droplets	Probably airborne
Initial site of infection	Periphery of lung	Nose and nasopharynx
Cutaneous infection	Uncommon	Typical, very common
Infection of peripheral nerves	No	Yes
Infection is curable	Yes	Yes
CMI	Mainly 2 polar types; strong and weak CMI	Full spectrum from strong to none
Outcome if untreated	High mortality	Very low mortality; high disability rate from peripheral neuropathy
Vaccine	BCG (variable protection)	BCG (variable protection)

dendritic cells, facilitating phagocytosis.[1] Innate immunity to mycobacteria is mediated by macrophages and dendritic cells, including Langerhans cells in the skin, and may be sufficient to prevent further progression of the infection.

If innate immunity is insufficient, mycobacterial antigens are presented to CD4+ T cells, initiating the acquired CMI.[2] Based largely on inherited immunologic capabilities, CMI in most individuals will be driven by activated CD4+ T lymphocytes

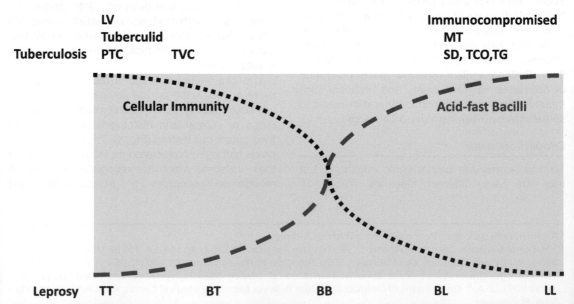

Fig. 1. Immunopathologic patterns of cutaneous tuberculosis and leprosy. The cellular immune status and bacterial load of different forms of cutaneous tuberculosis compared with the broad, continuous spectrum in leprosy. Cutaneous tuberculosis: MT, miliary tuberculosis; PTC, primary tuberculous chancre; SD, scrofuloderma; TCO, tuberculosis cutis orificialis; TG, tuberculous gumma.

elaborating tumor necrosis factor-α (TNF-α) and interleukin-2 (IL-2), stimulating macrophage release of interferon-γ (IFN-γ), the TH1 pattern of cytokines.[3] TH1 responses are associated with the formation of well-organized granulomas. The epithelioid macrophage is a specialized cell producing large quantities of cytokines, with enhanced microbicidal activity. Such granulomas are associated with limited proliferation of mycobacteria.[4,5] Caseous necrosis is thought to be a result of the death and regeneration of the epithelioid cells within the granuloma, a process mediated by TNF-α and proteases.[6]

Although granuloma formation has been understood as a host-protective strategy to limit spread of the mycobacteria, recent studies suggest that M tuberculosis may use the granuloma to shield itself from the host's immunologic killing mechanisms and antimicrobial agents.[7] Therapies targeting granuloma formation are being studied as adjunctive therapies for the treatment of TB.[8]

Such a shielding effect of granulomas may play a role in the human tuberculosis and leprosy, but it is also apparent that in these 2 infections the well-organized epithelioid granuloma is associated with a high degree of CMI and a limited bacterial load. When CMI is weak or absent, a TH-2 response to mycobacterial infection results, characterized by the production of IL-4 and IL-10. In such individuals, well-organized granulomas do not develop, and mycobacteria proliferate and may reach large numbers, such as in lepromatous leprosy or tuberculosis in immunosuppressed individuals.

Antibodies play no role in protective immunity to M tuberculosis or M leprae. Negligible antibody production is elicited by either agent in individuals who have strong CMI and granulomatous responses. In general, therefore, tests for antibodies are not useful in the diagnosis of these infections, whereas assays for CMI mediators such as IFN-γ[9] are sensitive and specific for tuberculosis, and measurements of CXCL-10 show promise for use in leprosy.[10,11]

CUTANEOUS TUBERCULOSIS
Epidemiology

TB remains the second leading cause of death worldwide, despite concerted measures to improve detection and treatment. The World Health Organization (WHO) estimates that 8.6 million people were diagnosed with TB in 2012 (122 cases per 100,000 population) and 1.3 million died of the disease.[12] Although the incidence of TB has decreased 2% over the last decade, global efforts to reach the 2015 Millennium Development Goal of decreasing TB-related mortality by 50%

are unlikely to succeed,[12] and the increase in multidrug-resistant TB (MDR-TB) raises concerns of an epidemic of untreatable cases.[6]

Skin involvement is a relatively rare extrapulmonary manifestation of systemic TB, comprising less than 1% to 2% of all cases.[13–18] However, cutaneous TB is still an important differential diagnosis to consider in the age of HIV/AIDS, MDR-TB, and immunosuppressive therapies.[19]

Etiopathogenesis

Cutaneous TB in humans is primarily caused by M tuberculosis, although rarely this is due to Mycobacterium bovis.[20–24] The development of cutaneous TB depends on multiple factors, including the route of infection, duration of exposure and previous sensitization, and the individual's CMI.[22]

Cutaneous manifestations of TB are immunologically driven; individuals without effective CMI face a higher risk of active disease with exudative lesions and disseminated miliary TB.[5] The tuberculin skin test (purified protein derivative [PPD]), reflecting delayed hypersensitivity to M tuberculosis antigens, becomes positive 3 to 8 weeks after infection.[6]

Histopathology

Typically, 3 to 6 weeks after infection, the classic tuberculoid granuloma develops, with a central focus of epithelioid histiocytes and Langhans giant cells surrounded by a mantle of lymphocytes. Caseation necrosis occurs in the center of the granuloma, often with calcification and fibrosis. The number of bacilli is roughly proportional to the amount of necrosis present. The histopathological features of different forms of cutaneous TB depend on source of infection (exogenous vs endogenous) and the host's CMI.

Both sarcoidosis and lupus vulgaris (LV) are characterized by granulomas, but sarcoidal granulomas typically have minimal lymphocytic inflammation and no caseation necrosis. Perineural involvement helps to distinguish tuberculoid leprosy from cutaneous TB (see later discussion). The causative organism must be identified in other infections with a prominent granulomatous infiltrate (ie, atypical mycobacteria, leishmaniasis, blastomycosis, and chromomycosis). Tertiary syphilis can also be granulomatous; however, increased plasma cells and endothelial swelling help differentiate it from TB. Rosacea and panniculitis can exhibit a nonspecific nodular granulomatous infiltrate, but typical tuberculoid granulomas are absent.[6] Rare cases of lupus miliaris disseminatus faceii, a controversial entity generally understood as a rosacea variant, have shown evidence of TB.[6,13]

Classification and Clinical Presentations

The classification of cutaneous TB has evolved from a model based on clinical morphology to one incorporating the route of transmission and immune status (**Table 2**).[13,25] In an individual with high CMI, few bacilli are noted histologically, and they are difficult to culture. Patients with low CMI have many mycobacteria, easily seen in Ziehl-Neelsen–stained sections and cultured.[26] The presence of numerous acid-fast bacilli (AFB) indicates impaired CMI and suggests consideration of other entities such as leprosy (see **Fig. 1**).

High immune forms

Tuberculosis verrucosa cutis (TVC) is a warty plaquelike form occurring most commonly on the extremities as a result of direct cutaneous inoculation in a previously sensitized individual (**Fig. 2**). TVC can occur by accidental inoculation (ie, "prosector's wart"), by autoinoculation from sputum in a patient with active TB, and in children with some immunity exposed to infected sputum.[6] Clinically, TVC starts as an asymptomatic indurated papule, gradually evolving into a brownish-red verrucous plaque with a soft center, sometimes with keratinous discharge; this may spontaneously involute, forming a hypopigmented and atrophic scar, or it can become a large, exophytic, keloidal plaque, with rare sporotrichoid spread or lymphadenitis.[6] Histologically, TVC shows epidermal hyperplasia with a mixed dermal infiltrate of neutrophils, lymphocytes, and some giant cells. Bacilli may or may not be identified. The differential diagnosis is broad, including fungal infections (sporotrichosis, blastomycosis, and chromomycosis) as well as leishmaniasis, tertiary syphilis, hypertrophic lichen planus, psoriasis, and squamous cell carcinoma.[27]

LV is a chronic and progressive form of cutaneous TB that occurs in patients with moderate to high CMI. Historically, LV has been the most common presentation of cutaneous TB in Asia and South Africa.[15,28–30] It presents with multiple red-brown papules coalescing into plaques (**Fig. 3**), developing a gelatinous quality centrally; its appearance on diascopy resembles "apple jelly."[6,13] Lesions run a variable course and may cause significant tissue destruction, heal with atrophic scarring, or have a prolonged course with minimal cutaneous damage.[6,26] The most commonly affected areas were the head and neck in Europe,[31] and the extremities, trunk, and buttocks in Asia.[15,32] LV may originate from an underlying focus of TB in a lymph node, bone, or joint, by direct contiguous extension, or via lymphatic spread.[6] It may result from reactivation of latent cutaneous TB or after exogenous inoculation, including Bacille Calmette-Guérin (BCG) vaccination.[21] Involvement of the face may result from hematogenous spread, and acral lesions may result from reinoculation.[13] Clinical variants include classic plaque-type, ulcerative, vegetating, tumorlike, papular, and nodular forms.[6] Histologic findings often include typical tuberculoid granulomas surrounded by numerous lymphocytes, sparse caseation necrosis, and fibrosis (**Figs. 4** and **5**). Bacilli may or may not be identified by acid-fast staining.

LV is morphologically diverse and can mimic a plethora of cutaneous conditions, such as Spitz nevus and lupus erythematosus,[6] in early stages as well as rosacea[33] and port-wine stains[34] in chronic disease. Verrucous and vegetating lesions (**Fig. 6**) can resemble deep fungal infections or other mycobacterial infections. Differentiating the "apple-jelly" lesions of LV from those of sarcoidosis and leprosy can be challenging, and subtle nuances such as the firm texture of leprosy nodules versus the more grainlike quality of sarcoid lesions may be the only clinical clues.[6]

Tuberculids, first described by Darier in 1896,[35] are hypersensitivity reactions to *M tuberculosis* or other mycobacterial antigen in a person with strong CMI against TB. Tuberculids classically include lichen scrofulosorum (**Fig. 7**), papulonecrotic tuberculid (**Fig. 8**), nodular tuberculid, erythema induratum (Bazin disease), and the more recently described nodular granulomatous phlebitis.[17,36–38] Tuberculids tend to run a relapsing and remitting course, appearing in crops and healing with scarring. Although the histology of tuberculids can vary, they generally show granulomatous inflammation (**Fig. 9**) and some degree of necrosis and vasculitis (**Figs. 10** and **11**), suggesting that they are the result of released mycobacterial antigens from concurrent or distant TB.[38] Tuberculids fail to show evidence of mycobacteria with special stains or cultures, but polymerase chain reaction (PCR) has detected mycobacterial DNA in some specimens.[6,39]

Low immune forms

A tuberculous chancre results from cutaneous or mucosal inoculation in a person with a low level of CMI. It most commonly presents in children as an inflammatory papule at the site of inoculation on the face or extremities; after 2 to 4 weeks, this develops into a firm, shallow solitary ulcer with regional lymphadenopathy. Histologically, abundant neutrophils and numerous AFB are seen, with necrosis involving skin and lymph nodes. Later, lesions demonstrate more granulomatous inflammation with fewer bacilli. The

Table 2
Clinical and histologic classification of cutaneous tuberculosis

TB Type	Host Immunity to *M tuberculosis*	Clinical Presentation	Histologic Features	PPD
TVC	High	Hyperkeratotic papule or plaque, resolves spontaneously with scarring, often with lymphadenopathy	Pseudoepitheliomatous hyperplasia of epidermis with intense dermal infiltrate of neutrophils, lymphocytes, and some giant cells; ± bacilli	+
LV	Moderate to high	Plaque: gelatinous Hypertrophic: soft nodules Ulcerative: necrotic Vegetative: papule with ulceration or necrosis Commonly involving face/neck; "apple-jelly" appearance on diascopy	Tuberculoid granulomas embedded in sheets of lymphocytes, sparse or absent caseation, extensive fibrosis with healing; increased risk of developing nonmelanoma skin cancer in lesions; ± bacilli	±
Tuberculids	Moderate to high	Papulonecrotic tuberculid, dusky small papules with central necrosis Lichen scrofulosorum, multiple grouped lichenoid papules Erythema induratum (Bazin), painful ulcerated nodules on posterior legs Nodular tuberculid, bluish-red nontender, nonulcerating nodules on legs Nodular granulomatous phlebitis, nonulcerating, subcutaneous nodules along leg veins of anterior and medial leg	Superficial granulomatous infiltrate, wedge-shaped necrosis, granulomatous vasculitis Variable dermal granulomas Granulomatous vasculitis at junction of deep dermis/subcutis Septal and lobular panniculitis with granulomatous vasculitis Epithelioid granulomas with Langhan giant cells in walls of cutaneous veins No bacilli	+
Scrofuloderma	Low	Nodule over affected cervical lymph node, suppurates and ulcerates with fistulae progressing to scarring	Ulcerated dermal abscess with scattered histiocytes, few lymphocytes, marked caseation necrosis containing numerous bacteria in the deeper structures; ++ bacilli	+
Tuberculosis cutis orificialis	Low	Painful papule that ulcerates with "punched-out" borders; usually oral cavity or genitourinary	Ulceration with underlying caseating granulomas; ++ bacilli	±
Miliary tuberculosis	Low	Numerous discrete minute red to violaceous papulopustules, umbilication, hemorrhagic necrosis, crusting; heal with atrophic scarring	Focal necrosis with microabscesses surrounded by chronic inflammation; in HIV patients more pustular with numerous neutrophils; ++ bacilli	±
Tuberculous gumma (metastatic tuberculous abscess)	Low	Indurated deep nodule(s) on trunk, face, extremities, becoming fluctuant with draining sinuses, ± ulceration	Tuberculous granulation tissue, massive necrosis, and abscess formation; ++ bacilli	±
Tuberculous chancre	Naïve host	Usually follows penetration injury; inflammatory papule progresses to nontender, shallow, undermined ulcer with painless lymphadenopathy	Acute neutrophilic inflammation with necrosis in skin and affected lymph nodes. Granulomatous inflammatory infiltrate in later lesions; ++ bacilli (early), ± late	±

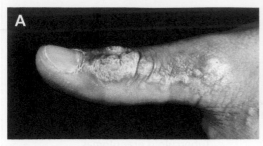

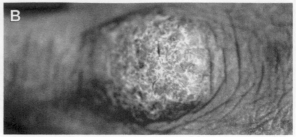

Fig. 2. (A,B) TVC ("prosector's wart") occurring on the hand.

differential diagnosis includes tularemia, other mycobacterial infections (especially *Mycobacterium marinum*), sporotrichosis, and actinomycosis.[6]

Scrofuloderma results from breakdown of skin overlying a contiguous tuberculous focus, most commonly a lymph node, bone, or joint, or a lacrimal gland or duct (**Fig. 12**).[6] It has been reported as the most common form in children,[28] but is also seen in adults.[14] Clinically, an abscess or fistula draining purulent material forms from an underlying focus of infection with subsequent induration and ulceration of the site. Histologically, an ulcerated dermal abscess with marked caseation necrosis is present, with scattered histiocytes, lymphocytes, and numerous AFB. The differential diagnosis includes sporotrichosis, hidradenitis suppurativa, actinomycosis, and syphilitic gumma.[6,27]

Tuberculosis cutis orificialis (**Fig. 13**) is a form of autoinoculation TB occurring in mucosal or orificial sites after local trauma. Patients are typically immunocompromised and are often severely ill with advanced visceral TB.[6] Lesions present on the nose, mouth, tongue, lips, and infrequently, on the vulva, as small erythematous papules that rapidly break down, forming undermined and painful ulcers with violaceous edges. Histology demonstrates ulceration with underlying caseating granulomas. The clinical differential diagnosis is broad and includes herpes simplex, Crohn disease, malignancy, aphthous ulcers, paracoccidioidomycosis, and the Melkersson-Rosenthal syndrome.[27,40]

Cutaneous miliary TB is a rare manifestation due to hematogenous spread of mycobacteria to the skin, usually from a pulmonary or meningeal focus.[41] It primarily affects young children and immunocompromised patients.[32,41] Lesions present as crops of widespread, minute (1–4 mm) papulopustules and vesicles on the trunk and extremities. The initial diagnosis of systemic TB may sometimes be made from a skin biopsy in this form,[41] showing focal necrosis and microabscesses. Lesions can mimic folliculitis[42] as well as lymphomatoid papulosis, disseminated herpes infection, bacterial endocarditis, disseminated cryptococcosis, and papulopustular syphilis.[27,41]

Tuberculous gumma (metastatic tuberculous abscess) occurs as a result of hematogenous spread of TB from a primary focus that remains latent until a period of lowered resistance (ie, malnutrition, immune compromise).[13] Lesions begin as solitary or multiple subcutaneous nodules or abscesses, usually on the extremities, which break down forming an ulcer with draining sinuses.[6] Histology shows granulation tissue, massive necrosis, and abscess formation with

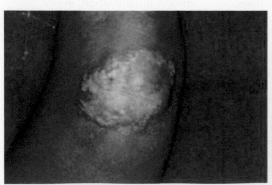

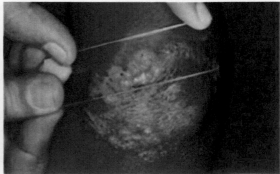

Fig. 3. LV, classic plaque-type, which demonstrated a classic "apple-jelly" appearance on diascopy.

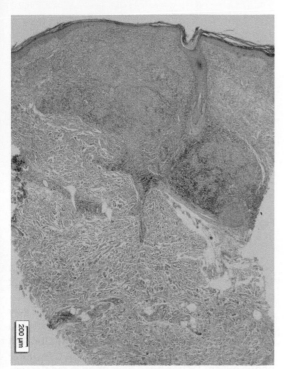

Fig. 4. Histology of LV, showing dermal granulomas accompanied by a dense lymphocytic infiltrate (H&E, ×20).

numerous AFB. Histologically, the differential diagnosis includes deep fungal infections, syphilitic gumma, and leishmaniasis.[27]

Systemic Associations

Transmission of *M tuberculosis* is primarily via respiratory droplets; therefore, the most common site of primary infection is the pulmonary system. Although primary inoculation of the skin with tuberculosis is possible, most cases of cutaneous TB are related to tuberculous disease of other organs.[13]

Extrapulmonary disease occurs more commonly in immunocompromised patients and may affect

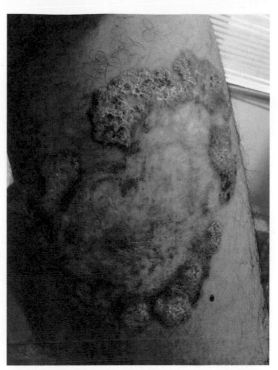

Fig. 6. Hyperkeratotic lesions of LV may clinically resemble a deep fungal infection or other mycobacterial infection.

lymph nodes, meninges, eyes, peritoneal cavity, and intra-abdominal organs.[5,43–45] Kivanç-Altunay and colleagues[46] observed that spread of visceral TB to skin was rare.

Comorbidities that increase the risk of both systemic and cutaneous TB include HIV/AIDS, young age, solid organ transplantation, poorly controlled diabetes mellitus, intravenous drug abuse, renal failure, underlying systemic malignancy, vitamin D or A deficiency, and chronic immunosuppressive therapies.[4,5,47,48] In a patient with diabetes mellitus

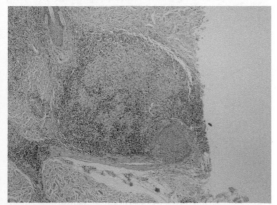

Fig. 5. LV with well-formed epithelioid granulomas in the papillary and reticular dermis (H&E, ×40).

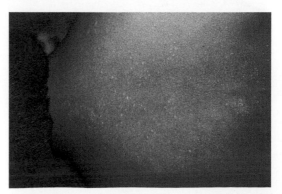

Fig. 7. Lichen scrofulosorum with scattered lichenoid papules, characteristically healing with varioliform scarring.

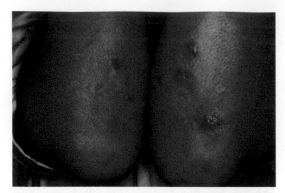

Fig. 8. Papulonecrotic tuberculid from a TB hypersensitivity reaction in a person with strong immunity.

and taking corticosteroids, atypical gangrenous or vegetating forms of TB and tuberculous cellulitis-like lesions have been seen.[49] Cutaneous TB in immunodeficient patients often elicits a less granulomatous inflammatory response, and more bacilli are identified.[6]

Cutaneous tuberculosis in immunocompromised patients

The frequency of extrapulmonary TB in patients with advanced HIV infection is high when there is concomitant pulmonary TB; the incidence of coinfection is up to 20% in the United States.[43,50,51] Despite this, the coexistence of cutaneous TB and HIV is relatively rare.[41] However, the clinical features of cutaneous TB in HIV+ patients are highly variable and unusual. In India, scrofuloderma and LV were the most common presentations of cutaneous TB in HIV+ patients[51]; LV has also presented with erythematous plaques on the cheek and pinna,[51] ulcerated lesions, cellulitis-like lesions, subcutaneous abscesses, and tuberculids.[42,49,52] These patients are more likely to

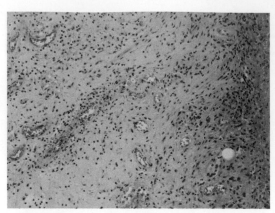

Fig. 10. Chronic granulomatous small-vessel vasculitis in a papulonecrotic tuberculid (H&E, ×100).

develop acute fulminant miliary TB in the skin,[42,53,54] often associated with drug-resistant strains[55] and carrying a poor prognosis.[42]

Renal transplant patients are 5 times more likely to acquire TB, with an incidence of 0.5% to 1% in the United States, most commonly during the first year after transplantation.[56,57] Although rare, cutaneous miliary TB has been described in renal transplant recipients presenting with multiple erythematous papules on the lower extremities[47,57] or with erythematous and violaceous lesions on the legs, subcutaneous nodules, and necrotizing tuberculous fasciitis of the gluteus muscle.[42]

Evaluation and Management

Definitive diagnosis of TB requires a positive culture of M tuberculosis or identification of mycobacterial DNA by PCR.[6,22] Skin biopsy, smear, and acid-fast stains should be performed in all suspicious cases. Notably, recent data suggest that in latent infection with distinct cell-wall alterations, M

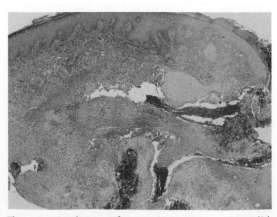

Fig. 9. Histology of papulonecrotic tuberculid. Epidermal ulceration, necrosis, and palisading histiocytes in the dermis. No AFB are identified (H&E, ×20).

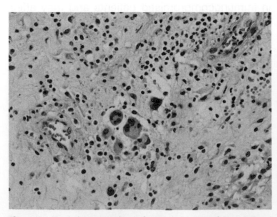

Fig. 11. Papulonecrotic tuberculid. Langhans giant cells and a mixed inflammatory infiltrate adjacent to a small blood vessel (H&E, ×200).

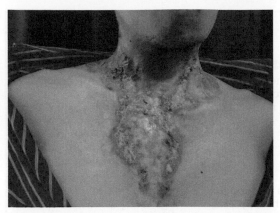

Fig. 12. Late-stage scrofuloderma of the neck and anterior chest.

tuberculosis may lose Ziehl-Neelsen staining, and tissue samples with negative AFB stains may be positive by culture and PCR analysis.[58]

A positive PPD reaction is helpful in diagnosis, but different degrees of induration are significant in different groups, (eg, immunocompetent individuals, young children, immigrants, injection drug users, immunosuppressed patients, or those who have chest radiograph findings of prior TB).[13,59] Serum QuantiFERON-TB Gold (QFT-G; Cellestis Inc, Valencia, CA, USA), which measures IFN-γ release by sensitized lymphocytes in vitro, is highly specific and has been recommended by the Centers for Disease Control and Prevention (CDC) for use in all circumstances in which the PPD skin test is used.[59]

PCR techniques are highly sensitive and specific and are helpful in detecting *M tuberculosis* when the bacterial load is extremely low.[6] Mycobacterial DNA has also been identified in papulonecrotic tuberculid and erythema induratum.[39] Because PCR can be positive due to bacteremia and not necessarily cutaneous disease, it must be interpreted within the clinical context.[60]

Treatment of cutaneous TB consists of multiple drug treatment (MDT) to prevent the emergence of bacterial resistance, for a length of time sufficient to eliminate the mycobacteria (**Table 3**). Because many patients with skin findings also have simultaneous systemic TB, the treatment regimens are identical.[61] The CDC recommends a 2-phase regimen: (1) initial intensive bactericidal treatment for 8 weeks with daily isoniazid, rifampin, pyrazinamide, and either ethambutol or streptomycin; and (2) maintenance for 16 weeks with isoniazid and rifampin given daily or 2 or 3 times weekly.[62] Surgical excision may be effective in cases of LV, scrofuloderma, and TVC. Plastic surgery can be helpful when cutaneous TB is complicated by severe scarring and disfigurement.[6,22,23]

Clinical results/outcomes in the literature

Cutaneous TB usually responds well to MDT, and clinical improvement should be expected after 4 to 6 weeks.[63] It is important to individualize the therapy, taking into account overall health, immune status, type and degree of cutaneous involvement, stage of disease, patient compliance with medication administration, and side effects.[27] Although MDR-TB and extensively drug-resistant TB pose serious threats to management,[64,65] it is extremely rare for resistant strains to develop in the context of cutaneous TB.

Summary

Although cutaneous TB is relatively rare, the increase in new cases of pulmonary TB has led to an increase in incidence of cutaneous TB. This increase in incidence is especially true in high-risk populations, such as in endemic and resource-poor areas and in patients with HIV coinfection or other forms of immunosuppression. A diagnosis of cutaneous TB warrants a rigorous search for systemic disease and concurrent immunosuppression such as HIV infection. Given its often-elusive clinical and histopathological findings, physicians must maintain a high level of diagnostic suspicion to accurately recognize, diagnose, and manage cutaneous TB.

LEPROSY (HANSEN DISEASE)
Epidemiology

Leprosy remains one of the important neglected tropical diseases. The WHO estimates that approximately 220,000 new cases occur annually,[66] based on passive case-finding; active case finding studies have indicated that the actual number may be 6-fold greater than this.[67] India and Brazil report the greatest number of new cases each year. Approximately 200 new cases are diagnosed annually in the United States.[68] Most new cases in the United States are in patients with a history of foreign birth or travel.

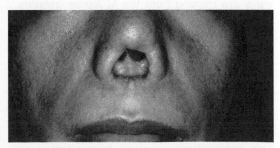

Fig. 13. Tuberculosis cutis orificialis of bilateral nares with violaceous papules and plaques that ulcerate and heal with atrophic scarring.

Table 3
First-line medications for tuberculosis

Agent	Interval and Doses	Adverse Reactions	Monitoring
Isoniazid	Initial phase: 5 mg/kg daily, max 300 mg 5 mg/kg daily, BIW or TIW, max 900 mg	Paresthesias, peripheral neuropathy, elevated LFTs, nausea, vomiting	Baseline CMP; monthly LFTs for patients >35 y old, history of hepatic disease or alcoholism, or IV drug abuse; women in postpartum period; optional ophthalmologic examination
Rifampin	10 mg/kg daily, BIW or TIW, max 600 mg	Nausea and vomiting, diarrhea, pyrexia, abdominal pain, orange/red discoloration of bodily fluids, flulike symptoms, elevated LFTs	Baseline CBC, CMP; LFTs every 2–4 wk if hepatic impairment
Pyrazinamide	20–25 mg/kg daily, max 2 g Recommended adult dosages by weight, using whole tablets (MMWR)	Malaise, joint pain, rash, photosensitivity, anorexia, hyperuricemia, gout, elevated LFTs	Baseline uric acid and CMP, then periodically
Ethambutol	15–20 mg/kg daily, Recommended adult dosages by weight, using whole tablets (MMWR)	Blurred vision, blindness, flulike symptoms, nausea, vomiting, anorexia, pruritus, rash, elevated LFTs	Baseline CBC, CMP; baseline ophthalmologic examination, then periodically

Abbreviations: BIW, 2 times weekly; CBC, complete blood count; CMP, comprehensive metabolic panel; LFT, liver function test; TIW, 3 times weekly.

Data from Treatment of Tuberculosis, American Thoracic Centers for Disease Control and Prevention. Society, CDC, and Infectious Diseases Society of America. MMWR 2003;52(No. RR-11):3–5;19–25.

However, 20% to 24% of new cases each year are seen in persons who have never traveled outside the United States. Most of these are in the Gulf coast states, and substantial evidence now indicates that leprosy is a zoonosis in North America, carried by the 9-banded armadillo (*Dasypus novemcinctus*).[69] Preliminary evidence indicates that this may also be true in other regions in the Western hemisphere.

Prolonged, close contact seems to be the greatest risk factor for infection.[70] Most individuals have native immunity to *M leprae* and will not develop disease when exposed. Transmission of *M leprae* is probably via airborne droplets expelled from the nasopharynx[71]; this site is also suspected of being the major route of entry as well. Some evidence indicates that skin-to-skin transmission may also occur.[71]

Etiopathogenesis

M leprae, the causative agent of leprosy, is a noncultivable, obligate intracellular pathogen that has a very slow division time of approximately 13 days. In contrast with *M tuberculosis*, *M leprae* is weakly acid fast: Ziehl-Neelsen stains may be negative, whereas Fite stains will demonstrate abundant organisms (**Fig. 14**). *M leprae* has optimal growth in cool skin sites (32–34°C) (**Fig. 15**) and is the only bacterial pathogen capable of infecting peripheral nerves, where it inhabits Schwann cells and intraneural macrophages (**Fig. 16**).

The genome of *M leprae* has only half as many coding genes as *M tuberculosis*, and a large percentage of these are pseudogenes (see **Table 1**).[72] Genes for key enzymes of several metabolic pathways are missing from the *M leprae* genome,[73] consistent with its obligatory intracellular existence. The precise details of this metabolic dependency are not clear and this is a topic of continuing investigation.

Most individuals have native immunity to infection with *M leprae*, but among susceptible individuals, this pathogen elicits an extraordinarily broad spectrum of CMI in man based on the immunologic mechanisms described in the Introduction. This immunologic spectrum is manifested clinically as a wide range of lesions ranging from macules to nodules to diffuse infiltration, and

ZN Stain   Fite Stain

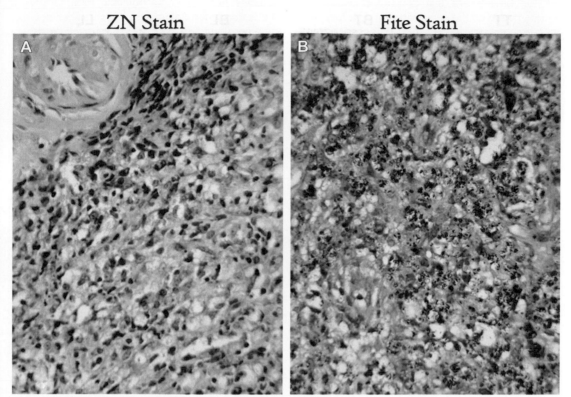

Fig. 14. Comparison of Ziehl-Neelsen (Z-N) and Fite stains. *M leprae* is weakly acid-fast, and a standard Z-N stain revealed few or no bacilli in this specimen (*A*). Fite staining of another section of the same specimen revealed abundant *M leprae* (*B*) (A, B: original magnification, ×1000).

histologically as a correspondingly wide range of appearances in the skin (**Fig. 17**). Based on clinical and pathologic criteria, this spectrum is divided into 5 types: polar tuberculoid (TT), borderline tuberculoid (BT), mid-borderline (BB), borderline lepromatous (BL), and polar lepromatous (LL).[74] Most patients are classified into the BT, BL, and LL groups. Because the immunologic underpinnings of this spectrum are genetically determined, the classification in any individual patient does *not* typically start at TT and then "slide down" in the

spectrum. Rather, the established infection in any one patient will generally remain in a particular portion of the spectrum; slight upgrading or downgrading may occur and present as clinical reactions (see later discussion).

Classification and Clinical Presentations

Clinically, hypoesthesia or anesthesia within or adjacent to skin lesions is highly suggestive of leprosy. Associated findings include enlarged or

TT   BT   BB   BL   LL

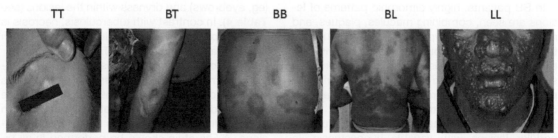

Fig. 15. Variations in leprosy lesions across the spectrum. Cutaneous lesions in leprosy are usually found at cool sites of the face, torso, and extremities. Lesions range from well-defined macules in tuberculoid disease to elevated plaques and "target" lesions in the BB leprosy, to diffuse infiltration and nodular lesions in lepromatous patients. (Abbreviations as in **Fig. 1.**) (*Courtesy of* Stryjewska B, MD, Baton Rouge, LA; and *From* Joyce MP. Leprosy. In: Walker PF, Barnett ED, editors. Immigrant medicine. Philadelphia: Elsevier; 2007. p. 460; with permission.)

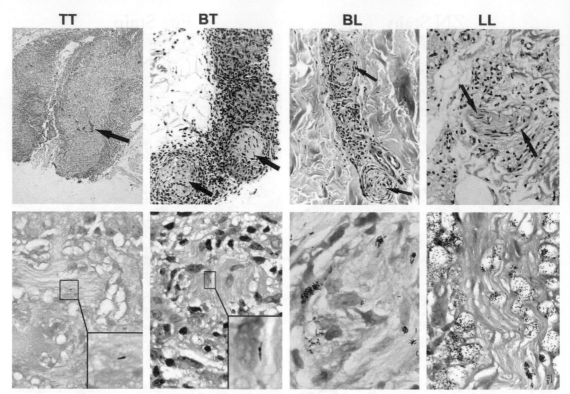

Fig. 16. *M leprae* in cutaneous nerves. Perineural inflammation (*upper panel*) and intraneural AFB (*lower panel*) are shown in cutaneous nerves from lesions ranging from TT to LL. Severe granulomatous inflammation in TT lesions may render nerves difficult to detect. *M leprae* may be difficult to demonstrate within nerves in TT-BT lesions, but are abundant in nerves in LL-BL lesions. (*Arrows* in upper panel indicate cutaneous nerves). (*Upper panel*, TT: S-100, ×20; BT, BL, LL: H&E, ×20. *Lower panel*: Fite stain, ×1000. Abbreviations as in **Fig. 1**.)

tender peripheral nerves, or history of painless cuts or burns on the hands or feet. In individual patients, across the spectrum from TT to LL, there is a progressive increase in the number of lesions and a gradual change from flat, sharply defined macules in tuberculoid lesions to diffuse infiltration and indurated plaques and nodules in lepromatous lesions (**Table 4**). Macules also characterize BT leprosy, but they are more numerous and usually distributed asymmetrically on the face, trunk, and limbs.

In BB patients, highly dimorphic patterns of lesions are seen, combining macules, plaques, and nodules. BL patients typically have numerous infiltrated macular and papular or nodular lesions, with poorly defined margins. They are seen on both sides of the body, often somewhat symmetric. Hypoesthesia may be present but is not seen as consistently as in tuberculoid lesions.

Polar LL patients have numerous, diffuse or nodular lesions with variable hypoesthesia. In advanced disease, diffuse thickening and wrinkling of the skin of the face may produce classic "leonine facies," but in less advanced disease, thickening of the skin may be subtler. Madarosis

and nodular thickening of the earlobes are typical in LL and BL leprosy but may not be evident in early cases.

Histologically, across the leprosy spectrum, there is a concomitant decrease in organization of the infiltrates, from well-organized epithelioid granulomas in TT lesions to totally disorganized aggregates of foamy histiocytes in LL lesions (see **Fig. 16** and **Table 4**). Perineural inflammation is characteristic in all types. The infiltrates can also destroy dermal appendages, leading to loss of hair (eg, eyebrows) and dryness within the lesions (see **Table 4**). In contrast with tuberculosis, necrosis is rare in leprosy and is seen almost exclusively in granulomas in nerves in TT-BT lesions.

The bacterial load increases across this spectrum, from rare AFB in TT lesions to enormous numbers of bacilli in LL lesions (see **Fig. 17**). The papillary dermis is an especially favorable site in which to find the rare bacilli in both TT and BT lesions. A Fite stain should be performed in all biopsies with perineural inflammation to try to identify acid-fast organisms. *M leprae* is the only bacterium to infect peripheral nerves, and the finding of AFB within nerves is pathognomonic of

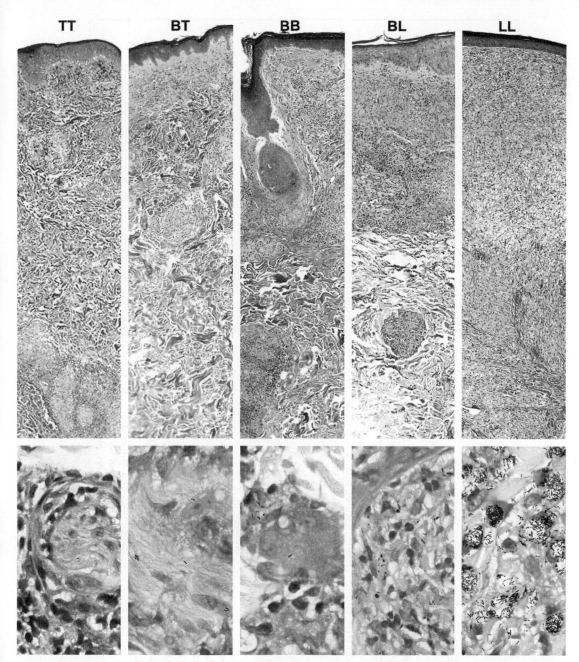

Fig. 17. The immunopathological spectrum of leprosy. Representative fields from each of the histopathological types of leprosy in the Ridley-Jopling classification are presented in the upper panel, in H&E stained sections (original magnification, ×63), and in the Fite-stained sections in the lower panel (original magnification, ×1000). TT leprosy is so named because the well-formed epithelioid granulomas are virtually identical to those seen in tuberculosis; acid-fast organisms are rare and difficult to demonstrate. In BT lesions, the granulomas are not as highly organized as in TT lesions, but acid-fast organisms are rare. In BB lesions, some foci of inflammation show epithelioid granulomatous organization, while other foci are disorganized and contain foamy histiocytes. Acid fast organisms are readily demonstrated but may not be abundant. BL infiltrates are composed of poorly organized aggregates of lymphocytes and foamy histiocytes, many of which have foamy cytoplasm. Numerous AFB can be found in any field. Polar LL lesions reveal confluent aggregates of foamy histiocytes. (Abbreviations as in **Fig. 1.**) (*From* Scollard DM, Adams LB, Gillis TP, et al. The continuing challenges of leprosy. Clin Microbiol Rev 2006;19:341; with permission.)

Table 4
Classification of leprosy

Leprosy Type	Cellular Immunity to *M leprae*	Clinical Presentation	Histologic Features	AFB (Fite Stain)	Frequency[a] (%)
Indeterminate[b]	Uncertain	Single lesion, often pale macule	Nonspecific perineural inflammation	Rare	2.9
TT	High degree of delayed hypersensitivity (DTH); strong Th-1 immune response	One to 3 macules (may be large), pale or erythematous, dry, sharply defined margins; sensation often reduced	Well-organized epithelioid granulomas involving nerves, occasional giant cells, necrosis is rare	Rare	3.2
BT	Moderately strong DTH; strong Th-1 immune response	Many macules, bilateral, pale or erythematous, dry, sharply defined margins; sensation often reduced	Moderately organized epithelioid granulomas involving nerves, occasional giant cells, necrosis is rare	Rare, but often in small cluster when found	24.3
BB	Weak DTH; weak Th-1 type immune response, some antibody production	"Dimorphic": mixed macules, plaques, "target lesions"; some margins sharp, others diffuse; sensation often reduced	"Dimorphic": epithelioid granulomas as well as aggregates of foamy histiocytes; nerves involved	Some bacilli in most fields	3.2
BL	Very weak delayed hypersensitivity; Th-2 type immune response; polyclonal antibody response	Multiple plaques and nodules, diffuse margins, bilateral and often widespread; sensory loss in some but not all lesions	Disorganized aggregates of lymphocytes and foamy histiocytes; nerves involved	Many bacilli in all fields; some globi	31.4
LL	Absent DTH to *M leprae*; Th-2 immune response; strong polyclonal antibody response	Multiple plaques, papules, and nodules, diffuse margins; sometimes diffuse thickening; bilateral and often widespread; sensory loss in some but not all lesions	Disorganized aggregates of lymphocytes and foamy histiocytes, sometimes confluent sheets of histiocytes; nerves involved	Very large number of bacilli in all fields; many globi	34.9

[a] Frequency (%) in 678 biopsies of new cases of leprosy. Biopsies processed at the NHDP from 2004 to 2013.
[b] Indeterminate means that a *definite diagnosis of leprosy* is made, but histologically the infiltrate is small and classification is uncertain.

leprosy. PCR can be used to identify *M leprae* in biopsies. PCR for *M leprae* is very specific but is not appreciably more sensitive than Fite staining and examination by an experienced microscopist.

Disorders commonly mistaken clinically and histologically for tuberculoid leprosy include sarcoidosis, granuloma annulare, and various superficial fungal infections. The diffuse infiltrates and macules of lepromatous leprosy are sometimes mistaken clinically for cutaneous lymphoma, and histologically for histiocytic neoplasms.

Considerable information has been gained regarding the immunologic status of leprosy lesions,[75,76] but there is still no single unifying hypothesis that can explain the wide spectrum of this disease. At the tuberculoid end of the spectrum, a Th-1 cytokine profile is present, similar to that in tuberculous granulomas,[3,5] while at the lepromatous pole, a Th-2 profile is seen.[77]

Current evidence suggests that the immunologic responses to *M leprae* are controlled genetically at 2 levels: native and acquired immunity. Most people have native immunity to *M leprae*, determined by several genes, such as PAKRG,[78,79] and mediated by Langerhans cells and dendritic cells.[3,80] Individuals who do not express native immunity may become infected with *M leprae* if sufficiently exposed, and an acquired immune response develops. This acquired immune response is regulated and determined by several genes, including many that are HLA-linked and expressed largely through T-cell functions, as indicated by cytokine profiles.[81] Although genetic determinants of both native and acquired immunity have been identified in many studies, at this time there are no clinically available genetic tests that can identify who is susceptible, nor what type of T-cell response a susceptible individual will develop if infected.

Lepromatous patients, who generate little or no CMI to *M leprae*, do produce a strong polyclonal antibody response. This strong polyclonal antibody response is the basis of attempts to develop serologic tests for leprosy,[82] but such methods do not detect most TT-BT patients and so they are not useful as general diagnostic tests.[83] However, this polyclonal antibody response may result in false positive serologic tests for syphilis, HIV, and other similar diseases.

Systemic Associations

Leprosy reactions represent the major burden of leprosy today, complicating the course of disease in 40% to 50% of patients. These reactions are spontaneous immunologic phenomena occurring as part of the natural course of infection in some patients; they are not drug reactions and are not caused by MDT. Two major types of reactions occur: "reversal" (type 1, T1R) reactions and *erythema nodosum leprosum* (type 2, T2R).

T1Rs occur in borderline patients (BT, BB, and BL) and are a manifestation of spontaneously enhanced cellular immunity, with expression of Th-1 cytokines and the chemokine, CXCL10.[10,84] Clinically, T1R presents as increased erythema and induration of pre-existing lesions, often with acute neuritis as well as acral edema, joint pain, and systemic symptoms that often suggest an autoimmune disease. Although they often present with severe, dramatic cutaneous lesions, the skin biopsy may show only subtle, nonspecific pathologic changes, such as edema or an increased number of giant cells. Clinical diagnosis is paramount, because there are no reliable histologic criteria for diagnosis. If the underlying diagnosis of leprosy is not recognized, such patients are frequently referred to rheumatologists and may be given corticosteroid regimens for many months. This regimen may provide transient relief of symptoms, but also enhances the growth of *M leprae*.

T2Rs present as crops of tender, erythematous nodules on any part of the body, not necessarily related to pre-existing lesions. This reaction occurs among lepromatous (LL-BL) patients, who have a high bacterial load and also have abundant circulating anti-*M leprae* antibodies. The pathogenesis of T2R is not understood. Although widely considered to be an antigen-antibody complex phenomenon,[85] the evidence supporting this is not fully convincing. Acute inflammatory infiltrates are characteristic of T2R, however, and the mechanisms of neutrophil recruitment are under investigation.[86] Clinically, in addition to the typical nodules, these patients experience acute neuritis, fever, leukocytosis (leukocyte counts sometimes ranging from 15,000 to 20,000/mm^3), and moderate to severe malaise. Skin biopsy of a lesion less than 24 hours old may reveal focal infiltrates of polymorphs superimposed on the disorganized lymphohistiocytic infiltrate of lepromatous leprosy (**Fig. 18**). Circulating C-reactive protein is also usually elevated.[87] Patients with T2R sometimes present to emergency rooms so acutely ill that they are evaluated for sepsis, if the underlying diagnosis of leprosy is not recognized.

Both types of reactions respond well to corticosteroids, but if the reaction is severe, high doses may be required. Tapering of corticosteroids is often difficult, because the reaction may reappear as the dose is lowered. There are no reliable laboratory tests to evaluate regression of the underlying immunologic phenomena. Thalidomide is

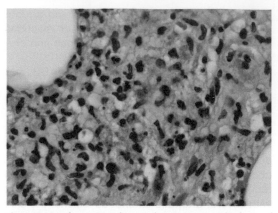

Fig. 18. Erythema nodosum leprosum, with foci of polymorphonuclear leukocytes superimposed on the disorganized, chronic inflammatory infiltrates of lepromatous leprosy (H&E, original magnification, ×400).

remarkably effective in the treatment of T2R[88]; it was this single benefit of thalidomide that kept the drug from being totally banned from all formularies for nearly 20 years, until newer uses for it were recognized. Medically, thalidomide is the drug of choice for T2R. However, because of its cost and the many precautions necessary to avoid the risk of phocomelia, in practice thalidomide is usually used for T2R only when corticosteroids do not control the reaction or if they cannot be tapered satisfactorily. Thalidomide has no beneficial effect in T1R.

All of the clinical-histopathological types of leprosy pose serious consequences for the patient who is not treated. Although the granulomatous inflammation in tuberculoid types of disease is associated with greatly limited bacterial growth and thus makes these patients far less infectious to others, the granulomas can destroy tissue. Because bacilli localize to peripheral nerves, these slender structures are especially vulnerable to damage and destruction by the granulomatous inflammation of TT-BT leprosy.[89] Thus, even though acid-fast organisms are rare in Fite-stained sections of TT-BT disease, signs and symptoms of clinical sensory and motor neuropathy are often observed earlier in tuberculoid patients than in lepromatous ones. In BB, BL, and LL forms of the disease, an increasing bacterial load is observed within nerves. Although the immune responses to *M leprae* in these patients are ineffective and are less damaging to nerves in the short term, eventually the combined effects of chronic infection and inflammation result in nerve injury, demyelination, and fibrous scarring.

These nerve injuries, if untreated, may progress functionally from slight sensory loss to complete anesthesia of hands or feet, or of the cornea. Motor weakness follows and ultimately may result in paralysis affecting fingers and toes as well as the musculature of the eye. Such nerve injury occurs to some degree in all cases of leprosy (ie, reduced sensory perception in skin lesions), and this may be seriously aggravated by leprosy reactions.

AFB and characteristic histopathological lesions of leprosy are usually *not* seen in the affected hand or foot or eye; these clinical findings are distal effects of nerve injury *proximal* to the affected site. The pathogenesis of the anesthetic foot, and the pressure ulcers that may result, was worked out in studies of neuropathy in leprosy[90] and has now been widely applied to the management of neuropathic injuries in diabetes mellitus.[91]

Evaluation and Management

Uncomplicated leprosy is treated with a MDT regimen of dapsone, rifampin, and clofazimine. For tuberculoid (TT-BT) disease, daily dapsone and rifampin are recommended for 1 year in the United States (**Table 5**). For lepromatous disease, daily clofazimine is added to this regimen, and the 3 drugs are given for 2 years. The WHO distributes these drugs in blister packs, but rifampin is provided only once monthly (see **Table 5**). These basic recommendations were made empirically by a WHO committee in 1982,[92] but in 1998 the WHO recommended reducing the duration of treatment by half[93,94] (see **Table 5**); many experienced physicians prefer the longer duration of treatment.

Clofazimine is not available commercially; it is distributed globally by the WHO in blister packs with dapsone and rifampin. In the United States, clofazimine is currently classified by the Food and Drug Administration as an investigational drug. The National Hansen's Disease Programs (NHDP) holds the Investigational New Drug Application for the use of clofazimine to treat leprosy, and the NHDP is the sole distributor of this drug in the United States. Additional information is available at www.hrsa.gov/hansensdisease.

Alternative drugs that are known to be effective against *M leprae*, both in laboratory tests and in clinical trials, are minocycline, clarithromycin, ofloxacin/levofloxacin, and moxifloxacin. Any of these can be substituted for any of the first-line drugs if necessary because of intolerance or interaction with other drugs the patient is taking.

Dapsone, rifampin, and clofazimine have been used extensively and are safe and well-tolerated in the vast majority of patients. Dapsone may cause mild anemia in many patients and should not be used at all in patients with G6PD deficiency.

Table 5
Treatment of leprosy: US and World Health Organization regimens

Agent	USA/NHDP[a]	WHO[b]
Tuberculoid (paucibacillary)		
Dapsone	100 mg/d for 12 mo	100 mg/d for 6 mo
Rifampin	600 mg/d for 12 mo	600 mg once monthly under supervision for 6 mo
Lepromatous (multibacillary)		
Dapsone	100 mg/d for 24 mo	100 mg/d for 12 mo
Rifampin	600 mg/d for 24 mo	600 mg once monthly given under supervision for 12 mo
Clofazimine	50 mg/d for 24 mo (if refused, may substitute daily Minocycline)	50 mg/d, plus 300 mg each month given under supervision for 12 mo

[a] The US-recommended MDT protocol has been evaluated in a retrospective study.[92]
[b] The MDT drug combination was recommended by a WHO committee in 1982[86]; no randomized controlled trial has been performed. In 1998, the WHO recommended reducing the duration of MDT treatment by half.[87,88]

From Scollard DM, Joyce MP. Leprosy (Hansen's disease). In: Rakel RE, Bope ET, editors. Conn's current therapy. St Louis (MO): Elsevier Science; 2003. p. 103; with permission.

Hemoglobin and hematocrit values should be checked during treatment. Possible hepatotoxicity with rifampin should be evaluated with periodic tests of liver function, and it may be necessary to avoid this drug in patients with hepatitis or other liver disease. Clofazimine causes bluish-black pigmentation of lesions as well as diffuse darkening of the skin in sun-exposed areas, and compliance with this drug is sometimes poor as a result of patients' cosmetic concerns.

Clinical Results/Outcomes

Notably, because *M leprae* is not cultivable, it is not possible to demonstrate killing of bacilli by routine culture or other methods. The bacteriostatic and bacteriocidal effects of antimycobacterial agents against *M leprae* have been documented in laboratory studies (reviewed in Ref.[69]). Recent reports indicate that measurements of RNA from *M leprae* extracted directly from biopsies may be used to assess viability,[95,96] but these assays are still only available in research settings. MDT for leprosy was recommended by a WHO committee in 1981, but has not been studied in a randomized, controlled trial.[97] The clinical efficacy of MDT has been demonstrated by clinical experience in patients in the United States[98] and in hundreds of thousands of patients globally over the last 3 decades.[97]

Lesions of Hansen's disease respond slowly to treatment, and the primary means of evaluation is clinical observation. In the early decades of treatment, slit skin smears were often performed. The minute amount of fluid obtained from the dermis was smeared onto slides and stained for AFB, and the number of bacteria was estimated by manual counting. This method was promoted as a means to demonstrate the decline in the bacterial load. The difficulty of standardizing this technique clinically, as well as the variability of staining quality and of counting accuracy in different laboratories, has resulted in the discontinuation of this method in most clinics and national programs. A more complete and accurate assessment can be obtained by annual biopsy of skin lesions.

Even after *M leprae* have been killed by MDT, dead organisms remain in tissues for months or years (**Fig. 19**), their numbers declining very slowly, to the great consternation of many physicians unfamiliar with the management of leprosy. The removal of dead bacilli by physiologic processes is not enhanced by extending MDT; continuing to treat until no organisms can be seen in biopsies or skin smears was recommended in the early days of dapsone monotherapy, but with MDT this is unnecessary and costly and risks long-term side effects of the medications.

Drug resistance in *M leprae* occurs but is rare.[99] Mutations associated with resistance to dapsone, rifampin, and fluoroquinolones are the same as those seen in *M tuberculosis*.[100] These mutations can be identified in *M leprae* DNA extracted from formalin-fixed, paraffin-embedded biopsies if the bacterial load is great enough to provide sufficient DNA.

Relapses or reinfection with *M leprae* is possible but is also rare[101] and usually occurs more than 10 years after completion of treatment. The development of "new" lesions during or after treatment is not unusual and is almost always due to leprosy reactions, not relapse.

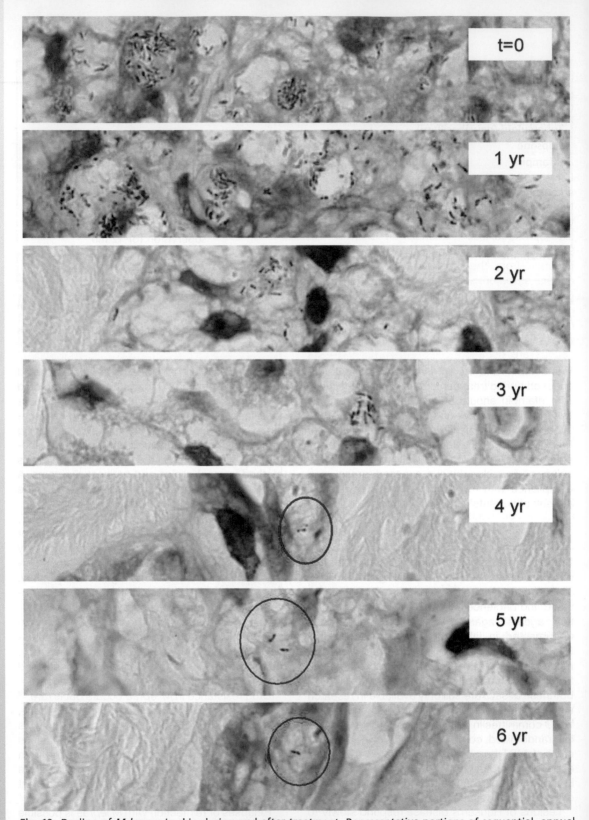

Fig. 19. Decline of *M leprae* in skin during and after treatment. Representative portions of sequential, annual biopsies of skin lesions from one lepromatous patient are shown, starting with the initial, pretreatment biopsy (t = 0). The patient was treated with the NHDP-recommended MDT regimen of daily rifampin, dapsone, and clofazimine for 2 years. At 1 year, organisms are still numerous but show evidence of degeneration. Treatment was discontinued at the time of the biopsy taken at 2 years. The bacterial load continued to decline slowly after MDT was discontinued, but rare organisms could still be observed after 6 years. Circles locate rare bacilli. Clinically, the cutaneous lesions resolved and did not relapse (Fite stains, ×1000). (*From* Scollard DM, Stryjewska B, MD, Leprosy. In: Rose BD, editor. UpToDate. Wellesley (MA): UpToDate; 2013; Graphic 74309, with permission.)

Coinfection with *M tuberculosis* and *M leprae* was common before the availability of good antimycobacterial treatment, but is uncommon today.[102] Coinfection is usually seen in immunocompromised or immunosuppressed patients.

Summary

Leprosy remains an important disease worldwide and, although rare, continues to be seen in the United States. Globally, untreated persons constitute the main reservoir of infection; in North America, leprosy is also a zoonotic infection among 9-banded armadillos, and people can acquire the infection from them. Uncomplicated infections appear as chronic, indolent lesions that not are painful, but systemic immunologic reactions occurring during the course of the disease may be so severe as to suggest sepsis, with fever, prostration, and an elevated leukocyte count. Reactions are common; relapse is rare. *M leprae* infection is curable, requiring 1 to 2 years of MDT. Neuropathy resulting from the infection may be permanent and disabling if the disease is not diagnosed and treated early. An extraordinarily broad spectrum of cellular immunity and granuloma formation in leprosy results in a wide range of clinical appearances. Hypoesthesia in or near lesions, or concomitant nerve enlargement or tenderness, aids in differentiating leprosy from superficial fungal infection, sarcoidosis, granuloma annulare, cutaneous lymphoma, and histiocytosis. Skin biopsies of suspicious lesions, diffuse histiocytic processes, or granulomas of uncertain cause should be evaluated for AFB using a Fite stain. The finding of AFB within cutaneous nerves is pathognomonic of leprosy. *M leprae* can also be identified by PCR in biopsies; this is highly specific but is not significantly more sensitive than a Fite stain and careful histologic examination.

ACKNOWLEDGMENTS

The authors gratefully acknowledge Abelaine A. Venida, MD, DPDS and Ma. Teresita G. Gabriel MD, FPDS for their invaluable technical assistance and contribution of clinical images.

REFERENCES

1. Killick KE, Ni Cheallaigh C, O'Farrelly C, et al. Receptor-mediated recognition of mycobacterial pathogens. Cell Microbiol 2013;15:1484–95.
2. Harding CV, Boom WH. Regulation of antigen presentation by Mycobacterium tuberculosis: a role for Toll-like receptors. Nat Rev Microbiol 2010;8: 296–307.
3. Ottenhoff TH. New pathways of protective and pathological host defense to mycobacteria. Trends Microbiol 2012;20:419–28.
4. Hernandez C, Cetner AS, Jordan JE, et al. Tuberculosis in the age of biologic therapy. J Am Acad Dermatol 2008;59:363–80 [quiz: 382–4].
5. Frieden TR, Sterling TR, Munsiff SS, et al. Tuberculosis. Lancet 2003;362:887–99.
6. Burns T, Breathnach S, Cox N, et al, editors. Cutaneous tuberculosis in: Rook's textbook of dermatology. 8th edition. Oxford: Blackwell Publishing; 2010. Sections 31.37–31.10.
7. Guirado E, Schlesinger LS. Modeling the mycobacterium tuberculosis granuloma—the critical battlefield in host immunity and disease. Front Immunol 2013;4:98.
8. Paige C, Bishai WR. Penitentiary or penthouse condo: the tuberculous granuloma from the microbe's point of view. Cell Microbiol 2010;12: 301–9.
9. Oxlade O, Pinto M, Trajman A, et al. How methodologic differences affect results of economic analyses: a systematic review of interferon gamma release assays for the diagnosis of LTBI. PLoS One 2013;8:e56044.
10. Scollard DM, Chaduvula MV, Martinez A, et al. Increased CXC ligand 10 levels and gene expression in type 1 leprosy reactions. Clin Vaccine Immunol 2011;18:947–53.
11. Bobosha K, Tjon Kon Fat EM, van den Eeden SJ, et al. Field-evaluation of a new lateral flow assay for detection of cellular and humoral immunity against Mycobacterium leprae. PLoS Negl Trop Dis 2014;8:e2845.
12. World Health Organization. Global tuberculosis report 2013 (WHO/HTM/TB/2013/11). Geneva (Switzerland): WHO; 2013.
13. Bravo FG, Gotuzzo E. Cutaneous tuberculosis. Clin Dermatol 2007;25:173–80.
14. Zouhair K, Akhdari N, Nejjam F, et al. Cutaneous tuberculosis in Morocco. Int J Infect Dis 2007;11: 209–12.
15. Macarayo M, Abad-Venida ML. The spectrum of cutaneous tuberculosis: local experience of Jose R. Reyes Memorial Medical Center Department of Dermatology. Part I: cutaneous tuberculosis: a ten-year descriptive analysis (1979–1988). Journal of the Philippine Society of Cutaneous Medicine 2000;1(1):61–7.
16. Sehgal VN, Srivastava G, Khurana VK, et al. An appraisal of epidemiologic, clinical, bacteriologic, histopathologic, and immunologic parameters in cutaneous tuberculosis. Int J Dermatol 1987;26: 521–6.
17. Kumar B, Muralidhar S. Cutaneous tuberculosis: a twenty-year prospective study. Int J Tuberc Lung Dis 1999;3:494–500.

18. Farina MC, Gegundez MI, Pique E, et al. Cutaneous tuberculosis: a clinical, histopathologic, and bacteriologic study. J Am Acad Dermatol 1995;33:433–40.

19. Semaan R, Traboulsi R, Kanj S. Primary Mycobacterium tuberculosis complex cutaneous infection: report of two cases and literature review. Int J Infect Dis 2008;12:472–7.

20. Enhanced surveillance of Mycobacterium bovis in humans. Commun Dis Rep CDR Wkly 1998;8: 281–4.

21. Farsinejad K, Daneshpazhooh M, Sairafi H, et al. Lupus vulgaris at the site of BCG vaccination: report of three cases. Clin Exp Dermatol 2009;34: e167–9.

22. Barbagallo J, Tager P, Ingleton R, et al. Cutaneous tuberculosis: diagnosis and treatment. Am J Clin Dermatol 2002;3:319–28.

23. Lai-Cheong JE, Perez A, Tang V, et al. Cutaneous manifestations of tuberculosis. Clin Exp Dermatol 2007;32:461–6.

24. Lupi O, Madkan V, Tyring SK. Tropical dermatology: bacterial tropical diseases. J Am Acad Dermatol 2006;54:559–78 [quiz: 578–80].

25. Tigoulet F, Fournier V, Caumes E. Clinical forms of the cutaneous tuberculosis. Bull Soc Pathol Exot 2003;96:362–7.

26. Hay RJ. Cutaneous infection with Mycobacterium tuberculosis: how has this altered with the changing epidemiology of tuberculosis? Curr Opin Infect Dis 2005;18:93–5.

27. Frankel A, Penrose C, Emer J. Cutaneous tuberculosis: a practical case report and review for the dermatologist. J Clin Aesthet Dermatol 2009;2: 19–27.

28. Kumar B, Rai R, Kaur I, et al. Childhood cutaneous tuberculosis: a study over 25 years from northern India. Int J Dermatol 2001;40:26–32.

29. Bhutto AM, Solangi A, Khaskhely NM, et al. Clinical and epidemiological observations of cutaneous tuberculosis in Larkana, Pakistan. Int J Dermatol 2002;41:159–65.

30. Visser AJ, Heyl T. Skin tuberculosis as seen at Ga-Rankuwa Hospital. Clin Exp Dermatol 1993;18: 507–15.

31. Marcoval J, Servitje O, Moreno A, et al. Lupus vulgaris. Clinical, histopathologic, and bacteriologic study of 10 cases. J Am Acad Dermatol 1992;26: 404–7.

32. Sehgal VN. Cutaneous tuberculosis. Dermatol Clin 1994;12:645–53.

33. Warin AP, Jones EW. Cutaneous tuberculosis of the nose with unusual clinical and histological features leading to a delay in the diagnosis. Clin Exp Dermatol 1977;2:235–42.

34. Cotterill JA. Lupus vulgaris simulating a port-wine stain. Br J Dermatol 1988;119:127–8.

35. Darier MJ. Des "tuberculides" cutanees. Ann Dermatol Syphilol 1896;7:1431–6.

36. Beyt BE Jr, Ortbals DW, Santa Cruz DJ, et al. Cutaneous mycobacteriosis: analysis of 34 cases with a new classification of the disease. Medicine 1981; 60:95–109.

37. Mataix J, Botella R, Herrero A, et al. Tuberculous primary complex of the skin. Int J Dermatol 2008; 47:479–81.

38. Jordaan HF, Van Niekerk DJ, Louw M. Papulonecrotic tuberculid. A clinical, histopathological, and immunohistochemical study of 15 patients. Am J Dermatopathol 1994;16:474–85.

39. Victor T, Jordaan HF, Van Niekerk DJ, et al. Papulonecrotic tuberculid. Identification of Mycobacterium tuberculosis DNA by polymerase chain reaction. Am J Dermatopathol 1992;14:491–5.

40. Weedon D. "Tuberculoisis" in: Weedon's skin pathology. 3rd edition. London: Churchill Livingstone Elsevier; 2010. p. 556–9.

41. Libraty DH, Byrd TF. Cutaneous miliary tuberculosis in the AIDS era: case report and review. Clin Infect Dis 1996;23:706–10.

42. Grossman ME, Fox LP, Kovarik C, et al. Mycobacterium tuberculosis. In: Cutaneous manifestations of infection in the immunocompromised host, Chapter 5—Mycobacteria. 2nd edition. New York: Springer; 2012. p. 109–10.

43. Kingkaew N, Sangtong B, Amnuaiphon W, et al. HIV-associated extrapulmonary tuberculosis in Thailand: epidemiology and risk factors for death. Int J Infect Dis 2009;13:722–9.

44. Yang Z, Kong Y, Wilson F, et al. Identification of risk factors for extrapulmonary tuberculosis. Clin Infect Dis 2004;38:199–205.

45. Mehta S, Suratkal L. Ophthalmoscopy in the early diagnosis of opportunistic tuberculosis following renal transplant. Indian J Ophthalmol 2007;55: 389–91.

46. Kivanç-Altunay I, Baysal Z, Ekmekçi TR, et al. Incidence of cutaneous tuberculosis in patients with organ tuberculosis. Int J Dermatol 2003;42: 197–200.

47. Yodmalai S, Chiewchanvit S, Mahanupab P. Cutaneous miliary tuberculosis in a renal transplant patient: a case report and literature review. Southeast Asian J Trop Med Public Health 2011;42:674–8.

48. Wilkinson RJ, Llewelyn M, Toossi Z, et al. Influence of vitamin D deficiency and vitamin D receptor polymorphisms on tuberculosis among Gujarati Asians in west London: a case-control study. Lancet 2000;355:618–21.

49. Lee NH, Choi EH, Lee WS, et al. Tuberculous cellulitis. Clin Exp Dermatol 2000;25:222–3.

50. Barnes PF, Bloch AB, Davidson PT, et al. Tuberculosis in patients with human immunodeficiency virus infection. N Engl J Med 1991;324:1644–50.

51. Varshney A, Goyal T. Incidence of various clinico-morphological variants of cutaneous tuberculosis and HIV concurrence: a study from the Indian sub-continent. Ann Saudi Med 2011;31:134–9.

52. Friedman PC, Husain S, Grossman ME. Nodular tuberculid in a patient with HIV. J Am Acad Dermatol 2005;53:S154–6.

53. Inwald D, Nelson M, Cramp M, et al. Cutaneous manifestations of mycobacterial infection in patients with AIDS. Br J Dermatol 1994;130:111–4.

54. High WA, Evans CC, Hoang MP. Cutaneous miliary tuberculosis in two patients with HIV infection. J Am Acad Dermatol 2004;50:S110–3.

55. Regnier S, Ouagari Z, Perez ZL, et al. Cutaneous miliary resistant tuberculosis in a patient infected with human immunodeficiency virus: case report and literature review. Clin Exp Dermatol 2009;34: e690–2.

56. Higgins RM, Cahn AP, Porter D, et al. Mycobacterial infections after renal transplantation. Q J Med 1991;78:145–53.

57. Sakhuja V, Jha V, Varma PP, et al. The high incidence of tuberculosis among renal transplant recipients in India. Transplantation 1996;61:211–5.

58. Vilcheze C, Molle V, Carrere-Kremer S, et al. Phosphorylation of KasB regulates virulence and acid-fastness in Mycobacterium tuberculosis. PLoS Pathog 2014;10:e1004115.

59. National Tuberculosis Controllers Association, Centers for Disease Control and Prevention. Guidelines for the investigation of contacts of persons with infectious tuberculosis. Recommendations from the National Tuberculosis Controllers Association and CDC. MMWR Recomm Rep 2005;54:1–47.

60. Penneys NS, Leonardi CL, Cook S, et al. Identification of Mycobacterium tuberculosis DNA in five different types of cutaneous lesions by the polymerase chain reaction. Arch Dermatol 1993;129:1594–8.

61. Tappeiner G, Wolff K. Tuberculosis and other mycobacterial infections. In: Fitzpatrick TB, Eisen AZ, Wolff K, et al, editors. Dermatology in general medicine. 5th edition. New York: McGraw Hill; 1999. p. 2274–92.

62. American Thoracic Society, Centers for Disease Control and Prevention, Infectious Diseases Society of America. American Thoracic Society/Centers for Disease Control and Prevention/Infectious Diseases Society of America: controlling tuberculosis in the United States. Am J Respir Crit Care Med 2005;172:1169–227.

63. Ramam M, Mittal R, Ramesh V. How soon does cutaneous tuberculosis respond to treatment? Implications for a therapeutic test of diagnosis. Int J Dermatol 2005;44:121–4.

64. Chiang CY, Centis R, Migliori GB. Drug-resistant tuberculosis: past, present, future. Respirology 2010;15:413–32.

65. Gandhi NR, Moll A, Sturm AW, et al. Extensively drug-resistant tuberculosis as a cause of death in patients co-infected with tuberculosis and HIV in a rural area of South Africa. Lancet 2006;368:1575–80.

66. World Health Organization. Leprosy elimination. 2014. Available at: http://www.who.int/lep. Accessed June 14, 2014.

67. Moet FJ, Schuring RP, Pahan D, et al. The prevalence of previously undiagnosed leprosy in the general population of northwest bangladesh. PLoS Negl Trop Dis 2008;2:e198.

68. U.S. Department of Health and Human Services (HRSA). National Hansen's Disease (Leprosy) Program. 2001. Available at: http://www.hrsa.gov/hansensdisease/. Accessed June 14, 2014.

69. Truman RW, Singh P, Sharma R, et al. Probable zoonotic leprosy in the southern United States. N Engl J Med 2011;364:1626–33.

70. Sales AM, Ponce de Leon A, Duppre NC, et al. Leprosy among patient contacts: a multilevel study of risk factors. PLoS Negl Trop Dis 2011;5:e1013.

71. Job CK, Jayakumar J, Kearney M, et al. Transmission of leprosy: a study of skin and nasal secretions of household contacts of leprosy patients using PCR. Am J Trop Med Hyg 2008;78:518–21.

72. Cole ST, Eiglmeier K, Parkhill J, et al. Massive gene decay in the leprosy bacillus. Nature 2001;409: 1007–11.

73. Wheeler PR. The microbial physiologist's guide to the leprosy genome. Lepr Rev 2001;72:399–407.

74. Ridley DS, Jopling WH. Classification of leprosy according to immunity. A five-group system. Int J Lepr Other Mycobact Dis 1966;34:255–73.

75. Scollard DM, Adams LB, Gillis TP, et al. The continuing challenges of leprosy. Clin Microbiol Rev 2006;19:338–81.

76. Montoya D, Modlin RL. Learning from leprosy: insight into the human innate immune response. Adv Immunol 2010;105:1–24.

77. Salgame P, Abrams JS, Clayberger C, et al. Differing lymphokine profiles of functional subsets of human CD4 and CD8 T cell clones. Science 1991;254:279–82.

78. Mira MT, Alcais A, Nguyen VT, et al. Susceptibility to leprosy is associated with PARK2 and PACRG. Nature 2004;427:636–40.

79. Misch EA, Berrington WR, Vary JC Jr, et al. Leprosy and the human genome. Microbiol Mol Biol Rev 2010;74:589–620.

80. Schenk M, Krutzik SR, Sieling PA, et al. NOD2 triggers an interleukin-32-dependent human dendritic cell program in leprosy. Nat Med 2012;18:555–63.

81. Yamamura M, Uyemura K, Deans RJ, et al. Defining protective responses to pathogens: cytokine profiles in leprosy lesions. Science 1991;254:277–9.

82. Duthie MS, Raychaudhuri R, Tutterrow YL, et al. A rapid ELISA for the diagnosis of MB leprosy

based on complementary detection of antibodies against a novel protein-glycolipid conjugate. Diagn Microbiol Infect Dis 2014;79:233–9.

83. Oskam L, Slim E, Buhrer-Sekula S. Serology: recent developments, strengths, limitations and prospects: a state of the art overview. Lepr Rev 2003; 74:196–205.

84. Stefani MM, Guerra JG, Sousa AL, et al. Potential plasma markers of Type 1 and Type 2 leprosy reactions: a preliminary report. BMC Infect Dis 2009;9:75.

85. Kahawita IP, Lockwood DN. Towards understanding the pathology of erythema nodosum leprosum. Trans R Soc Trop Med Hyg 2008;102:329–37.

86. Lee DJ, Li H, Ochoa MT, et al. Integrated pathways for neutrophil recruitment and inflammation in leprosy. J Infect Dis 2010;201:558–69.

87. Silva EA, Iyer A, Ura S, et al. Utility of measuring serum levels of anti-PGL-I antibody, neopterin and C-reactive protein in monitoring leprosy patients during multi-drug treatment and reactions. Trop Med Int Health 2007;12:1450–8.

88. Sheskin J. The treatment of lepra reaction in lepromatous leprosy. Fifteen years' experience with thalidomide. Int J Dermatol 1980;19:318–22.

89. Scollard DM. The biology of nerve injury in leprosy. Lepr Rev 2008;79:242–53.

90. Hall OC, Brand PW. The etiology of the neuropathic plantar ulcer: a review of the literature and a presentation of current concepts. J Am Podiatry Assoc 1979;69:173–7.

91. Boulton AJ. Diabetic foot–what can we learn from leprosy? Legacy of Dr Paul W. Brand. Diabetes Metab Res Rev 2012;28(Suppl 1):3–7.

92. Chemotherapy of leprosy for control programmes. World Health Organ Tech Rep Ser 1982;675:1–33.

93. WHO Expert Committee on Leprosy. World Health Organ Tech Rep Ser 1998;874:1–43.

94. Ji B. Why multidrug therapy for multibacillary leprosy can be shortened to 12 months. Lepr Rev 1998;69:106–9.

95. Martinez AN, Lahiri R, Pittman TL, et al. Molecular determination of Mycobacterium leprae viability by use of real-time PCR. J Clin Microbiol 2009;47: 2124–30.

96. Davis GL, Ray NA, Lahiri R, et al. Molecular assays for determining Mycobacterium leprae viability in tissues of experimentally infected mice. PLoS Negl Trop Dis 2013;7:e2404.

97. Lockwood D. Leprosy. Clin Evid 2002;8:709–20.

98. Dacso MM, Jacobson RR, Scollard DM, et al. Evaluation of multi-drug therapy for leprosy in the United States using daily rifampin. South Med J 2011;104:689–94.

99. Williams DL, Hagino T, Sharma R, et al. Primary multidrug-resistant leprosy, United States. Emerg Infect Dis 2013;19:179–81.

100. Williams DL, Scollard DM, Gillis TP. PCR-based diagnosis of leprosy in the United States. Clin Microbiol Newsl 2003;25:57–61.

101. Shen J, Liu M, Zhang J, et al. Relapse in MB leprosy patients treated with 24 months of MDT in south west China: a short report. Lepr Rev 2006; 77:219–24.

102. Trindade MA, Miyamoto D, Benard G, et al. Leprosy and tuberculosis co-infection: clinical and immunological report of two cases and review of the literature. Am J Trop Med Hyg 2013;88:236–40.

Nontuberculous Mycobacteria
Skin and Soft Tissue Infections

Tania M. Gonzalez-Santiago, MD, Lisa A. Drage, MD*

KEYWORDS

- Nontuberculous mycobacteria • Atypical mycobacteria • Skin and soft tissue infections
- Rapidly growing mycobacteria • *Mycobacterium chelonae* • *Mycobacterium fortuitum*
- *Mycobacterium abscessus* • *Mycobacterium marinum*

KEY POINTS

- Skin and soft tissue infections caused by nontuberculous mycobacteria (NTM), especially the rapidly growing mycobacteria, appear to be increasing in incidence.
- Consider NTM as a cause of skin and soft tissue infection after trauma, surgery, or a cosmetic procedure, especially if the infection is not responding to typical antibiotic regimens.
- Skin signs can include abscesses, sporotrichoid nodules, or ulcers, but may not be distinctive, necessitating a high index of clinical suspicion.
- Obtain tissue cultures and susceptibility studies specifically for mycobacteria.
- Management is via prolonged antibiotic treatment that is species specific, generally based on antimicrobial susceptibility studies and may include surgical intervention.

INTRODUCTION
Definition and Classification

Mycobacteria species other than those of the *Mycobacterium tuberculosis* complex or *Mycobacterium leprae* are known as nontuberculous mycobacteria (NTM), environmental mycobacteria, or atypical mycobacteria. NTM are a diverse group of ubiquitous, environmental, acid-fast organisms that can produce a wide range of diseases, including infections of the skin and soft tissues. More than 170 species of NTM have been identified, most of which have been incriminated in skin and soft tissue infections (SSTI).[1,2] Traditionally, NTM have been classified into Runyon groups based on colony morphology, growth rate, and pigmentation.[3,4] As technology moves

forward, this classification system has become less useful and identification is now made using rapid molecular diagnostic systems.[5] Nonetheless, growth rates continue to provide practical means for grouping species of NTM. On this basis, NTM can be categorized into rapidly growing mycobacteria (RGM) and slowly growing mycobacteria (SGM).

RGM include species that produce mature growth on media plated within 7 days. These are subdivided into 5 groups based on pigmentation and genetic similarity: *Mycobacterium fortuitum, Mycobacterium chelonae/abscessus, Mycobacterium mucogenicum, Mycobacterium smegmatis*, and early pigmenting RGM. SGM include species of mycobacteria that require more than 7 days to reach mature growth. Examples of SGM

Disclosures: Drs T.M. Gonzalez-Santiago and L.A. Drage have no disclosures.
Department of Dermatology, Mayo Clinic College of Medicine, Mayo Clinic, 200 First Street Southwest, Rochester, MN 55905, USA
* Corresponding author.
E-mail address: drage.lisa@mayo.edu

Dermatol Clin 33 (2015) 563–577
http://dx.doi.org/10.1016/j.det.2015.03.017
0733-8635/15/$ – see front matter © 2015 Elsevier Inc. All rights reserved.

are *Mycobacterium marinum, Mycobacterium ulcerans, Mycobacterium kansasii, Mycobacterium haemophilum,* and *Mycobacterium scrofulaceum.* Some species require nutritional supplementation of routine mycobacteria media, grow best at lower/higher temperatures or require prolonged incubation.

Most NTM species are easily isolated from the environment, including water (both natural and municipal systems), soil, plants, animals, and birds.[6] Exceptions to this include *M haemophilum* and *M ulcerans,* which are rarely isolated. Tap water is considered the major reservoir for NTM pathogens in humans and as such is of increasing public health concern.[7] Species typically recovered from tap water include *Mycobacterium gordonae, M kansasii, Mycobacterium xenopi, Mycobacterium simiae, Mycobacterium* avium complex (MAC), and the RGM. NTM develop and are protected within biofilms, the filmy layer between the solid and liquid interface, in municipal water systems. Carson and colleagues[8,9] showed that 83% of the incoming city water in hemodialysis centers throughout the United States contained NTM. The presence of mycobacteria in up to 90% of samples taken from piped water systems has been described.[10] Furthermore, biofilms may make the mycobacteria resistant to common disinfectants. NTM are difficult to eradicate with common decontamination techniques and are relatively resistant to standard disinfectants such as chlorine, glutaraldehyde, gigasept, and virkon.[11–13] They can grow in hot and cold water systems. In some cases, temperatures of up to 70°C are required to inhibit the organism.[14,15] Importantly, no evidence of person-to-person spread has been reported with NTM.[16]

Clinical Syndromes

Four clinical syndromes account for most infections with NTM: pulmonary disease, lymphadenitis, disseminated disease, and SSTIs.[17]

Pulmonary disease

The most common form of localized NTM infection is chronic pulmonary disease in human immunodeficiency virus (HIV)-negative hosts. Signs and symptoms of NTM lung disease are often nonspecific, making this a challenging diagnosis that requires extensive laboratory and imaging workup. MAC followed by *M kansasii,* and *M abscessus* are the most common pathogens in the United States.

Lymphadenitis

Localized cervical lymphadenitis is the most common NTM disease in children and is typically caused by MAC and *M scrofulaceum.*[18] It occurs in children between 1 and 5 years of age. The cervicofacial nodes, particularly the submandibular nodes, are most frequently involved.[10] These can enlarge rapidly with the formation of fistulas to the skin, and prolonged drainage may occur. As with all other NTM infections, definitive diagnosis of lymphadenitis is made by recovery of the etiologic organism from cultures.[7]

Disseminated Disease

Disseminated NTM infections occur almost exclusively in immunocompromised patients.

Disseminated disease in patients with human immunodeficiency virus

Although *M tuberculosis* continues to be the most prevalent mycobacterial disease in HIV-AIDS, disseminated NTM is well documented and is associated with increased mortality in this patient population.[19] The most commonly implicated NTM is MAC and although the incidence has decreased significantly with the introduction of highly active antiretroviral therapy, it remains an important complication of AIDS.[20] *M kansasii, Mycobacterium genavense, M scrofulaceum, M xenopi, M fortuitum,* and *M gordonae* are among many other NTM responsible for disseminated disease in patients with HIV.[21] Symptoms are not specific and in most cases resemble those seen in disseminated tuberculosis. These include intermittent or persistent fever, night sweats, weight loss, fatigue, malaise, and anorexia.[22]

Disseminated disease in the severely immunocompromised

Disseminated disease in patients without HIV is rare and seen in the setting of significant immunosuppression (eg, transplant recipients, chronic corticosteroid use, leukemia). Systemic dissemination of a primary cutaneous NTM can occur. In most cases, disseminated disease presents with disseminated cutaneous lesions. The RGM species *M chelonae* is the most commonly isolated organism, presenting with multiple, red, draining, subcutaneous nodules or abscesses. *M kansasii, M haemophilum, M fortuitum, M abscessus,* and others have also been reported.[23]

Skin and soft tissue infections

The increasing reports of SSTI NTM infections in recent years have attracted significant attention in the medical community. Initially thought to reflect the increased immunosuppressed population, numerous reports document infection in healthy individuals. The exact incidence of SSTI NTM infections is yet to be determined. The largest population-based study on the incidence of NTM, from Olmsted County, Rochester, MN, showed an incidence of 2.0 per 100,000 person-years, and a nearly threefold increase in the incidence of cutaneous NTM infections over a 30-year period.[24] RGM were more predominant in the last decade of the study. This is supported by multiple publications that show an upward trend in all forms of NTM infections.[25,26] In recent studies, NTM account for 15% of total isolates of acid-fast bacilli (AFB) with the remaining 85% *M tuberculosis*. Population-based studies in Spain showed that NTM infections represented 0.64% to 2.29% of all mycobacterial infections.[23]

SSTIs caused by NTM include 2 distinctive species-specific clinical disorders: "fish-tank" granuloma and Buruli ulcer (BU), caused by *M marinum* and *M ulcerans*, respectively. However, most SSTIs caused by NTM are nonspecific in their clinical presentations and may present with abscesses, cellulitis, nodules, sporotrichoid nodules, ulcers, panniculitis, draining sinus tracts, folliculitis, papules, and plaques. The polymorphous manifestations of cutaneous NTM make the diagnosis difficult and a high index of suspicion in the appropriate clinical setting (**Table 1**) is necessary to make a prompt diagnosis.[27] NTM infections should be considered in all patients with "therapy resistant" SSTIs. Cutaneous NTM infections typically develop after traumatic injury, surgery, or cosmetic procedures. As reviewed previously, they also can occur secondarily as a consequence of a disseminated mycobacterial

disease, especially among immunosuppressed patients. Although RGM have a weaker pathogenicity than SGM, they also can cause disseminated diseases in immunocompromised hosts.[3] The etiopathogenesis, clinical presentation, evaluation, and management (**Table 2**) of the NTM commonly responsible for SSTI are discussed in detail herein.

SLOW-GROWING MYCOBACTERIA
Mycobacterium marinum

Etiopathogenesis
The primary risk factors for infection with *M marinum* are exposure to aquatic environments or marine animals. Thus, *M marinum* infections are commonly known as "fish-tank granuloma," "aquarium granuloma," or "swimming pool granuloma." *M marinum* is a slow-growing *Mycobacterium* with an intermediate incubation period of 16 days.[28] Infections are typically seen in immunocompetent patients who have jobs or hobbies related to exposure to fresh or salt water. Up to 45% of cases with confirmed *M marinum* infection have a history of a fish-related activity.[29] The main form of inoculation is trauma followed by exposure to water/fish environments. Most of the preceding lesions are superficial abrasions or negligible wounds.[29,30] The duration from the onset of the symptoms to visiting a doctor varies from 15 days to as long as 3 years. Patients usually do not seek medical attention until their symptoms worsen.[31,32]

Table 1
Clinical settings for skin and soft tissue infections caused by nontuberculous mycobacteria

Type of Mycobacteria	Clinical Setting
Slow-growing mycobacteria	
Mycobacterium marinum	• Generally seen in immunocompetent patients with minor trauma followed by exposure to fresh or salt water jobs and/or hobbies related to marine environment or aquatic animals (fish, shells, aquariums)
Mycobacterium ulcerans	• Endemic to West Africa and Australia • Affects communities associated with aquatic environments
Mycobacterium kansasii	• Typically seen after local trauma followed by exposure to contaminated water or in the severely immunocompromised
Mycobacterium haemophilum	• Generally seen in severe immunosuppression
Rapid-growing mycobacteria	
Mycobacterium fortuitum *Mycobacterium abscessus* *Mycobacterium chelonae*	• Direct inoculation (trauma, surgery, or cosmetic procedures) • Linked to use of nonsterile water in nosocomial settings • Trauma, surgery, injections (botulinum toxin, biologics, dermal fillers), liposuction, laser resurfacing, skin biopsy, Mohs surgery, tattoos, acupuncture, body piercing, pedicures, mesotherapy, and so forth

Table 2
Treatment for skin and soft tissue infections caused by nontuberculous mycobacteria

Type of Mycobacteria	Treatment	Level of Evidence
Slow-growing mycobacteria		
Mycobacterium marinum	• Limited skin and soft tissue infections: clarithromycin, doxycycline, minocycline, and trimethoprim-sulfamethoxazole monotherapy for 3 mo • Severe infections: combination of rifampin and ethambutol	D, E
Mycobacterium ulcerans	• Combination of rifampin and streptomycin for 8 wk • Surgical intervention for lesions that continue to enlarge despite 4 wk of antibiotic therapy • Treatment of superimposed bacterial infection • Skin grafting to accelerate healing of large ulcers	E
Mycobacterium kansasii	• Regimens with antituberculous and traditional antibiotics have been described • Treatment based on susceptibility studies	C, E
Mycobacterium haemophilum	• No standard guidelines are available • Multidrug regimen, such as clarithromycin, ciprofloxacin, and rifabutin, guided by susceptibility studies	D, E
Rapid-growing mycobacteria		
Mycobacterium fortuitum *Mycobacterium abscessus* *Mycobacterium chelonae*	• Monotherapy is not recommended • Culture results and antimicrobial sensitivity studies guide therapy • Limited skin and soft tissue infection: oral therapy with 2 agent to which the isolate is susceptible for a minimum of 4 mo, such as clarithromycin or azithromycin in combination with ciprofloxacin, levofloxacin, doxycycline, minocycline, or trimethoprim-sulfamethoxazole • For severe or disseminated disease: initial parenteral treatment with 2–3 agents to which the isolate is susceptible, followed by oral treatment for 6–12 mo	E

C, case-control study or retrospective study; D, case series or case reports; E, expert opinion.

Clinical presentation

Initially, a solitary, erythematous papule or nodule is seen at the site of inoculation, often on an extremity. This can progress to a verrucous violaceous plaque and/or ulcerate producing a serosanguineous discharge. Proximal extension of the infection may occur through lymphatic spread and 20% of patients present with a sporotrichoid distribution (**Fig. 1**).[33,34] *M marinum* invades deeper tissues, such as tendon sheaths, bursae, bones, and joints in up to 29% of cases. Deeper soft tissue invasion can be seen in all patients regardless of their immunologic state.[29,35] Because of the organism's poor growth at 37°C, however, systemic dissemination is rare and has been reported to occur only in immunocompromised patients.[36,37]

Evaluation

Evaluation should include a detailed history, including risk factors, duration of disease, site and morphology of lesions, and previous medical history. Biopsies for tissue cultures and routine

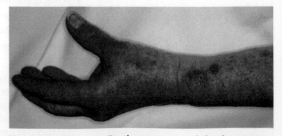

Fig. 1. *M marinum.* Erythematous nodules in a sporotrichoid distribution.

histopathologic examination are required for an accurate diagnosis. Diagnosis is confirmed with tissue cultures. *M marinum* colonies are usually seen after 10 to 28 days of incubation,[34] but cultures should be observed for at least 6 weeks. On histopathologic sections (routine hematoxylin and eosin), *M marinum* shows prominent epidermal changes, such as acanthosis, pseudoepitheliomatous hyperplasia, and exocytosis. Common histopathologic patterns include granulomatous inflammatory infiltrate with tuberculoid granuloma formation, sarcoidlike granulomas, or rheumatoidlike nodules.[37] However, less-specific findings also are encountered, such as lichenoid granulomatous dermatitis, interstitial granulomatous dermatitis, and dermal small vessel proliferation with granulation tissue–like changes.[38] AFB may be seen in small quantities but may not be detected by regular microscopy.[39] In one study, only 33% of the acid-fast staining on drainage material or tissue was positive.[31]

Management
Antimicrobials are the mainstays of successful treatment for *M marinum*. In superficial cutaneous infections, clarithromycin, doxycycline, minocycline, and trimethoprim-sulfamethoxazole as monotherapy are effective treatment options. Multidrug therapy is recommended for more significant infections, especially if deeper structures are involved. In contrast to other NTM, routine antimicrobial susceptibility testing of isolates of *M marinum* is not required unless treatment failure is observed.[40–42] In cases of severe infections, including those with a sporotrichoid distribution pattern, the most effective drugs seem to be a combination of rifampicin and ethambutol.[43] Spontaneous remission has been reported in untreated infections and in immunocompetent hosts.[44] Surgical treatment is not usually recommended and is usually reserved for deeper infections of subcutaneous tissue, such as tendons and bone.[45,46]

Mycobacterium ulcerans

Etiopathogenesis
M ulcerans is the causative agent of Buruli ulcer, also known as Bairnsdale ulcer. A major pathogen in West Africa and Australia, BU is one of the neglected emerging diseases and is the third most frequent mycobacterial disease in humans after tuberculosis and leprosy.[47–49] *M ulcerans* infection is found in communities associated with rivers, swamps, wetlands, and human-linked changes in the aquatic environment, particularly those created as a result of environmental disturbance, such as deforestation, dam construction, and agriculture. Although likely transmitted via skin trauma,

some studies suggest living agents, such aquatic insects, mosquitoes, or other biting arthropods, as transmissive agents of *M ulcerans*.[50] Cultivation of this species is difficult, requiring up to several months to grow, so molecular detection and identification are more practical than culture. The unique virulence factor of *M ulcerans* is the toxin mycolactone, which causes extensive necrosis and local immunosuppression. Because of the immunosuppressive properties of the mycolactone toxin, the disease can progress with minimal to no pain or fever.[51] Of note, patients with HIV have an increased risk for all other NTM except for *M ulcerans*.[52]

Clinical presentation
M ulcerans infection typically begins as a painless, small nodule less than 5 cm in diameter. Other initial clinical presentations include papules, plaques, and subcutaneous edema. Although the extremities are most frequently involved, less commonly reported areas include the head, neck, trunk, and genital regions. After a few days to weeks, the initial lesion ulcerates, develops an undermined border, and progresses slowly and painlessly. Unless secondary bacterial infections occur, the patient usually remains asymptomatic during the progression of the disease.[53] Although involvement of multiple organs is rare, osteomyelitis can develop in up to 15% of cases.[54]

Evaluation
Diagnosis of BU is usually based on clinical presentation because of limited access to laboratory services. According to the World Health Organization (WHO), there is no diagnostic test that can be used in the field. Research is progressing to develop one. Polymerase chain reaction is the common method for confirmation because it is fast and has a sensitivity of 70% to 80%.[55] Acid-fast staining from the edge of an undermined ulcer also can help in the diagnosis. This has a lower sensitivity of 40% to 60% and does not rule out other mycobacterial infections. Nonetheless, this is probably the most readily available laboratory technique in the field.[56] Culture sensitivity is low and at least 6 weeks of incubation is required. Samples should be obtained from the edge of an ulcer or alternatively from the center of a nonulcerated lesion.[55] Ideally, for transportation, the samples should be kept cool at 4°C.[57]

BU has a characteristic histopathology with a high sensitivity.[58] In the initial phase of infection there are large numbers of extracellular AFB with striking subcutaneous edema and necrosis. Some of the more classic features include vascular occlusion, hemorrhage, and, unlike other mycobacterial infections, a lack of granulomatous inflammation. In later stages of BU (typically 6 months after the onset), granulomas are formed. Additional features, more typical for an untreated BU lesion, include fat cell ghosts and minimal perivascular infiltration.[58,59]

Management

Although spontaneous healing of BU can be seen in up to one-third of cases, this can take months and lead to deep scarring, contractions, and disfiguring scars (**Fig. 2**). In addition, extensive tissue destruction may lead to amputation. Patients who are not treated early may suffer long-term permanent functional disabilities. Early diagnosis and treatment are the only ways to minimize morbidity.[60,61]

The current recommended antibiotic therapy per WHO guidelines is an 8-week course of rifampin and streptomycin. Surgical intervention should be reserved only for lesions that continue to enlarge despite 4 weeks of antibiotic therapy, for debridement of superimposed bacterial infection, or for skin grafting to accelerate healing of large ulcers.[62]

OTHER IMPORTANT SLOW-GROWING MYCOBACTERIA CAUSING SKIN AND SOFT TISSUE INFECTIONS
Mycobacterium kansasii

M kansasii typically causes pulmonary disease that resembles pulmonary tuberculosis. It has been recovered consistently from tap water in endemic areas in the United States, including the southeastern and southern coastal states and the central plains states.[63] Unlike other NTM, it

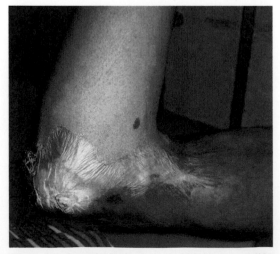

Fig. 2. *M ulcerans.* Healed ulcer with deep scarring and contractions.

has not been recovered from soil or natural water supplies.[64] Primary cutaneous lesions have been described in patients exposed to contaminated water, particularly after local trauma. Disseminated disease can occur in immunosuppressed patients but it typically remains as a localized, indolent, lesion confined to the skin in the immunocompetent.[65] Cutaneous lesions can have a sporotrichoid distribution,[66] and present as nonhealing ulcers, nodules, and cellulitis.[67,68] Treatment with a variety of agents, including traditional antituberculous agents as well as erythromycin, minocycline, and doxycycline, has been successful. Because of resistance, antibiotic selection should always be based on specific sensitivities.[69]

Mycobacterium haemophilum

M haemophilum is a fastidious organism that has a unique culture requirement for iron supplementation and a lower growth temperature of 28° to 30°C. The natural habitat and how an infection is acquired remain unknown.[70] The 2 main clinical settings for infection with *M haemophilum* are severe immunosuppression and healthy children who present with lymphadenopathy. The clinical spectrum of cutaneous infections is broad and varies from localized disease to systemic disease with cutaneous dissemination.[71,72] Cutaneous lesions include erythematous papules, plaques (**Fig. 3**), nodules, necrotic abscesses, or chronic ulcers. The skin lesions are usually painless at first, but as they evolve grow painful. *M haemophilum* skin infections tend to occur on the extremities.

No standard guidelines are available for the treatment of *M haemophilum* skin disease. General recommendations include use of multiple antibiotics, such as clarithromycin, ciprofloxacin, and rifabutin guided by susceptibility studies. The duration of therapy is not well defined and should be tailored based on the immune state, clinical presentation, and course.[70] Surgical excision should be considered for localized and limited infection. Patients with localized cutaneous infection often have a good prognosis with no major sequelae.

RAPIDLY GROWING MYCOBACTERIA

SSTIs with RGM are primarily caused by 3 species: *M fortuitum, M abscessus,* and *M chelonae.* Other mycobacteria implicated in SSTIs include the *M smegmatis* group. The incidence of RGM infections has increased over time and they are recognized as common contaminants of water and cosmeceuticals.[24] Nonsterile water is a frequent source of infection by RGM in nosocomial infections. RGM have been encountered in an

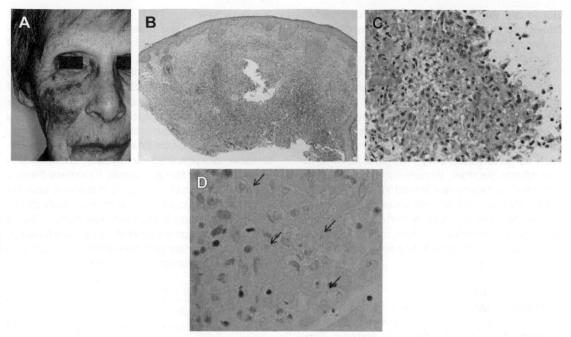

Fig. 3. *M haemophilum*. (*A*) Confluent, erythematous papules with focal erosions on the right cheek. Patient had a history of surgical resection of squamous cell carcinoma of the tongue. (*B*) Hematoxylin-eosin stains showed granulomatous and suppurative mixed inflammation (×5). (*C*) Closer view showing numerous histiocytes (×40). (*D*) AFB stain showed filamentous bacilli (×100) (*arrows*).

ever-increasing number of clinical settings associated with trauma, surgery, and cosmetic procedures (see **Table 1**). The clinical presentation can be nonspecific, therefore a high index of suspicion is necessary for diagnosis. Reported skin findings are diverse and include subcutaneous nodules, abscesses, cellulitis, ulcers, sporotrichoid nodules, sinus tracts, drainage from chronic wounds, erythema, papules, pustules, and folliculitis. Initial signs and symptoms for the RGM can also vary depending on the offending species. Immunosuppressed patients may present with multifocal disease regardless of the species.

Diagnosis of these infections is often delayed, as mycobacterial cultures are not routinely performed on surgical wound infections or skin biopsy specimens. Mycobacterial cultures from tissue biopsy or drainage material are required for the accurate diagnosis of RGM, especially because treatment varies depending on the species and its sensitivities. *M fortuitum, M abscessus,* and *M chelonae* are all resistant to tuberculosis drugs, but variably susceptible to a number of traditional antibiotics. Antimicrobial susceptibility studies should be requested on all isolates and repeated when faced with evidence of treatment failure. Unfortunately, there are no randomized, controlled clinical trial results to guide therapy of RGM infections. General treatment recommendations for

limited SSTIs with these RGM include the use of 2 oral antibiotics (to which the isolate is susceptible) for 4 to 6 months. Severe skin disease may require initial use of parenteral therapy, followed by oral therapy continued for 6 to 12 months. Surgical therapy can be an important adjunctive treatment in select cases. Consultation with an infectious disease specialist should be considered to aid in management of RGM infections.

The specific differences among these species are discussed in detail in the following sections.

Mycobacterium fortuitum

Etiopathogenesis
M fortuitum is the most common RGM encountered in clinical practice. Similar to other RGM, it is isolated from environmental sources, such as water, soil, and dust, and from nosocomial sources. Human infection is sporadic and is primarily caused by direct inoculation of the bacterium via trauma or an invasive procedure. In comparison with the other RGM, *M fortuitum* is less frequently linked with cosmetic procedures. Nonetheless, cutaneous infections secondary to tattooing, pedicures, and mesotherapy are described.[73–76] A large outbreak of pedicure-associated *M fortuitum* furunculosis from whirlpool footbaths was documented in California. This affected healthy

individuals and was attributed to inappropriate cleaning of the whirlpool baths and contaminated tap water.[74] Shaving the legs before the procedure appears to be one of the main risk factor for infection.[73–77] Of note, other subspecies, such as *M chelonae, Mycobacterium massiliense,* and *Mycobacterium bolletii,* also should be considered when pedicure-related mycobacterial infection is suspected, especially because these often require different diagnostic techniques, such as gene sequencing.[77] In general, *M fortuitum* affects younger, immunocompetent patients who tend to experience limited infections associated with low mortality. However, *M fortuitum* is increasingly known as an opportunistic pathogen causing disseminated infection, mainly in patients with impaired cellular immunity or receiving glucocorticoid therapy.[78]

Clinical presentation

Classically, cutaneous infection with *M fortuitum* presents with a single subcutaneous nodule located at a site of trauma or surgery. Thus, compared with other RGM, patients recall experiencing trauma or a surgical procedure at the site. *M fortuitum* is typically seen in a younger patient population than either *M abscessus* or *M chelonae.* Patients are less likely to have significant systemic comorbidities or use an immunosuppressive medication.[79] Up to 89% of *M fortuitum* infections present as a single lesion and *M chelonae* and *M abscessus* are more likely to present as multiple lesions.[74] Disseminated disease has been documented in immunocompromised patients, particularly HIV/AIDS. In this patient population, infection due to *M fortuitum* can present with lymphadenopathy in the absence of skin lesions.[80]

Evaluation

Given the nonspecific clinical findings, a detailed history is necessary to identify the source of infection. Biopsies for mycobacterial tissue cultures and routine histopathology are essential for an accurate diagnosis. A detailed description of specific variations on cutaneous histopathology has not been established. Most cases present with a mixed suppurative-granulomatous inflammation with a minority of cases showing well-formed granulomas. Giant cells are rarely present, whereas focal abscesses and dermal and subcutaneous abscesses without granuloma formation are a rather common finding.[80] In most cases, mycobacterial stains, such as AFB, are negative. However, negative stains do not exclude the diagnosis and the physician should always base the medical management on culture isolates.

Management

Although optimal treatment is not defined, *M fortuitum* is generally more drug susceptible than are *M chelonae* or *M abscessus,* and often oral regimens can be devised. Nonetheless, an erythromycin methylase (*erm*) gene in *M fortuitum* is capable of inducing resistance to macrolides.[41] Monotherapy is not advised. *M fortuitum* has been shown to be sensitive in vitro to the oral antibiotics clarithromycin, azithromycin, ciprofloxacin, levofloxacin, moxifloxacin, doxycycline, minocycline, linezolid, and trimethoprim-sulfamethoxazole. Parenteral therapy options may include amikacin, imipenem, and cefoxitin.[40,81] Surgical therapy is an important adjunctive tool in treating *M fortuitum* infections; patients with a single lesion are more likely to undergo surgical treatment or surgical treatment in combination with antibiotic therapy (76%vs 40%).[79]

Mycobacterium abscessus

Etiopathogenesis

M abscessus subsp *abscessus* is part of the *M chelonae/abscessus* complex. It is found in soil, water, and dust, and is endemic in the southeastern United States from Florida to Texas.[82] Previously classified as a subspecies of *M chelonae, M chelonae* subsp *abscessus,* it was named as its own species in 1992.[79] After *M fortuitum, M abscessus* is the second most common RGM species isolated from clinical specimens. It is the most pathogenic of the 3 common RGM and can cause lung disease in addition to significant skin disease. In one study, nonpulmonary infections with *M abscessus* were associated with postsurgical or postinjection wounds (43%), localized community-acquired wound infections (23%), disseminated cutaneous infections (20%), and miscellaneous types of infections (13%). As expected, of the 23% of cases resulting in localized infection, disease developed after a break in the skin surface and subsequent direct contact with contaminated water or soil.[79,83] Recently, multiple reports have shown outbreaks of *M abscessus* infections caused by nonsterile techniques or contaminated materials, after Mohs surgery, liposuction, soft tissue augmentation, mesotherapy, and acupuncture.[84–89]

Clinical presentation

Infection by *M abscessus* usually follows penetrating trauma in immunocompetent individuals. Initial presentation includes the formation of a tender, fluctuant, subcutaneous abscess at the inoculation site. Other presentations include ulcerations, draining sinuses, or nodules. The primary lesion is often followed by a sporotrichoid appearance of ascending lymphadenitis.[90] Although not common, *M abscessus* can cause disseminated disease in the immunocompromised population. Patients present with systemic symptoms and often have multiple, red to violaceous, subcutaneous nodules, and lymphadenopathy.[91,92] Although most disseminated cutaneous disease is due to *M chelonae*, disseminated disease due to *M abscessus* is typically very serious and difficult to treat.

Evaluation

A detailed history to identify potential sources of inoculation should be obtained in every patient presenting with clinical lesions suggestive of an RGM. This is important to identify outbreaks, especially in hospital settings. Patients also should be aware to note any evidence of infection at a site where they received procedures, such as surgery or injections. Lesional biopsies for tissue culture and routing histopathologic examination are required for an accurate diagnosis and treatment. Three main histopathologic patterns have been described for cutaneous infection with *M abscessus*: (1) deep dermal and subcutaneous granulomatous inflammation (see **Fig. 5**C, D), (2) abscess with mild granulomatous reaction, and (3) deep dermal and subcutaneous granulomatous inflammation with no neutrophil component. In this study, acid-fast stains were positive in 27% of cases. Interestingly, atypical mycobacterial when identified on tissue cultures using acid-fast stains are typically clumped and surrounded by a vacuole.[93]

Management

Currently, there are no standard guidelines for the treatment of cutaneous *M abscessus* infection. Treatment should be mainly based on in vitro sensitivities of the culture isolates. However, in vivo efficacy does not always reflect in vitro sensitivity; it also depends on general host defenses against the infection. *M abscessus* is often difficult to treat. *M abscessus* is usually susceptible only to clarithromycin, azithromycin, linezolid, and clofazimine.[40,41] *M abscessus* may also carry a macrolide resistance (*erm*) gene.[94] Although clarithromycin is generally a recommended drug of choice, it should be given in a combination with another antibiotic for 4 to 6 months.[95] Parental medications may be necessary initially, such as amikacin, cefoxitin, tigecycline, or imipenem.[40] Removal of foreign bodies and/or incision and drainage of abscesses is essential to management.[7]

Mycobacterium chelonae

Etiopathogenesis

M chelonae is an RGM isolated from environmental, nonhuman animal and human sources. Severe and sometimes disseminated cutaneous disease is most frequently seen with *M chelonae* and has been commonly reported in association with immunosuppression with drugs, such as corticosteroids or underlying disease states, such as leukemia or solid organ transplantation.[96–98] Infection also has been linked to the use of biologics that have specific T-cell–directed activity, such as adalimumab.[99] Most cases involving *M chelonae* are sporadic, but outbreaks secondary to the use of contaminated water and injections is an emerging problem. *M chelonae* infection has been linked to some cosmetic procedures, such as injection sites of botulinum toxin, liposuction, breast augmentation, and under skin flaps.[100–103] There have been reports associated with the use of contaminated footbaths in a beauty salon and tattoo parlors.[73,104–106] Although *M fortuitum* is the most common culprit, *M chelonae* also has been shown to cause pedicure-associated infection. Recent reports showed *M chelonae* to be endemic in 2 North Carolina counties where suboptimal footbath cleaning during pedicures led to numerous cases of furunculosis.[77] *M chelonae* also can colonize skin wounds, such as hidradenitis suppurativa lesions.[107]

Clinical presentation

The clinical presentation of SSTIs with *M chelonae* varies. In one series, the clinical disease included disseminated cutaneous infection in 53% of cases; localized cellulitis, abscess, or osteomyelitis in 35% of cases; and catheter infections in 12%.[108] The classic cutaneous presentation is disseminated disease with multiple lesions (**Fig. 4**) in the form of tender, erythematous, draining nodules. Some patients present with a chronic, nonhealing cellulitis or skin ulcers (**Fig. 5**). This is usually painful and spreads slowly. Areas of cellulitis associated with the infection are frequently hyperpigmented. Infections associated with surgical procedures may present as wound infections,

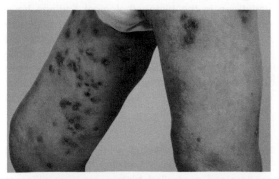

Fig. 4. *M chelonae.* Multiple, punched out, ulcerated nodules with associated erythema and a mild exudate in an immunosuppressed patient.

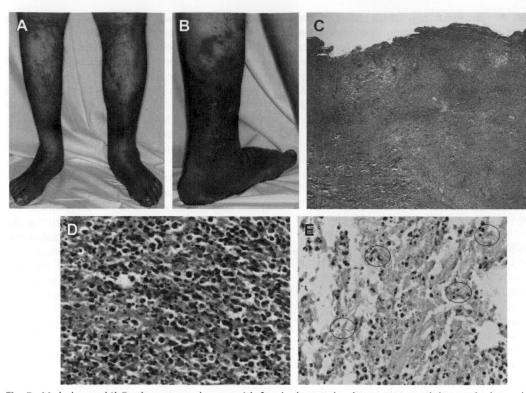

Fig. 5. *M chelonae.* (*A*) Erythematous plaques with focal, ulcerated, subcutaneous nodules on the lower legs of a nonimmunosuppressed patient. (*B*) Proximal extension of erythema. (*C*) Hematoxylin-eosin stain showing granulomatous and suppurative mixed inflammation (×10). (*D*) Mixed dermal inflammation (×40). (*E*) Acid-fast stain with filamentous bacilli (×40) (*circled*).

draining fistulae/sinus tracts, or inflamed and/or dysfunctional prosthetic devices.[109] Patients can present with skin nodules, sinus tracts, and abscess formation.

Evaluation

Similar to all other RGM, a detailed history is critical to trace any potential environmental sources and identify outbreaks. Biopsies are essential for tissue culture and routine histopathologic analysis. Histopathology may show neutrophilic abscesses along with granulomatous inflammation. Specific variations in the histopathological findings have not been described in the literature. *M chelonae* can be acid-fast positive, although the staining may be weak, and in some cases it can be negative. A negative acid-fast smear does not eliminate the possibility of any mycobacterial infections, and cultures are always needed to establish the diagnosis.

Management

To date, no specific guidelines for the treatment of *M chelonae* have been published and there are no randomized controlled trials comparing different therapeutic regimens. Identification of antimicrobial susceptibility through culture is essential.[110]

M chelonae is usually susceptible or intermediate in susceptibility to clarithromycin, moxifloxacin, linezolid, clofazimine, doxycycline, ciprofloxacin, or levofloxacin.[111,112] Parenteral antibiotics include tobramycin, amikacin, imipenem, and tigecycline.[40,41] Acquired resistance to clarithromycin has been documented with monotherapy; therefore, in agreement with the evidence thus far, the use of monotherapy should be avoided. Adjunctive surgical treatment may be indicated.

SUMMARY

- NTM are ubiquitous, environmental, AFB.
- SSTIs by NTM are increasing in incidence.
- Water is a common source of these infections. The use of nonsterile tap water in surgical and cosmetic procedures is frequently cited as the source of nosocomial infection.
- NTM cause SSTIs primarily after traumatic inoculation, surgery, and cosmetic procedures.
- Because of their varied clinical presentation, a high index of suspicion is necessary to diagnose SSTIs caused by NTM. NTM should be suspected in infections at sites of previous trauma, surgery, or cosmetic procedures

than are not responding to typical antibiotic treatment. Tissue samples and drainage material should be cultured for mycobacteria, as well as typical bacteria and fungi.

- Histopathologic examination, although often nonspecific, can trigger consideration of an NTM infection if a granulomatous pattern is present. AFB stains are often negative.
- *M marinum* is associated with a distinct clinical pattern: the "Fish-tank granuloma."
- *M ulcerans* causes the slow-growing, painless, and destructive Buruli ulcer. It is a significant health problem in western Africa and other parts of the world.
- The rapidly growing *Mycobacterium* include 3 clinically relevant species (*M fortuitum*, *M abscessus*, and *M chelonae*) and are causing an increasing number of SSTIs.
  - *M fortuitum* generally causes a single nodule at the site of trauma or surgery, in a young, immunocompetent patient and is responsive to many oral antibiotics.
  - *M abscessus* and *M chelonae* are more likely to occur in older, immunosuppressed patients, present with multiple nodules or abscesses, and be more difficult to treat.
- Treatment of limited SSTIs by NTM is generally based on antimicrobial susceptibility studies and often includes the use of 2 or more antibiotics for several months. In select cases, surgery is an important adjunct.
- Further research to define the optimal treatment for SSTIs caused by NTM is needed.

REFERENCES

1. Falkinham JO 3rd. Surrounded by mycobacteria: nontuberculous mycobacteria in the human environment. J Appl Microbiol 2009;107(2):356–67.
2. Euzeby JP. Mycobacterium. 1997. Available at: http://www.bacterio.net. Accessed May 1, 2014.
3. Yu JR, Heo ST, Lee KH, et al. Skin and soft tissue infection due to rapidly growing mycobacteria: case series and literature review. Infect Chemother 2013;45(1):85–93.
4. Runyon EH. Anonymous mycobacteria in pulmonary disease. Med Clin North Am 1959;43(1): 273–90.
5. Bicmen C, Gunduz AT, Coskun M, et al. Molecular detection and identification of mycobacterium tuberculosis complex and four clinically important nontuberculous mycobacterial species in smear-negative clinical samples by the genotype mycobacteria direct test. J Clin Microbiol 2011;49(8): 2874–8.
6. van Ingen J, Blaak H, de Beer J, et al. Rapidly growing nontuberculous mycobacteria cultured from home tap and shower water. Appl Environ Microbiol 2010;76(17):6017–9.
7. Bennett JE, Dolin R, Douglas RG, et al, editors. Mandell, Douglas, and Bennett's principles and practice of infectious diseases, vol. 2, 7th edition. Philadelphia: Elsevier, Churchill Livingstone; 2009.
8. Carson LA, Bland LA, Cusick LB, et al. Prevalence of nontuberculous mycobacteria in water supplies of hemodialysis centers. Appl Environ Microbiol 1988;54(12):3122–5.
9. Carson LA, Cusick LB, Bland LA, et al. Efficacy of chemical dosing methods for isolating nontuberculous mycobacteria from water supplies of dialysis centers. Appl Environ Microbiol 1988;54(7): 1756–60.
10. Schulze-Robbecke R, Janning B, Fischeder R. Occurrence of mycobacteria in biofilm samples. Tuber Lung Dis 1992;73(3):141–4.
11. Steed KA, Falkinham JO. Effect of growth in biofilms on chlorine susceptibility of *Mycobacterium avium* and *Mycobacterium intracellulare*. Appl Environ Microbiol 2006;72(6):4007–11.
12. Griffiths PA, Babb JR, Bradley CR, et al. Glutaraldehyde-resistant *Mycobacterium chelonae* from endoscope washer disinfectors. J Appl Microbiol 1997;82(4):519–26.
13. Griffiths PA, Babb JR, Fraise AP. Mycobactericidal activity of selected disinfectants using a quantitative suspension test. J Hosp Infect 1999;41(2): 111–21.
14. Selvaraju SB, Khan IU, Yadav JS. Biocidal activity of formaldehyde and nonformaldehyde biocides toward *Mycobacterium immunogenum* and *Pseudomonas fluorescens* in pure and mixed suspensions in synthetic metalworking fluid and saline. Appl Environ Microbiol 2005;71(1):542–6.
15. Carter G, Wu M, Drummond DC, et al. Characterization of biofilm formation by clinical isolates of *Mycobacterium avium*. J Med Microbiol 2003; 52(Pt 9):747–52.
16. Falkinham JO. The changing pattern of nontuberculous mycobacterial disease. Can J Infect Dis 2003;14(5):281–6.
17. Diagnosis and treatment of disease caused by nontuberculous mycobacteria. This official statement of the American Thoracic Society was approved by the Board of Directors, March 1997. Medical Section of the American Lung Association. Am J Respir Crit Care Med 1997;156(2 Pt 2):S1–25.
18. Swanson DS, Pan X, Musser JM. Identification and subspecific differentiation of *Mycobacterium scrofulaceum* by automated sequencing of a region of the gene (hsp65) encoding a 65-kilodalton heat shock protein. J Clin Microbiol 1996;34(12): 3151–9.
19. Thomsen VO, Andersen AB, Miorner H. Incidence and clinical significance of non-tuberculous

mycobacteria isolated from clinical specimens during a 2-y nationwide survey. Scand J Infect Dis 2002;34(9):648–53.

20. Karakousis PC, Moore RD, Chaisson RE. Mycobacterium avium complex in patients with HIV infection in the era of highly active antiretroviral therapy. Lancet Infect Dis 2004;4(9):557–65.

21. Phillips MS, von Reyn CF. Nosocomial infections due to nontuberculous mycobacteria. Clin Infect Dis 2001;33(8):1363–74.

22. Nightingale SD, Byrd LT, Southern PM, et al. Incidence of Mycobacterium-avium-intracellulare complex bacteremia in human-immunodeficiency-virus positive patients. J Infect Dis 1992;165(6):1082–5.

23. Ferreira RM, Saad MH, Silva MG, et al. Non-tuberculous mycobacteria I: one year clinical isolates identification in tertiary hospital aids reference center, Rio de Janeiro, Brazil, in pre highly active antiretroviral therapy era. Mem Inst Oswaldo Cruz 2002;97(5):725–9.

24. Wentworth AB, Drage LA, Wengenack NL, et al. Increased incidence of cutaneous nontuberculous mycobacterial infection, 1980 to 2009: a population-based study. Mayo Clin Proc 2013;88(1):38–45.

25. Morimoto K, Iwai K, Uchimura K, et al. A steady increase in nontuberculous mycobacteriosis mortality and estimated prevalence in Japan. Ann Am Thorac Soc 2013;11(1):1–8.

26. Leung JM, Olivier KN. Nontuberculous mycobacteria: the changing epidemiology and treatment challenges in cystic fibrosis. Curr Opin Pulm Med 2013; 19(6):662–9.

27. Bendl BJ, Ongley RC. Cutaneous nontuberculous mycobacterial infections. Can Fam Physician 1978;24:269–73.

28. AlKhodair R, Al-Khenaizan S. Fish tank granuloma: misdiagnosed as cutaneous leishmaniasis. Int J Dermatol 2010;49(1):53–5.

29. Ang P, Rattana-Apiromyakij N, Goh CL. Retrospective study of Mycobacterium marinum skin infections. Int J Dermatol 2000;39(5):343–7.

30. Kullavanijaya P, Sirimachan S, Bhuddhavudhikrai P. Mycobacterium marinum cutaneous infections acquired from occupations and hobbies. Int J Dermatol 1993;32(7):504–7.

31. Wu TS, Chiu CH, Yang CH, et al. Fish tank granuloma caused by Mycobacterium marinum. PLoS One 2012;7:e41296.

32. Etuaful S, Carbonnelle B, Grosset J, et al. Efficacy of the combination rifampin-streptomycin in preventing growth of Mycobacterium ulcerans in early lesions of Buruli ulcer in humans. Antimicrob Agents Chemother 2005;49(8):3182–6.

33. Gombert ME, Goldstein EJ, Corrado ML, et al. Disseminated Mycobacterium marinum infection after renal transplantation. Ann Intern Med 1981; 94(4 pt 1):486–7.

34. Gluckman SJ. Mycobacterium marinum. Clin Dermatol 1995;13(3):273–6.

35. Aubry A, Chosidow O, Caumes E, et al. Sixty-three cases of Mycobacterium marinum infection: clinical features, treatment, and antibiotic susceptibility of causative isolates. Arch Intern Med 2002;162(15): 1746–52.

36. Holmes GF, Harrington SM, Romagnoli MJ, et al. Recurrent, disseminated Mycobacterium marinum infection caused by the same genotypically defined strain in an immunocompromised patient. J Clin Microbiol 1999;37(9):3059–61.

37. Lacaille F, Blanche S, Bodemer C, et al. Persistent Mycobacterium marinum infection in a child with probable visceral involvement. Pediatr Infect Dis J 1990;9(1):58–60.

38. Abbas O, Marrouch N, Kattar MM, et al. Cutaneous non-tuberculous mycobacterial infections: a clinical and histopathological study of 17 cases from Lebanon. J Eur Acad Dermatol Venereol 2011; 25(1):33–42.

39. Gray SF, Smith RS, Reynolds NJ, et al. Fish tank granuloma. BMJ 1990;300(6731):1069–70.

40. Griffith DE, Aksamit T, Brown-Elliott BA, et al. An official ATS/IDSA statement: diagnosis, treatment, and prevention of nontuberculous mycobacterial diseases. Am J Respir Crit Care Med 2007;175(4):367–416.

41. Brown-Elliott BA, Nash KA, Wallace RJ Jr. Antimicrobial susceptibility testing, drug resistance mechanisms, and therapy of infections with nontuberculous mycobacteria. Clin Microbiol Rev 2012; 25(3):545–82.

42. Rallis E, Koumantaki-Mathioudaki E. Treatment of Mycobacterium marinum cutaneous infections. Expert Opin Pharmacother 2007;8(17):2965–78.

43. Aubry A, Jarlier V, Escolano S, et al. Antibiotic susceptibility pattern of Mycobacterium marinum. Antimicrob Agents Chemother 2000;44(11):3133–6.

44. Dorronsoro I, Sarasqueta R, González AI, et al. Cutaneous infections by Mycobacterium marinum. Description of 3 cases and review of the literature. Enferm Infecc Microbiol Clin 1997;15(2):82–4 [in Spanish].

45. Young-Afat DA, Dayicioglu D, Oeltjen JC, et al. Fishing-injury-related flexor tenosynovitis of the hand: a case report and review. Case Rep Orthop 2013;2013:587176.

46. Flondell M, Ornstein K, Bjorkman A. Invasive Mycobacterium marinum infection of the hand. J Plast Surg Hand Surg 2013;47(6):532–4.

47. Sopoh GE, Johnson RC, Chauty A, et al. Buruli ulcer surveillance, Benin, 2003-2005. Emerg Infect Dis 2007;13(9):1374–6.

48. Debacker M, Aguiar J, Steunou C, et al. Mycobacterium ulcerans disease (Buruli ulcer) in rural hospital, Southern Benin, 1997-2001. Emerg Infect Dis 2004;10(8):1391–8.

49. Amofah G, Bonsu F, Tetteh C, et al. Buruli ulcer in Ghana: results of a national case search. Emerg Infect Dis 2002;8(2):167–70.

50. Silva MT, Portaels F, Pedrosa J. Aquatic insects and *Mycobacterium ulcerans*: an association relevant to Buruli ulcer control? PLoS Med 2007;4:e63.

51. Deshayes C, Angala SK, Marion E, et al. Regulation of mycolactone, the *Mycobacterium ulcerans* toxin, depends on nutrient source. PLoS Negl Trop Dis 2013;7:e2502.

52. Stienstra Y, van der Graaf WT, te Meerman GJ, et al. Susceptibility to development of *Mycobacterium ulcerans* disease: review of possible risk factors. Trop Med Int Health 2001;6(7):554–62.

53. Hospers IC, Wiersma IC, Dijkstra PU, et al. Distribution of Buruli ulcer lesions over body surface area in a large case series in Ghana: uncovering clues for mode of transmission. Trans R Soc Trop Med Hyg 2005;99(3):196–201.

54. Pszolla N, Sarkar MR, Strecker W, et al. Buruli ulcer: a systemic disease. Clin Infect Dis 2003;37: e78–82.

55. Phillips R, Horsfield C, Mangan J, et al. Cytokine mRNA expression in *Mycobacterium ulcerans*-infected human skin and correlation with local inflammatory response. Infect Immun 2006;74(5): 2917–24.

56. Walsh DS, Meyers WM, Portaels F, et al. High rates of apoptosis in human *Mycobacterium ulcerans* culture-positive buruli ulcer skin lesions. Am J Trop Med Hyg 2005;73(2):410–5.

57. WHO. Treatment of *Mycobacterium ulcerans* disease (Buruli ulcer). 2014. Available at: http://www.who.int/mediacentre/factsheets/fs199/en/. Accessed January 1, 2014.

58. Guarner J, Bartlett J, Whitney EA, et al. Histopathologic features of *Mycobacterium ulcerans* infection. Emerg Infect Dis 2003;9(6):651–6.

59. Ruf MT, Sopoh GE, Brun LV, et al. Histopathological changes and clinical responses of Buruli ulcer plaque lesions during chemotherapy: a role for surgical removal of necrotic tissue? PLoS Negl Trop Dis 2011;5:e1334.

60. Stienstra Y, van Roest MH, van Wezel MJ, et al. Factors associated with functional limitations and subsequent employment or schooling in Buruli ulcer patients. Trop Med Int Health 2005;10(12): 1251–7.

61. Schunk M, Thompson W, Klutse E, et al. Outcome of patients with buruli ulcer after surgical treatment with or without antimycobacterial treatment in Ghana. Am J Trop Med Hyg 2009;81(1):75–81.

62. WHO. Treatment of *Mycobacterium ulcerans* disease (Buruli ulcer). Available from: htpp://apps.who.int/iris/bitstream/10665/77771/1/9789241503402_eng.pdf. Accessed January 10, 2014.

63. Chapman J. The atypical mycobacteria. New York: Plenum Publishing; 1977.

64. Steadham JE. High-catalase strains of *Mycobacterium-kansasii* isolated from water in Texas. J Clin Microbiol 1980;11(5):496–8.

65. Stengem J, Grande KK, Hsu S. Localized primary cutaneous *Mycobacterium kansasii* infection in an immunocompromised patient. Am Acad Dermatol 1999;41(5):854–6.

66. Czelusta A, Moore AY. Cutaneous *Mycobacterium kansasii* infection in a patient with systemic lupus erythematosus: case report and review. Am Acad Dermatol 1999;40(2):359–63.

67. Razavi B, Cleveland MG. Cutaneous infection due to *Mycobacterium kansasii*. Diagn Microbiol Infect Dis 2000;38(3):173–5.

68. Chaves A, Torrelo A, Mediero IG, et al. Primary cutaneous *Mycobacterium kansasii* infection in a child. Pediatr Dermatol 2001;18(2):131–4.

69. Wu TS, Leu HS, Chiu CH, et al. Clinical manifestations, antibiotic susceptibility and molecular analysis of *Mycobacterium kansasii* isolates from a university hospital in Taiwan. J Antimicrob Chemother 2009;64(3):511–4.

70. Lindeboom JA, Bruijnesteijn van Coppenraet LE, van Soolingen D, et al. Clinical manifestations, diagnosis, and treatment of *Mycobacterium haemophilum* infections. Clin Microbiol Rev 2011; 24(4):701–17.

71. Tangkosakul T. *Mycobacterium haemophilum* cutaneous infection in immunocompromised patients, 5-case report from a tertiary hospital, Bangkok, Thailand. Int J Infect Dis 2012;16:E297.

72. Straus WL, Ostroff SM, Jernigan DB, et al. Clinical and epidemiologic characteristics of *Mycobacterium-haemophilum*, an emerging pathogen in immunocompromised patients. Ann Intern Med 1994;120(2):118–25.

73. Redbord KP, Shearer DA, Gloster H, et al. Atypical *Mycobacterium furunculosis* occurring after pedicures. Am Acad Dermatol 2006;54(3):520–4.

74. Winthrop KL, Abrams M, Yakrus M, et al. An outbreak of *Mycobacterial furunculosis* associated with footbaths at a nail salon. N Engl J Med 2002; 346(18):1366–71.

75. Suvanasuthi S, Wongpraparut C, Pattanaprichakul P, et al. *Mycobacterium fortuitum* cutaneous infection from amateur tattoo. J Med Assoc Thai 2012;95(6): 834–7.

76. Quinones C, Ramalle-Gómara E, Perucha M, et al. An outbreak of *Mycobacterium fortuitum* cutaneous infection associated with mesotherapy. J Eur Acad Dermatol Venereol 2010;24(5):604–6.

77. Stout JE, Gadkowski LB, Rath S, et al. Pedicure-associated rapidly growing mycobacterial infection: an endemic disease. Clin Infect Dis 2011; 53(8):787–92.

78. Sungkanuparph S, Sathapatayavongs B, Pracharktam R. Rapidly growing mycobacterial infections: spectrum of diseases, antimicrobial susceptibility, pathology and treatment outcomes. J Med Assoc Thai 2003;86(8):772–80.

79. Uslan DZ, Kowalski TJ, Wengenack NL, et al. Skin and soft tissue infections due to rapidly growing mycobacteria—Comparison of clinical features, treatment, and susceptibility. Arch Dermatol 2006; 142(10):1287–92.

80. Smith MB, Schnadig VJ, Boyars MC, et al. Clinical and pathologic features of Mycobacterium fortuitum infections. An emerging pathogen in patients with AIDS. Am J Clin Pathol 2001;116(2):225–32.

81. Wallace RJ Jr, Swenson JM, Silcox VA, et al. Treatment of nonpulmonary infections due to Mycobacterium fortuitum and Mycobacterium chelonei on the basis of in vitro susceptibilities. J Infect Dis 1985;152(3):500–14.

82. Brown-Elliott BA, Wallace RJ Jr. Clinical and taxonomic status of pathogenic nonpigmented or late-pigmenting rapidly growing mycobacteria. Clin Microbiol Rev 2002;15(4):716–46.

83. Wallace RJ Jr, Swenson JM, Silcox VA, et al. Spectrum of disease due to rapidly growing mycobacteria. Rev Infect Dis 1983;5(4):657–79.

84. Fisher EJ, Gloster HM Jr. Infection with Mycobacterium abscessus after Mohs micrographic surgery in an immunocompetent patient. Dermatol Surg 2005;31(7 Pt 1):790–4.

85. Murillo J, Torres J, Bofill L, et al. Skin and wound infection by rapidly growing mycobacteria: an unexpected complication of liposuction and liposculpture. The Venezuelan Collaborative Infectious and Tropical Diseases Study Group. Arch Dermatol 2000;136(11):1347–52.

86. Ryu HJ, Kim WJ, Oh CH, et al. Iatrogenic Mycobacterium abscessus infection associated with acupuncture: clinical manifestations and its treatment. Int J Dermatol 2005;44(10):846–50.

87. Toy BR, Frank PJ. Outbreak of Mycobacterium abscessus infection after soft tissue augmentation. Dermatol Surg 2003;29(9):971–3.

88. Garcia-Navarro X, Barnadas MA, Dalmau J, et al. Mycobacterium abscessus infection secondary to mesotherapy. Clin Exp Dermatol 2008;33(5):658–9.

89. Wongkitisophon P, Rattanakaemakorn P, Tanrattanakorn S, et al. Cutaneous Mycobacterium abscessus infection associated with mesotherapy injection. Case Rep Dermatol 2011;3(1):37–41.

90. Lee WJ, Kim TW, Shur KB, et al. Sporotrichoid dermatosis caused by Mycobacterium abscessus from a public bath. J Dermatol 2000;27(4): 264–8.

91. Liu R, To KK, Teng JL, et al. Mycobacterium abscessus bacteremia after receipt of intravenous infusate of cytokine-induced killer cell therapy for body beautification and health boosting. Clin Infect Dis 2013;57(7):981–91.

92. Su SH, Chen YH, Tsai TY, et al. Catheter-related Mycobacterium abscessus bacteremia manifested with skin nodules, pneumonia, and mediastinal lymphadenopathy. Kaohsiung J Med Sci 2013; 29(1):50–4.

93. Rodriguez G, Ortegón M, Camargo D, et al. Iatrogenic Mycobacterium abscessus infection: histopathology of 71 patients. Br J Dermatol 1997; 137(2):214–8.

94. Tebas P, Sultan F, Wallace RJ Jr, et al. Rapid development of resistance to clarithromycin following monotherapy for disseminated Mycobacterium chelonae infection in a heart transplant patient. Clin Infect Dis 1995;20(2):443–4.

95. Esteban J, Ortiz-Perez A. Current treatment of atypical mycobacteriosis. Expert Opin Pharmacother 2009;10(17):2787–99.

96. Jankovic M, Zmak L, Krajinovic V, et al. A fatal Mycobacterium chelonae infection in an immunosuppressed patient with systemic lupus erythematosus and concomitant Fahr's syndrome. J Infect Chemother 2011;17(2):264–7.

97. Bark CM, Traboulsi RS, Honda K, et al. Disseminated Mycobacterium chelonae infection in a patient receiving an epidermal growth factor receptor inhibitor for advanced head and neck cancer. J Clin Microbiol 2012;50(1):194–5.

98. Sbidian E, Kramkimel N, Routier E, et al. Nosocomial disseminated Mycobacterium chelonae infection in an immunocompromised patient. Eur J Dermatol 2010;20(3):407.

99. Diaz F, Urkijo JC, Mendoza F, et al. Mycobacterium chelonae infection associated with adalimumab therapy. Scand J Rheumatol 2008;37(2): 159–60.

100. Saha M, Azadian BS, Ion L, et al. Mycobacterium chelonae infection complicating cosmetic facial surgery. Br J Dermatol 2006;155(5):1097–8.

101. Latorre-Gonzalez G, García-García M, Martínez Martínez-Colubi M, et al. Disseminated cutaneous infection by Mycobacterium chelonae after botulinic toxin injection in an immunosuppressed patient. Med Clin (Barc) 2005;125(11):439 [in Spanish].

102. Dessy LA, Mazzocchi M, Fioramonti P, et al. Conservative management of local Mycobacterium chelonae infection after combined liposuction and lipofilling. Aesthetic Plast Surg 2006;30(6):717–22.

103. Brickman M, Parsa AA, Parsa FD. Mycobacterium cheloneae infection after breast augmentation. Aesthetic Plast Surg 2005;29(2):116–8.

104. Drage LA, Ecker PM, Orenstein R, et al. An outbreak of mycobacterium chelonae infections in tattoos. J Am Acad Dermatol 2010;62(3):501–6. http://dx.doi.org/10.1016/j.jaad.2009.03.034.

105. Drage LA, Ecker PM, Orenstein R, et al. An outbreak of *Mycobacterium chelonae* infections in tattoos. Am Acad Dermatol 2010;62(3):501–6.

106. Kennedy BS, Bedard B, Younge M, et al. Outbreak of *Mycobacterium chelonae* infection associated with tattoo ink. N Engl J Med 2012; 367(11):1020–4.

107. Patnaik S, Mohanty I, Panda P, et al. Disseminated *Mycobacterium chelonae* infection: Complicating a case of hidradenitis suppurativa. Indian Dermatol Online J 2013;4(4):336–9.

108. Wallace RJ Jr, Brown BA, Onyi GO. Skin, soft tissue, and bone infections due to *Mycobacterium chelonae chelonae*: importance of prior corticosteroid therapy, frequency of disseminated infections, and resistance to oral antimicrobials other than clarithromycin. J Infect Dis 1992;166(2): 405–12.

109. Unai S, Miessau J, Karbowski P, et al. Sternal wound infection caused by *Mycobacterium chelonae*. J Cardiovasc Surg 2013;28(6):687–92.

110. Regnier S, Cambau E, Meningaud JP, et al. Clinical management of rapidly growing mycobacterial cutaneous infections in patients after mesotherapy. Clin Infect Dis 2009;49(9):1358–64.

111. Swenson JM, Wallace RJ Jr, Silcox VA, et al. Antimicrobial susceptibility of five subgroups of *Mycobacterium fortuitum* and *Mycobacterium chelonae*. Antimicrob Agents Chemother 1985; 28(6):807–11.

112. Brown BA, Wallace RJ Jr, Onyi GO, et al. Activities of four macrolides, including clarithromycin, against *Mycobacterium fortuitum*, *Mycobacterium chelonae*, and *M. chelonae*-like organisms. Antimicrob Agents Chemother 1992;36(1):180–4.

New World and Old World Leishmania Infections
A Practical Review

Ines Kevric, MD[a], Mark A. Cappel, MD[a], James H. Keeling, MD[b],*

KEYWORDS

- Leishmania infection • Leishmaniasis • Cutaneous leishmaniasis • Mucocutaneous leishmaniasis

KEY POINTS

- Leishmaniasis is a parasitic infection transmitted by the bite of a sandfly, which is endemic to tropical and subtropical regions.
- The incidence of cases is rising with increased travel to these areas.
- Polymerase chain reaction is emerging as the diagnostic test of choice, because it quickly and accurately identifies the infecting species.
- Treatment recommendations vary, but pentavalent antimonials remain the preferred choice in most centers.
- Travelers to endemic countries should be counseled appropriately, because there is no vaccine to prevent this infection.

INTRODUCTION/OVERVIEW

Leishmaniasis is a tropical disease caused by an intracellular parasite of the genus *Leishmania*. The vector of transmission is the sandfly, which deposits one of the 20 disease-causing protozoan species during a blood meal. Clinical presentation depends on the complex interplay between the host cell-mediated immune response, and the specific protozoa and vector species. There are four generally accepted classifications of clinical disease: (1) cutaneous leishmaniasis (CL), (2) diffuse CL (DCL), (3) mucocutaneous leishmaniasis (ML), and (4) visceral leishmaniasis (VL). This disease is also often classified according to the world regions in which it occurs. Old World (OW) leishmaniasis exists in the Eastern Hemisphere and is endemic in Asia, Africa, and southern Europe. New World (NW) leishmaniasis is endemic to the Western Hemisphere, extending from south-central Texas to Central and South America

(except Chile and Uruguay). The disease is not found in Australia, Antarctica, or the Pacific islands.

It is difficult to obtain accurate numbers on disease incidence. It is believed to be underreported because it can be subclinical and is a disease primarily affecting the impoverished parts of the world. Estimates suggest that there are 12 million people infected, with 2 million new cases annually, most of which are cutaneous and mucocutaneous infections.[1–3] Leishmaniasis is the second leading cause of parasite-related death (after malaria) causing 20,000 to 30,000 deaths annually.[2]

Although this disease historically is limited to the tropics and subtropics, there are several factors contributing to its dissemination to new areas. These include climate change, urbanization, deforestation, increased travel for tourist and work-related reasons, immigration from endemic countries, and military operations.[4–8] In the United States, leishmaniasis is typically

[a] Department of Mayo Clinic, 4500 San Pablo Rd, Jacksonville, FL 32224, USA; [b] Department of Dermatology, Mayo Clinic, 4500 San Pablo Road South, Jacksonville, FL 32224, USA
* Corresponding author.
E-mail address: Keeling.James@mayo.edu

Dermatol Clin 33 (2015) 579–593
http://dx.doi.org/10.1016/j.det.2015.03.018
0733-8635/15/$ – see front matter © 2015 Elsevier Inc. All rights reserved.

diagnosed among travelers to endemic areas, military personnel, and immigrants. However, CL acquired in Texas and Oklahoma has been reported.[3,9] Long-term stay in endemic countries is a risk factor, but travelers may become infected in 12 hours in an endemic area.[10] The lack of familiarity with this disease in nonendemic countries leads to delays in its diagnosis and selection of proper treatment.[6–8,11]

ETIOPATHOGENESIS

Leishmania infection is acquired through the bite of the female sandfly of the genera *Phlebotomus* (OW) and *Lutzomyia* (NW). At the time of the blood meal, the flagellated motile promastigote form of leishmania is deposited and quickly phagocytosed by macrophages, dendritic cells, and neutrophils. Inside the host cells, the promastigote transforms into the aflagellate amastigote form. It then multiplies by binary fission and proceeds to infect other cells. The cycle is completed when the sandfly feeds again consuming the amastigotes, which transform back into the promastigote form in the gut of the sandfly. The promastigotes then migrate to the proboscis of the sandfly and are ready to repeat the cycle with the subsequent bite.

The major reservoirs of this disease are animals, such as dogs and rodents. The female sandfly is most active from dusk to dawn, and bites typically occur on the exposed skin of the arms, legs, neck, and face. The sandfly is smaller than a mosquito, has a painless bite, and does not make an audible noise. Infection also can be transmitted through needle sharing, blood transfusion with infected blood products,[12] or transplacentally.[13]

The major infecting species of OW and NW leishmaniasis and the associated clinical disease classification are included in **Table 1**.[2,3,14–17] It is generally regarded that OW species cause self-limiting disease and may not require treatment, whereas some NW species have a propensity to affect mucosal surfaces and thus necessitate more aggressive parenteral treatment (**Fig. 1**).[18,19]

IMMUNOLOGY

The health status of the individual, the species of *Leishmania*, and the vector of transmission are thought to be factors in determining the clinical presentation resulting from infection. It is the interplay of these elements that fashions the individual immunologic response and generates the clinical picture. The current understanding of the complex overlapping immunologic regulatory pathways is imperfect but is growing and is the subject of more detailed reviews.[16,20–22] This article provides a limited overview of key factors involved in the immunologic response.

A classic simple T-helper (Th) cell type 1/2 model has been used for years to explain the disease. Promastigotes transmitted by the sandfly bite are processed by dendritic cells and presented to naive T-cells, which in turn produce a pattern of cytokines resulting in the formation of differentiated and expanded T-cell populations: Th1, Th2, and T-reg cells. Th1 CD4$^+$ cells are activated and produce interleukin-2, interferon-γ, and tumor necrosis factor. Interferon-γ activates macrophages, which then engulf and kill the protozoa. T-reg cells then are activated and modulate the ongoing antimicrobial response thereby limiting damage to the host. However, should the Th2 CD4$^+$ response predominate, Th1 response would be inhibited and infection would persist and spread.

Table 1
Leishmania taxonomy

Region	Complex	Species	Clinical Manifestation
Old World	Leishmania donovani	L donovani	CL, VL, PKLD, ML (rare)
		L infantum	CL, VL (children), PKLD, ML (rare)
		L chagasi	CL, VL (children), PKLD, ML (rare)
	Leishmania tropica	L tropica	CL, ML (rare), VL (rare)
		L major	CL, ML (rare)
		L aethiopica	CL, DCL
New World	Leishmania mexicana	L mexicana	CL, DCL (rare)
		L amazonensis	CL, DCL, ML, VL (rare), PKLD (rare)
		L venezuelensis	CL, DCL (rare)
	Leishmania (Viannia) braziliensis	L braziliensis	CL, ML, VL
		L guyanensis	CL, ML
		L panamensis	CL, ML
		L peruviana	CL

Abbreviation: PKLD, post–kala-azar dermal leishmaniasis.

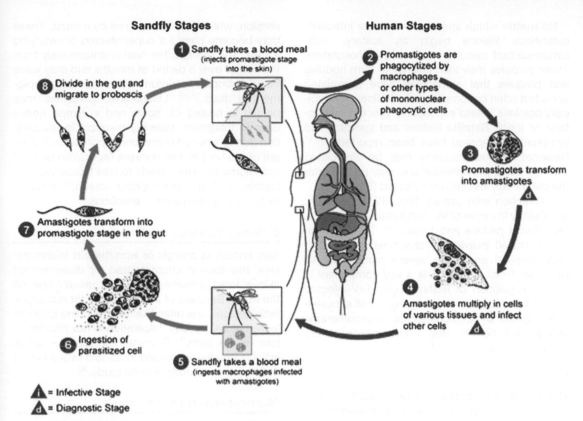

Sandfly Stages

1 Sandfly takes a blood meal
(injects promastigote stage
into the skin)

8 Divide in the gut and
migrate to proboscis

7 Amastigotes transform into
promastigote stage in the gut

6 Ingestion of
parasitized cell

5 Sandfly takes a blood meal
(ingests macrophages infected
with amastigotes)

Human Stages

2 Promastigotes are
phagocytized by
macrophages,
or other types
of mononuclear
phagocytic cells

3 Promastigotes transform
into amastigotes

4 Amastigotes multiply in cells
of various tissues and infect
other cells

i = Infective Stage

d = Diagnostic Stage

Fig. 1. Life cycle of the *Leishmania* parasite. (*Courtesy of* CDC/DPDx. Available at: http://www.cdc.gov/dpdx/leishmaniasis/index.html.)

The disease process is more complex. In addition to leishmania, some sandflies also may carry bacteria and viruses that can be transmitted with the bite and precipitate a proinflammatory response possibly enabling disease persistence.[23,24] The best example is the recent discovery that ML-causing species harbor leishmania RNA virus-1, which may facilitate evasion of host protective immune response.[25] Infected monocytes and fibroblasts may permit organisms to elude immune-mediated disease control.[16] The heavily parasitized cells noted in DCL caused by *L amazonensis* infection occur in the setting of antigen-specific impaired cell activation.[20] This organism seems to be unique in its ability to resist host-derived toxic molecules and drugs used in the treatment of leishmaniasis. The recently identified Th17 CD4$^+$ cell population produced by the primed naive T cells is known to be important in protection against infections and participate in inflammatory and autoimmune diseases. Although interleukin-17 produced in a regulated manner by Th17 CD4$^+$ cells may prevent *L donovani* from progressing to kala-azar, excessive interleukin-17 production can be associated with the destructive presentation and features of ML in patients

infected with *L braziliensis*.[20] With respect to impact of overall host health, patients with coexisting human immunodeficiency virus (HIV) infection are at increased risk of VL.[20]

In that most leishmania infections are subclinical or self-limited, the immune system is well designed to control disease. Nevertheless the various expressions and manifestations of the disease demonstrate that a weak immune response is permissive with respect to disease progression, whereas an exuberant immune response can produce destructive results. Research sorting out this interplay of vector, organism, and host parameters is ongoing.

CLINICAL PRESENTATIONS

The clinical manifestations of leishmaniasis occur on a full spectrum ranging from asymptomatic to lethal. This depends on the infecting species, vector, immune status of the host, age, nutritional status, inoculation site and dose, and genetic background of the host.[14,18,26] Fortunately, subclinical and self-healing CL is common. However, an inappropriate immune response leads to uncontrolled parasite replication and subsequent nonhealing forms.

No matter which species causes the infection, cutaneous lesions begin as solitary, well-circumscribed papules at the site of inoculation. These papules may then enlarge to form nodules and plaques that sometimes have associated scale but often become ulcerated. Ulcers are typically painless unless secondarily infected by bacteria or fungi. Satellite lesions and sporotrichoid (lymphangitic) spread have been reported.[7,10,11] Regional lymphadenopathy may be associated with the initial presentation and may persist after the cutaneous lesions have cleared (**Figs. 2–7**).

Coinfection with pre-existing HIV is common, particularly in cases of VL, and further complicates the clinical picture and treatment.[11,27] Immunocompromised individuals have been reported to have atypical and more severe manifestations. Because T-cell activation is a key component in immunoregulation of leishmaniasis, HIV-infected patients and those with iatrogenic T-cell suppression caused by corticosteroids, chemotherapy, anticytokine agents, and transplant drugs are most vulnerable.[27–29]

Cutaneous Leishmaniasis

This is the most common form of leishmaniasis and is characterized by one or more lesions that develop weeks to months after a bite. Ulcers often have raised indurated borders with central erosion, which may be covered by a crust. These may become painful if superinfected or overlying a joint. The ulcers often heal spontaneously from the center over a period of months and may leave behind atrophic, cribriform scars with a hyperpigmented halo.[14,18] Leishmania parasites may persist in healed CL scars and in lymph nodes despite treatment, possibly resulting in reactivation during a period of immunosuppression.[26] Failure of the host to limit parasite replication by local granuloma formation leads to less typical presentations, such as sporotrichoid spread,[23] erysipeloid,[24] and psoriasiform[25] eruptions.

Diffuse Cutaneous Leishmaniasis

Also known as anergic or lepromatous leishmaniasis, this form is characterized by disseminated skin-colored papules or nodules usually sparing the trunk. Because of its propensity for numerous facial lesions, it is often likened to leonine facies of lepromatous leprosy. Ulceration is not characteristic of this form.[17] Reported incidence in Brazil is 2.4% and has increased three-fold over a period of 20 years according to one study.[30]

Mucocutaneous Leishmaniasis

ML, often regarded as "metastatic" CL, develops as an uncommon sequela of NW cutaneous

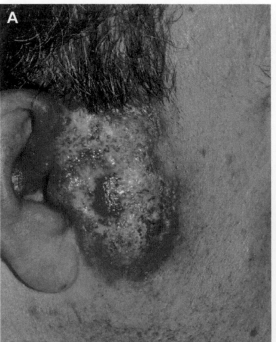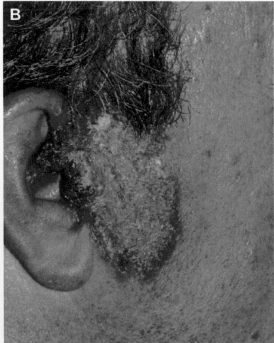

Fig. 2. (*A*) *Leishmania mexicana* infection of the right preauricular region. (*B*) *L mexicana* infection of the right preauricular region, responding after 1 month of treatment with oral fluconazole. (*By permission* of the Mayo Foundation for Medical Education and Research. All rights reserved.)

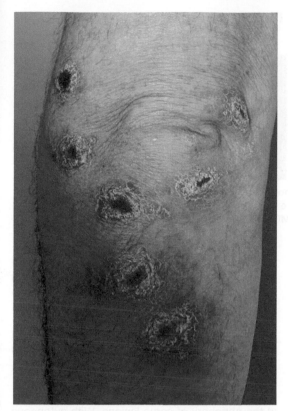

Fig. 3. *Leishmania panamensis* infection on the left elbow. Note that the pattern of the lesions suggests multiple sandfly bites in this exposed region of the arm. (*By permission* of the Mayo Foundation for Medical Education and Research. All rights reserved.)

disease 1 to 2 years or more after clinical healing of primary lesions. Progression to ML is generally not seen with OW infection, but the reasons for this remain unclear. Early manifestations include persistent nasal congestion and bleeding, and pharyngeal symptoms, such as hoarseness.

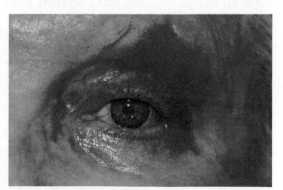

Fig. 4. *Leishmania infantum* infection of the left peri-orbital region. Note the granulomatous appearance of this apply-jelly–colored, indurated plaque. (*By permission* of the Mayo Foundation for Medical Education and Research. All rights reserved.)

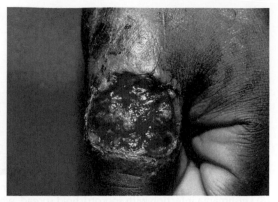

Fig. 5. Cutaneous leishmaniasis demonstrating a typical-appearing primary ulceration on the left thumb. (*Courtesy of* J. Keeling, MD, Jacksonville, FL; with permission.)

Visualization reveals erythema and edema that eventually progresses to ulceration with a muco-purulent exudate. The mucosa of the eyes or genitals is rarely involved.[17,18] Ultimately ML leads to mutilating destruction of mucous membranes of the nose, mouth, throat, and surrounding tissues. There is a paucity of data on the risk of progression to ML, but literature indicates it may develop in about 1% to 10% of NW CL cases.[30,31] Associated risk factors seem to be male gender, incomplete or missed antimony treatments, large and multiple lesions particularly above the waist, HLA-DR2 and HLA-DQx3 genetic background, and malnutrition.[32,33] Adequate treatment of the primary CL infection likely prevents ML. Complete ear, nose, and throat examination is indicated in confirmed cases of ML-causing strains.

Visceral Leishmaniasis

Also known as kala-azar (black sickness), this type of leishmaniasis develops months to years following

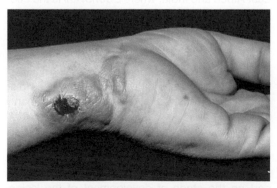

Fig. 6. Leishmaniasis acquired in south Texas presenting as a granulomatous-appearing plaque with a central ulceration on the left wrist. (*Courtesy of* J. Keeling, MD, Jacksonville, FL; with permission.)

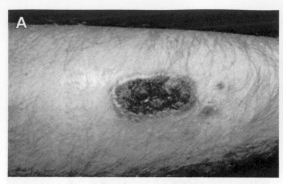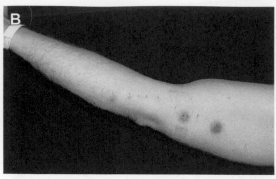

Fig. 7. (*A*) Leishmania infection with the primary cutaneous lesion occurring on the dorsum of the right forearm. (*B*) Leishmania infection with sporotrichoid spread, where subsequent lesions have tic marks indicating the presence of subcutaneous nodules. (*Courtesy of* J. Keeling, MD, Jacksonville, FL; with permission.)

inoculation and is a result of infected macrophages disseminating through the reticuloendothelial system. It is characterized by fevers, significant weight loss, anorexia, weakness, pallor, cough, diarrhea, epistaxis, hepatosplenomegaly, lymphadenopathy, and growth retardation in children. In certain patient population, significant hyperpigmentation can be noted which accounts for the name "black sickness". Laboratory abnormalities include normocytic anemia, thrombocytopenia, neutropenia, transaminitis, hypoalbuminemia, and hypergammaglobulinemia.[34] If left untreated, it is usually lethal within 2 years.[2] Death usually results from infection, severe anemia, or hemorrhage. It exists both in the NW and OW, but six countries (Bangladesh, Brazil, Ethiopia, India, Sudan, and South Sudan) account for greater than 90% of cases.

A possible sequela of subclinical and untreated VL is post–kala-azar dermal leishmaniasis, which appears as diffuse hypopigmented macules, malar rash, papules, nodules, and plaques in all parts of the body. It is regarded as an active source of kala-azar infection and is almost exclusively found in East Africa and India, where *L donovani* is the etiologic agent.[2,14,35]

SYSTEMIC ASSOCIATIONS

Aside from lymphadenopathy, systemic manifestations are generally only found with VL, as discussed previously. Fevers are not commonly reported.

HISTOPATHOLOGY

The histopathologic finding of CL depends in large part on the stage of development of the lesion. Acute lesions have a dense dermal infiltrate of parasitized histiocytes, lymphocytes, plasma cells, and variable numbers of neutrophils. With

increased lesion chronicity, small tuberculoid granulomas begin to replace the reducing number of parasitized histiocytes and decreased lymphoplasmactytic infiltrate. The overlying epidermis may show ulceration, neutrophil microabscesses, acanthosis, or atrophy, also depending on the lesion stage and biopsy site. Mucosal lesions may show nonspecific chronic inflammation and only a few parasitized histiocytes. Pseudoepitheliomatous hyperplasia may be prominent, particularly at the periphery of some lesions. With cutaneous involvement of visceral leishmaniasis (post–kala-azar dermal leishmaniasis), the epidermis is atrophic and nonulcerated, and follicular plugging is frequently present in lesions on the face. This form of dermal leishmaniasis demonstrates a nodular to diffuse dermal lymphohistiocytic infiltrate with variable numbers of organisms present.

The histopathologic features also depend greatly on the host response and degree of cellular immunity. Similar to the leprosy, large numbers of organisms and a primarily histiocytic infiltrate indicates an anergic response (DCL), whereas small numbers of organisms are associated with necrosis and a granulomatous response (self-healing CL). The recidivans or lupoid form of chronic CL represents an exaggerated tuberculoid response to very few organisms, and resembles lupus vulgaris with tubercles surrounded by lymphocytes but no necrosis and only sparse plasma cells. When leishmania organisms are sparse, the granulomatous infiltrate may be histologically misdiagnosed as sarcoidosis, foreign body granuloma, granuloma annulare, or granulomatous rosacea.

In all variants of leishmaniasis, the amastigote form of the organism multiples within the histiocytes of the human host. Amastigotes are round-to-ovoid structures and measure approximately 2 to 4 μm in impression smears or touch preparations, but may be only 1 to 3 μm in histologic sections because of shrinkage during tissue processing. Although the morphologic features may be better appreciated with a Giemsa stain, the organisms appear as basophilic dotlike structures within the vacuolated cytoplasm of histiocytes in hematoxylin-eosin–stained sections and tend to localize to the periphery of the parasitized histiocytes, the so-called marquee sign. *Leishmania* amastigotes have a prominent nucleus and an eccentric rod-shaped kinetoplast. They are termed Leishman-Donovan bodies and must be differentiated from other organisms that are parasitized by histiocytes, including histoplasmosis, granuloma inguinale, and rhinoscleroma. In particular, histoplasma organisms are of similar size, but the cytoplasm of the cell is retracted from the thick poorly staining cell wall to produce a halolike appearance. Additionally unlike leishmania amastigotes, histoplasmosis does not have a kinetoplast and stains positively with fungal stains, such as Gomori methenamine silver and periodic acid–Schiff.

Leishmania promastigotes are not seen in the human host, but may be found in the sandfly vector or in culture media. The promastigote form is more elongated, measuring 10 to 15 μm long. Promastigotes have a prominent central nucleus with an anterior kinetoplast and a single long flagellum that emerges from the anterior end of the organism (Figs. 8–11).

EVALUATION AND MANAGEMENT

There are several diagnostic modalities currently in use, and selection of the proper method is based on convenience and availability. In the United States, the Centers for Disease Control and

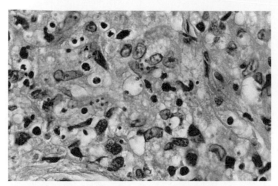

Fig. 9. Histopathology of biopsy specimen showing leishmania amastigotes within the cytoplasm of histiocytes. Note the associated plasma cell infiltrate and that the identifying feature of the kinetoplast is visible in some of the organisms (hematoxylin-eosin, original magnification ×1000). (*Courtesy of* J. Keeling, MD, Jacksonville, FL; with permission.)

Prevention can offer assistance with diagnosis and treatment (**Table 2**).

Direct observation of the intracellular parasites can be accomplished by Giemsa-stained tissue smear, biopsy, or scraping of a new ulcer at its active edge. This should be the first step because results are available in minutes; however, sensitivity is highly variable (19%–77%) and requires experience for optimal diagnosis.[36,37] Skin biopsy with tissue culture in biphasic media (eg, Novy-Macneal-Nicole or chick embryo media) is another direct method and is positive in about 40% of patients. The sensitivity of these methods decreases as lesions age and number of parasites decreases.[3,17,38]

Polymerase chain reaction has quickly emerged as the diagnostic method of choice because it rapidly provides the most reliable speciation,

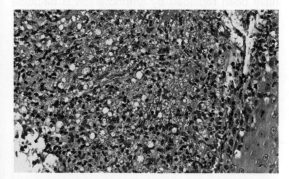

Fig. 8. Histopathology of biopsy specimen showing numerous intrahistiocytic leishmania organisms. Note that the amastigotes tend to distribute around the periphery of the cytoplasm, the so-called marquee sign (hematoxylin-eosin, original magnification ×400). (*By permission* of the Mayo Foundation for Medical Education and Research. All rights reserved.)

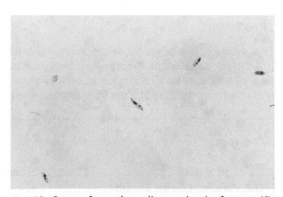

Fig. 10. Smear from the salivary gland of a sandfly showing the promastigote form of leishmania. (*Courtesy of* J. Keeling, MD, Jacksonville, FL; with permission.)

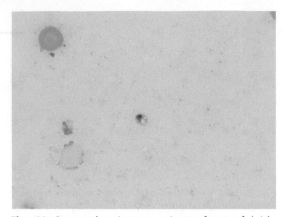

Fig. 11. Smear showing amastigote form of leishmania with a prominent kinetoplast. (*Courtesy of CDC.*)

with sensitivity around 97% to 100%.[6,39] An adequate sample can be obtained from a biopsy or a needle aspirate.

Immunoassays, such as enzyme-linked immunosorbent assay, Western blot, and flow cytometry, can be used to detect the presence of antileishmania antibodies but are often negative in cutaneous forms of the disease. Also, because of their cross-reactivity with Chagas disease, they are not very specific.[17,38]

The Montenegro (leshmanin) skin test is a delayed hypersensitivity-type reaction produced by injecting phenol-killed promastigotes into the dermis. An induration greater than 5 mm after 48 to 72 hours indicates exposure to *Leishmania* but is not diagnostic of active disease. It is negative early in infection process (<3 months), but turns positive in almost all patients with leishmaniasis and remains positive for life. Sensitivity ranges from less than 50% to 85%.[40,41] It is not approved by the Food and Drug Administration and not routinely available in many nonendemic countries.[6,7]

TREATMENT

The available therapies for leishmaniasis are far from ideal because of their toxicity, high costs, lack of efficacy, lack of access in certain areas, and emerging drug resistance. Furthermore, there

is a paucity of data from well-designed, well-reported trials regarding effective treatments.[42,43] It is important to note that reported schedules of treatment are variable in different studies and centers. Systemic therapy is recommended for all NW species to prevent progression to ML (except *L mexicana*, where the risk of progression is nearly zero).[19,44] Otherwise, goals of treating CL are to expedite healing, reduce recurrence, and minimize disfiguring scars. Treatment of purely CL may be accomplished with topical or local therapy only, and no one local modality has been proven to be superior. Prompt treatment is recommended in any immunocompromised patient; those with more than three lesions; lesions greater than 2.5 cm; and lesions on the joints, face, hands, or feet.[45]

Four drugs obtainable in the United States are believed to be active against all forms of leishmaniasis in children and adults and can be obtained through the Centers for Disease Control and Prevention (404-718-4745) with institutional review board approval: (1) intravenous (IV) sodium stibogluconate, (2) IV amphotericin B deoxycholate, (3) IV liposomal amphotericin B, and (4) oral miltefosine.[46] When the infecting species is identified, the clinician should choose the most appropriate treatment based on likelihood to progress to ML. If no species is identified, patients should undergo complete treatment with one of the previously mentioned agents. Improvement is usually observed within 6 to 12 weeks, but the patient should be followed for 1 year to observe a full response because of propensity of the lesions to recur.[47]

Pentavalent antimonials (IV sodium stibogluconate and intramuscular [IM] meglumine antimoniate) remain the standard first-line treatment. The exceptions to this are India, where antimonials have been replaced by amphotericin B because of resistance,[48] and French Guiana, where greater than 90% of CL is caused by *L guyanensis* and the treatment of choice is pentamidine.[49] The currently recommended regimen for both drugs is 20 mg/kg/d IV or IM for 3 to 4 weeks with cure rates upward of 90%.[45,50,51] Common adverse effects reported with antimonials include gastrointestinal symptoms, fatigue, musculoskeletal pain,

Table 2
CDC contact information for US physicians

CDC Branch	Contact	Services
CDC Parasitic Disease Division www.cdc.gov/parasites/contactus.html	404-718-4745	Assistance with diagnosis and treatment options obtainable
CDC Laboratories	770-488-4475	Request media for culture, PCR

Abbreviations: CDC, Centers for Disease Control and Prevention; PCR, polymerase chain reaction.

transaminitis, elevated lipase, leukopenia, thrombocytopenia, reversible T-wave changes on electrocardiogram (ECG), and cardiotoxicity.[51–54] Therefore, an ECG, complete blood count, complete metabolic panel, and pancreatic enzymes should be checked before starting therapy and biweekly during therapy. Intralesional therapy with these drugs can be an option in species that typically only result in CL. Injection site pain is usually the only adverse event. Pregnancy category is unknown.

Conventional amphotericin B deoxycholate is considered second-line therapy in cases that do not respond to antimonials, and it is the only drug that has not induced resistance despite its use for nearly 60 years.[17] It is typically recommended as a slow infusion of 0.5 to 1.0 mg/kg. It has been demonstrated to be very effective against VL (>90% cure rate) when the previously mentioned suggested dosing is used for 15 days.[55] However, it is difficult to tolerate, and common adverse events include fever and rigors with infusion, nephrotoxicity, hypokalemia, and anemia. Biweekly complete blood count and complete metabolic panel should be checked in patients undergoing therapy. This drug is pregnancy category B.

Liposomal amphotericin B is now first-line treatment of VL in most industrialized countries because of its shorter regimen, decreased toxicity, and greater than 95% cure rate. Dosing regimens are varied, but literature suggests that cumulative dose of 10–15 mg/kg over 3–5 days is effective in achieving >90% cure rate.[56] It is very expensive ($5000–$6000 for 70-kg person), and therefore inaccessible in parts of the world with the greatest disease burden.[47] There are limited data on liposomal amphotericin B use with CL. However, despite the cost and paucity of data, liposomal amphotericin B is being increasingly used as first-line treatment of CL and ML in nonendemic counties.[57]

Pentamidine is another alternative treatment for those intolerant of or unresponsive to antimonials. It has been successfully used to treat L guyanensis, where it is first-line treatment, and L braziliensis, with a reported cure rate ranging from 35% to 90%.[49,50,58,59] The suggested dosing regimen is 2–4 mg/kg IM injections every other day for a total of 2–7 doses, depending on study. Hyperglycemia persisting after long-term administration, elevated creatine kinase, cardiotoxicity (ECG changes, tachycardia), hypotension, nephrotoxicity, and hepatotoxicity are the reported adverse events in the aforementioned studies. Evaluation of these systems with appropriate laboratory studies before initiation of therapy and before each administration is recommended. This drug is pregnancy category C.

Miltefosine, a chemotherapy agent, is the only oral treatment with demonstrated in vivo efficacy against CL, ML, and VL, and is well-liked because of its more convenient oral dosing of 2.5 mg/kg/d for 4 weeks. It has previously been demonstrated to be very effective against VL and has a 95% cure rate[60] and a 60% to 80% cure rate with ML.[61] In CL, it seems to be efficacious against L panamensis with a 91% cure rate, but it is significantly less effective for the treatment of L mexicana (53%) and L braziliensis (21%).[62] Common adverse events include nausea, vomiting, motion sickness, headache, diarrhea, and creatinine elevation. It is contraindicated in pregnant or breastfeeding women, and contraception should be used in women of child-bearing potential. This drug is pregnancy category D.

Paromomycin is an old aminoglycoside agent most currently marketed for oral treatment of enteric parasites and for topical treatment of leishmaniasis. For the latter indication, it is typically used in a topical formulation of 15% paromomycin/12% methylbenzethonium in white soft paraffin applied twice daily for 3 to 6 weeks. Cure rates vary considerably from 17% to 86%.[63–65] Adverse events are usually limited to local irritation and pruritus, but do not usually lead to discontinuation of treatment. As such this may be a good option to certain strains because of its ease of administration, few adverse events, and low cost. Pregnancy category is unknown.

Ketoconazole has successfully treated select strains of leishmania according to small studies done in the 1980 and 1990s; however, more recent studies show inconsistent results, and its use has been questioned. More recently a fluconazole regimen of 200 mg daily (or 2.5–5 mg/kg/d) for 6 weeks has been used and well tolerated. Cure rates range from 44% to 88%.[66–69] Other newer-generation oral triazoles, such as fluconazole, itraconazole, and posaconazole, may also be considered because of the lower risk of hepatotoxicity than with ketoconazole.[70,71] This drug is pregnancy category C.

Azithromycin has been shown to have limited antileishmanial effects and is typically only recommended for patients with contraindications to more traditional therapies or for patients who have failed them. It is used in a dosing regimen of 500 mg daily for 5 to 10 days, often with repeat monthly cycles. Reported response and cure rates in CL are about 25% and 10%, respectively.[72,73] One study of three elderly patients with MCL demonstrated healing in all three patients.[74] It is well tolerated; the most common adverse events are found in the gastrointestinal system. This drug is pregnancy category B.

Table 3
Old World leishmaniasis treatment and outcomes

Study Group	Level of Evidence	Study Type	Species/Clinical	Treatment Regimen	Follow-up	Outcomes (Complete Cure)
Alrajhi (2002)	A	Randomized, double-blind clinical trial	L major/CL	A. Fluconazole, 200 mg, 6 wk B. Placebo, 6 wk	3 mo	A. 63/106 B. 22/103
Asilian (2003)	A	Randomized, double-blind clinical trial	L major/CL	A. Paromomycin, 4 wk B. Paromomycin, 2 wk (plus 2 wk placebo)	105 days	A. 62/117 B. 46/116
Asilian (2006)	A	Randomized clinical trial	L major/CL	A. Photodynamic therapy weekly, 4 wk B. Paromomycin (15% + 12% MBCL), BID 28 d C. Placebo ointment, BID 28 d	2 mo	A. 29/31 B. 14/34 C. 4/30
Firooz (2006)	A	Randomized, assessor-blind clinical trial	L tropica/CL	A. Imiquimod 5%, 3 times/wk, 28 d plus meglumine antimoniate, IM 20 mg/kg/d, 14 d B. Placebo cream 28 d plus meglumine antimoniate, 20 mg/kg/d, 14 d	20 weeks	A. 30/59 B. 32/60
Mohebali (2007)	A	Randomized, open-label clinical trial	L major/CL	A. Miltefosine, 2.5 mg/kg/d, 28 d B. Meglumine antimoniate, IM 20 mg/kg/d, 14 d	3 mo	A. 26/32 B. 25/31
Mosleh (2008)	B	Unrandomized cohort	L major/CL	Liquid nitrogen applied at 2 cm range for 10–15 sec × 2 cycles, q 1 wk, 1–7 treatments	Up to 3 y	Lesions <1 cm: 94% cure Lesions 1–2 cm: 78% cure Lesions >2 cm: 53% cure
Reithinger (2005)	A	Randomized controlled trial	L tropica/CL	A. Thermotherapy 50°C, 30 sec B. Sodium stibogluconate, IM 20 mg/kg/d, 21 d C. Sodium stibogluconate, IL 2–5 mL every 5–7 d, 5 injections	100 days	A. 75/139 B. 26/144 C. 70/148
Sadeghian (2006)	A	Randomized, double-blind clinical trial	L major/CL	A. Pentoxifylline, 400 mg TID plus meglumine antimoniate 20 mg/kg/d, 20 d B. Placebo TID plus meglumine antimoniate, 20 mg/kg/d, 20 d	3 mo	A. 26/32 B. 16/32

A, high-quality randomized controlled trial (RCT) or prospective study; B, lesser-quality RCT or prospective study.

Abbreviations: IL, intralesional; MBCL, methylbenzethonium chloride.

Data from Refs.[66,81–86,89]

Table 4
New World leishmaniasis treatment and outcomes

Study Group	Level of Evidence	Study Type	Species/Clinical	Treatment Regimen	Follow-up	Outcomes: Complete Cure (n/N)
Andersen (2005)	A	Double-blind clinical trial	L braziliensis/CL	A. Pentamidine, 2 mg/kg QOD, 7 injections B. IV meglumine antimoniate, 20 mg/kg/d, 20 d	6 mo	A. 14/40 B. 31/40
Martinez (1997)	A	Randomized controlled trial	L braziliensis/CL	A. Allopurinol, (20 mg/kg/d divided over 4 doses), 15 d, plus IV stibogluconate, 20 mg/kg/d, 15 d B. IV stibogluconate, 20 mg/kg/d, 15 d	1 y	A. 36/51 B. 19/49
Miranda-Verastegui (2005)	A	Randomized, double-blind clinical trial	L braziliensis, L peruviana CL with clinical resistance to antimony	A. Meglumine antimoniate, IV or IM 20 mg/kg/d plus imiquimod 5% cream "QOD", 20 d B. Meglumine antimoniate, 20 mg/kg/d plus vehicle, "QOD" 20 d	1 y	A. 13/20 (faster healing, less scarring) B. 15/20
Oliveira-Neto (1997)	A	Prospective cohort	L braziliensis/CL	Meglumine antimoniate, IL 425 mg in 5 mL (amount injected depends on lesion size)	Up to 10 y	59/74 patients
Saenz (1990)	A	Randomized controlled trial	L panamensis, L mexicana, L braziliensis/CL	A. Ketoconazole, 600 mg/d, 28 d B. Sodium stibogluconate, IM 20 mg/kg/d, 20 d C. Placebo, 28 d	3 mo	A. 16/21 B. 13/19 C. 0/11
Soto (2004)	A	Randomized, double-blind clinical trial	L panamensis/CL	A. Generic sodium stibogluconate, IM 20 mg/kg/d, 20 d B. Branded SSG (Pentostam, Glucantime) 20 mg/kg/d, 20 d	6 mo	A. 40/48 B. 50/56
Soto (2004)	A	Randomized, double-blind clinical trial	Colombia (L panamensis), Guatemala (L braziliensis, L mexicana) CL	A. Miltefosine, PO 2.5 mg/kg/d, 28 d B. Placebo, 28 d	6 mo	A. Colombia 40/49, Guatemala 20/40 B. Columbia 9/24, Guatemala 4/20
Soto (2007)	B	Unrandomized cohort	Bolivia ML	A. Miltefosine, PO 2.5 mg/kg/d, 28 d B. Amphotericin B, 1 mg/kg qOD, 45 d	12 mo	A. 51/72 B. 7/19
Velez (1997)	A	Randomized controlled trial	84% L panamensis, 16% L braziliensis, CL	A. Allopurinol, 300 mg QID, 28 d B. Placebo pills, QID, 28 d C. IM meglumine antimoniate, 20 mg/kg/d, 20 d	3 mo, 1 y	A. 18/55 B. 17/46 C. 52/56

A, high-quality randomized controlled trial (RCT) or prospective study; B, lesser-quality RCT or prospective study.
Abbreviation: SSG, sodium stibogluconate.
Data from Refs.[50,61,62,76,78,80,87,88,90]

Imiquimod seems to stimulate antileishmanial activity inside macrophages, and when used in combination with pentavalent antimonials, it may augment the treatment response.[75] The 5% to 7.5% ointment is used topically every other day for 20 days in conjunction with IV antimonials, and treatment responses range from 72% to 100%.[76,77] Some studies demonstrate a better response when the drugs are used in combination compared with antimonials alone, whereas others demonstrate only a faster healing time and better cosmetic results.[75–77] Other immunomodulators also have been tried (pentoxifylline, granulocyte-macrophage colony–stimulating factor, cyclosporine, monoclonal antibodies), but further studies are needed on all of these to optimize recommendations. This drug is pregnancy category C.

Allopurinol has been demonstrated as a useful adjunct to pentavalent antimonials but its mechanism of action remains unclear. When used in a regimen of 20 mg/kg given over 4 doses for 15 days with antimonials, cure rates range from 71% to 74%.[78,79] However, it is ineffective on its own.[80] This drug is pregnancy category C.

Local and physical therapy may be useful when there is no risk for more advanced disease. Local methods include paromomycin ointment, imiquimod ointment, and intralesional pentavalent antimonials. Physical methods include cryotherapy, heat, surgical excision, laser, and tattooing. Overall there is a paucity of data using these methods, and only centers with experience tend to implement them. With all of these methods caution should be exercised to avoid scarring, especially if lesions are large or on delicate areas, such as the face.

PREVENTION

There are currently no effective vaccines available for any form of leishmaniasis. Travelers need to be advised that the best way to prevent infection is to protect themselves from sandfly bites. Travelers should wear protective clothing; minimize exposed skin and outdoor activity in the dusk to dawn hours; use DEET on the skin and clothing; remain in air-conditioned and ventilated areas (sandflies cannot fly against wind resistance); and use permethrin-treated bed nets, curtains, and clothing. In endemic countries, efforts may be focused on eliminating the reservoirs and the vector.[2,3]

CLINICAL RESULTS

Clinical results can be found in **Tables 3** and **4**.

SUMMARY

Leishmaniasis is an important cutaneous disease affecting an estimated 12 million people worldwide. As travel to endemic areas increases, dermatologists need to keep this entity in the differential for any chronic skin lesion in persons who may have had a possible exposure for any duration. It can be difficult to diagnose because manifestations are varied and sometimes subclinical. Treatment options are diverse but far from ideal because of toxicity, lack of access, low care rates, and emerging resistance. We recommend that physicians practicing in the United States consult the CDC for current treatment guidelines. Further basic and clinical research is needed to better elucidate the complex host-species relationship resulting in different clinical manifestations and for development of more effective therapies.

REFERENCES

1. den Boer M, Argaw D, Jannin J, et al. Leishmaniasis impact and treatment access. Clin Microbiol Infect 2011;17(10):1471–7.
2. Leishmaniasis. 2014. Available at: http://www.who.int/topics/leishmaniasis/en/. Accessed April 02, 2014.
3. Parasites. Leishmaniasis. 2013. Available at: http://www.cdc.gov/parasites/leishmaniasis/index.html. Accessed April 02, 2014.
4. Sutherst RW. Global change and human vulnerability to vector-borne diseases. Clin Microbiol Rev 2004;17(1):136–73.
5. Pavli A, Maltezou HC. Leishmaniasis, an emerging infection in travelers. Int J Infect Dis 2010;14(12): e1032–9.
6. Lawn SD, Whetham J, Chiodini PL, et al. New World mucosal and cutaneous leishmaniasis: an emerging health problem among British travellers. QJM 2004; 97(12):781–8.
7. El Hajj L, Thellier M, Carrière J, et al. Localized cutaneous leishmaniasis imported into Paris: a review of 39 cases. Int J Dermatol 2004;43(2):120–5.
8. Malik AN, John L, Bruceson AD, et al. Changing pattern of visceral leishmaniasis, United Kingdom, 1985-2004. Emerg Infect Dis 2006;12(8):1257–9.
9. Wright NA, Davis LE, Aftergut KS, et al. Cutaneous leishmaniasis in Texas: a northern spread of endemic areas. J Am Acad Dermatol 2008;58(4):650–2.
10. Melby PC, Kreutzer RD, McMahon-Pratt D, et al. Cutaneous leishmaniasis: review of 59 cases seen at the National Institutes of Health. Clin Infect Dis 1992;15(6):924–37.
11. Weitzel T, Mühlberger N, Jelinek T, et al. Imported leishmaniasis in Germany 2001-2004: data of the

SIMPID surveillance network. Eur J Clin Microbiol Infect Dis 2005;24(7):471–6.

12. Cardo LJ. Leishmania: risk to the blood supply. Transfusion 2006;46(9):1641–5.

13. Figueiro-Filho EA, Duarte G, El-Beitune P, et al. Visceral leishmaniasis (kala-azar) and pregnancy. Infect Dis Obstet Gynecol 2004;12(1):31–40.

14. Akilov OE, Khachemoune A, Hasan T. Clinical manifestations and classification of Old World cutaneous leishmaniasis. Int J Dermatol 2007;46(2):132–42.

15. Banuls AL, Hide M, Prugnolle F. Leishmania and the leishmaniases: a parasite genetic update and advances in taxonomy, epidemiology and pathogenicity in humans. Adv Parasitol 2007;64:1–109.

16. Kaye P, Scott P. Leishmaniasis: complexity at the host-pathogen interface. Nat Rev Microbiol 2011; 9(8):604–15.

17. Lupi O, Bartlett BL, Haugen RN, et al. Tropical dermatology: tropical diseases caused by protozoa. J Am Acad Dermatol 2009;60(6):897–925 [quiz: 926–8].

18. Schwartz E, Hatz C, Blum J. New world cutaneous leishmaniasis in travellers. Lancet Infect Dis 2006; 6(6):342–9.

19. Blum J, Desjeux P, Schwartz E, et al. Treatment of cutaneous leishmaniasis among travellers. J Antimicrob Chemother 2004;53(2):158–66.

20. Soong L, Henard CA, Melby PC. Immunopathogenesis of non-healing American cutaneous leishmaniasis and progressive visceral leishmaniasis. Semin Immunopathol 2012;34(6):735–51.

21. Nylen S, Eidsmo L. Tissue damage and immunity in cutaneous leishmaniasis. Parasite Immunol 2012; 34(12):551–61.

22. Awasthi A, Mathur RK, Saha B. Immune response to Leishmania infection. Indian J Med Res 2004;119(6): 238–58.

23. Iftikhar N, Bari I, Ejaz A. Rare variants of cutaneous leishmaniasis: whitlow, paronychia, and sporotrichoid. Int J Dermatol 2003;42(10):807–9.

24. Salmanpour R, Handjani F, Zerehsaz F, et al. Erysipeloid leishmaniasis: an unusual clinical presentation. Eur J Dermatol 1999;9(6):458–9.

25. Rubio FA, Robayna G, Herranz P, et al. Leishmaniasis presenting as a psoriasiform eruption in AIDS. Br J Dermatol 1997;136(5):792–4.

26. Bogdan C. Leishmaniasis in rheumatology, haematology and oncology: epidemiological, immunological and clinical aspects and caveats. Ann Rheum Dis 2012;71(Suppl 2):i60–6.

27. Alvar J, Aparicio P, Aseffa A, et al. The relationship between leishmaniasis and AIDS: the second 10 years. Clin Microbiol Rev 2008;21(2):334–59. table of contents.

28. Xynos ID, Tektonidou MG, Pikazis D, et al. Leishmaniasis, autoimmune rheumatic disease, and anti-tumor necrosis factor therapy, Europe. Emerg Infect Dis 2009;15(6):956–9.

29. Antinori S, Cascio A, Parravicini C, et al. Leishmaniasis among organ transplant recipients. Lancet Infect Dis 2008;8(3):191–9.

30. Jirmanus L, Glesby MJ, Guimarães LH, et al. Epidemiological and clinical changes in American tegumentary leishmaniasis in an area of Leishmania (Viannia) braziliensis transmission over a 20-year period. Am J Trop Med Hyg 2012;86(3):426–33.

31. Perez-Ayala A, Norman F, Pérez-Molina JA, et al. Imported leishmaniasis: a heterogeneous group of diseases. J Travel Med 2009;16(6):395–401.

32. Machado-Coelho GL, Caiaffa WT, Genaro O, et al. Risk factors for mucosal manifestation of American cutaneous leishmaniasis. Trans R Soc Trop Med Hyg 2005;99(1):55–61.

33. Petzl-Erler ML, Belich MP, Queiroz-Telles F. Association of mucosal leishmaniasis with HLA. Hum Immunol 1991;32(4):254–60.

34. Maltezou HC, Siafas C, Mavrikou M, et al. Visceral leishmaniasis during childhood in southern Greece. Clin Infect Dis 2000;31(5):1139–43.

35. Berman JD. Human leishmaniasis: clinical, diagnostic, and chemotherapeutic developments in the last 10 years. Clin Infect Dis 1997;24(4):684–703.

36. Seaton RA, Morrison J, Man I, et al. Out-patient parenteral antimicrobial therapy: a viable option for the management of cutaneous leishmaniasis. QJM 1999;92(11):659–67.

37. Weigle KA, de Dávalos M, Heredia P, et al. Diagnosis of cutaneous and mucocutaneous leishmaniasis in Colombia: a comparison of seven methods. Am J Trop Med Hyg 1987;36(3):489–96.

38. Bolognia J, Jorizzo J, Schaffer J. Protozoa and worms: leishmaniasis. In: Nelson S, Warschaw K, editors. Dermatology. Philadelphia, PA: Elsevier; 2012. p. 1391–7.

39. Oliveira JG, Novais FO, de Oliveira CI, et al. Polymerase chain reaction (PCR) is highly sensitive for diagnosis of mucosal leishmaniasis. Acta Trop 2005;94(1):55–9.

40. Convit J, Ulrich M, Fernández CT, et al. The clinical and immunological spectrum of American cutaneous leishmaniasis. Trans R Soc Trop Med Hyg 1993;87(4):444–8.

41. Arana BA, Roca M, Rizzo NR, et al. Evaluation of a standardized leishmanin skin test in Guatemala. Trans R Soc Trop Med Hyg 1999;93(4):394–6.

42. Gonzalez U, Pinart M, Rengifo-Pardo M, et al. Interventions for American cutaneous and mucocutaneous leishmaniasis. Cochrane Database Syst Rev 2009;(2):CD004834.

43. Gonzalez U, Pinart M, Reveiz L, et al. Interventions for Old World cutaneous leishmaniasis. Cochrane Database Syst Rev 2008;(4):CD005067.

44. Andrade-Narvaez FJ, Vargas-González A, Canto-Lara SB, et al. Clinical picture of cutaneous leishmaniases due to Leishmania (Leishmania) mexicana

in the Yucatan peninsula, Mexico. Mem Inst Oswaldo Cruz 2001;96(2):163–7.

45. Hepburn NC. Cutaneous leishmaniasis: an overview. J Postgrad Med 2003;49(1):50–4.

46. Murray HW, Berman JD, Davies CR, et al. Advances in leishmaniasis. Lancet 2005;366(9496):1561–77.

47. Murray HW. Leishmaniasis in the United States: treatment in 2012. Am J Trop Med Hyg 2012;86(3):434–40.

48. Maltezou HC. Visceral leishmaniasis: advances in treatment. Recent Pat Antiinfect Drug Discov 2008;3(3):192–8.

49. Nacher M, Carme B, Sainte Marie D, et al. Influence of clinical presentation on the efficacy of a short course of pentamidine in the treatment of cutaneous leishmaniasis in French Guiana. Ann Trop Med Parasitol 2001;95(4):331–6.

50. Andersen EM, Cruz-Saldarriaga M, Llanos-Cuentas A, et al. Comparison of meglumine antimoniate and pentamidine for Peruvian cutaneous leishmaniasis. Am J Trop Med Hyg 2005;72(2):133–7.

51. Herwaldt BL, Berman JD. Recommendations for treating leishmaniasis with sodium stibogluconate (Pentostam) and review of pertinent clinical studies. Am J Trop Med Hyg 1992;46(3):296–306.

52. Aronson NE, Wortmann GW, Johnson SC, et al. Safety and efficacy of intravenous sodium stibogluconate in the treatment of leishmaniasis: recent U.S. military experience. Clin Infect Dis 1998;27(6):1457–64.

53. Davidson RN. Practical guide for the treatment of leishmaniasis. Drugs 1998;56(6):1009–18.

54. Antezana G, Zeballos R, Mendoza C, et al. Electrocardiographic alterations during treatment of mucocutaneous leishmaniasis with meglumine antimoniate and allopurinol. Trans R Soc Trop Med Hyg 1992;86(1):31–3.

55. Sundar S, Chakravarty J, Rai VK, et al. Amphotericin B treatment for Indian visceral leishmaniasis: response to 15 daily versus alternate-day infusions. Clin Infect Dis 2007;45(5):556–61.

56. Olliaro PL, Guerin PJ, Gerstl S, et al. Treatment options for visceral leishmaniasis: a systematic review of clinical studies done in India, 1980-2004. Lancet Infect Dis 2005;5(12):763–74.

57. Harms G, Schonian G, Feldmeier H. Leishmaniasis in Germany. Emerg Infect Dis 2003;9(7):872–5.

58. de Paula CD, Sampaio JH, Cardoso DR, et al. A comparative study between the efficacy of pentamidine isothionate given in three doses for one week and N-methil-glucamine in a dose of 20 mg SbV/day for 20 days to treat cutaneous leishmaniasis. Rev Soc Bras Med Trop 2003;36(3):365–71 [in Portuguese].

59. Soto-Mancipe J, Grogl M, Berman JD. Evaluation of pentamidine for the treatment of cutaneous leishmaniasis in Colombia. Clin Infect Dis 1993;16(3):417–25.

60. Jha TK, Sundar S, Thakur CP, et al. Miltefosine, an oral agent, for the treatment of Indian visceral leishmaniasis. N Engl J Med 1999;341(24):1795–800.

61. Soto J, Toledo J, Valda L, et al. Treatment of Bolivian mucosal leishmaniasis with miltefosine. Clin Infect Dis 2007;44(3):350–6.

62. Soto J, Arana BA, Toledo J, et al. Miltefosine for new world cutaneous leishmaniasis. Clin Infect Dis 2004;38(9):1266–72.

63. Faghihi G, Tavakoli-kia R. Treatment of cutaneous leishmaniasis with either topical paromomycin or intralesional meglumine antimoniate. Clin Exp Dermatol 2003;28(1):13–6.

64. Arana BA, Mendoza CE, Rizzo NR, et al. Randomized, controlled, double-blind trial of topical treatment of cutaneous leishmaniasis with paromomycin plus methylbenzethonium chloride ointment in Guatemala. Am J Trop Med Hyg 2001;65(5):466–70.

65. Armijos RX, Weigel MM, Calvopiña M, et al. Comparison of the effectiveness of two topical paromomycin treatments versus meglumine antimoniate for New World cutaneous leishmaniasis. Acta Trop 2004;91(2):153–60.

66. Alrajhi AA, Ibrahim EA, De Vol EB, et al. Fluconazole for the treatment of cutaneous leishmaniasis caused by Leishmania major. N Engl J Med 2002;346(12):891–5.

67. Morizot G, Delgiudice P, Caumes E, et al. Healing of Old World cutaneous leishmaniasis in travelers treated with fluconazole: drug effect or spontaneous evolution? Am J Trop Med Hyg 2007;76(1):48–52.

68. Aerts O, Duchateau N, Willemse P, et al. Cutaneous leishmaniasis: treatment with low-dose oral fluconazole with an excellent cosmetic result. Pediatr Dermatol 2014;32(1):154–5.

69. Daly K, De Lima H, Kato H, et al. Intermediate cutaneous leishmaniasis caused by Leishmania (Viannia) braziliensis successfully treated with fluconazole. Clin Exp Dermatol 2014;39(6):708–12.

70. de Macedo-Silva ST, Urbina JA, de Souza W, et al. In vitro activity of the antifungal azoles itraconazole and posaconazole against Leishmania amazonensis. PLoS One 2013;8(12):e83247.

71. Khazaeli P, Sharifi I, Talebian E, et al. Anti-leishmanial effect of itraconazole niosome on in vitro susceptibility of Leishmania tropica. Environ Toxicol Pharmacol 2014;38(1):205–11.

72. Teixeira AC, Paes MG, Guerra Jde O, et al. Low efficacy of azithromycin to treat cutaneous leishmaniasis in Manaus, AM, Brazil. Rev Inst Med Trop Sao Paulo 2007;49(4):235–8.

73. Layegh P, Yazdanpanah MJ, Vosugh EM, et al. Efficacy of azithromycin versus systemic meglumine antimoniate (Glucantime) in the treatment of cutaneous leishmaniasis. Am J Trop Med Hyg 2007;77(1):99–101.

74. Silva-Vergara ML, Silva Lde A, Maneira FR, et al. Azithromycin in the treatment of mucosal leishmaniasis. Rev Inst Med Trop Sao Paulo 2004;46(3):175–7.

75. Buates S, Matlashewski G. Treatment of experimental leishmaniasis with the immunomodulators imiquimod and S-28463: efficacy and mode of action. J Infect Dis 1999;179(6):1485–94.

76. Miranda-Verastegui C, Llanos-Cuentas A, Arévalo I, et al. Randomized, double-blind clinical trial of topical imiquimod 5% with parenteral meglumine antimoniate in the treatment of cutaneous leishmaniasis in Peru. Clin Infect Dis 2005;40(10):1395–403.

77. Arevalo I, Tulliano G, Quispe A, et al. Role of imiquimod and parenteral meglumine antimoniate in the initial treatment of cutaneous leishmaniasis. Clin Infect Dis 2007;44(12):1549–54.

78. Martinez S, Gonzalez M, Vernaza ME. Treatment of cutaneous leishmaniasis with allopurinol and stibogluconate. Clin Infect Dis 1997;24(2):165–9.

79. Martinez S, Marr JJ. Allopurinol in the treatment of American cutaneous leishmaniasis. N Engl J Med 1992;326(11):741–4.

80. Velez I, Agudelo S, Hendrickx E, et al. Inefficacy of allopurinol as monotherapy for Colombian cutaneous leishmaniasis. A randomized, controlled trial. Ann Intern Med 1997;126(3):232–6.

81. Asilian A, Jalayer T, Nilforooshzadeh M, et al. Treatment of cutaneous leishmaniasis with aminosidine (paromomycin) ointment: double-blind, randomized trial in the Islamic Republic of Iran. Bull World Health Organ 2003;81(5):353–9.

82. Asilian A, Davami M. Comparison between the efficacy of photodynamic therapy and topical paromomycin in the treatment of Old World cutaneous leishmaniasis: a placebo-controlled, randomized clinical trial. Clin Exp Dermatol 2006;31(5):634–7.

83. Firooz A, Khamesipour A, Ghoorchi MH, et al. Imiquimod in combination with meglumine antimoniate for cutaneous leishmaniasis: a randomized assessor-blind controlled trial. Arch Dermatol 2006;142(12):1575–9.

84. Mohebali M, Fotouhi A, Hooshmand B, et al. Comparison of miltefosine and meglumine antimoniate for the treatment of zoonotic cutaneous leishmaniasis (ZCL) by a randomized clinical trial in Iran. Acta Trop 2007;103(1):33–40.

85. Reithinger R, Mohsen M, Wahid M, et al. Efficacy of thermotherapy to treat cutaneous leishmaniasis caused by *Leishmania tropica* in Kabul, Afghanistan: a randomized, controlled trial. Clin Infect Dis 2005;40(8):1148–55.

86. Sadeghian G, Nilforoushzadeh MA. Effect of combination therapy with systemic glucantime and pentoxifylline in the treatment of cutaneous leishmaniasis. Int J Dermatol 2006;45(7):819–21.

87. Saenz RE, Paz H, Berman JD. Efficacy of ketoconazole against *Leishmania braziliensis* panamensis cutaneous leishmaniasis. Am J Med 1990;89(2):147–55.

88. Soto J, Valda-Rodriquez L, Toledo J, et al. Comparison of generic to branded pentavalent antimony for treatment of new world cutaneous leishmaniasis. Am J Trop Med Hyg 2004;71(5):577–81.

89. Mosleh IM, Geith E, et al. Efficacy of a weekly cryotherapy regimen to treat Leishmania major cutaneous leishmaniasis. Am J Acad Dermatol 2008;58(4):617–24.

90. Oliveira-Neto MP, Schuback A, et al. Intralesional therapy of American cutaneous leishmaniasis with pentavalent antimony in Rio de Janeiro, Brazil - an area of leishmania (V.) braziliensis transmission. Int J Derm 1997;36:463–8.

Deep Fungal Infections, Blastomycosis-Like Pyoderma, and Granulomatous Sexually Transmitted Infections

CrossMark

Jacqueline A. Guidry, MD[a], Christopher Downing, MD[a,*],
Stephen K. Tyring, MD, PhD[a,b]

KEYWORDS

- Granulomatous disease • Deep mycoses • Fungal infection • Blastomycosis-like pyoderma
- Granuloma inguinale • Donovanosis • Lymphogranuloma venereum

KEY POINTS

- Deep fungal infections have similar skin findings and are therefore differentiated by laboratory testing.
- The mainstay of treatment of these diseases is azoles for mild to moderate disease and amphotericin B for severe disease.
- Blastomycosis-like pyoderma (BLP) is clinically indistinguishable from deep fungal infections and responds best to treatment with the vitamin A analog, acitretin.
- Granuloma inguinale and lymphogranuloma venereum (LGV) are 2 sexually transmitted granulomatous diseases that create ulcerative lesions. Both are treated with doxycycline.

A granuloma is a nonspecific histologic finding that can indicate a wide range of diseases from vasculitis or other autoimmune processes to leukocyte oxidase deficiency, hypersensitivity, chemical exposure, malignancy, or infection.[1] Histologically, granulomas have a nodular appearance with a central area of breakdown that is surrounded by a circular or horseshoe-shaped ring of hallmark multinucleated giant cells.[1,2] Giant cells, also called epithelioid cells, begin as normal macrophages that fuse and transform in the presence of inflammatory and immune cytokines.[1]

The pathogenesis of granuloma formation is mediated by the immune system. Initially, immune cells are drawn to the area because of injury to the tissue through either infection or foreign body reaction.[1,2] The presence of a nondegradable product continuously stimulates the immune system via T_H1 cells, B-cell activity, and circulating immune complexes.[1] Infections can act as stimuli for both arms of granuloma development because the infectious organism is recognized as an antigen and a foreign body simultaneously.[2]

Three specific types of granuloma-forming infections are reviewed in this article, including deep fungal infections, BLP, and granulomatous sexually transmitted infections (STI).

Disclosure statement: the authors have no disclosures.
[a] Center for Clinical Studies, 1401 Binz, Suite 200, Houston, TX 77004, USA; [b] Department of Dermatology, University of Texas Health Science Center, 6655 Travis, Suite 600, Houston, TX 77003, USA
* Corresponding author.
E-mail address: cdowning@ccstexas.com

Dermatol Clin 33 (2015) 595–607
http://dx.doi.org/10.1016/j.det.2015.03.019
0733-8635/15/$ – see front matter © 2015 Elsevier Inc. All rights reserved.

ETIOPATHOGENESIS
Deep Fungal Infections

Blastomycosis, coccidioidomycosis, cryptococcus, histoplasmosis, and sporotrichosis are granulomatous deep fungal infections with cutaneous manifestations. The pathogens are dimorphic fungi that infect both immunocompetent and immunocompromised hosts; however, a patient's immune status (in addition to the volume or intensity of the exposure) often affects the severity of the infection.[3]

All these diseases present as localized or systemic infections.[2] Aside from sporotrichosis, the granulomatous deep fungal infections are most commonly acquired via inhalation into the respiratory tract, although direct inoculation into the skin is also possible.[4] Generally, these fungal infections have no notable preponderance for one age group or gender. **Table 1** compares the infectious organism and common clinical presentations of granulomatous deep fungal infections.

Blastomycosis is caused by *Blastomyces dermatitidis*, shown in **Fig. 1**. The organism is prevalent in North America, most notably in the Ohio and Mississippi river valleys, and certain countries in Africa (Zimbabwe, South Africa).[4] Travel to and habitation in an endemic area are the primary risk factors for acquiring blastomycosis.[5] Although *B dermatitidis* can affect almost every organ, the lung is the most common site of infection (91%), followed by the skin (18%) and bones (4%).[6]

Coccidioidomycosis was the first of the major mycoses to be recognized.[3] The disease is caused by 2 separate species. *Coccidioides immitis* is found specifically in the San Joaquin Valley in California, whereas *Coccidioides posadasii* is found in Texas, Arizona, Mexico, and Central and South America.[3,4] There has been an increase in incidence of disease in the United States in the past 15 years. In 2011, the incidence was 42.6 cases per 100,000 population, which increased from 5.3 cases per 100,000 population in 1998.[7] The 2 organisms are not distinguishable phenotypically and cause disease primarily by inhalation of spores (98% of cases).[3,4]

Coccidioides species are quite ubiquitous in the aforementioned areas, yet clinically relevant infections from the fungi are less common. Infections are reported slightly more often in men than in women, but it is unclear if this is intrinsic to the organism or is based on a higher exposure rate in men because of cultural occupation roles.[4] There is no difference in acquisition of coccidioidomycosis between races; however, disseminated disease is seen with much higher prevalence in Filipino and African American populations.[3] In addition, immunosuppression and pregnancy are both risk factors for developing clinically relevant disease.[3]

Cryptococcal infection is caused by 4 serotypes (A–D) of the fungi *Cryptococcus neoformans*, shown in **Fig. 2**.[8] The serotypes have unique infectious etiologies. Most cryptococcal infections in the United States are caused by serotype A, which is commonly found in pigeon droppings and soil.[8] However, individuals with previous exposure to pigeons or pigeon breeders have not been found to have increased incidence of the disease.[8] Serotypes B and C have an unknown ecological reservoir, yet are the most frequent causes of cryptococcal infection in southern California.[8] This disease does occur more frequently in immunocompromised individuals.[8]

Also known as Darling disease, histoplasmosis is a fungal infection caused by *Histoplasma capsulatum*.[3,4] The infection is common in temperate climates across the globe and, like coccidioidomycosis, is reported slightly more frequently in men than in women.[3,4] The fungus has a high preponderance in soil contaminated with bat or bird droppings, especially chickens, turkeys, and geese.[3,4] Therefore, individuals who have visited caves or who are involved in cleaning or construction work at sites contaminated with *H capsulatum* are at the highest risk of contracting the disease.[3] Infection can occur at the time of exposure or on reactivation, especially in the setting of immunosuppression.[3] Immunocompetent individuals who are exposed to *H capsulatum* are often asymptomatic or have a clinically insignificant infection.[3] Patients with human immunodeficiency virus (HIV) infection are at higher risk of developing histoplasmosis, especially if their CD4 lymphocyte count is below 200.[3] Histoplasmosis is considered an AIDS-defining illness.[3] There is a variant of histoplasmosis, called African histoplasmosis, which is caused by *Histoplasma duboisii* and is primarily found in patients who reside in Africa.[9]

Sporotrichosis is caused by the dimorphic fungus *Sporothrix schenckii*, named after the medical student Benjamin Schenk who discovered the organism in 1898.[3] It is the most common and least severe of all the granulomatous diseases.[10] *Sporothrix schenckii* is highly prevalent in both temperate and tropical climates.[3] Organisms are most often found in the soil or on plants but have been isolated from wood, grain, animals, and insects.[3,10]

Unlike the other granulomatous mycoses, sporotrichosis most often develops after direct inoculation into the skin. Inoculation can occur from thorns, splinters, or any other sharp objects

Table 1
Causes and presentation of granulomatous deep fungal infections

Clinical Condition	Fungal Species	Presentation and Systemic Symptoms
Blastomycosis	*Blastomyces dermatitidis*	Primary pulmonary • Most common • Asymptomatic to acute or chronic pneumonia • Skin findings in 70%–80% of patients • Always treat Primary cutaneous: see Clinical Presentation section Disseminated • 25% osteomyelitis • 10%–20% genitourinary (prostatitis or epididymoorchitis) • 5%–10% CNS (meningitis or cranial abscess)
Coccidioidomycosis	*Coccidioides immitis* *Coccidioides posadasii*	Primary pulmonary • Most common, also called valley fever • Majority asymptomatic or with mild symptoms • Significant pulmonary illness rare but can disseminate • Skin findings in 15% of patients Primary cutaneous: see Clinical Presentation section Disseminated • Bony involvement most common after lungs and skin • CNS involvement rare, but high fatality
Cryptococcus	*Cryptococcus neoformans*	Primary pulmonary • Typically caused by separate species, *Cryptococcus gattii* Primary cutaneous: see Clinical Presentation section Disseminated • CNS most common, as meningitis or meningoencephalitis • Skin most common extraneural site (10%–20%) • Osteomyelitis and genital ulcerations, but rarely
Histoplasmosis	*Histoplasma capsulatum*	Primary pulmonary • Brief malaise to severe respiratory illness • Most cases resolve spontaneously Primary cutaneous: see Clinical Presentation section Disseminated • Chronic, indolent course in immunocompetent • Acute, rapidly fatal in infants and immunosuppressed • Hepatosplenomegaly, pancytopenia from bone marrow involvement, polyarthritis, or CNS
Sporotrichosis	*Sporothrix schenckii*	Lymphocutaneous: see Clinical Presentation section Fixed cutaneous: see Clinical Presentation section Disseminated • Rare, associated with immunosuppression • Due to hematogenous spread from primary skin lesions • Bone and lung involvement most common • High mortality in pulmonary and CNS disease Extracutaneous • Most rare, associated with immunosuppression • Usually due to inhalation and hematogenous spread • Osteoarticular involvement in 80% of cases

Abbreviation: CNS, central nervous system.

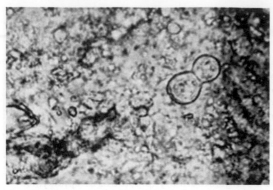

Fig. 1. Microscopic appearance of *B dermatitidis*. (*Courtesy of* Centers for Disease Control and Prevention, Atlanta, GA; with permission.)

that have come into contact with vegetative matter, including a scratch or bite from an infected animal.[3,11] Therefore gardening, farming, and participation in other outdoor activities place individuals at higher risk for developing sporotrichosis.[3] Infection occurs after inhalation, although infrequently, and tends to lead to more serious disease.[10] Immunocompromised individuals typically also experience more severe illness; however, limited infections in healthy, young adults are more common.[10] Early reports suggested that sporotrichosis was more frequent in men, but this seems to be more related to cultural differences in exposure than a true preponderance in the male population.[3,10,12]

Blastomycosis-Like Pyoderma

First named by Brown and Klingman in 1957, BLP is a slow-growing, large vegetative lesion that is clinically indistinguishable from cutaneous blastomycosis or a bromoderma.[13] The cause is likely a combination of immunosuppression and an

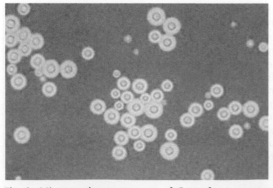

Fig. 2. Microscopic appearance of *C neoformans* species. (*Courtesy of* Centers for Disease Control and Prevention, Atlanta, GA; with permission.)

abnormal reaction of skin tissue to a bacterial infection (**Box 1**).[14] The lesions occur in men and women with no clear gender predominance and can be located on the face, scalp, axilla, trunk, or distal extremities.[15,16] Elderly patients are more commonly affected.[17]

There is no single cause of BLP. Instead, the disease is thought to be an exaggerated tissue reaction to an underlying primary or secondary bacterial infection, most frequently *Staphylococcus aureus*, in patients with some form of immunosuppression.[13,14,17,18] Organisms are isolated from cultures of pus by draining skin lesions or from cultures of tissue by a skin biopsy.[17,19] Immune suppression can be systemic, such as in patients with leukemia or those on chemotherapy or in malnourished individuals, or localized from trauma, sun exposure, or even underlying dermatologic diseases such as eczema.[17,19–22] Rarely, BLP develops at the site of a tattoo, which may cause relative immunosuppression because of increased mercury and iodine levels in that area.[23,24] A list of bacterial pathogens and causes of immunosuppression of BLP are listed in **Box 1**.

Granulomatous Sexually Transmitted Diseases

Granuloma inguinale, also referred to as donovanosis, is an STI that results in chronic, ulcerative lesions located in the genital or perianal region.[25] The infection is caused by the intracellular gram-negative bacillus or coccobacillus *Klebsiella granulomatis* (previously known as *Calymmatobacterium granulomatis*).[25–27] The disease is quite rare in North America and Europe but has a high prevalence in certain geographic hot spots, predominantly in tropical regions.[25,28] Papua New Guinea, South Africa, parts of India and Brazil, Zambia, Vietnam, Japan, and Australia (specifically among the aboriginal populations of Australia) are particularly affected.[25,28]

LGV is an STI caused by specific serovars (L1, L2, or L3) of *Chlamydia trachomatis*.[27] Infections can be seen in any population, although the presentation is frequently different in heterosexual versus homosexual populations as discussed in clinical presentations.[27] LGV is most frequently found in tropical locations and has been commonly reported in Africa, India, Southeast Asia, and the Caribbean.[29] However, outbreaks of serotype L2 of LGV in men who have sex with men (MSM) have occurred in Europe, Australia, and the United States in the twenty-first century.[29] Risk factors for the disease include HIV, other ulcerative infections or STIs, travel abroad, anal intercourse, and meeting sexual partners online.[29]

Box 1
Etiopathogenesis of BLP

Bacteria
  Gram positive
    Staphylococcus aureus (most common)
    Beta-hemolytic streptococci
  Gram negative
    Escherichia coli
    Proteus
    Pseudomonas
  Anaerobes
    Clostridium perfringens
    Prevotella
Immune suppression
  Systemic
    HIV/AIDS
    Long-term prednisone or other immunosuppressive medications
    Malignancies (especially leukemia or lymphoma)
    Poor nutrition status
    Others (alcoholism, obesity, diabetes mellitus, granulomatous disease, congenital immunodeficiency, autoimmune disease)
  Local
    Sun-damaged skin
    Radiation therapy
    Others (mercurial sensitivity from prior tattooing, underlying dermatologic condition)

CLINICAL PRESENTATIONS
Deep Fungal Infections

Cutaneous manifestations of fungal infections are widely variable and for the most part are almost impossible to differentiate based on clinical appearance alone. Each of the 5 deep fungal infections is commonly reported to cause nodular, papular, ulcerative, and verrucous lesions.[4,30] The lesions are slow growing and usually start as small nodules or papules, which progress to larger verrucous or plaquelike lesions that often ulcerate.[3–5,30] Gummas, abscesses, fistulas, pustules, chancres, and lymphadenitis are also frequently described.[3–5,9] Significant scarring in the site of prior or healed lesions is common to all deep mycoses.[4,9]

Sporotrichosis may be the easiest of the granulomatous mycoses to distinguish clinically in its most classic and common form, lymphocutaneous disease, because of the pattern of lesion development (**Fig. 3**).[3,11,12] The initial lesion appears at the site of inoculation, and at or around the time it heals, another lesion develops proximally along the same lymphatic tract.[10] This

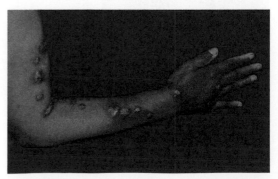

Fig. 3. Clinical appearance of lymphocutaneous form of sporotrichosis. (*Courtesy of* Penvadee Pattanaprichakul, MD, Bangkok, Thailand.)

pattern continues until multiple lesions have developed that track up the extremity, as seen in **Fig. 4**. Not surprisingly, regional lymphadenopathy is also common.[10] Upper extremity lesions are most common in adults; however, facial lesions are frequently seen in children.[10,12] The characteristics of the individual lesions seen in sporotrichosis do not differ significantly from those of the other fungal infections with cutaneous manifestations. As mentioned, the lymphocutaneous form of sporotrichosis is most common and represents 75% to 80% of infections.[3] The second form of cutaneous sporotrichosis is fixed or localized cutaneous disease.[10,12] Infection in this form is limited to 1 or 2 lesions at the site of inoculation.[12]

Cutaneous involvement in blastomycosis, coccidioidomycosis, and histoplasmosis is most frequently because of disseminated disease.[3,4] About 15% of patients with primary pulmonary coccidioidomycosis and 70% to 80% of patients with primary pulmonary blastomycosis have cutaneous manifestations.[9,30,31] Conversely, primary skin involvement is rare in these 3 entities and occurs only after direct inoculation.[4,9] Laboratory workers handling the fungi are most at risk, although primary cutaneous disease can also be acquired from the bite of an infected dog in blastomycosis or in farm workers in coccidioidomycosis.[9] The presentation of the primary cutaneous forms may be more easily confused with sporotrichosis, because they mimic its progression with lesions, which ulcerate, and scar followed by new lesions along the same lymphatic tract.[4,9] Because of the mechanism of entry for sporotrichosis and primary cutaneous forms of blastomycosis, coccidioidomycosis, and histoplasmosis, bilateral disease is rare.[10]

Erythema multiforme (EM) and erythema nodosum (EN) are also seen as skin manifestations in coccidioidomycosis and histoplasmosis.[9] **Fig. 5** shows a case of EN in a patient with coccidioidomycosis. EM and EN are thought to develop because of hypersensitivity to the fungi.[9] In patients with coccidioidomycosis, EM is reported more frequently in children, whereas EN is more often reported in women.[9]

Cryptococcal infections primarily involve the central nervous system (CNS); however, 10% to 15% of patients have cutaneous lesions that develop before their CNS symptoms (**Fig. 6**).[9] Isolated cutaneous cryptococcus has been described but is exceptionally rare and can present as cellulitis.[8] CNS-related cutaneous lesions tend to develop first on the head and neck and can precede the diagnosis by 2 to 8 months.[9] Lesions on the head and neck are also seen in histoplasmosis in HIV-infected patients, in addition to involvement of the trunk, extremities, and mucosal surfaces (oral, anal, or genital).[4,9] Cutaneous involvement of histoplasmosis is more frequent in HIV-infected patients.[4] Both cryptococcus and histoplasmosis may present with typical lesions described above or with more specific molluscum-like papules, which are not seen in the other granulomatous mycoses.[4,8] African histoplasmosis, caused by *H duboisii*, results in similar cutaneous manifestations and osteomyelitis.[9]

Blastomycosis-Like Pyoderma

The lesions of BLP can be singular or multiple and can occur almost anywhere on the body, although

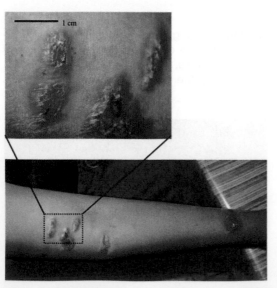

Fig. 4. lymphocutaneous sporotrichosis. (*Courtesy of* Centers for Disease Control and Prevention, Atlanta, GA; with permission.)

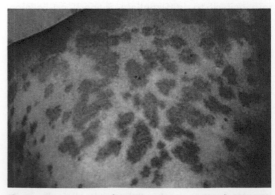

Fig. 5. EN due to infection with coccidioidomycosis. (*Courtesy of* Centers for Disease Control and Prevention, Atlanta, GA; with permission.)

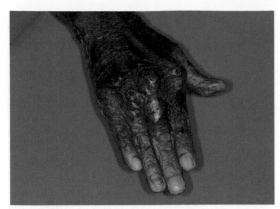

Fig. 6. Cutaneous cryptococcal findings on the hands. (*Courtesy of* Penvadee Pattanaprichakul, MD, Bangkok, Thailand.)

they have been reported most frequently in the extremities.[32] The lesions appear as indolent, gradually expanding vegetative plaques with multiple pustules and often with multiple sinus tracts with purulent drainage.[17,20,33] Skin biopsy of the lesion reveals subcorneal pustules and spongiotic psoriasiform changes with exaggerated invaginations from the epidermis to the dermis and perivascular and interstitial inflammation.[19,33] Perhaps the most specific finding on skin biopsy is the presence of multiple polymorphonuclear leukocytes arranged in microabscesses.[23]

BLP has a cutaneous appearance similar to that of granulomatous fungal infections, especially blastomycosis, although squamous cell carcinoma should also been on the differential and thus a skin biopsy is necessary to rule out this more malignant possibility.[15] BLP can be differentiated from deep fungal infections by negative results of fungal culture.[15] Bromoderma can be ruled out based on history or bromide blood levels.[15]

Granulomatous STDs

Granuloma inguinale most often presents as a papule that progresses slowly to a characteristic beefy-red or velvety ulcerative appearance (described as ulceratogranulomatous); however, hypertrophic, necrotic, and sclerotic variants are also seen.[25,26,28,34] The ulcerogranulomatous form is highly vascular and bleeds easily.[26,27] Lymphadenopathy is uncommon, and lesions are typically painless but may be pruritic.[26–28] The timing of sexual contact preceding the development of lesions is highly variable; incubation periods from 3 days to 12 weeks have been reported.[28,34] Lesions are most commonly on the distal part of penis in men and the introitus for

women but can also be seen in the inguinal folds, as shown in **Fig. 7**.[28]

The initial lesion of LGV is relatively asymptomatic and self-limited, most commonly a small, painless ulceration that frequently resolves before being detected by the patient (**Fig. 8**).[28,34] The initial lesion presents in the urethra, vagina, or rectum between 3 and 30 days after infection.[34] LGV can be complicated by secondary bacterial infection of lymphatic obstruction and possibly elephantiasis if left untreated.[34] Although the primary lesion is painless, LGV is associated with unilateral and tender lymphadenopathy of the femoral or inguinal lymph nodes.[34,35] Often, a patient's painful lymphadenopathy is the first recognized symptom; this is especially true in heterosexual patients.[27] In MSM or women with rectal exposure, proctitis or proctocolitis with or without hemorrhage is frequently the alerting symptom.[27]

SYSTEMIC ASSOCIATIONS
Deep Fungal Infections

For blastomycosis, coccidioidomycosis, cryptococcus, and histoplasmosis, disease occurs under 3 different umbrellas: primary pulmonary, primary cutaneous (discussed in the preceding section), and disseminated. Primary pulmonary disease presents in each as a pneumonia-like illness, which may have associated fatigue, cough, chest pain, or dyspnea, as well as infiltrates or opacities on chest radiography.[31] Disseminated disease is usually because of hematogenous spread of the primary pulmonary infection.[30] Sporotrichosis has 4 different forms: lymphocutaneous, fixed cutaneous, disseminated, and extracutaneous.[10] **Table 1** discusses specific clinical presentations

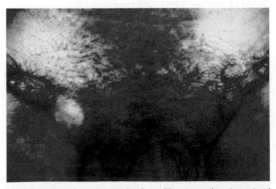

Fig. 7. Granuloma inguinale affecting the inguinal folds in a male patient. Both acute and healed lesions are seen. (*Courtesy of* Centers for Disease Control and Prevention, Atlanta, GA; with permission.)

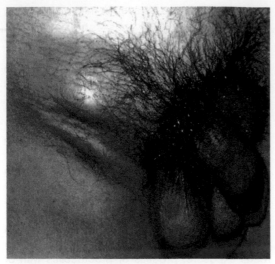

Fig. 8. Bubo lesion in LGV. (*Courtesy of* Angkana Charoenwatanachokchai, MD, Bangkok, Thailand.)

and systemic associations for each of the deep mycoses.

Granulomatous STDs

Extragenital infection in granuloma inguinale is rare, but it can occur. Extension of the infection into the pelvis or hematogenous spread to liver or other intra-abdominal organs, lung, bone, and oral mucosa has been reported.[26–28] Dissemination is more often seen in pregnant patients.[28] Manifestations outside the skin are more common in LGV. Untreated infections quickly spread to involve the gastrointestinal (GI) tract and cause proctocolitis and colorectal fistulas or strictures.[27] Symptoms of secondary spread from the skin may be the initial complaint of the patient, because the manifestations can cause tenesmus, constipation, and rectal bleeding or pain.[34]

EVALUATION AND MANAGEMENT
Deep Fungal Infections

Culture on Sabouraud agar is the gold standard diagnosis for each of the deep fungal infections.[3,4,10,30,36] Direct microscopy with staining can also be used to diagnose each of these infections by identifying the causative organism but is less sensitive.[3,30] In sporotrichosis, visualization of fungal organisms is rare; however, sometimes characteristic asteroid bodies can be observed, especially in lymphocutaneous disease.[3,12] Drainage from a wound, pus drained from an abscess, sputum, or bronchial lavage washings can all be used for this technique.[4,30] **Table 2** lists the characteristic microscopic appearance of each fungus.[2,4,11,30,37,38]

Table 2	
Microscopic appearance of the deep mycoses	
Disease	Microscopic Appearance
Blastomycosis	Large yeast with unipolar budding and thick cell walls
Coccidioidomycosis	Thick-walled, nonbudding spherule with endospores
Cryptococcus	Single, narrow-based budding yeast
Histoplasmosis	Narrow-based budding, intracellular yeast
Sporotrichosis	Round to cigar-shaped yeast with single or multiple buds

Serologic testing exists for coccidioidomycosis, cryptococcus, histoplasmosis, and sporotrichosis.[3,11,37] There may be some delay in positivity with initial infection, but serial results can give clinicians an idea of the patient's response to treatment and high titers make disseminated disease more likely and may prompt more intensive clinical investigation.[3] Patients with *Coccidioides* infection typically exhibit eosinophilia.[39]

Antigen testing for histoplasmosis has the highest sensitivity in the urine, especially in cases of disseminated disease.[3] The latex agglutinin serology test for cryptococcus is over 90% sensitive and specific and may be the most clinically relevant diagnostic test for cryptococcal infection.[37] India ink is another cryptococcus-specific diagnostic tool, which may be especially helpful in resource-limited environments where agglutinin testing is unavailable.[37]

A skin test has been developed for blastomycosis and histoplasmosis; however, the efficacy of this test is unclear because of positive results associated with exposure only and not active infection.[4,30] When the skin test is combined with antibody levels, it may add some prognostic value.[4]

Blastomycosis-Like Pyoderma

In 1979, Su and colleagues[15] proposed a set of 5 diagnostic criteria listed in **Box 2**. More recently, the literature suggests that a diagnosis of BLP based on only the first 3 criteria is sufficient.[17]

Granulomatous STDs

Definitive diagnosis of granuloma inguinale is based on visualization of pathognomonic Donovan bodies in infected tissue.[34] Tissues treated with either Wright or Giemsa stain can reveal the deep purple bacteria inside the cytoplasm of mononuclear phagocytes and can be present in up to 80% of cases (**Fig. 9**).[25,28] This method of diagnosis is rapid and reliable.[26] Because of the intracellular location, granuloma inguinale cannot be diagnosed by culture and polymerase chain reaction diagnosis is possible, but not commercially available.[26]

LGV can be definitively diagnosed by (1) detection of *C trachomatis* serotype L1, L2, or L3 on culture, (2) positive result of immunofluorescence showing inclusion bodies in leukocytes in an inguinal lymph node aspirate, or (3) positive result of microimmunofluorescence for LGV strain of *C trachomatis*.[34] Nucleic acid amplification testing can also be diagnostic, although this assay is not approved by the US Food and Drug Administration for rectal lesions.[27,34] In addition, serologic testing, especially complement fixation

titers more than 1:64, can support the diagnosis in the appropriate clinical scenario.[27,35] If LGV testing is not available, then patients whose symptoms fit the clinical picture should be treated empirically.[27]

CLINICAL RESULTS/OUTCOMES IN THE LITERATURE
Deep Fungal Infections

The backbone of treatment of each of these diseases is azoles for mild or limited disease and amphotericin B for severe or disseminated disease.[3,10,30,37] Itraconazole tends to be the favored azole therapy because it is efficacious while having a low side effect profile.[3,10] Fluconazole is less effective and relapse of disease is more common; however, it may be particularly useful as an adjunct therapy in CNS disease because it penetrates the blood-brain barrier, whereas itraconazole does not.[3] **Table 3** demonstrates the preferred treatments for each deep fungal infection specifically.[3,30,37]

Standard dosing for fluconazole and itraconazole is 200 to 400 mg daily.[3] Newer azoles, voriconazole and posaconazole, are dosed at 800 mg daily.[3] Amphotericin B is used in its regular or lipid formulation: dosing of 0.25 to 1 mg/kg for the regular formulation and 3 to 6 mg/kg for the liposomal formulation.[3,37] Often, amphotericin is switched to an oral azole after a few weeks of treatment as long as the patient is clinically improving.[3] In CNS disease, liposomal amphotericin B is preferred because it has higher concentration in brain tissue and the reduced side effect profile, when compared with the standard formulation, allows for more aggressive dosing.[3]

Patients with coccidioidomycosis and histoplasmosis can sometimes recover spontaneously; therefore, in the right clinical scenario, clinicians may choose to forgo treatment and only follow-up the patients clinically for resolution of the infection.[3] This decision would be appropriate only in patients with limited, mild disease without risk factors for developing severe disease.[3] In general, the duration of treatment can be based on clinical improvement.[3] Titers can also be followed up to monitor disease resolution.[3] However, treatment of cryptococcus in patients with HIV infection or AIDS must be continued for at least 12 months or until their CD4 count is more than 100.[37] This protocol does not hold for patients with CNS involvement from coccidioidomycosis or *Cryptococcus*; they require lifelong treatment.[3,37]

Mild sporotrichosis with only cutaneous lesions can be treated with oral potassium iodide.[3,10] Initial dosing is 1 to 1.4 g daily, which can

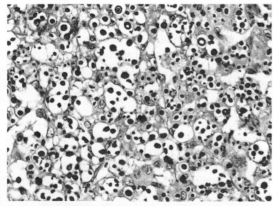

Fig. 9. Periodic acid-Schiff stain (PAS) stain of *Cryptococcus* species. (*Courtesy of* Penvadee Pattanaprichakul, MD, Bangkok, Thailand.)

Table 3
Recommended treatment of deep fungal mycoses

Fungal Disease		Treatment
Blastomycosis	Mild, cutaneous only, or maintenance	Itraconazole (B)
	Severe	Amphotericin B (C)
Coccidioidomycosis	Limited or cutaneous	No treatment, follow-up clinically until resolved
		Itraconazole (A)
		Voriconazole, posaconazole (C)
	Severe or disseminated	Amphotericin B (D) ± itraconazole or fluconazole
		Surgical debridement
	CNS involvement	Lifelong treatment
Cryptococcus	Mild or moderate	Fluconazole (B)
	Severe or CNS involvement	Amphotericin B+ flucytosine (B) followed by fluconazole then lifelong maintenance
Histoplasmosis	Asymptomatic	Symptomatic treatment
		Itraconazole (B)
	Chronic or progressive	Trimethoprim/sulfamethoxazole (D)
		Itraconazole or fluconazole (B)
		Voriconazole or posaconazole (D)
	Severe, disseminated, or in patient with HIV infection	Amphotericin B (B)
	African variant	Same as above
Sporotrichosis	Mild, cutaneous	Potassium iodide solution (B)
	Moderate, severe, or immunosuppressed	Itraconazole or terbinafine (A)
	Disseminated	Amphotericin B followed by itraconazole (E)

Level of evidence: A, high-quality randomized controlled trial (RCT) or prospective study; B, lesser-quality RCT or prospective study; C, case-control study or retrospective study; D, case series or case reports; E, expert opinion.

be titrated up as tolerated by the patient to a maximum of 5 g daily.[12] GI side effects are common but usually do not require cessation of treatment.[10,12] Potassium iodide therapy should be continued for 4 weeks after clinical findings have resolved.[11] Terbinafine has also been used in the treatment of sporotrichosis with good outcomes.[11] In one case report of 9 patients with cutaneous sporotrichosis, local hyperthermia using pocket warmers or infrared ray was used with 100% efficacy and minimal side effects.[40]

Blastomycosis-Like Pyoderma

Based on the hypothesis that BLP is partly due to an overreaction of native tissue to a bacterial infection in the skin, treatment with multiple antibiotics has been tried over the past several decades. However, despite the fact that bacteria are thought to play a large role in the development and progression of BLP, the response of the disease to antibiotics is highly variable.[16] Despite this, antibiotics are still used and should be tailored based on the sensitivities of culture results from the pus or skin.[33] Often, successful treatments require multiple modalities, including

antibiotics, topical dressings, physical destruction with cryotherapy, curettage or lasers, and the vitamin A analog, acitretin. Detailed results from the literature are given in **Table 4**. Correcting the patient's underlying immunosuppression, when possible, may improve outcomes.[23]

The following treatments have been reported in the literature with no improvement: topical, intralesional, or systemic steroids; ketoconazole, doxycycline, or minocycline; extended courses of oral erythromycin and dicloxacillin; ascorbic acid and zinc sulfate; parenteral penicillin or cefazolin; permanganate soaks; topical antibiotic power; potassium iodide or boric acid solution; and superficial exposure to X-ray.[13,17,19,33,41]

Granulomatous STDs

The Centers for Disease Control and Prevention recommend that both granuloma inguinale and LGV be treated first with doxycycline for 14 and 21 days, respectively.[27] **Table 5** shows treatment options. For granuloma inguinale, treatment needs to be continued until all lesions have healed, which may prolong the course.[27] Alternative regimens for granuloma inguinale are azithromycin (which

Table 4
Treatment regimens and responses for BLP reported in the literature

Drug Regimen	Dosing	Duration	No. of Patients	Outcome	Reference	Evidence Level
Acitretin alone	25 mg × 10 wk 10 mg × 4 mo	10 wk 4 mo	3/3	Resolved	20,22	D
Acitretin Ciprofloxacin Clindamycin	25 mg daily × 15 d 500 mg daily Topical gel	15 d	1/1	Improved but recurred	20	D
Acitretin Mequitazine Bepotastine γ-Linoleic acid Urea cream	20 mg daily 10 mg daily 20 mg daily 80 mg daily Topical	8 mo	1/1	Resolved	16	D
Augmentin	Unknown dosing	Unknown	1/1	Responded	19	D
Augmentin Ketoconazole	Unknown dosing	3 wk	1/1	No improvement	13	D
Carbon dioxide laser Minocycline	N/A 100 mg twice daily	Unknown	1/1	Resolved	41	D
Cefdinir Terbinafine	Unknown dosing	Unknown	1/1	Resolved	21	D
Ciprofloxacin Gentamicin	500 mg every 12 h Topical 3 times daily	2 wk	1/1	Resolved	13	D
Clindamycin Meropenem	Unknown dosing	Unknown	1	Recurred	21	D
Clotrimazole	Unknown dosing	7 d	1/1	Resolved	32	D
Cryotherapy with liquid nitrogen	20-s freeze-thaw cycle	5 per week for 3 wk	1/1	Resolved	33	D
Curettage Salicylazosulfapyridine	N/A 2 g daily	10 d	4/6	Resolved	18	D
Systemic antibiotics Topical dressing[a]	Unknown dosing	Unknown	4/6	Resolved	15	D

D, case series or case reports.

Acitretin only after checking liver enzymes and lipids.

[a] Copper sulfate or aluminum subacetate.

Data from Refs. 13,15,16,19–22,18,32,33,41

Table 5
Treatment of granuloma inguinale and LGV

	Treatment Regimen	Evidence Level
First line	Doxycycline 100 mg twice daily[a]	C for GI, B for LGV
Second line	Azithromycin 1 g weekly or 500 mg daily (GI only)	B
	Erythromycin 400 mg, 4 times daily	C for GI, B for LGV

B, lesser-quality RCT or prospective study; C, case-control study or retrospective study.

[a] If no improvement within 2 to 3 days, add gentamicin 1 mg/kg every 8 hours.

some investigators recommend as first line), ciprofloxacin, trimethoprim-sulfamethoxazole, or erythromycin.[26,27] If granuloma inguinale lesions are not responding within 2 to 3 days to appropriate treatment, an aminoglycoside should be added.[27,34] Erythromycin can be used as second-line treatment of LGV.[34] Despite effective therapy, the condition may relapse 6 to 18 months after treatment.[27] For both granuloma inguinale and LGV, significant scarring can persist after treatment and resolution of the disease.[27] Large infected nodes in LGV may require incision and drainage to prevent recurrent ulceration after treatment.[27]

SUMMARY

Granulomatous disease has many different causes: deep fungal infections, BLP, and granulomatous STIs. Clinical presentations of the deep mycoses and BLP are very similar, and diagnostic testing must be done to determine the underlying cause. Treatment is always targeted to the underlying cause.

REFERENCES

1. James DG. A clinicopathological classification of granulomatous disease. Postgrad Med J 2000;76: 457–65.
2. Zumla A, James DG. Granulomatous infections: etiology and classification. Clin Infect Dis 1996;23: 146–58.
3. Laniado-Laborín R. Coccidioidomycosis and other endemic mycoses in Mexico. Rev Iberoam Micol 2007;24:249–58.
4. Bonifaz A, Vázquez-González D, Perusquía-Ortiz AM. Endemic systemic mycoses: coccidioidomycosis, histoplasmosis, paracoccidioidomycosis and blastomycosis. J Dtsch Dermatol Ges 2011;9:705–15.
5. Bradsher RW. Clinical features of blastomycosis. Semin Respir Infect 1997;12(3):229–34.
6. Chapman SW, Lin AC, Hendricks KA, et al. Endemic blastomycosis is Mississippi: epidemiological and clinical studies. Semin Respir Infect 1997;12(3):219.
7. Centers for Disease Control and Prevention (CDC). Increase in reported coccidioidomycosis – United States, 1998-2011. MMWR Morb Mortal Wkly Rep 2013;62(12):217.
8. Hernandez AD. Cutaneous cryptococcosis. Dermatol Clin 1989;7(2):269–74.
9. Trent JT, Kirsner RS. Identifying and treating mycotic skin infections. J Wound Care 2003;16:122–9.
10. Ramos-e-Silva M, Vasconcelos C, Carneiro S, et al. Sporotrichosis. Clin Dermatol 2007;25:181–7.
11. Davis BA. Sporotrichosis. Dermatol Clin 1996;14(1): 69–76.
12. Michel da Rosa AC, Scroferneker ML, Vettorato R, et al. Epidemiology of sporotrichosis: a study of 304 cases in Brazil. J Am Acad Dermatol 2005;52: 451–9.
13. Trygg KJ, Madison KC. Blastomycosis-like pyoderma caused by pseudomonas aeruginosa: report of a case responsive to ciprofloxacin. J Am Acad Dermatol 1990;23(4 Pt 1):750–2.
14. Crowley JJ, Kim YH. Blastomycosis-like pyoderma in a man with AIDS. J Am Acad Dermatol 1997;36: 633–4.
15. Su WP, Duncan SC, Perry HO. Blastomycosis-like pyoderma. Arch Dermatol 1979;115:170–3.
16. Lee YS, Jung SW, Sim HS, et al. Blastomycosis-like pyoderma with good response to acitretin. Ann Dermatol 2011;23(3):365–8.
17. Nguyen RT, Beardmore GL. Blastomycosis-like pyoderma: successful treatment with low dose acitretin. Australas J Dermatol 2005;46:97–100.
18. Williams HM, Stone OJ. Blastomycosis-like pyoderma: case report of unusual entity with response to curettage. Arch Dermatol 1996;93:226–8.
19. Sawalka SS, Phiske MM, Jerajani HR. Blastomycosis-like pyoderma. Indian J Dermatol 2007;73(2):117–9.
20. Cecchi R, Bartoli L, Brunetti L, et al. Blastomycosis-like pyoderma in association with recurrent vesicular eczema: good response to acitretin. Dermatol Online J 2011;17(3):9.
21. Ouchi T, Tamura M, Nishimoto S, et al. A case of blastomycosis-like pyoderma caused by mixed infection of Staphylococcus epidermidis and Trichophyton rubrum. Am J Dermatopathol 2011;33(4):397–9.
22. Kobraei KB, Wesson SK. Blastomycosis-like pyoderma: response to systemic retinoid therapy. Int J Dermatol 2010;49:1336–8.
23. Stone OJ. Hyperinflammatory proliferative (blastomycosis-like) pyodermas: review, mechanisms, and therapy. J Dermatol Surg Oncol 1986;12(3):271–3.
24. Yaffee HS. Localized blastomycosis-like pyoderma occurring in a tattoo. Arch Dermatol 1960;82:153–4.

25. Lagergård T, Bölin I, Lindholm L. On the evolution of the sexually transmitted bacteria *Haemophilus ducreyi* and *Klebsiella granulomatis*. Ann N Y Acad Sci 2011;1230:e1–10.

26. O'Farrell N. 2010 European guideline on donovanosis. IUSTI/WHO European STD Guidelines Editorial Board. Int J STD AIDS 2010;21(9):609–10.

27. Workowski KA, Berman S, Centers for Disease Control and Prevention (CDC). Sexually Transmitted Disease Treatment Guidelines 2010. MMWR Recomm Rep 2010;59(RR12):1–116.

28. Richens J. The diagnosis and treatment of donovanosis (granuloma inguinale). Genitourin Med 1991; 67:441–52.

29. Markle W, Conti T, Kad M. Sexually transmitted diseases. Prim Care Clin Office Pract 2013;40:557–87.

30. Motswaledi HM, Monyemangene FM, Maloba BR, et al. Blastomycosis: a case report and review of the literature. Int J Dermatol 2012;51:1090–3.

31. Kanne JP, Yandow DR, Haemel AK, et al. Beyond skin deep: thoracic manifestations of systemic disorders affecting the skin. Radiographics 2011;31(6): 1651–68.

32. Dutta TK, James J, Baruah MC, et al. Blastomycosis-like pyoderma in a case of chronic myeloid leukemia. Postgrad Med J 1992;68.363–5.

33. Su Ö, Demirkesen C, Onsun N. Localized blastomycosis-like pyoderma with good response to cotrimoxazole and cryotherapy. Int J Dermatol 2004; 43:388–90.

34. Roett MA, Mayor MT, Uduhiri KA. Diagnosis and management of genital ulcers. Am Fam Physician 2012;85(3):254–62.

35. Centers for Disease Control and Prevention. Appendix: STD surveillance case definitions. Atlanta: US Department of Health and Human Services STD Surveillance. 2010. p. 152.

36. Saldanha Dominic RM, Prashanth HV, Shenoy S, et al. Diagnostic value of latex agglutination in cryptococcal meningitis. J Lab Physicians 2009;1(2):67–8.

37. Warkentien T, Crum-Cianflone NF. An update on cryptococcosis among HIV-infected persons. Int J STD AIDS 2010;21(10):679–84.

38. Chang P, Rodas C. Skin lesions in histoplasmosis. Clin Dermatol 2012;30:592–8.

39. Saubolle MA, McKellar PP, Sussland D. Epidemiologic, clinical, and diagnostic aspects of coccidioidomycosis. J Clin Microbiol 2007;45(1):26.

40. Hiruma M, Kawada A, Noguchi H, et al. Hyperthermic treatment of sporotrichosis: experimental use of infrared and far infrared rays. Mycoses 1992; 35(11–12):293.

41. Sawchuk WS, Heald PW. Residents' corner: blastomycosis-like pyoderma – report of a case responsive to combination therapy utilizing minocycline and carbon dioxide laser debridement. J Dermatol Surg Oncol 1986;12:1041–4.

Clinical Atlas of Granulomatous Disorders

Joseph C. English III, MD*

KEYWORDS

- Granuloma annulare • Reactive granulomatosis dermatitis • Sarcoidosis
- Granulomatous periorifacial dermatitis • Atypical mycobacterium

KEY POINTS

- Granulomatous disorders present with unique clinical morphologies.
- Visual recognition of granulomatous disorders is an important skill to be developed by the Health care provider.
- Visual recognition should be confirmed with histopathological evaluation.

Because dermatologists are classically visual learners and trained with many Kodachrome (now digital image) teaching sessions during residency and at continuing medical education conferences, I thought adding digital images would be ideal. Therefore, to further the reader's experience with granulomatous disorders that were reviewed in great detail in this issue of *Dermatology Clinics*, I have added a "Clinical Atlas of Granulomatous Disorder" from cases that I have encountered over my career. I initially intended to include dermatopathology, but being a clinician-educator I wanted to focus on the unique clinical morphologies that these diseases present. How-ever, with that being stated, dermatopathology plays a crucial role in differentiating these entities (ie, the best example is mucin staining to differentiate granuloma annulare from all other palisading granulomas). As one can tell, some images are scanned Kodachromes as my career has evolved from Kodak film to .jpg images, so I apologize for some horizontal lines in a few images. I want to thank all the patients that allowed me to image their skin disease and all the past, present, and future residents and colleagues who have and will work tirelessly in managing these patients with me. I hope you enjoy this collection as much as I enjoyed putting this section together for you.

No financial associations.
No conflicts of interest.
University of Pittsburgh, Department of Dermatology, UPMC North Hills Dermatology, 9000 Brooktree Rd, Suite 200, Wexford, PA 15090, USA
* 9000 Brooktree Road, Suite 200, Wexford, PA 15090.
E-mail address: englishjc@upmc.edu

Dermatol Clin 33 (2015) 609–630
http://dx.doi.org/10.1016/j.det.2015.03.020
0733-8635/15/$ – see front matter © 2015 Elsevier Inc. All rights reserved.

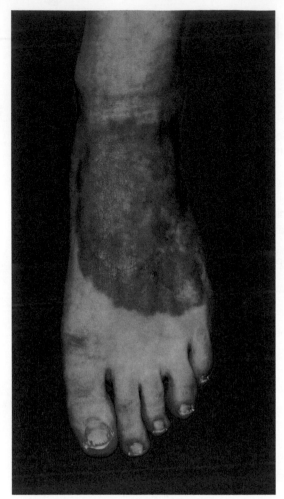

Fig. 1. Granuloma annulare – macular.

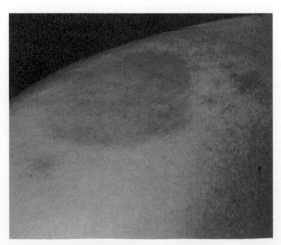

Fig. 2. Granuloma annulare – macular.

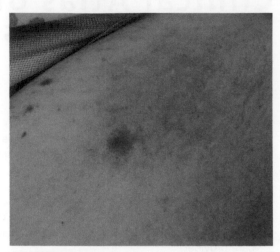

Fig. 3. Granuloma annulare – Fig. 2 lesion resolved with punch biopsy.

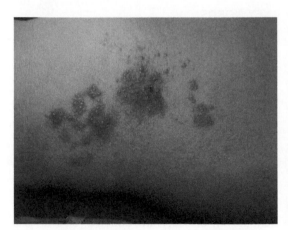

Fig. 4. Granuloma annulare – localized papular.

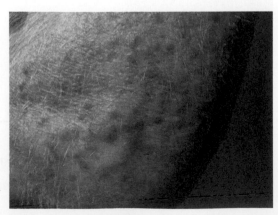

Fig. 5. Granuloma annulare – disseminated.

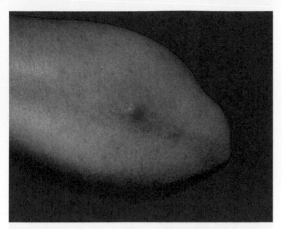

Fig. 6. Granuloma annulare – subcutaneous.

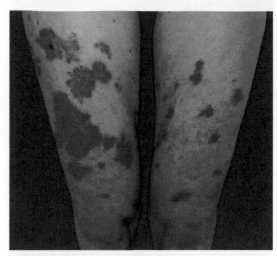

Fig. 9. Granuloma annulare – atypical.

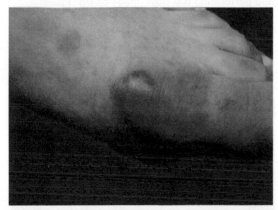

Fig. 7. Granuloma annulare – subcutaneous and macular.

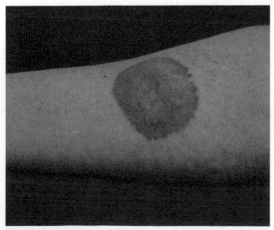

Fig. 8. Granuloma annulare – necrobiosis lipoidica/sarcodosis-like.

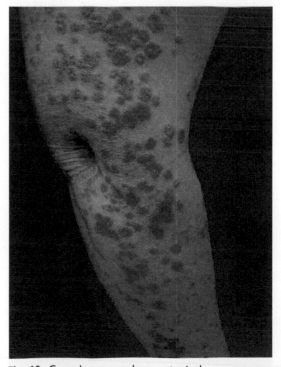

Fig. 10. Granuloma annulare – atypical.

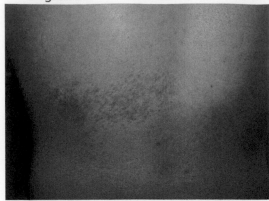

Fig. 11. Granuloma annulare – atypical zosteriform.

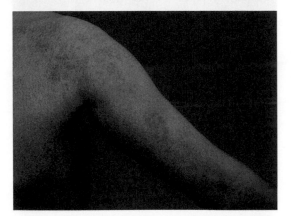

Fig. 12. Granuloma annulare – atypical zosteriform (arm of patient in Fig. 11).

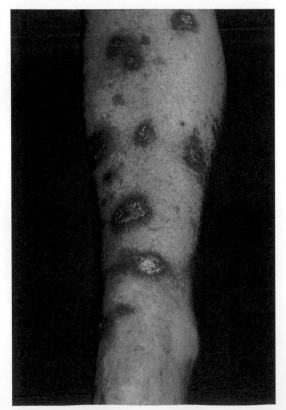

Fig. 13. Granuloma annulare – atypical unilateral leg.

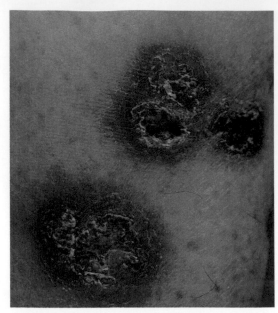

Fig. 14. Granuloma annulare – atypical unilateral leg and perforating (up close image of Fig. 13).

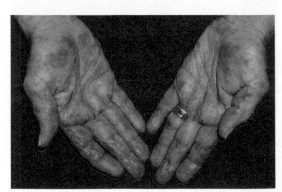

Fig. 15. Granuloma annulare – palmar.

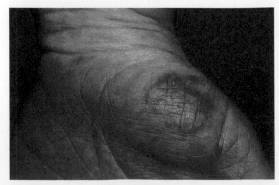

Fig. 16. Granuloma annulare – palmar.

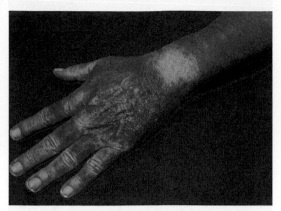

Fig. 17. Elastolytic actinic giant cell granuloma.

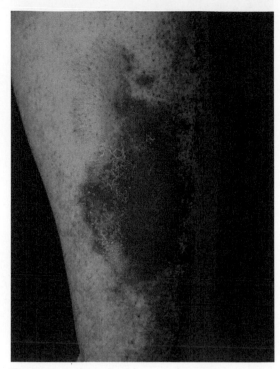

Fig. 20. Necrobisos lipoidica – early stage.

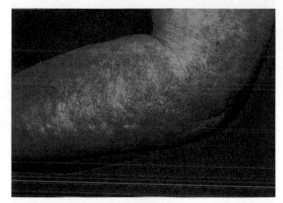

Fig. 18. Elastolytic actinic giant cell granuloma (elbow of patient in Fig.17).

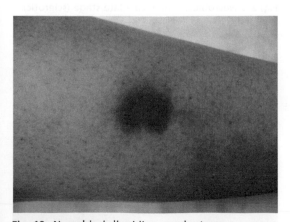

Fig. 19. Necrobiosis lipoidica – early stage.

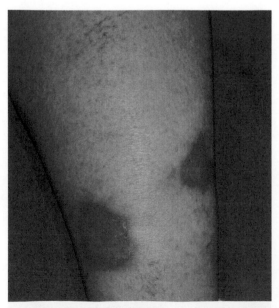

Fig. 21. Necrobiosis lipoidica – early stage (xanthomatous).

614

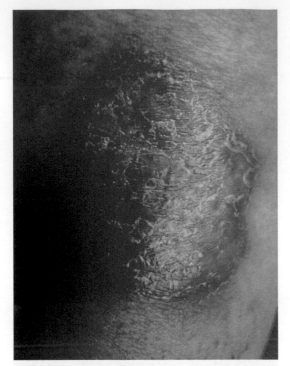

Fig. 22. Necrobiosis lipoidica – early stage (xanthomatous and up close image of Fig. 21).

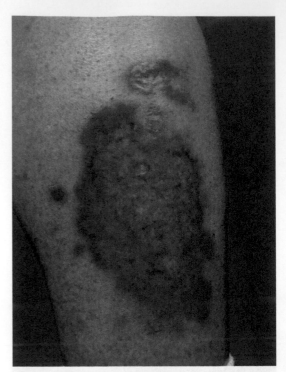

Fig. 24. Necrobiosis lipoidica – late stage (xanthomatous).

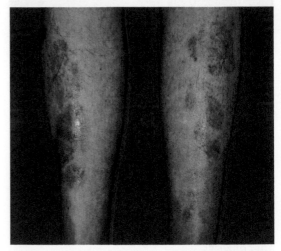

Fig. 25. Necrobiosis lipoidica – late stage (sclerotic).

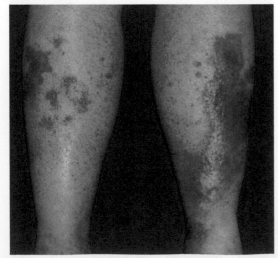

Fig. 23. Necrobiosis lipoidica – middle stage (xanthomatous).

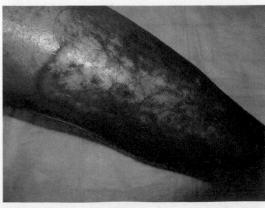

Fig. 26. Necrobiosis lipoidica – late stage (sclerotic).

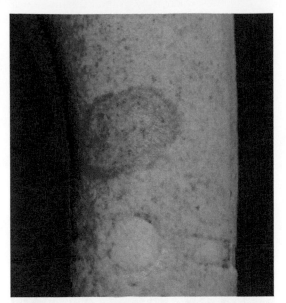

Fig. 27. Necrobiosis lipoidica – upper extremity.

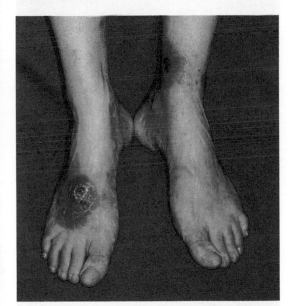

Fig. 28. Necrobiosis lipoidica – ulcerative.

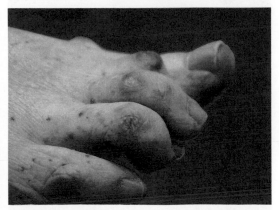

Fig. 29. Rheumatoid nodules – with coexisting rheumatoid vasculitis.

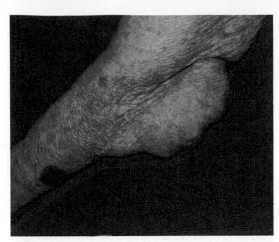

Fig. 30. Rheumatoid nodule – massive.

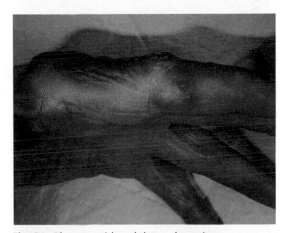

Fig. 31. Rheumatoid nodules – ulcerating.

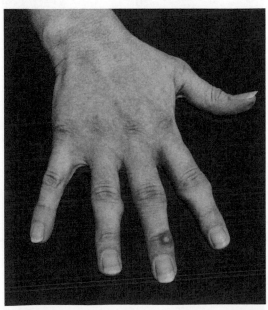

Fig. 32. Accelerated rheumatoid nodulosis – methotrexate induced.

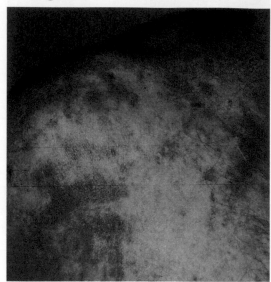

Fig. 33. Reactive granulomatous dermatitis – interstitial granulomatous dermatitis type.

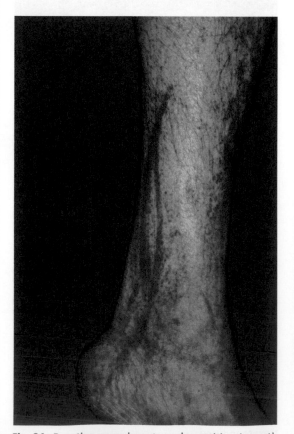

Fig. 34. Reactive granulomatous dermatitis – interstitial granulomatous dermatitis type.

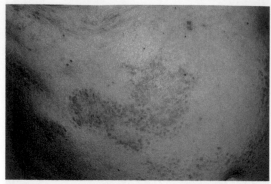

Fig. 35. Reactive granulomatous dermatitis – granuloma annulare type.

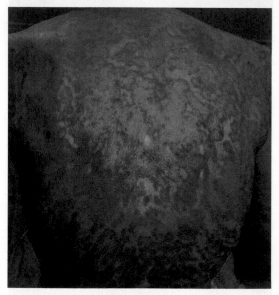

Fig. 36. Reactive granulomatous dermatitis – granuloma annulare type.

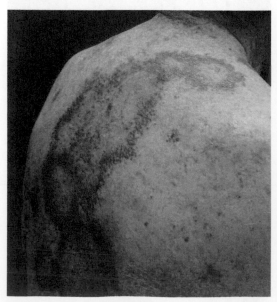

Fig. 37. Reactive granulomatous dermatitis – granuloma annulare type.

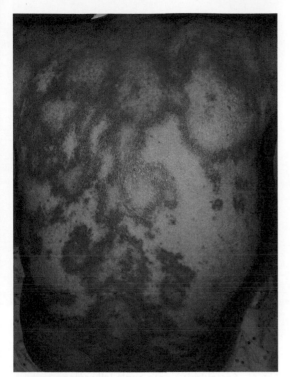

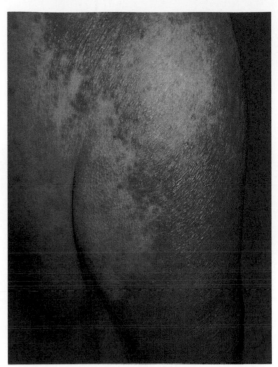

Fig. 38. Reactive granulomatous dermatitis – granu loma annulare type.

Fig. 40. Reactive granulomatous dermatitis – granuloma annulare type (upper arm of patient in Fig. 39).

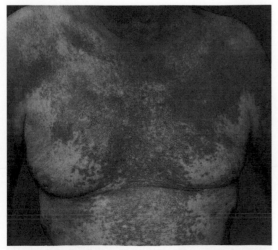

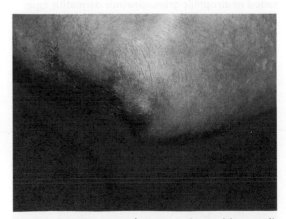

Fig. 39. Reactive granulomatous dermatitis – granuloma annulare type.

Fig. 41. Reactive granulomatous dermatitis – palisaded neutrophilic granulomatous dermatitis type.

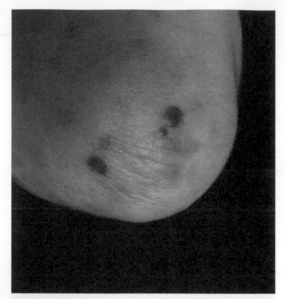

Fig. 42. Reactive granulomatous dermatitis – palisaded neutrophilic granulomatous dermatitis type.

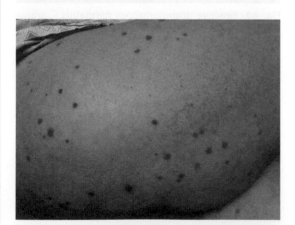

Fig. 43. Reactive granulomatous dermatitis – palisaded neutrophilic granulomatous dermatitis type.

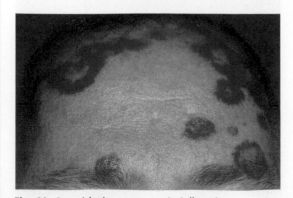

Fig. 44. Sarcoidosis – note apple jelly color.

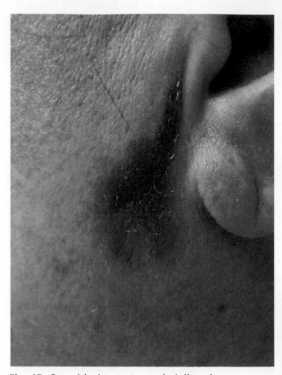

Fig. 45. Sarcoidosis – note apple jelly color.

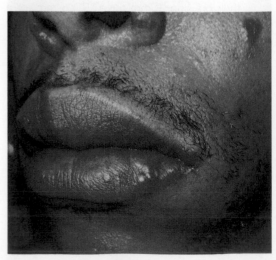

Fig. 46. Sarcoidosis – lip.

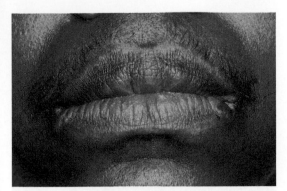

Fig. 47. Sarcoidosis – split papules at commissure.

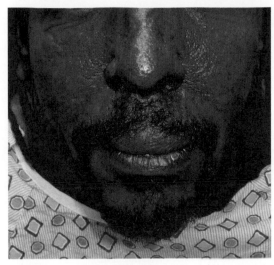

Fig. 50. Sarcoidosis – Fig. 49 resolved lupus pernio after treatment with azathioprine.

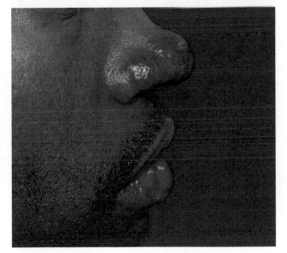

Fig. 48. Sarcoidosis – early lupus pernio.

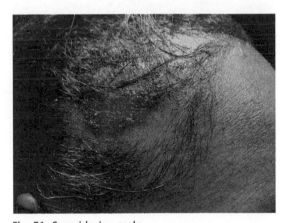

Fig. 51. Sarcoidosis – scalp.

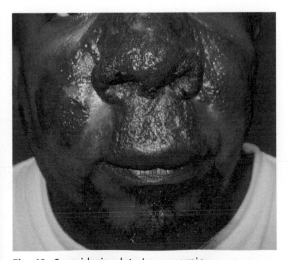

Fig. 49. Sarcoidosis – late lupus pernio.

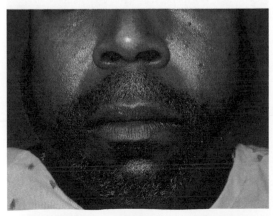

Fig. 52. Sarcodiosis – parotid gland involvement.

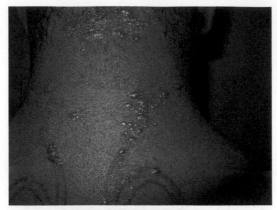

Fig. 53. Sarcoidosis – papular and tattoo associated.

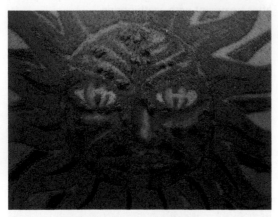

Fig. 54. Sarcoidosis – tattoo associated.

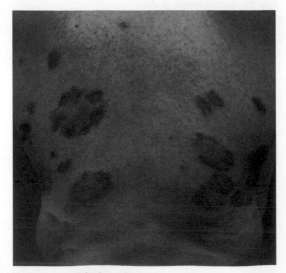

Fig. 55. Sarcoidosis – plaques.

Fig. 56. Sarcoidosis – plaques/psoriasiform.

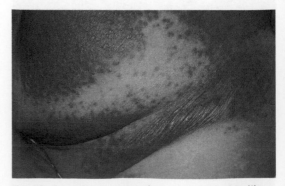

Fig. 57. Sarcodiosis – granulomatous slack skin-like.

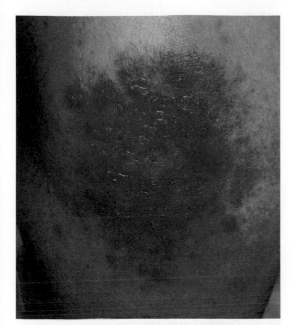

Fig. 58. Sarcoidosis – necrobiosis lipoidica-like.

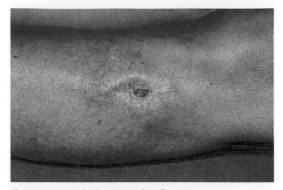

Fig. 61. Sarcoidosis – morpheaform.

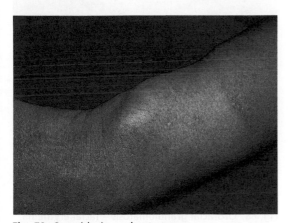

Fig. 59. Sarcoidosis – subcutaneous.

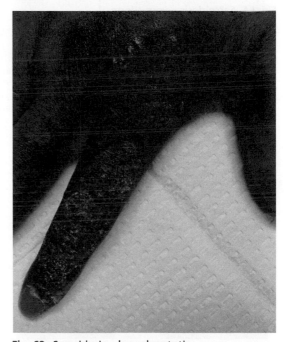

Fig. 62. Sarcoidosis – hyperkeratotic.

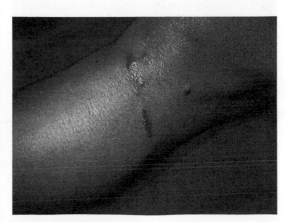

Fig. 60. Sarcoidosis – scar.

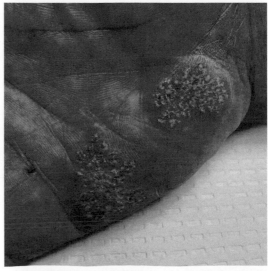

Fig. 63. Sarcoidosis – hyperkeratotic (palm of patient in Fig. 62).

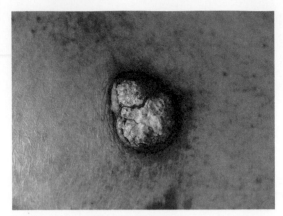

Fig. 64. Sarcoidosis – verruciform.

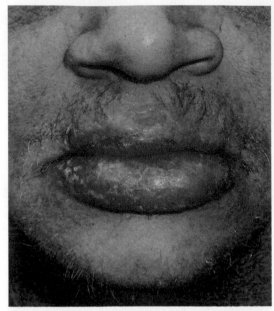

Fig. 67. Orofacial granulomatosis.

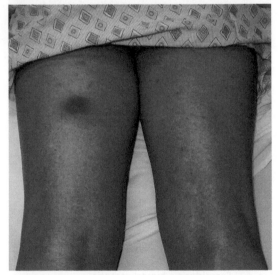

Fig. 65. Cutaneous Crohn's – metastatic.

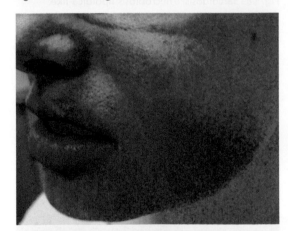

Fig. 68. Orofacial granulomatosis – facial erythema.

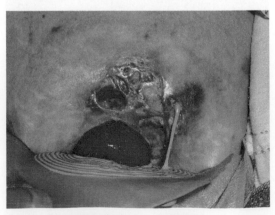

Fig. 66. Cutaneous Crohn's – peristomal.

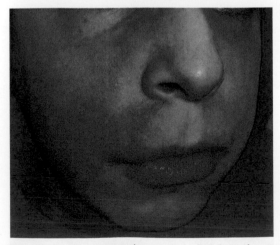

Fig. 69. Orofacial granulomatosis – facial erythema and angular cheilitis.

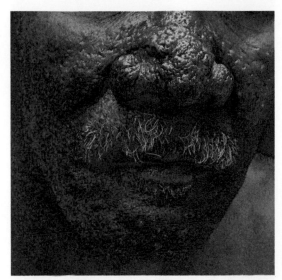

Fig. 70. Granulomatous rosacea – chin lesion with background rhinophyma.

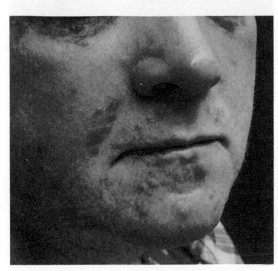

Fig. 73. Granulomatous periorifical dermatitis.

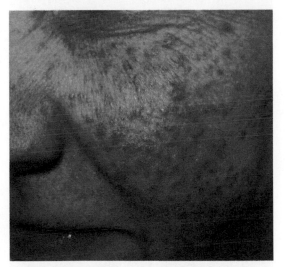

Fig. 71. Granulomatous periorifical dermatitis.

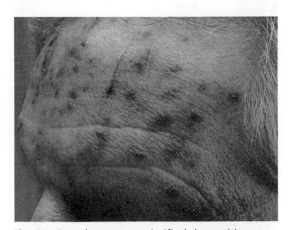

Fig. 74. Granulomatous periorifical dermatitis.

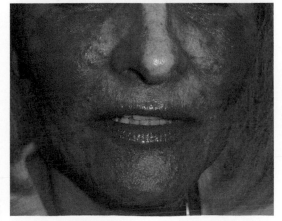

Fig. 72. Granulomatous perioroficial dermatitis – topical steroid induced.

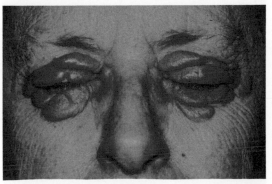

Fig. 75. Adult-onset orbital with periorbital xanthogranulomas.

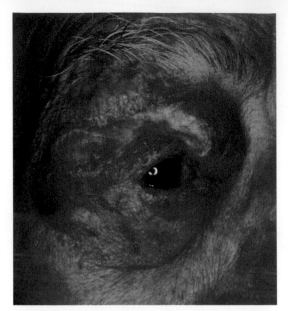

Fig. 76. Adult onset asthma with periorbital xanthogranulomas status-post treatment.

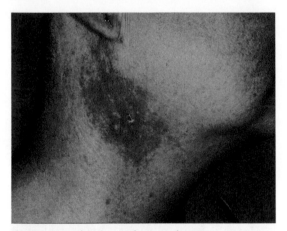

Fig. 77. Necrobiotic xanthogranuloma.

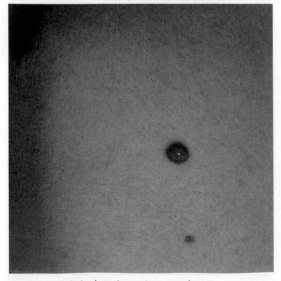

Fig. 78. Adult isolated xanthogranuloma.

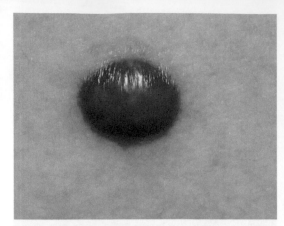

Fig. 79. Adult isolated xanthogranuloma (up close image of Fig. 78).

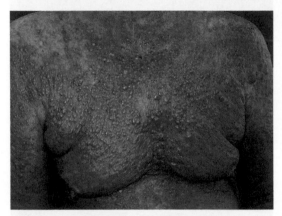

Fig. 80. Adult disseminated/eruptive xanthogranulomas.

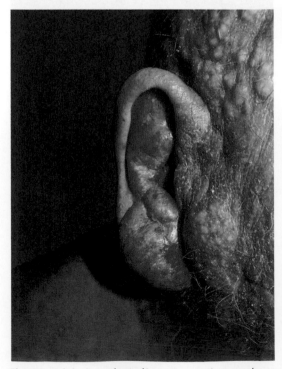

Fig. 81. Adult disseminated/eruptive xanthogranuloma (ear of patient in Fig.80).

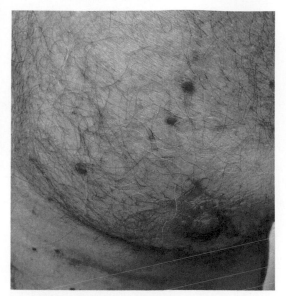

Fig. 82. Rosi–Dorfman syndrome.

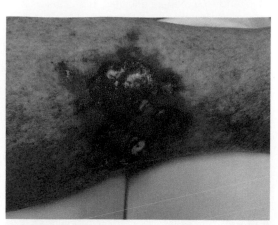

Fig. 85. Granulomatosis with polyangiitis – Fig. 84 lesion resolving with azathioprine treatment.

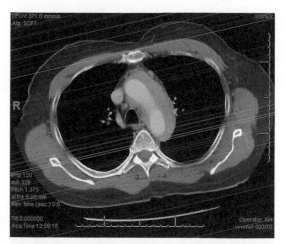

Fig. 83. Rosi–Dorfman syndrome – limited skin in Fig. 82 had extensive periaortic involvement.

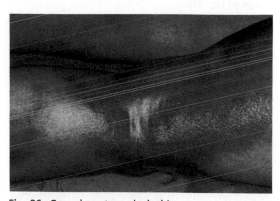

Fig. 86. Granulomatous slack skin.

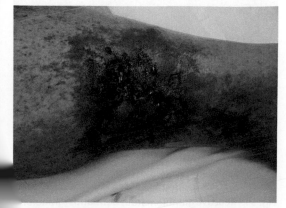

. 84. Granulomatosis with polyangiitis.

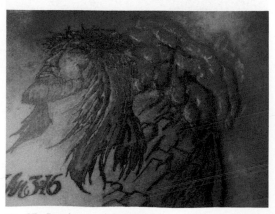

Fig. 87. Foreign body granuloma – tattoo.

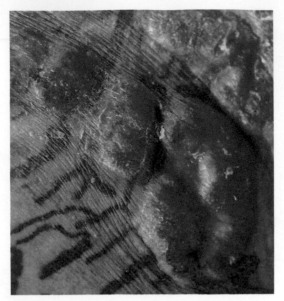

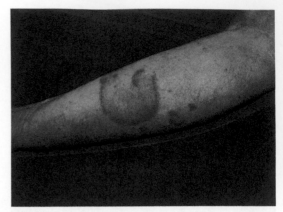

Fig. 90. Reactive granulomatous dermatitis (granuloma annulare type) drug reaction – cholesterol-lowering agent.

Fig. 88. Foreign body granuloma – tattoo (up close image of Fig. 87).

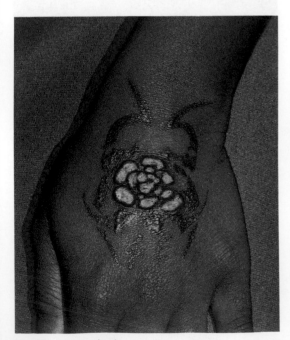

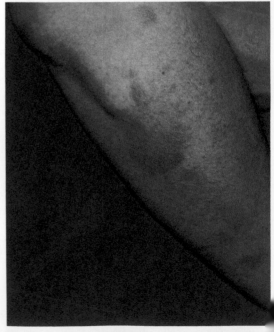

Fig. 89. Foreign body granuloma – tattoo.

Fig. 91. Reactive granulomatous dermatitis (granuloma annulare type) drug reaction – antihypertensive age

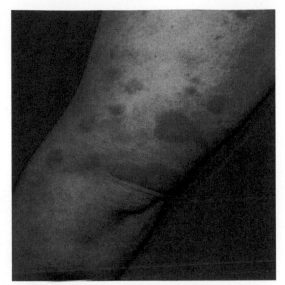

Fig. 92. Reactive granulomatous dermatitis (granuloma annulare type) drug reaction – antihypertensive agent.

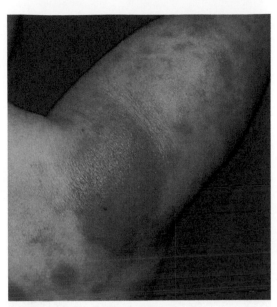

Fig. 95. Leprosy – lepromatous.

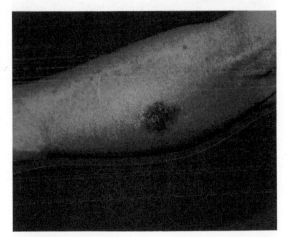

Fig. 93. Necrotic tuberculin purified protein derivative (PPD) site reaction.

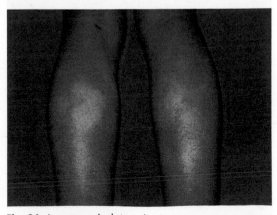

Fig. 94. Leprosy – indeterminate.

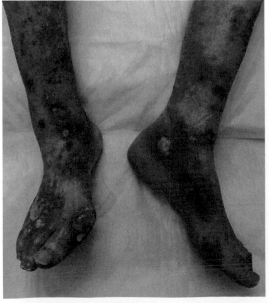

Fig. 96. Atypical mycobacterium (*Mycobacterium chelonae*).

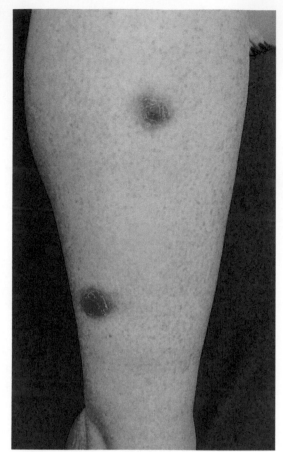

Fig. 97. Atypical mycobacterium (*Mycobacterium fortuitum*).

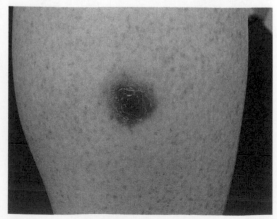

Fig. 98. Atypical mycobacterium (*Mycobacterium fortuitum* – up close image of Fig. 97)).

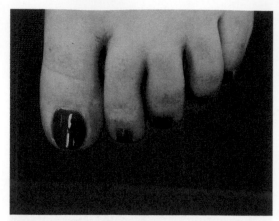

Fig. 99. Atypical mycobacterium (*Mycobacterium fortuitum*) – pedicure that induced Figs. 97 and 98.

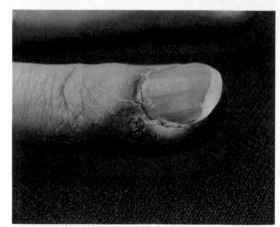

Fig. 100. Atypical mycobacterium (*Mycobacterium marinum*).

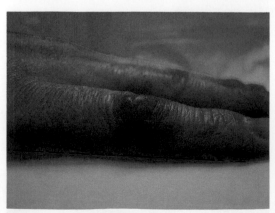

Fig. 101. Atypical mycobacterium (*Mycobacterium marinum*).

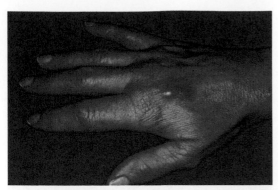

Fig. 102. Atypical mycobacterium (*Mycobacterium marinum*).

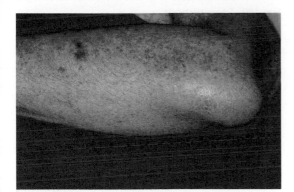

Fig. 103. Atypical mycobacterium (*Mycobacterium marinum*) – skin and bursitis.

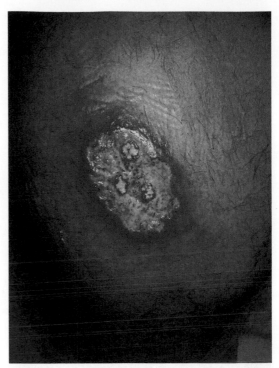

Fig. 105. Leishmaniasis.

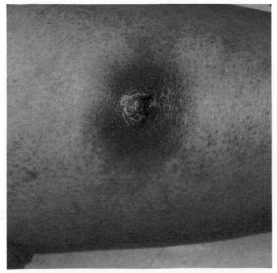

Fig. 104. Atypical mycobacterium (*Mycobacterium avium intracellulare*).

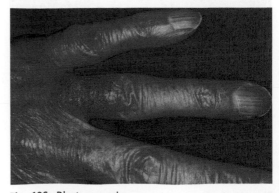

Fig. 106. Blastomycosis.

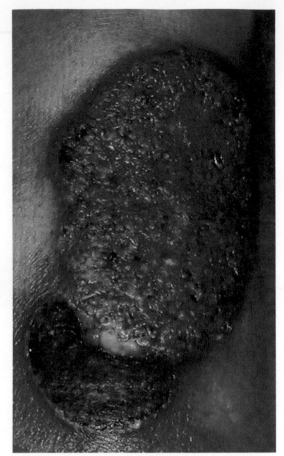

Fig. 107. Blastomycosis-like pyoderma.

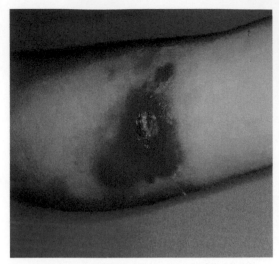

Fig. 109. Sporotrichosis.

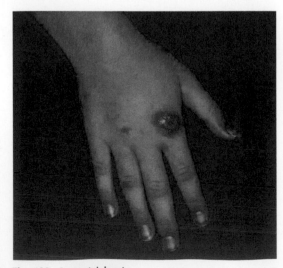

Fig. 108. Sporotrichosis.

Index

Note: Page numbers of article titles are in **boldface** type.

A

AAPOX. See *Adult-onset asthma and periocular xanthogranuloma.s*

Accelerated nodulosis
  and rheumatoid nodules, 367

Acid-fast bacilli
  and cutaneous tuberculosis, 544, 546, 549
  and leprosy, 552–554, 556, 557, 559

Acrochordae
  and Crohn disease, 418

Adult-onset asthma
  and periocular xanthogranuloma, 457–462
  and periorbital xanthogranulomas, 624

Adult orbital xanthogranulomatous disease
  clinical presentation of, 458, 459
  etiopathogenesis of, 457, 458
  evaluation of, 460, 461
  and systemic associations, 459, 460
  treatment of, 461, 462

Adult orbital xanthogranulomatous disease: A review with emphasis on etiology, systemic associations, diagnostic tools, and treatment, **457–463**

Adult xanthogranuloma
  clinical presentation of, 465, 466
  etiopathogenesis of, 465
  evaluation of, 466
  management of, 466
  and systemic associations, 466

Adult xanthogranuloma, reticulohistiocytosis, and Rosai-Dorfman disease, **465–473**

AFB. See *Acid-fast bacilli.*

Alcoholic liver cirrhosis
  and elastolytic actinic giant cell granuloma, 337

Allergy
  and orofacial granulomatosis, 437

Alopecia areata
  and Crohn disease, 426

Aluminum
  and foreign body granulomas, 511–513

American College of Rheumatology
  and rheumatoid nodules, 361, 362

Animal collagen
  and cosmetic implants, 502–504, 506

Antibiotics
  and granuloma annulare, 320
  for sarcoidosis, 409

Antileprotic agents
  for orofacial granulomatosis, 440

Antimalarials
  and granuloma annulare, 321
  and necrobiosis lipoidica, 356
  for sarcoidosis, 407

Antineutrophil cytoplasmic antibody–associated vasculitis
  clinical features of, 477–479
  and eosinophilic granulomatosis with polyangiitis, 478, 479
  etiopathogenesis of, 476, 477
  evaluation of, 479, 480
  and granulomatosis with polyangiitis, 477, 478
  management of, 479, 480
  and microscopic polyangiitis, 479
  and remission induction, 480
  and remission maintenance, 480
  and systemic associations, 477–479

Anti–tumor necrosis factor
  and orofacial granulomatosis, 439, 440

Anti–tumor necrosis factor-α
  and granuloma annulare, 321

AOXGD. See *Adult orbital xanthogranulomatous disease.*

Arthropod bite
  and foreign body granulomas, 515

Atrophic sarcoidosis, 398, 399

Atypical mycobacterium
  and *Mycobacterium avium intracellulare,* 629
  and *Mycobacterium chelonae,* 627
  and *Mycobacterium fortuitum,* 628
  and *Mycobacterium marinum,* 628, 629

B

BB. See *Mid-borderline leprosy.*

BC. See *Bovine collagen.*

Benign nodulosis
  and rheumatoid nodules, 368

Beryllium
  and foreign body granulomas, 513

Biologics
  and necrobiosis lipoidica, 356

BL. See *Borderline lepromatous leprosy.*

Blastomycosis, 629
  and deep fungal infections, 596, 597, 600–602, 604

Blastomycosis-like pyoderma, 630
  clinical presentation of, 600–601
  diagnostic criteria for, 603
  etiopathogenesis of, 598, 599

Dermatol Clin 33 (2015) 631–641
http://dx.doi.org/10.1016/S0733-8635(15)00067-4
0733-8635/15/$ – see front matter © 2015 Elsevier Inc. All rights reserved.

Moving?

Make sure your subscription moves with you!

To notify us of your new address, find your **Clinics Account Number** (located on your mailing label above your name), and contact customer service at:

Email: journalscustomerservice-usa@elsevier.com

800-654-2452 (subscribers in the U.S. & Canada)
314-447-8871 (subscribers outside of the U.S. & Canada)

Fax number: 314-447-8029

**Elsevier Health Sciences Division
Subscription Customer Service
3251 Riverport Lane
Maryland Heights, MO 63043**

*To ensure uninterrupted delivery of your subscription, please notify us at least 4 weeks in advance of move.

Printed and bound by CPI Group (UK) Ltd, Croydon, CR0 4YY

03/10/2024

01040382-0002